Pediatric Urology

Pediatric Urology
Surgical Complications and Management

EDITED BY

Duncan T. Wilcox MBBS MD FEAPU

Associate Professor, Pediatric Urology
Rose Mary Haggar Professorship in Urology
University of Texas Southwestern
Dallas, TX, USA

Prasad P. Godbole FRCS FRCS (PAED)

Consultant Paediatric Urologist
Sheffield Children's NHS Trust
Sheffield, UK

Martin A. Koyle MD FAAP FACS

Professor of Urology and Pediatrics
University of Washington;
Chief, Division of Urology
Children's Hospital and Regional Medical Center
Seattle, WA, USA

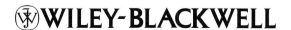

WILEY-BLACKWELL

A John Wiley & Sons, Ltd., Publication

This edition first published 2008, © 2008 by Blackwell Publishing Ltd

Blackwell Publishing was acquired by John Wiley & Sons in February 2007. Blackwell's publishing program has been merged with Wiley's global Scientific, Technical and Medical business to form Wiley-Blackwell.

Registered office: John Wiley & Sons Ltd, The Atrium, Southern Gate, Chichester, West Sussex, PO19 8SQ, UK

Editorial offices: 9600 Garsington Road, Oxford, OX4 2DQ, UK
The Atrium, Southern Gate, Chichester, West Sussex, PO19 8SQ, UK
111 River Street, Hoboken, NJ 07030-5774, USA

For details of our global editorial offices, for customer services and for information about how to apply for permission to reuse the copyright material in this book please see our website at www.wiley.com/wiley-blackwell

Library of Congress Cataloguing-in-Publication Data

Pediatric urology: surgical complications and management/edited by Duncan T. Wilcox, Prasad P. Godbole, Martin A. Koyle.
    p.;cm
    Includes bibliographical references and index.
    ISBN:978-1-4051-6268-5 (alk.paper)
    1. Genitourinary organs—Surgery—Complications. 2. Pediatric urology. I. Wilcox, Duncan T. II. Godbole, Prasad III, Koyle, Martin A. [DNLM: 1. Urologic Diseases—surgery. 5. Infant. 6. Intraoperative Complications—prevention & control. 7. Male Urogenital Diseases—surgery. 8. Postoperative Complications—prevention & control. WS 320 P3756 2008]
RD571.P45 2008
617.4′601—dc22

ISBN: 978-1-4051-6268-5   2007050631

A catalogue record for this book is available from the British Library.

Set in 9.25/11 Minion by Charon Tec Ltd (A Macmillan Company), Chennai, India
Printed and bound in Singapore by Markono Print Media Pte Ltd

1 2008

Contents

Contributors, viii

Foreword, xii

Preface, xiv

Part I Principles of Surgical Audit

1 How to Set Up a Prospective Surgical Audit, 3
Andrew Sinclair and Ben Bridgewater

2 Evaluating Personal Surgical Audit and What to Do If Your Results Are Outside the "Mean", 8
Andrew Sinclair and Ben Bridgewater

3 The Implications of a Poor Surgical Outcome, 12
Robert Wheeler

Part II General Principles

4 The Metabolic and Endocrine Response to Surgery I, 21
Laura Coates and Joe I. Curry

5 The Metabolic and Endocrine Response to Surgery II: Management, 29
Benjamin P. Wisner, Douglas Ford and Martin A. Koyle

6 Perioperative Anesthetic and Analgesic Risks and Complications, 36
Philippa Evans and Mark Thomas

Part III Open Surgery of the Upper Urinary Tract

7 Nephrectomy, 47
Paul Crow and Mark Woodward

8 Partial Nephrectomy, 52
Marc-David Leclair and Yves Héloury

9 Ureteropelvic Junction Obstruction, 58
Jenny Yiee and Duncan T. Wilcox

10 Ureteral Reimplant Surgery, 67
Laurence S. Baskin and Gerald Mingin

11 Ureteroureterostomy, 73
Job K. Chacko and Martin A. Koyle

Part IV Surgery of the Bladder

12 Epispadias–Exstrophy Complex, 83
Ahmad A. Elderwy and Richard Grady

13 Umbilical and Urachal Anomalies, 92
Paul F. Austin

Part V Endoscopic Surgery of the Urinary Tract

14 Cystoscopy and Cystoscopic Interventions, 101
Divyesh Y. Desai

15 Vesicoureteric Reflux, 111
Christian Radmayr

16 Interventional Procedures, 117
Korgun Koral

17 Minimally Invasive Interventions for Stone Disease, 125
H. Serkan Dogan and Serdar Tekgül

18 General Laparoscopy, 132
Chris Kimber and Neil McMullin

19 Laparoscopy for the Upper Urinary Tract, 138
J.S. Valla

20 Robotics in Pediatric Urology: Pyeloplasty, 145
L. Henning Olsen and Yazan F. Rawashdeh

21 Lower Urinary Tract Laparoscopy in Pediatric Patients, 152
Rakesh P. Patel, Benjamin M. Brucker and Pasquale Casale

Part VI Genitalia

22 Hernia and Hydrocele Repair, 163
Henrik Steinbrecher

23 Orchidopexy and Orchidectomy, 170
Kim A.R. Hutton and Indranil Sau

24 Laparoscopic Orchidopexy, 183
Derek J. Matoka, Michael C. Ost, Marc C. Smaldone and Steven G. Docimo

25 Varicocele, 193
Ramnath Subramaniam and Eva Macharia

26 Hypospadias Urethroplasty, 201
Warren T. Snodgrass

27 Phalloplasty for the Biological Male, 212
Piet Hoebeke, Nicolaas Lumen and Stan Monstrey

28 Female Genital Reconstruction I, 218
Sarah M. Creighton

29 Female Genital Reconstruction II, 224
Jeffrey A. Leslie and Richard C. Rink

30 Persistent Cloaca, 232
Stephanie Warne and Duncan T. Wilcox

Part VII Renal Impairment Surgery

31 Hemodialysis and Peritoneal Dialysis, 241
    Alun Williams

32 Kidney Transplantation, 247
    Alun Williams

Part VIII Urogenital Tumors

33 Wilms Tumor and Other Renal Tumors, 257
    Michael Ritchey and Sarah Conley

34 Rhabdomyosarcoma, 262
    Barbara Ercole, Michael Isakoff and Fernando A. Ferrer

35 Testicular Tumors, 269
    Jonathan H. Ross

36 Adrenal Tumors, 278
    Bruce Broecker and James Elmore

Part IX Trauma

37 Genital Trauma, 289
    Vijaya Vemulakonda and Richard W. Grady

38 Urinary Tract Trauma, 296
    Ashok Rijhwani, W. Robert DeFoor, Jr, and Eugene Minevich

Part X Surgery for Urinary and Fecal Incontinence

39 Augmentation Cystoplasty, 307
    Prasad P. Godbole

40 Appendicovesicostomy and Ileovesicostomy, 315
    Martin Kaefer

41 Surgical Management of the Sphincter Mechanism, 324
    Juan C. Prieto and Linda A. Baker

42 Surgery for Fecal Incontinence, 337
    W. Robert DeFoor, Jr, Eugene Minevich, Curtis A. Sheldon and Martin A. Koyle

Index, 344

Contributors

Paul F. Austin MD, FAAP
Director of Pediatric Urology Research
Associate Professor of Urologic Surgery
St. Louis Children's Hospital
Washington University School of Medicine
St. Louis, MO, USA

Linda A. Baker MD
Director of Pediatric Urology Research
Associate Professor of Urology
University of Texas Southwestern Medical Center at Dallas;
Pediatric Urologist
Children's Medical Center at Dallas
Dallas, TX, USA

Laurence S. Baskin MD
Professor of Urology and Pediatrics
Chief of Pediatric Urology
UCSF Children's Hospital
University of California
San Francisco, CA, USA

Ben Bridgewater MBBS, PhD, FRCS (CTh)
Consultant Cardiac Surgeon
Clinical Director and Director of Clinical Audit
University Hospital of South Manchester NHS Foundation Trust
Manchester, UK

Bruce Broecker MD
Clinical Associate Professor of Pediatric Urology
Emory University School of Medicine
Atlanta, GA, USA

Benjamin M. Brucker MD
Children's Hospital of Philadelphia
Hospital of the University of Pennsylvania
Philadelphia, PA, USA

Pasquale Casale MD
Division of Pediatric Urology
Children's Hospital of Philadelphia
Philadelphia, PA, USA

Job K. Chacko MD
Fellow, Pediatric Urology
A.I. duPont Hospital for Children
Thomas Jefferson University
Wilmington, DE, USA

Laura Coates MBBS, MRCS
Paediatric Surgery Registrar
Department of Paediatric Surgery
Bristol Royal Hospital for Children
Bristol, UK

Sarah Conley MD
Resident, Urology
Mayo Clinic College of Medicine
Phoenix, AZ, USA

Sarah M. Creighton MD, FRCOG
Consultant Gynaecologist
Elizabeth Garrett Anderson Hospital
University College Hospital
London, UK

Paul Crow MbChb, MD, FRCS (Urol)
Specialist Registrar in Paediatric Urology
Department of Paediatric Urology
Bristol Royal Hospital for Children
Bristol, UK

Joe I. Curry MBBS, FRCS (Eng), FRCS (Paed Surg)
Consultant Neonatal and Paediatric Surgeon
The Hospital for Sick Children
Great Ormond Street
London, UK

W. Robert DeFoor, Jr, MD, MPH
Assistant Professor
Division of Pediatric Urology
Cincinnati Children's Hospital
Cincinnati, OH, USA

Divyesh Desai MB MS, MChir (Urology), FEAPU
Paediatric Urologist and Director, Urodynamics Unit
Great Ormond Street Hospital for Children NHS Trust;
Honorary Lecturer, Institute of Child Health
London, UK

Steven G. Docimo MD
Vice President of Medical Affairs
Professor and Director, Pediatric Urology
The Children's Hospital of Pittsburgh of UPMC;
Vice-Chairman, Department of Urology
The University of Pittsburgh Medical Center
Pittsburgh, PA, USA

H. Serkan Dogan MD
Division of Pediatric Urology
Department of Urology
Uludag University
Bursa, Turkey

Ahmad A. Elderwy MD
Visiting Fellow, Pediatric Urology
Children's Hospital and Regional Medical Center
Seattle, WA, USA;
Assiut University Hospital
Assiut, Egypt

James Elmore MD
Clinical Assistant Professor of Pediatric Urology
Emory University School of Medicine
Atlanta, GA, USA

Barbara Ercole MD
University of Connecticut
Hartford, CT, USA

Philippa Evans BA, MBBS, MRCP, FRCA
SpR Anaesthetics
Great Ormond Street Hospital
London, UK

Fernando A. Ferrer MD
Associate Professor
Pediatric Surgery (Urology) and Oncology
Connecticut Children's Medical Center
University of Connecticut
Hartford, CT, USA

Douglas Ford MD
Professor of Pediatrics
Section of Pediatric Nephrology
University of Colorado at Denver and Health Sciences Center
The Children's Hospital
Aurora, CO, USA

Prasad P. Godbole FRCS, FRCS (Paed)
Consultant Paediatric Urologist
Sheffield Children's NHS Trust
Sheffield, UK

Richard W. Grady MD
Associate Professor of Urology
Department of Urology
The University of Washington School of Medicine
Children's Hospital and Regional Medical Center
Seattle, WA, USA

Yves Héloury MD, FEAPU
Professor of Pediatric Surgery
Head of Department
Hôpital Mère-Enfant
Nantes, France

Piet Hoebeke MD, PhD
Department of Pediatric Urology and Urogenital Reconstruction
Ghent University Hospital
Gent, Belgium

Kim A.R. Hutton MBChB, ChM, FRCS (Paed)
Consultant Paediatric Surgeon and Urologist
University Hospital of Wales
Cardiff, Wales, UK

Michael Isakoff MD
Assistant Professor
Hematology and Oncology
Connecticut Children's Medical Center
University of Connecticut
Hartford, CT, USA

Martin Kaefer MD
Associate Professor of Urology
Department of Pediatric Urology
Indiana University School of Medicine
Indianapolis, IN, USA

Chris Kimber FRACS, FRCS, MAICD
Head of Paediatric Surgery and Urology
Southern Health;
Consultant Paediatric Urologist
Royal Children's Hospital
Melbourne, Australia

Korgun Koral MD
Associate Professor of Radiology
University of Texas Southwestern Medical Center at Dallas;
Children's Medical Center
Dallas, TX, USA

Martin A. Koyle MD, FAAP, FACS
Professor of Urology and Pediatrics
University of Washington;
Chief, Division of Urology
Children's Hospital and Regional Medical Center
Seattle, WA, USA

Marc-David Leclair MD, FEAPU
Consultant in Pediatric Urology
Pediatric Surgery Department
Hôpital Mère-Enfant
Nantes, France

Jeffrey A. Leslie MD
Fellow, Pediatric Urology
James Whitcomb Riley Hospital for Children
Indiana University Department of Urology
Indianapolis, IN, USA

Nicolaas Lumen MD
Department of Pediatric Urology and Urogenital Reconstruction
Ghent University Hospital
Gent, Belgium

Eva Macharia BA, MA (Oxon), MBBChir (Cantab)
Surgical Trainee
Department of Paediatric Urology
St. James University Hospital
Leeds, UK

Derek J. Matoka MD
Division of Pediatric Urology
Children's Hospital of Pittsburgh of UPMC
The University of Pittsburgh Medical Center
Pittsburgh, PA, USA

Neil McMullin MBBS, FRACS, FFin, MAICD
Director of Urology
Royal Children's Hospital;
Consultant Paediatric Urologist
Southern Health
Melbourne, Australia

Eugene Minevich MD
Associate Professor
Division of Pediatric Urology
Cincinnati Children's Hospital Medical Center
Cincinnati, OH, USA

Gerald Mingin MD
Assistant Professor of Surgery
The University of Vermont;
Attending Pediatric Urologist
Vermont Children's Hospital
Burlington, VT, USA

Stan Monstrey MD, PhD
Department of Plastic Surgery
Ghent University Hospital
Gent, Belgium

L. Henning Olsen MD, FEBU, FEAPU
Consultant Urological Surgeon
Pediatric Urologist
Clinical Associate Professor in Urology
Department of Urology, Section of Pediatric Urology
Aarhus University Hospital, Skejby;
Institute of Clinical Medicine
University of Aarhus
Aarhus, Denmark

Michael C. Ost MD
Assistant Professor of Pediatric Urology
Division of Pediatric Urology
Children's Hospital of Pittsburgh of UPMC
The University of Pittsburgh Medical Center
Pittsburgh, PA, USA

Rakesh P. Patel MD, MS, FRCS
Children's Hospital of Philadelphia
Hospital of the University of Pennsylvania
Philadelphia, PA, USA

Juan Carlos Prieto MD
Fellow, Pediatric Urology
University of Texas Southwestern Medical Center at Dallas;
Children's Medical Center at Dallas
Dallas, TX, USA

Christian Radmayr MD, PhD, FEAPU
Professor of Urology
Head, Department of Pediatric Urology
Medical University Innsbruck
Innsbruck, Austria

Yazan F. Rawashdeh MD, PhD
Department of Urology, Section of Pediatric Urology
Aarhus University Hospital, Skejby;
Institute of Clinical Medicine
University of Aarhus
Aarhus, Denmark

Ashok Rijhwani MS, MCh, FRCS, DNB
Consultant Pediatric Surgeon, Pediatric Urologist and
Transplant Surgeon
Columbia Asia Hospital
Bangalore, India

Richard C. Rink MD
Robert A. Garrett Professor of Pediatric Urology
Chief, Pediatric Urology
James Whitcomb Riley Hospital for Children
Indiana University School of Medicine
Indianapolis, IN, USA

Michael Ritchey MD
Professor of Urology
Mayo Clinic College of Medicine
Scottsdale, AZ, USA

Jonathan H. Ross MD
Head, Section of Pediatric Urology
Glickman Urological and Kidney Institute
The Children's Hospital at Cleveland Clinic;
Associate Professor of Surgery
Cleveland Clinic Lerner College of Medicine
Case Western Reserve University
Cleveland, OH, USA

Indranil Sau MBBS, MS, MRCS
Registrar in Paediatric Surgery
University Hospital of Wales
Cardiff, Wales, UK

Curtis A. Sheldon MD, FACS, FAAP
Professor and Director
Division of Pediatric Urology
Cincinnati Children's Hospital
Cincinnati, OH, USA

Andrew Sinclair FRCS (Urol)
Urology Registrar
Northwest England Regional Rotation
Cheshire, UK

Marc C. Smaldone MD
Division of Pediatric Urology
Children's Hospital of Pittsburgh of UPMC
The University of Pittsburgh Medical Center
Pittsburgh, PA, USA

Warren T. Snodgrass MD
Professor of Urology
Department of Urology, Pediatric Urology Section
Children's Medical Center and the University of Texas Southwestern
Medical Center
Dallas, TX, USA

Henrik Steinbrecher BSc (Hons), MBBS, MS, FRCS, FRCS (Paed)
Consultant Pediatric Urologist
Southampton General Hospital
Southampton, UK

Ramnath Subramaniam MBBS, FRCS (Paed), FEAPU
Consultant Pediatric Urologist
St. James University Hospital
Leeds, UK

Serdar Tekgül MD
Division of Pediatric Urology
Department of Urology
Hacettepe University
Ankara, Turkey

Mark Thomas BSc, MBBChir, FRCA
Consultant Paediatric Anaesthetist
Great Ormond Street Hospital
London, UK

J.S. Valla MD, FRCS, FEAPU
Chirurgie Pédiatrique
Fondation Lenval
Nice, France

Vijaya M. Vemulakonda MD, JD
Fellow, Pediatric Urology
The University of Washington School of Medicine
Children's Hospital and Regional Medical Center
Seattle, WA, USA

Stephanie Warne MD, MB BCh, FRCS
Paediatric Surgical Registrar
Royal Hospital for Sick Children
Edinburgh, UK

Robert Wheeler FRCS, MS, FRCPCH, LLB (Hons), LLM
Consultant Paediatric & Neonatal Surgeon
Honorary Senior Lecturer in Medical Law
Wessex Regional Centre for Paediatric Surgery
Southampton University Hospitals Trust
Southampton, UK

Duncan T. Wilcox MBBS, MD, FEAPU
Associate Professor, Pediatric Urology
Rose Mary Haggar Professorship in Urology
University of Texas Southwestern
Dallas, TX, USA

Alun Williams FRCS (Paed)
Consultant Paediatric Urologist
Nottingham University Hospitals NHS Trust
Nottingham, UK

Benjamin Wisner MD
Senior Resident, Division of Urology/Department of Surgery
The Children's Hospital
University of Colorado at Denver and Health Sciences Center
Aurora, CO, USA

Mark Woodward MD, FRCS (Paed)
Consultant Paediatric Urologist
Department of Paediatric Urology
Bristol Royal Hospital for Children
Bristol, UK

Jenny Yiee MD
Department of Urology
University of California Los Angeles
Los Angeles, CA, USA

Foreword

The readers of any book devoted to surgical complications will inevitably be looking for insights into how to avoid these complications in the first place. In this outstanding new textbook they will not be disappointed. Duncan Wilcox, Prasad Godbole and Martin Koyle and their impressive international team of contributors have extended their remit beyond a simple account of complications to produce a comprehensive and authoritative overview of what constitutes good practice in the specialty of pediatric urology.

As surgeons we tend to focus on factors such as technical error, inexperience and inadequate training. Nevertheless, it is important to recognise that many adverse outcomes are multifactorial in origin, reflecting system failures rather than the failings of an individual surgeon. Indeed, weak teamwork, poor communication and substandard overall care can conspire to undo the work of the most experienced and talented of surgical craftsmen. Decision making and clinical judgement are also fundamental to good surgical practice and no amount of technical mastery will guarantee success when an operation has been performed unnecessarily or for the wrong indications. For this reason the editors and contributors have also examined the broader factors contributing to poor surgical outcomes.

Surgeons in all specialties are rapidly having to adapt to the demands of greater accountability and the chapter on personal audit provides welcome guidance on this subject.

Post operative death, the most measurable of adverse outcomes, is thankfully a rare event in pediatric urological practice. But whilst many non lethal complications can be readily documented and compared between surgeons (hypospadias revision rates and testicular atrophy following orchidopexy being obvious examples) deriving meaningful and reproducible measures of the success of other procedures, such as continence rates after lower tract reconstruction, can be more problematic. In the face of these difficulties the editors and contributors have nevertheless succeeded in providing pediatric urologists

with the most comprehensive and authoritative overview of results and complications published to date.

Surgical advances and innovations inevitably bring risks as well as benefits. The chapters on minimally invasive treatments of stone disease, endoscopic correction of reflux and laparoscopic pediatric urology will be read with particular interest by those surgeons who are still on their personal learning curves with these new interventional procedures.

Despite the surgeon's best endeavors, almost every operation carries some risk of unavoidable complications and virtually no pediatric urological procedure can guarantee an outcome which will always meet the patient's (more often parents') expectations. One of the more undesirable aspects of modern surgical practice is the prevalence of malpractice lawyers ready to exploit these situations. In fact, many aggrieved parents may simply be seeking an explanation and a possible apology rather than punitive financial redress. It is to be hoped that that this excellent book may help to forestall some misguided litigation by enabling pediatric urologists to put occasional individual adverse outcomes into context – by reference to the results reported by other surgeons and within the speciality as a whole.

Surgical training has traditionally relied upon the apprenticeship model in which young surgeons benefited from the experience of their seniors, which in many instances included hard lessons learned "on the job." This approach to specialist training is now both unacceptable and outdated. Unacceptable because of a regulatory climate which dictates that experience should no longer be gained at the expense of patients. Outdated because the old apprenticeship model is increasingly difficult to reconcile with the reduction in trainees' working hours and their legitimate expectation of a better work/life balance.

As we move to a far more structured model of training the emphasis will shift to learning about complications, not at first or second hand, but through a collective experience disseminated via meetings, journals and the authoritative multi author format exemplified by this textbook. Duncan Wilcox, Prasad Godbole and Martin Koyle and their contributors are to be congratulated on this outstanding contribution to the training and continuing education of pediatric urologists at every stage in their careers. The role of this textbook in promoting higher standards of surgical practice is also destined to make an invaluable contribution to the future well being of pediatric urological patients and their families.

Professor David F.M. Thomas
Department of Paediatric Urology
Leeds Teaching Hospitals
Leeds, UK

Preface

In recent years there has been an increasing emphasis on evidenced-based medicine. To improve surgical-based specialties, it is essential to understand that complications occur and that honest reporting of complications is vital if we are to continue to develop. In the field of pediatric urology, there are a number of textbooks that concentrate on the diagnosis and treatment of conditions. The aim of this book, however, is to focus on surgical outcomes and hence complications in pediatric urology. In addition, ways to avoid and treat complications are discussed.

We are very grateful to our authors, who have drawn on their experience and the literature to give an honest account of the surgical outcomes and complications of pediatric urological procedures and are giving advice on how to avoid and treat such problems. Where possible this book has relied on evidenced-based information but where this is not available then surgical experience has been highlighted. As you will see there is plenty of room left in the field of pediatric urology for new evidenced-based practice.

We would like to thank Elisabeth Dodds of Wiley-Blackwell for all her advice with this project and trying to ensure we remained on schedule, and to the authors of the chapters who were understanding and timely with their submissions.

Most importantly, we wish to thank our families for all their support and patience with this project.

Duncan T. Wilcox
Prasad P. Godbole
Martin A. Koyle

Principles of
Surgical Audit

1

How to Set Up a Prospective Surgical Audit

Andrew Sinclair and Ben Bridgewater

Key points

- Clinical audit can be prospective and/or retrospective.
- Audit information can be obtained from national, hospital, and surgeon-specific data.
- A clinical department benefits from a clear audit plan.
- Clinical audit improves patient outcome.

Introduction

Clinical audit is one of the "keystones" of clinical governance. A surgical department that subjects itself to regular and comprehensive audit should be able to provide data to current and prospective patients about the quality of the services it provides, as well as reassurance to those who pay for and regulate health care. Well-organized audit should also enable the clinicians providing services to continually improve the quality of care they deliver.

There are many similarities between audit and research, but historically audit has often been seen as the "poor relation." For audit to be meaningful and useful, it must, like research, be methodologically robust and have sufficient "power" to make useful observations; it would be easy to gain false reassurance about the quality of care by looking at outcomes in a small or "cherry-picked" group of straightforward cases. Audit can be conducted retrospectively or prospectively and, again like research, prospective audit has the potential to provide the most useful data, and routine prospective audit provides excellent opportunities for patient benefit [1–4].

Pediatric Urology: Surgical Complications and Management. Edited by Duncan T. Wilcox, Prasad P. Godbole and Martin A. Koyle. © 2008 Blackwell Publishing, ISBN: 978-1-4051-6268-5.

Much of the experience we draw on comes from cardiac surgery, where there is a long history of structured data collection, both in the United States and in the United Kingdom. This was initially driven by clinicians [1–3,5], but more recently has been influenced by politicians and the media [6,7]. Cardiac surgery is regarded as an easy specialty to audit in view of the high volume and proportion of a single operation coronary artery bypass graft (CABG) in most surgeons practice set against a small but significant hard measurement end point of mortality (which is typically approximately 2%).

Why conduct prospective audit?

There are a number of reasons why clinicians might decide to conduct a clinical audit as given in Table 1.1.

Table 1.1 Possible reasons for conducting clinical audit.

As a result of local clinical interests
As a result of clinical incident reporting
To comply with regional or national initiatives
To inform patients about surgical results
To drive continuous quality improvement
For health care regulation

As a result of local clinical interests

Historically, many audit projects have been undertaken as a result of local clinical interests. This may reflect interest in a particular procedure by an individual or a group, or may reflect concern about specific outcomes for a particular operation.

As a result of clinical incident reporting

The major "disciplines" that ensure high quality care and patient safety are clinical risk management and audit. Most health care organizations should have sophisticated systems in place to report and learn from adverse incidents and near misses [8]. Reporting is usually voluntary and investigated according to a "fair and just culture" but it is unlikely that all incidents that occur are reported. If an adverse incident is recorded, this identifies that it has occurred, but gives no indication of how often it has happened previously, and only limited indication of the likelihood of recurrence. A mature organization should have clear links between risk reporting and audit, and choose topics for the latter based on data from the former.

To comply with regional or national initiatives

Increasingly, audits have been driven by organizations that exist outside a hospital. These may include audit led by professional societies, regulatory bodies, or regional/national quality improvement initiatives.

To inform patients about surgical results

Across the world, health care is becoming more patient-focussed. The modern health care consumer will sometimes look to choose their health care provider on the basis of that hospital or surgeon's outcomes and, even if patients are not choosing between different hospitals, recent data from the United Kingdom suggests that patients are interested in outcomes of surgery by their doctors [9]. Patients' views should inform decisions about what to audit, and they may be interested in many areas which will be dependent on the planned operation but may include data on mortality, success rates, length of stay, and the incidence of postoperative infection and other complications.

To drive continuous quality improvement

It has been shown quite clearly from cardiac surgery that structured data collection, analysis, and feedback to clinicians improve the quality of outcomes. This has been detected when data is anonymous [2,3] and where

named surgeon and hospital outcomes have been published [1,4]. The magnitude of this effect is large; in the United Kingdom a system of national reporting for surgical outcomes was introduced in 2001 and has led to a 40% reduction in risk-adjusted mortality [4]. The introduction of any drug showing a similar benefit would be heralded as a major breakthrough, but routine national audit has not been embraced by most surgical specialties. Simply collecting and reviewing data seems to drive improvement, but is likely that the magnitude of the benefits derived and the speed at which improvements are seen can be maximized by developing a clear understanding of what data to collect and using optimal managerial structures and techniques to deliver better care. There is some debate about whether publicly disclosing health care outcomes encourages clinicians to avoid taking on high-risk cases [1,4,7,10,11].

For health care regulation

Health care regulators have a responsibility to ensure that hospitals, and the clinicians working in them, are performing to a satisfactory standard. While some assurance can be gained from examining the systems and processes in place within an organization, the "proof of the pudding is in the eating" and demonstrating satisfactory clinical results is important and can only come from analyzing benchmarked outcomes data. Regulators of individual clinicians, such as the American Boards in the United States and the General Medical Council in the United Kingdom, are changing their emphasis so that it is becoming more important for clinicians to prove they are doing a good job, rather than this being assumed. Routine use of structured outcomes data is included in draft proposals for recertification by the American Board of Thoracic Surgery and the Society for Cardiothoracic Surgery of Great Britain and Ireland and will follow to other specialties in time [12].

What data can be used for audit?

Routine hospital data

Most health care systems are rich in data and poor in information. Medicare data in the United States and Hospital Episodes Statistics in the United Kingdom contain data on patient demographics, diagnoses, procedure, mortality, length of stay, day cases rates, and readmissions. These information systems are developed for administration or financial purposes rather than clinical ones, but may potentially contain much useful clinical data and will often have the capacity to provide some degree of adjustment for casemix. In the United Kingdom, this data has historically not been trusted by clinicians, but recently there has been increasing engagement between doctors and the data which is improving clinical data quality and increasing confidence. Many UK hospitals now have systems to benchmark their outcomes against national or other peer groups, flag up areas of good practice, detect outlying performance, and engage in quality improvement [13].

Ideally, hospitals should have clearly defined systems in place to use the data: for example, they should regularly compare their outcomes for chosen procedures against an appropriately selected group of other hospitals. Significant "good" practice should be celebrated and shared with others inside and outside the organization, and bad outcomes should be investigated. It is not infrequent that high mortality or other clinical indictor rates may have a clear explanation other than that of "bad" clinical practice. The data may be incorrect, or there may be issues about classification or attribution that explain away an apparent alert, but structured investigation should improve the organization's and the clinician's knowledge about their data systems and may lead to impressions that necessitate improvements in patient care.

Specialty-specific multicenter data

A number of surgical disciplines in the United States and the United Kingdom have embarked upon national programs to collect prospective disease- or operation-specific datasets. These are usually clinically driven and have benefits above routine hospital data in that a more useful dataset can be designed for specific purposes and in particular can look in more detail at subtleties of casemix and specific clinical outcomes in a way that is more robust and sensitive than that derived from routine hospital administration systems. Contemporary cardiac surgical datasets collect variables on preoperative patient characteristics, precise operative data and postoperative mortality, ICU stay, hospital stay, reexplorations, infection, renal failure, tracheostomy, blood usage, stroke rate, and intraaortic balloon pump use. The preoperative and operative data allow outcomes to be adjusted for case complexity to prevent comparison of "apples and oranges" by various algorithms such as the EuroSCORE [14].

Setting up specialty-specific multicenter audit raises a number of challenges including defining clarity of purpose, gaining consensus, agreeing a dataset, securing resource, overcoming information technology issues, and clarifying ownership of data, information policies,

and governance arrangements. In cardiac surgery, there is now increasing international dialogue between professional organizations to move toward the collection of standardized data to allow widespread comparisons.

Locally derived data

Individual hospital departments will often decide to audit a specific theme that may be chosen because of clinical risk management issues, subspecialist interest, or other concerns. In the UK National Health Service (NHS), dedicated resource for audit was historically "top sliced" from the purchasers of health care to generate a culture of clinical quality improvement, but commentators are divided about whether significant benefits have been realized from this approach [9]. In the early stages, large amounts of audit activity were undertaken, but there were significant failures in subsequently delivering appropriate change. To maximize the chances of improving care as a result of audit, the following should be considered. Will the sample size be big enough to be useful? What dataset is needed? Will that data be accessible from existing hospital casenotes or will prospective data collection be necessary? Is there an existing robust benchmark to which the results of the audit can be compared? How will the "significance" of the results be analyzed? Does conducting the audit have financial implications? Will the potential results of the audit have financial implications? Are all stakeholders who may need to change their behavior as a result of the audit involved in the process?

Techniques of data collection

Historically, the majority of audit activity was conducted from retrospective examination of casenotes, which was labour intensive and relied on the accuracy and completeness of previously recorded data. There has subsequently been increasing use of prospective data collection, much of which has been based on paper forms. This obviously improves the quality of data, but again requires time and effort from clinical or administrative staff for completion. The development of care pathways whereby multidisciplinary teams manage clinical conditions in predefined ways are thought to improve patient outcomes and will generate structured data that is readily amenable to audit. The use of modern information technology to support care pathways is the "holy grail" of effective audit – all data is generated for clinical use and the relevant subset of that data can then be examined for any relevant purpose. The care pathway can be adapted to include new or alternative variables as required. All data collection can be networked and wireless, assuming issues about data access, confidentiality, and security are resolved. Variations on this theme are now available in many hospitals and it is these principles that underpin a major IT investment in the UK NHS [15]. Maximizing benefits from this approach raises a number of challenges including producing major changes in clinical practice and medical culture.

Good practice in audit

A clinical department should benefit from a clear forward plan about its audit activity that should be developed by the multidisciplinary team in conjunction with patients and their carers. The audit activity should include an appropriate mix of national, local, and risk management driven issues, and the specifics should depend on the configuration of services and local preferences. The plan should include thoughts about dissemination of results to users and potential users of the services. The multidisciplinary team should include doctors, professionals allied to medicine, and administration staff. Adherence to the audit plan should be monitored through the departmental operational management structures. For the department to be successful in improving care as a result of audit, there should be clear understanding of effective techniques of change management.

Arguments against audit

In the United Kingdom, audit has been an essential part of all doctors' job plans for a number of years, but audit activity remains sporadic. In some high-profile specialties such as cardiac surgery, comprehensive audit has been led by clinicians and driven by politicians and the media. In other areas there has been little or no coordinated national audit activity. This may be due to a perceived lack of benefits from audit from clinicians along with failure to meet challenges in gaining consensus or difficulties in securing adequate resource. The experience from cardiac surgery is that structured national audit improves the quality of mortality outcomes [1–4]. It is likely that other issues such as complication rates are also reduced with associated costs savings, and as such effective audit may well pay for itself.

Summary

In modern health care, patients are increasingly looking to be reassured about the quality of care they receive and doctors are being driven toward demonstrating their competence, rather than this being assumed. Hospital departments should have a robust clinical governance strategy that should include "joined-up" clinical risk management and audit activity. There are strong arguments that structured audit activity improves the quality of outcomes and for these benefits to be maximized there should be involvement of multidisciplinary teams supported by high-quality operational management.

References

1 Hannan EL, Kilburn H, Jr., Racz M, Shields E, Chassin MR. Improving the outcomes of coronary artery bypass surgery in New York State. *JAMA* 1994;271:761–6.
2 Grover FL, Shroyer LW, Hammermeister K, Edwards FH, Ferguson TB, Dziuban SW *et al*. A decade of experience with quality improvement in cardiac surgery using the Veterans Affairs and Society of Thoracic Surgeons national databases. *Ann Surg* 2001;234:464–74.
3 Hammermeister KE, Johnson R, Marshall G, Grover FL. Continuous assessment and improvement in quality of care. A model from the Department of Veterans Affairs Cardiac Surgery. *Ann Surg* 1994;219:281–90.
4 Bridgewater B, Grayson AD, Brooks N, Grotte G, Fabri B, Au J *et al*. Has the publication of cardiac surgery outcome data been associated with changes in practice in Northwest England: An analysis of 25,730 patients undergoing CABG surgery under 30 surgeons over 8 years. *Heart* 2007; January 19; [Epub ahead of print]. PMID: 17237128.
5 Keogh BE, Kinsman R. Fifth national adult cardiac surgical database report 2003.
6 Available at http://society.guardian.co.uk/nhsperformance/story/0,,1439210,00.html accessed on 25.01.2008 .
7 Marshal M, Sheklle P, Brook R, Leatherman S. Dying to know: Public release of information about quality of healthcare. *Nuffield Trust and Rand* 2000.
8 An organisation with a memory. Report of an expert group on learning from adverse events in the NHS chaired by the Chief Medical Officer accessed on 25.01.2008. http://www.dh.gov.uk/en/Publicationsandstatistics/Publications/PublicationsPolicyAndGuidance/DH_4065083.
9 Good Doctors, safer patients. Proposals to strengthen the system to assure and improve the performance of doctors and to protect the safety of patients. A report by the Chief Medical Officer accessed on 25.01.2008. http://www.dh.gov.uk/en/Publicationsandstatistics/Publications/PublicationsPolicyAndGuidance/DH_4065083.

10 Chassin MR, Hannan EL, DeBuono BA. Benefits and hazards of reporting medical outcomes publicly. *N Engl J Med* 1996;334:394–8.

11 Dranove D, Kessler D, McCellan M, Satterthwaite M. Is more information better? The effects of report cards on healthcare providers. *J Polit Econ* 2003;111:555–88.

12 *Trust, assurance and safety. The regulation of health professionals in the 21st Century*. The Stationary Office: London, February 2007. http://www.dh.gov.uk/en/Publicationsandst atistics/Publications/PublicationsPolicyAndGuidance/DH_ 065946.

13 Available at www.drfoster.co.uk. accessed on 25.01.2008 .

14 Roques F, Nashef SA, Michel P *et al*. Risk factors and outcome in European cardiac surgery; analysis of the EuroSCORE multinational database of 19,030 patients. *Eur J Cardiothorac Surg* 1999;15:816–23.

15 Available at www.connectingforhealth.nhs.uk/. accessed on 25.01.2008.

2

Evaluating Personal Surgical Audit and What to Do If Your Results Are Outside the "Mean"

Andrew Sinclair and Ben Bridgewater

Key points

- Audit is the comparison of surgical results against a previously defined and accepted standard.
- Published results may be better than the normal surgeon's.
- Complexity specific audit is important.

- Dealing with outlying performance can be "directive" or "collaborative" depending on the surgeon.
- Surgeons are responsible for ensuring satisfactory quality of care.

Introduction

Any well-conducted audit should give information about systems and outcomes related to patient care. Data collection that generates new information about patient outcomes should be classified as research and to be regarded as audit, results need to be compared against a previously defined and accepted standard. Often an audit will demonstrate satisfactory outcomes and this in itself may be a useful finding which should be of interest to patients, clinicians, managers, commissioners, and regulators of health care. It is hoped that structured and regular audit data collection will lead to ongoing improvements in quality as described in the previous chapter. On occasions audit results will be unacceptable and it is essential that this is recognized and acted upon.

Pediatric Urology: Surgical Complications and Management. Edited by Duncan T. Wilcox, Prasad P. Godbole and Martin A. Koyle. © 2008 Blackwell Publishing, ISBN: 978-1-4051-6268-5.

Presentation and analysis of data

Effective audit requires clarity of purpose. When an audit is conceived the clinical question should be clearly stated and the data required to generate an answer should be defined. It is also important to be sure to what outcomes you will compare yourself, and there may be a number of options. Data on mortality or complication rates may be available from pooled national or regional registries [1–4]. Results of specific series of cases may be published through peer review journals for individual hospitals or individuals, but these outcomes may often be better than the "norm" because of submission and publication bias. False reassurance may be gained from comparing outcomes with outdated historical results; in cardiac surgery in the United Kingdom a widely accepted risk-adjustment algorithm, the EuroSCORE [5], has been used to benchmark hospitals and surgeons in recent years. This was developed in a multicenter study in Europe in 1997 and improvements in overall quality of care in the United Kingdom are such that it no longer reflects current practice [6]. In the United Kingdom, any cardiac surgeon who is not currently performing significantly better than predicted by the EuroSCORE would have a mortality rate that was higher than that of their peer group. It is unclear whether it still accurately predicts mortality elsewhere in Europe. This concept of "calibration drift" for cardiac surgery has been seen in both the United Kingdom and the United States.

It is possible to compare outcomes between units or surgeons simply by using "crude" or nonrisk-adjusted data. Cardiac surgeons have focussed on mortality, as it is a robust primary end point. In pediatric urology, mortality is not frequent enough to provide a meaningful measure and more appropriate end points need to be developed.

Using nonrisk-adjusted data has simplicity and transparency on its side but is not embraced with enthusiasm by the majority of surgeons. It is clear that there are quite marked differences in patients' characteristics between different units in cardiac surgery and this variability is probably greater between surgeons who have different subspecialist interests [7]. These issues will surely apply to other areas of surgery. Many surgeons are concerned that any attempt to produce comparative performance using nonrisk-adjusted data will stimulate a culture whereby higher risk patients are denied surgery to help maintain good results – the so-called risk averse behavior. To make data comparable between individual surgeons and units, there have been a number of attempts to adjust for operative risk in cardiac surgery [8–10]. Other specialties will need to develop appropriate methodology, and ideal tools should be accurate numerical predictors of observed risk (i.e. be calibrated correctly) and be able to discriminate appropriately across the spectrum of risk (i.e. accurately differentiate between lower- and higher-risk patients).

In addition to the appropriate use of risk adjustment, some units have found graphical techniques of presenting outcomes data useful to monitor performance. Various techniques have been used to help analyze results and detect trends or outlying performance at an early stage, such as cumulative summation or variable life-adjusted display plots. These curves may be adapted to include predicted mortality to enable observed and expected mortality to be compared. These techniques are well described by Keogh and Kinsman [2]. More recently interest is developing for measuring outcomes using statistical process control charts, which are widely used in manufacturing industry. These charts use units of time, typically months when institutions are under scrutiny and the outcome of interest is mortality, and display actual mortality against expected mortality, using control limits to define acceptable and unacceptable performance [11].

The use of funnel plots is becoming popular as a way of displaying hospital or individual mortality [12]. They are simply a plot of event rates against volume of surgery, and include exact binomial control limits, to allow excessive mortality to be easily detected. They give a "strong visual display of divergent performance" [2]. They have been used to analyze routine data to define clinical casemix and compare hospital outcomes in urology [13].

Classical statistical techniques may be used to compare individual outcomes with a benchmark. When analyzing data from an individual hospital or surgeon, it is probably appropriate to select 95% confidence intervals such that if significant differences are observed, there is a 1 in 20 probability that these are due to chance alone. Things become more difficult when many hospitals or surgeons are compared to a national benchmark. In the United Kingdom there are over 200 cardiac surgeons and any comparison of the group against the pooled mortality using 95% confidence intervals would raise a high probability of detecting outlying performance due to chance alone because of multiple comparisons, and it is appropriate to adjust for this. The choice of confidence intervals will always end up as a balance between ensuring that true outlying performance is detected without inappropriately creating stigma for surgeons with satisfactory outcomes. It may be useful to select different confidence limits for different purposes. Tight limits may be appropriate for local supportive clinical governance monitoring; one hospital in North West England launches an internal investigation into practice if a cardiac surgeon's results fall outside 80% confidence limits but wider limits of 99% have been used to report those surgeons' outcomes to the public [14].

Dealing with outlying performance

Detecting clinical outcomes that fall outside accepted limits does not necessarily indicate substandard patient care, but any analysis which indicates concern should trigger further validation of the data if appropriate and then, if indicated, an in-depth evaluation of clinical practice which may include analysis of subspecialty, casemix, and an exploration of the exact mechanisms of death or complications. This process may lead to reassurance that practice is satisfactory. Ideally this should be initiated by the concerned clinician who should be keen to learn from the experience to improve their practice. An excellent example comes from pediatric cardiac surgery where a surgeon developed concerns about his mortality outcomes following the arterial switch operation (which is complex, technically challenging, and congenital surgery) [15]. He studied his outcomes in detail using Cumulative Summation (CUSUM) methodology and determined that things were worse than he would have expected due to chance alone. He then underwent retraining with a colleague from another hospital with excellent outcomes, adapted his practice, and subsequently went on to demonstrate good outcomes in a further series of consecutive cases.

On occasion, the process of investigating outlying outcomes may be difficult for the individual hospital or surgeon involved. The investigation may raise significant methodological questions about the techniques of analysis and subsequent examinations. The cause of substandard results may be difficult to detect but may relate to failures in the systems of care in the hospital or department, or failures in the individual [16,7].

Clinical governance is an individual, departmental, and hospital responsibility. While the onus should be on the individual with unsatisfactory outcomes to investigate and change their practice, they may need support, advice, and direction from their clinical and managerial colleagues. Over recent years the roles of different organizations in clinical governance is becoming clearer. Most hospitals should now have increasingly effective management structures for promoting quality improvement and detecting suboptimal performance [17,18].

The investigation of unsatisfactory outcomes can be facilitated by an appropriate clinical leadership, and different techniques may be necessary for different circumstances with the concepts of "situational leadership" being useful to match the managerial intervention to the willingness and the readiness of the individual whose practice is being investigated [19]. Two examples make this point. A newly appointed cardiac surgeon had three adverse outcomes following the same type of operation that seemed to the colleagues to be due to a similar mechanism. Despite discussions the surgeon involved had little or no insight into the problem. No confidence intervals for performance were crossed because of the small volume of cases involved but, due to the clinical concerns, the surgeon was subjected to forced but supportive retraining of his intraoperative techniques, which led to re-introduction of full independent practice within a few months and excellent publicly reported results for that operation several years later. This would be described in a situational leadership model as a "directive" approach. A second example is that of a senior surgeon with a low volume mixed cardiothoracic practice

who had a "bad run" of cardiac results, which again led to outcomes that failed to generate statistically significant mortality outcomes. At his own initiation he involved his clinical managers and launched an in-depth analysis of his practice and detected that he was conducting very high-predicted risk surgery despite lower volumes of surgery than some single specialty colleagues. He was also suspicious of a potential common mechanism of adverse outcomes in several cases of mortality and some cases of morbidity. Along with colleagues he changed his referred practice to make it more compatible with low volume mixed cardiothoracic surgery and adapted his technique of surgery to avoid further problems. This again resulted in excellent subsequent outcomes. This would be described in a situational leadership model as a "collaborative" approach. From a managerial perspective both examples led to satisfactory ends, but adopting the appropriate leadership style was important in reaching the desired conclusions.

In addition to the roles of the individual and the hospital in ensuring satisfactory outcomes, other agencies should be acting to support the process. In the United Kingdom the Chief Medical Officer has recently produced a report entitled "Good Doctors, Safer Patients" about regulation of health care, where it is proposed that the General Medical Council will have overall responsibility for professional regulation, but will pass significant responsibilities down to employers [17]. It is suggested that professional societies should set clear unambiguous standards for care, and recertification of doctors should be dependent on achieving those standards. Patient consultation as part of this report has suggested that patients are keen to see that satisfactory outcomes of treatment by their doctors form part of this process. This direction of travel in the United Kingdom is similar to that proposed by the American Board of Medical Specialties and is a long way from the culture in which most doctors were trained. It will be a challenge for professional societies and the profession to deliver on this agenda.

Summary

Most audit projects will deliver results that demonstrate clinical practice is satisfactory. There is some evidence that scrutiny of results alone can contribute to improvements in quality. On occasions audit will flag up concern about clinical processes or outcome, but it is important that the data and the methods are "fit for purpose." The responsibility for ensuring that satisfactory quality of care is given and demonstrated is the responsibility of all involved in health care delivery including individual practitioners, employers, commissioners, professional societies, and regulators.

References

1 Grover FL, Shroyer LW, Hammermeister K, Edwards FH, Ferguson TB, Dziuban SW *et al*. A decade of experience with quality improvement in cardiac surgery using the veterans affairs and society of thoracic surgeons national databases. *Ann Surg* 2001;234:464–74.

2 Keogh BE, Kinsman R. Fifth national adult cardiac surgical database report 2003.

3 Available at http://www.nnecdsg.org/. Accessed 25.01.2008

4 Available at www.scts.org. Accessed 25.01.2008

5 Roques F, Nashef SA, Michel P *et al*. Risk factors and outcome in European cardiac surgery; analysis of the EuroSCORE multinational database of 19,030 patients. *Eur J Cardiothorac Surg* 1999;15:816–23.

6 Bhatti F, Grayson AD, Grotte GJ, Fabri BM, Au J, Jones MT *et al*. The logistic EuroSCORE in cardiac surgery: How well does it predict operative risk? *Heart* 2006;92:1817–20.

7 Bridgewater B, Grayson AD, Jackson M *et al*. Surgeon specific mortality in adult cardiac surgery: Comparison between crude and risk stratified data. *BMJ* 2003;327:13–7.

8 Parsonnet V, Dean D, Bernstein AD. A method of uniform stratification of risk for evaluating the results of surgery in acquired heart disease. *Circulation* 1989;79:I3–12.

9 Roques F, Michel P, Goldstone AR, Nashef SAM. The logistic EuroSCORE. *Eur Heart J* 2003;24:1–2.

10 Roques F, Nashef SA, Michel P *et al*. Risk factors and outcome in European cardiac surgery; analysis of the EuroSCORE multinational database of 19,030 patients. *Eur J Cardiothorac Surg* 1999;15:816–23.

11 Benneyan RC, Lloyd RC, Plsek PE. Statistical process control as a tool for research and healthcare improvement. *Qual Saf Health Care* 2003;12:458–64.

12 Speigelhalter D. Funnel plots for comparing institutional performance. *Stat Med* 2005;24:1185–202.

13 Mason A, Glodacre MJ, Bettley G, Vale J, Joyce A. Using routine data to define clinical case-mix and compare hospital outcomes in urology. *BJU Int* 2006;97:1145–7.

14 Bridgewater B on behalf of the adult cardiac surgeons on NW England. Mortality data in adult cardiac surgery for named surgeons: Retrospective examination of prospectively collected data on coronary artery surgery and aortic valve replacement. *BMJ* 2005;330:506–10.

15 de Leval MR, Francois K, Bull C *et al*. Analysis of a cluster of surgical failures. Application to a series of neonatal arterial switch operations. *J Thorac Cardiovasc Surg* 1994;107:914–23.

16 Learning from Bristol: The report of the public inquiry into children's heart surgery at the Bristol Royal Infirmary 1984–1995. Available at http://www.bristol-inquiry.org.uk/. http://www.dh.gov.uk/en/Publicationsandstatistics/Publications/PublicationsPolicyAndGuidance/DH_4002859   accessed 25.01.2008

17 Good Doctors, safer patients. Proposals to strengthen the system to assure and improve the performance of doctors and to protect the safety of patients. A report by the Chief Medical Officer. http://www.dh.gov.uk/en/Publicationsandstatistics/Publications/PublicationsPolicyAndGuidance/DH_4002859 accessed 25.01.2008

18 An organisation with a memory. Report of an expert group on learning from adverse events in the NHS chaired by the Chief Medical Officer. http://www.dh.gov.uk/en/Publicationsandstatistics/Publications/PublicationsPolicyAndGuidance/DH_4002859 accessed 25.01.2008

19 Hersey P, Blanchard KH. *Leadership and the One Minute Manager*. William Morrow, 1999. HarperCollins Business; New edition (1 Mar 2000).

3

The Implications of a Poor Surgical Outcome

Robert Wheeler

Introduction

One of the few stimuli prompting a unanimous response from any group of surgeons is the failure to produce the desired result, either from an operation or from a program of management. The response will be a mixture of empathy, regret, disappointment, frustration … and a lingering fear that litigation, or worse, may ensue. In the early 21st-century practice, a "poor outcome" can encompass anything from the irritation of a minor delay due to a misplaced ultrasound report, to the loss of the wrong kidney, or possibly a life. This chapter deals with how to approach a patient with a poor outcome while describing the legal pathways that can be taken. This chapter describes the situation from the viewpoint of the United Kingdom's legal system. Every country has slightly different laws but this chapter remains relevant for those surgeons practicing outside of the United Kingdom, as parallels can be drawn with most legal systems.

Disclosure of poor outcome

An apology

Doctors often debate the advisability of an apology in these circumstances, fearing that this could be construed as an admission of guilt, analogous to the advice given to motorists by their insurance companies if involved in a collision. The analogy is flawed. A poor outcome from

Pediatric Urology: Surgical Complications and Management. Edited by Duncan T. Wilcox, Prasad P. Godbole and Martin A. Koyle. © 2008 Blackwell Publishing, ISBN: 978-1-4051-6268-5.

treatment *may* be the result of mismanagement; but the final determination of fault, if present at all, will result from a complex investigation and logical assessment. While it could be argued that a fulsome apology may be seen as an indication of "guilt," this will have a minimal effect on the process that will establish whether a doctor's behavior has fallen below the reasonable standard (and if so, whether this lapse has caused the harm that is alleged). This effect has to be balanced against the undoubted good that an apology will do, i.e. benefiting the patient and reflecting well on the doctor's propriety and openness. An apology is therefore very strongly recommended; at the very least, failing this, an expression of regret is mandatory.

An explanation

An explanation as to how the suboptimal result has occurred is also necessary. Our society has chosen to regard a patient's autonomy, their right of self-determination, as the paramount consideration when dealing with their health. This manifests as a primacy for confidentiality and for the need to provide consent, both of which are sometimes put ahead of what may be in the (medical) best interests of the patient.

It therefore follows that any information that a doctor possesses concerning a patient must be shared with that patient, or the parents. There is a theoretical tension when considering children, since a child who is judged to be competent to provide consent is also entitled to decide whether their information should be shared with their parents. In practice, this entitlement should be honored by simply checking with the competent child that they have no objection to their parents being told; in the vast majority of cases, there will be none. So a full discussion should follow, to enlighten the family as to how the poor outcome has occurred.

An obligation to disclose errors that are not immediately obvious to the patient?

One particular difficulty is where an error has been made that is not immediately obvious to the patient, but has caused some tangible harm. There may be a temptation not to disclose. However, truth telling is a cornerstone of a trusting relationship, and trust between individuals is central to civilized life. Since "morality" pertains to character and conduct and has regard to the distinction between right and wrong, truth telling seems to be, inescapably, a moral activity. In families' moral education of their children, the universal duty adults impose on children to "own up" misdemeanors reflects this necessity to ensure that ordinary citizens are honest with each other. It also implies that "honesty" concerns the disclosure of hidden information, not simply the avoidance of the lie.

The relationship between doctors and their patients is not ordinary. It is described as a fiduciary relationship, emphasizing the necessity for mutual trust, confidence, and certainty (L. *fiderer*: to trust; *fides*: faith). In conclusion, considering the fiduciary relationship between doctors and their patients, and the lack of distinction between a lie and failing to disclose hidden information, there is a moral obligation to disclose.

Within the doctrine of behavioral ethics, the central "good" elements of human behavior rest upon honesty, probity, and truthfulness. From this perspective, disclosure of error would be considered as an ethical obligation.

How does the general public approach disclosure? In reality, generally, by ignoring the ethical and moral obligations outlined above. The man who owns up to scratching his neighbor's boat while it was unattended would be perceived to have done the "right thing," but such behavior might generate both mild surprise and congratulations on being "decent." Failure to report the damage would lead to a disconsolate but unsurprised owner, resigned to the fact that "no one ever owns up these days."

On a larger scale, viewing "acknowledging error" on Google reveals a robust avoidance of the obligation, "White House strategists conclude that acknowledging error is not an effective political tactic" [1]. Such comments recognize the moral obligation, but honor it in its avoidance. The general tenet of civil law is that the citizen should look after himself. There is no evidence of a civil obligation to report an error.

But the General Medical Council (GMC) [2] advises that doctors should report mistaken diagnoses. This advice is reiterated by the British Medical Association (BMA). Such advice does not specifically cover the area of operative error, although does include circumstances where patients "suffer harm."

Although this advice is not binding, it does represent the view of a recognizable body of medical opinion. Although civil judges do not invariably follow the GMC/BMA guidance, they may be influenced by it, and if they choose to, may reflect the guidance in any future judgements. What damage could flow from failure to know that something has gone wrong? The patient's eventual discovery may cause distress, but it could be difficult to claim that this distress equates to personal damage of a degree that a court would view as worthy of financial recompense. *Chester v. Afshar* [2004] made lawyers (briefly) believe that there was an appetite among senior judges for expanding the law [3], creating a new tort of "failure to report a medical error," a novel category of clinical negligence. Within a matter of weeks, a further House of Lords case (*Gregg v. Scott* [2005]) indicated that radical expansion was most unlikely.

Many NHS hospitals regard failure to report a serious untoward incident *to the hospital* as a disciplinary offence. However, there is no defined obligation to disclose the information to the patient, and one can see a potential conflict of interest on behalf of the hospital when deciding to disclose or not. However, should your hospital take a similar line, reporting a clinical error that could be construed as serious would seem prudent. But from a moral and ethical point of view, patients should also be told, before the hospital, because of the GMC's guidance and the fiduciary relationship a doctor has with the patient. Failing to disclose to the patient does not appear to create a liability in negligence, and even if the failure were admitted as falling below the reasonable standard of care, the claimant would have an uphill struggle in proving causation (*vide infra*). The National Patient Safety Authority's (NPSA) safer practice notice [4] advises health care staff to "apologize to patients, their families or carers if a mistake or error is made that leads to moderate or severe harm or death, explain clearly what went wrong and what will be done to stop the problem happening again." This consolidates the advice from the GMC/BMA, so the chances of being liable to civil actions will increase; but will only succeed if judges choose to follow the line of expanding the scope of clinical negligence.

From the professional point of view, given the GMC guidance, full disclosure is appropriate. In the rare case where disclosure would cause clinical harm, perhaps psychiatric injury, the doctrine of therapeutic privilege will protect the doctor who correctly applies it and withholds disclosure. As a clinical decision, disclosure of medical error puts the doctor in an unassailable position. The hospital may wish disclosure had not occurred, but will hardly make their displeasure visible. Paradoxically, there is evidence that disclosure of error reinforces, rather than diminishes, the relationship between doctor and patient. Even if the admission leads to litigation, the court is likely to view the voluntary disclosure much more favorably than apparent concealment.

From the perspective of the patient

Local resolution

If the patient complains of the outcome, the complaint will initially be dealt with locally, in the hope that resolution can be achieved. At the time of writing, this means that the claim is investigated by the hospital, which may involve experts from within or outwith the organization to take an initial view on whether the hospital should accept liability for the poor outcome. If this initial investigation and suggested remedy satisfies the patient, the matter is brought to a close. If not, then the complainant may request a convenor to appoint a panel to hear the case. The panel consists of a lay chairman and two members independent of the hospital. Clinical assessors are appointed to advise the panel when the complaint involves the exercise of clinical judgement. There is no provision for an appeal of the panel's decision.

The Ombudsman

If the complainant is refused panel review, he may refer that decision to the Health Service Commissioner [5] (Ombudsman), who may recommend that the decision to refuse a panel review be reconsidered. The Ombudsman is able to investigate complaints about clinical judgement, including those arising from independent providers of health services [6] and retired practitioners [7]. The Commissioner provides comments and recommendations, but has no power to award compensation, other than *ex gratia* payments for out of pocket expenses. Referral to the panel or the Ombudsman is not allowed if either civil or criminal proceedings have started.

NHS redress

Following a report [8] by the Chief Medical Officer (CMO) in 2003, there are now arrangements in England and Wales to create a scheme for redress [9] without civil proceedings. This scheme will cover injuries caused to patients by an act or omission concerned with diagnosis of illness, care, or treatment. Despite what some Parliamentarians may have believed during debates, this is not a no-fault compensation scheme. It is anticipated that it will cover treatment by the NHS, even if provided in private hospitals. However, the scheme cannot be engaged if civil proceedings have begun, and will terminate immediately if they commence.

The scheme must comprise: an explanation, an apology, a report on the action proposed to avoid future similar cases, and an offer of compensation. The latter may be monetary, or could take the form of a contract to provide restorative care and treatment. If monetary compensation is awarded for pain, suffering, and loss of amenity, there must be an upper limit on the amount to be offered. The implementation of such a scheme will be dependent on political will and the funding that is diverted to pay for it. If it is implemented in the described form, there may be a perverse incentive for the hospitals to settle low value claims irrespective of liability. If the complainant agrees to the offer, civil action will no longer be available to them. But even a relatively low guaranteed offer will seem attractive to both the hospital and the complainant, since it provides financial closure to both parties, a far cry from the uncertainty and expense of civil actions. What it fails to provide is the guarantee that the doctor who is not at fault will have their blamelessness and hence good reputation publicly acknowledged.

Litigation

If the local or extended resolution process fail, or the patient wish for redress in the civil courts, litigation will commence. The action will usually be directed against the NHS hospital; only naming the defending surgeon if the complaint arose from private practice. The purpose will be ostensibly to provide the claimant with the full facts relating to the case, and financial compensation. The claimant is likely to be suing on the grounds of the tort (civil wrong) of negligence. To establish this, several separate elements will need to be established. Firstly, the surgeon was responsible for the claimant's care at the time of the incident. In hospital practice this is usually straightforward. A doctor has a single and comprehensive duty to exercise reasonable care and skill in diagnosing, advising, and treating the patient [10]. The test is whether the surgeon's conduct was reasonable, and this will be determined in comparison to the objective standard, which is the standard of his or her peers; "it is sufficient if he exercises the ordinary skill of an ordinary competent man exercising that particular art" [11]. Therefore the claimant has to show that the surgeon's practice fell below the standard that would be set by his or her professional peer group [12]. It is this "standard of care" that is established by the expert witnesses who will be consulted concerning the case. However, the expert witnesses will also have to satisfy the judge that the standard they have identified can stand up to scrutiny, and be found to be coherent and logical [13]. Finally, the claimant has to show that the injury sustained was caused by the lapse in the standard of care, and that the damage must be such that the law regards it proper to hold the defendant responsible for it. The first of these two elements of causation is established on the basis of expert evidence, the latter by the court.

In private practice, the patient has the additional option of bringing an action in the law of contract, on the basis that they have purchased a service that has been imperfectly delivered. If a consent form has identified a particular surgeon, and the operation is performed by another; or if a surgeon fails to perform a promised procedure, then breach of contract will occur. An explicit and unequivocal guarantee, "I assure you that your vasectomy will be successful and you will never father children again" creates a contractual warranty on the basis of which action may be taken.

From the perspective of the surgeon

Local

The consequences for the surgeon are largely dependent on the magnitude of the damage caused. There is no doubt that close attention to and compliance with local procedures of incident reporting are vital to limit the negative consequences for the surgeon. The medical defense organizations emphasize the importance of alerting them to any potential claims as soon as a complaint has been made. If frequently repeated irritating inconveniences are being caused to patients, it is likely that the surgeon will be asked to play his or her part in eliminating any procedural errors responsible. Where serious injury has been caused, many hospitals will investigate the matter either through a system of Root Cause Analysis [14], or using some form of review group, usually composed of senior clinicians, risk managers, and executives. Should a serious breach of professional conduct be suspected, the Medical Director of the hospital will become involved and may refer the matter for local adjudication (the "three wise men" approach) or may refer on to the GMC. In the rare circumstance

when a patient's death may have been caused by gross incompetence, the possibility of a criminal charge may be considered. The police would interview all concerned, and the Crown Prosecution Service (in England) would then consider whether a conviction was likely on the basis of the written evidence, and whether it was in the interests of justice that the doctor should be charged with gross negligence manslaughter. It is noteworthy that the indemnity insurance that covers hospitals in England [15] is not available for criminal matters, reinforcing the importance of maintaining close contact with the medical defense organization.

General Medical Council (GMC)

Having been established as a result of lobbying by the BMA in 1858 [16], the GMC [17] sets standards for doctors and examines their performance and behavior against those standards. This important role acts as a safety net, allowing cases to be considered that are not actionable at law, but fall below the standard that should be expected of an ethical practitioner.

Having changed radically in recent times [18], further changes are suggested by the CMO [19], including the devolution of some powers to a local level. From the surgeon's point of view, it is the Fitness to Practise Panel that will determine whether his or her fitness to practice is impaired. If it is, a reprimand may be issued; conditions may be imposed on the doctor's registration, or suspension, or erasure ordered. An appeal mechanism to the courts is available to doctors throughout the United Kingdom. But an appeal is also available to complainants, if dissatisfied with CMC decision-making.

Council for Healthcare Regulatory Excellence

This organization exists to review the decisions of regulators, including those of the GMC. It has a duty to challenge the results of decisions that it considers to be excessively severe or lenient, although most of its challenges are on the latter grounds. The Council will review complaints about the GMC decisions and also scrutinizes decisions on its own behalf. The Council has the power to refer decisions to the High Court for reconsideration, if it is considered that their leniency was incompatible with adequate protection of the public. The effect of this process is that a complaint to the GMC may result in either an acquittal or reprimand falling short of suspension from the GMC, but the case being reopened by the Council for Healthcare Regulatory Excellence (CHRE) and a retrial being ordered in the High Court. This makes the process of professional regulation uncertain, and it is hard to imagine how a doctor who is acquitted by the GMC, only to have the judgement reversed by the High Court, would feel.

The media response

The feeding frenzy created when a poor surgical outcome is reported in the media needs no further description, but has to be acknowledged as a key element that needs to be considered and "managed" in the broadest sense. For reasons possibly derived from self-interest, hospitals are becoming more accustomed to dealing with the media, and it would make sense to shelter under any cover that may so be provided. It seems unlikely that many surgeons will "win" in a direct encounter with journalists, and there is ample evidence that neither adequate recompense nor retractions will follow unjust or misleading reporting. Bold public assertions are therefore inadvisable.

From the perspective of the hospital

Adverse event reporting and clinical governance

The response to failures at either end of this spectrum should be proportionate, but follow a surprisingly similar pattern. In each case, an apology and explanation is appropriate. In many institutions, all "adverse events" are collected into a central database, better to understand the systemic weaknesses that may have caused or contributed to the failure. These institutions in their turn share the database with those governing health care. In the context of the NHS, the data are collated with the NPSA, who in turn reports to the Healthcare Commission, providing the overarching control of "quality" within the national service.

NHS Act 1977 Practice Direction 2006

This legislation gives a Strategic Health Authority (SHA) the power to issue an "alert notice," naming an individual whom it considers poses "a significant risk of harm to patients, staff, or public, and who may seek work in the NHS" [20]. A draconian measure, the issue of such an alert may be requested by the chief executive or executive board member of an NHS body. The notice is sent to the National Clinical Assessment Service, the chief executive of each SHA in England, and the CMO for the other areas in Great Britain. It may then be sent to any NHS body that may be approached by the subject of the notice in search of work in the NHS. Such a notice must

be reviewed at intervals of no more than six months. Alert letters have been available since 2002 [21], but the new guidance is a timely reminder of the efforts being made to protect the public from harm.

What is alarming is that the qualifying criteria for the issue of an alert could be interpreted by an executive in an ill-considered way, at a time when they were feeling vulnerable, perhaps having attracted unwelcome media interest. Although there is provision for revocation of a notice, the damage to a clinician's reputation caused by a false allegation will be impossible fully to retract. Furthermore, the SHA is required to maintain a record of revoked notices for five years following revocation. It seems at least possible that this may disadvantage an "innocent" revokee who applies for work in the SHA area during the time period.

There is a requirement for the SHA to satisfy itself of the evidence supplied by the hospital, supporting the contention that there is a significant risk of harm. But it should be noted that it is the *risk of harm* that has to be significant, not the *degree of harm* itself. Should the climate develop in which unscrupulous health service managers behave aggressively toward clinical staff, it could be seen how a poor surgical result, from the practice of a "troublesome" clinician, could lead to a disproportionate and unjust outcome. It would be incorrect to leave the impression that such devastating consequences are likely to flow from a poor surgical outcome. Such an outcome would be disproportionate, and in the present climate, exceedingly unlikely. However, the NHS is going through an unprecedented transformation of such magnitude that the "old rules" can no longer be relied upon. Government thinking appears to be challenging all "core values," relating to where patients are treated, and what level of training needs to be achieved as a prerequisite for treating them. In this climate, it will be prudent to acknowledge the potential, as well as the probable, consequences of a poor surgical outcome.

Conclusion

A poor surgical outcome is a miserable business, for both patient and surgeon. Mercifully, few poor outcomes lead to litigation, and fewer still to the GMC or criminal courts. A prompt apology and full explanation will do a great deal more good than harm in the long term, and will make it more likely that the relationship between the surgeon and the family will recover and prosper. In many parts of the world, including England, there is a search for alternative modes of recompensing patients who claim to have suffered harm. This could lead to schemes that pay out small sums of money on the basis of scant evidence. Such schemes will flourish if they result in reducing the national financial burden of clinical negligence litigation, which is the reason for their existence. Hospitals may settle such claims irrespective of the effect on the surgeon's reputation, and we all need to consider how we will handle that. As governments become more aware of the voters' focus on the provision of health care, they are identifying measurable "quality" as a surrogate for success. In the United Kingdom, this scramble for the high ground of quality assurance has led government to provide itself with additional statutory tools of scrutiny and control. In this environment, careful compliance with local procedure in the event of an unwanted outcome becomes increasingly important.

References

1 Available at www.google.com.
2 Good Medical Practice London 2001, para 22.
3 House of Lords create new approach to causation Medical Law Monitor 2004, Vol. 11, No. 11, p. 1.
4 National Patient Safety Agency. *Being Open*. London, 2005.
5 Available at www.ombudsman.org.uk.
6 Health Services Commissioners (Amendments) Act 1996.
7 Health Services Commissioners (Amendments) Act 2000.
8 Department of Health. *Making Amends: A Consultation Paper Setting Out Proposals for Reforming the Approach to Clinical Negligence in the NHS*, 2003.
9 NHS Redress Act 2006.
10 Grubb A. *Principles of Medical Law*. Oxford University Press: Oxford, p. 323, 2004.
11 *Bolam v. Friern* HMC [1957] 2 All ER 118, 121.
12 *Bolam v. Friern* HMC [1957] 2 All ER 118.
13 *Bolitho v. City & Hackney* HA [1997] 4 All ER 771.
14 Available at www.npsa.nhs.uk/health/resources/root_cause_analysis.
15 Clinical Negligence Scheme for Trusts, NHS Litigation Authority.
16 Medical Act 1858.
17 Available at www.gmc-uk.org.
18 Mason JK, Laurie GT. *Law and Medical Ethics*. Oxford University Press: Oxford, 1.33, 2006.
19 Donaldson L. *Good doctors, Safer patients: Proposals to strengthen the system to assure and improve the performance of doctors and to protect the safety of patients*. DH: London, 2006.
20 Healthcare Professionals Alert Notices Directions 2006 S 1(3).
21 Health Service Circular 2002/011.

General Principles

The Metabolic and Endocrine Response to Surgery I

Laura Coates and Joe I. Curry

Key points

- After surgery, there is an initial catabolic stage followed by an anabolic stage.
- The catabolic response consists of secretion of cortisol, catecholamines, and glucagon.
- The anabolic response includes secretion of insulin and growth hormone.
- Fluid and electrolyte balance is mainly under the control of aldosterone and antidiuretic hormone.

- There is an immune component to the metabolic response that is not fully understood.
- Nonshivering thermogenesis plays a major role in neonatal thermoregulation.
- Studies comparing laparoscopic and open surgery have shown variable results with respect to the endocrine and metabolic response.

Introduction

The body's metabolic and endocrine responses to tissue damage follow similar pathways regardless of whether that tissue damage is accidental, for example as a result of trauma, or deliberate, as a result of surgery. There is, however, an inflammatory component which appears to vary with the type and size of the insult, and it seems that both the inflammatory factors and the changes in the metabolic state are simultaneously necessary to provide optimal healing and tissue repair. Trauma produces rapid changes in both hormone release and in the way that substrates are mobilized for energy, although the exact mechanisms are still being understood. Among the main changes that have been measured are increases in the concentrations of adrenocorticotrophic hormone (ACTH), cortisol, catecholamines, glucagon, insulin, growth hormone (GH), and in various substrates and their metabolites, for example glucose, lactate, and glycerol [1].

Pediatric Urology: Surgical Complications and Management. Edited by Duncan T. Wilcox, Prasad P. Godbole and Martin A. Koyle. © 2008 Blackwell Publishing, ISBN: 978-1-4051-6268-5.

The metabolic response

The end objectives of the metabolic response are to provide optimal cellular respiration and nutrition via:
- Increased oxygen availability
- Mobilization of protein and other body fuels
- Maintenance of fluid and electrolyte balance
- Disposal of the substrates produced by tissue damage [2].

The end product is the result of a complex interplay between physiological and biochemical functions, which appear to show great variation between patients and bring about rapid changes that do not seem to be totally predictable [1].

F.D. Moore in 1959 described four phases of the metabolic response which are still recognized today [2,3]:

1 The initial phase is related directly to the trauma and there are immediate physiological, hormonal, and biochemical changes within the body.

2 This describes the "turning point" when recovery begins and wound healing begins to mature. The initial changes noted in the metabolic and endocrine functions return to normal.

3 This phase usually takes place some time after the original insult and is characterized by the regaining of muscle strength. There is protein anabolism and a positive nitrogen balance.

4 The restoration of fat mass.

This is a more detailed description of what was previously described as the ebb and flow stages of trauma; more simply, it describes a catabolic ("hypometabolic") stage followed by an anabolic ("hypermetabolic") stage.

The catabolic response

Catabolic responses within the body are concerned with the breakdown of organic polymers and molecules into simpler molecules for the purpose of releasing energy. The catabolic hormones principally released as part of the response to trauma are cortisol, the catecholamines, and glucagon; their net result is to raise the basal metabolic rate, increase glucose concentrations, increase circulating insulin, and increase nitrogen excretion. The effect of these catabolic hormones is not only to increase the glucose concentration, but also to utilize less glucose for a given level of insulin.

Cortisol
Cortisol is a steroid hormone that accounts for approximately 95% of the glucocorticoid activity within the body. It is produced via the hypothalamo-pituitary axis (Figure 4.1).

Corticotrophin-releasing factor (CRF) is released from the hypothalamus under the influence of the body's circadian rhythm, stress, and the plasma levels of corticosteroids under a negative feedback system. CRF travels via the portal system to the anterior pituitary where it stimulates corticotrophs to produce ACTH, which in turn stimulates the adrenal cortex to produce cortisol.

The functions of cortisol are:
• Protein catabolism, primarily in muscle with the result of increasing plasma amino acids
• Promotion of gluconeogenesis
• Stimulating lipolysis
• Increasing sensitivity to vasoconstrictors, thereby raising blood pressure
• Anti-inflammatory and anti-immune effects. Glucocorticoids in general:
  – Have antihistamine effects by reducing mast cell concentration
  – Stabilize lysosomal membranes and thus slow the release of destructive enzymes

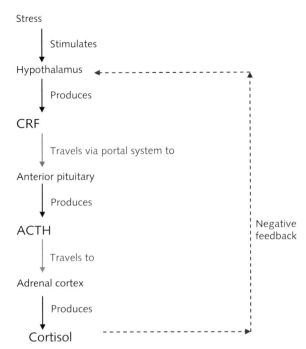

Figure 4.1 Regulation of cortisol secretion.

– Decrease capillary permeability
– Depress phagocytosis [4].

Immediately after trauma, ACTH levels increase rapidly and have been found to be far higher than those required for maximal stimulation of the adrenal cortex [2], although these excessive levels appear to be only transient [5]. Plasma cortisol levels, however, remain high for 2–3 days and cortisol breakdown products continue to be excreted in the urine for many days post-trauma.

Catecholamines
The major catecholamines, adrenaline and noradrenaline, are part of a group of neurotransmitters known as biogenic amines, which are modified decarboxylated amino acids. The axis through which they are produced and regulated is known as the sympatho-adrenal axis (Figure 4.2). They are the two principal hormones synthesized by the adrenal medulla, and are responsible for the sympathomimetic component of the "fight-or-flight" response.

The hypothalamus sends impulses to the sympathetic preganglionic neurons, which in turn stimulate the production of adrenaline and noradrenaline from the chromaffin cells of the adrenal medulla. The catecholamines then target their α- and β-adrenergic receptors on effectors innervated by sympathetic postganglionic axons. On the whole, α-receptors are excitatory, while β-receptors are variable in terms of their responses. Adrenaline stimulates both α- and β-adrenergic receptors and at low administered doses results in tachycardia with a simultaneous fall in systemic vascular resistance, mainly from its β effects. At higher doses, α effects predominate and vasoconstriction occurs. This has the effect of increasing perfusion pressure and thus maintaining renal blood flow and urine output, but only to a point – at much higher doses, cardiac output falls, and further vasoconstriction causes a decrease in renal perfusion.

Adrenaline is a highly effective promoter of gluconeogenesis by its action on hepatic and muscle phosphorylases [6]. The catecholamines inhibit insulin release and reduce peripheral glucose uptake, thus further increasing the plasma glucose and leading to the characteristic post-surgery hyperglycemia. Both adrenaline and noradrenaline increase free fatty acid mobilization and elevate oxygen consumption [2]. Plasma levels of the catecholamines are found to be raised immediately post stress and the levels are directly proportional to the extent of trauma. Again, as with cortisol, plasma levels are raised for a relatively short length of time but urinary excretion has been noted for a much longer period [7].

Glucagon

Glucagon is a peptide hormone produced by the α cells of the pancreatic islets. β-adrenergic activity stimulates these α cells to produce glucagon immediately post-trauma. The effects of glucagon are in direct contrast to the effects of insulin (Figure 4.3).

It raises plasma glucose levels by speeding up hepatic glycogenolysis and gluconeogenesis.

Glucagon release is also stimulated by:
• Increased sympathetic autonomic nervous system (ANS) activity, e.g. during exercise or trauma
• An increase in plasma amino acid concentration if the plasma glucose is low, e.g. following a protein-only meal and its release is inhibited by both insulin and somatostatin [4].

The anabolic response

The reactions within the body that combine simple molecules to form complex polymers are known as the anabolic reactions. Anabolism uses the energy created from catabolism to build the structural and functional

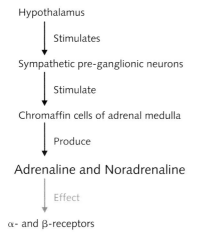

Figure 4.2 Production of catecholamines.

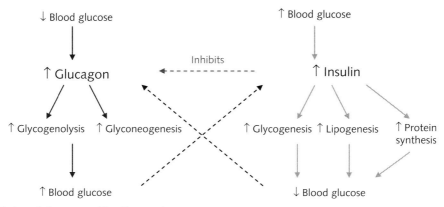

Figure 4.3 Regulation of glucagon and insulin secretion.

components of the body, for example the synthesis of proteins from amino acids or glycogen from glucose monomers. Insulin and GH are the two main hormones responsible for these synthesis reactions within the human body.

Insulin

Insulin is another peptide hormone produced by the pancreas – this time, from the β cells, which make up 70% of the total number of pancreatic islet cells. Insulin can be seen in Figure 4.3 to have contrasting actions to glucagon by ultimately decreasing blood glucose. Its other actions are to:
- Encourage diffusion of glucose into cells
- Accelerate glycogenesis
- Increase amino acid uptake and in turn increase protein synthesis
- Encourage lipogenesis
- Slow glycogenolysis and gluconeogenesis [4].

Insulin release is mainly stimulated by a rising blood glucose level, although many other substances also influence and regulate the plasma levels of insulin:
- Acetylcholine, via the vagal innervation of the pancreas
- Arginine and leucine – two amino acids
- Glucagon
- Gastric inhibitory peptide (GIP), a peptide released by the enteroendocrine cells of the small bowel in response to a postprandial glucose load
- GH and ACTH (indirectly) due to their effect of raising plasma glucose levels [4].

It can be seen that although glucagon stimulates insulin release, there is no reciprocal increase; insulin actually suppresses the release of glucagon. As blood glucose levels drop, and levels of insulin simultaneously decrease, more glucagon is released from the pancreas, which then increases blood glucose and stimulates once more the release of insulin, which then causes the glucose level to fall and the cycle begins once more.

Initially after trauma insulin levels are decreased [8], but these rise again after the first 24 h as the initial response to trauma stabilizes [9].

Growth hormone

GH is released from the anterior pituitary under the influence of growth hormone releasing hormone (GHRH) which is secreted into the portal system from the hypothalamus. Its release is inhibited by somatostatin, also known as growth hormone releasing inhibitory peptide (GHRIP). GH stimulates the production of insulin-like growth factor-1 (IGF-1) within the liver – and it is this which stimulates body and tissue growth in humans. The effects of this process are as follows:
- To increase protein and collagen synthesis
- To increase the basal metabolic rate
- To encourage the preservation of anabolic substrates, namely calcium, phosphorus, and nitrogen
- To increase fat oxidation
- To counter the effects of insulin.

The release of GH in the healthy individual is mainly nocturnal and pulsatile although injury and stress serve to stimulate its release, while hyperglycemia counteracts this and leads to suppression of the hormone.

GH levels have been shown to rise following trauma and gradually revert to normal within a few days. IGF-1 levels, similarly, decrease in 4–5 days following trauma [10].

Fluid balance

Sodium

Just as the glucocorticoids produced in the adrenal cortex influence glucose homeostasis in the body, so the mineralocorticoids influence mineral homeostasis; or more specifically, fluid and electrolyte balance. Approximately 95% of the mineralocorticoid activity is due to aldosterone, a steroid hormone manufactured in the zona glomerulosa of the adrenal cortex. This hormone targets the renal tubules to stimulate the reabsorption of sodium ions (Na^+). This in turn increases reabsorption of chloride and bicarbonate ions and leads to the retention of water. Aldosterone also promotes the excretion of potassium ions (K^+) and hydrogen ions (H^+) in the urine, thus helping to correct acidosis and restore pH.

Aldosterone control is under the influence of the renin–angiotensin system (Figure 4.4).

Hypotension, dehydration, or Na^+ loss stimulates the release of renin from the juxtaglomerular cells of the kidney. Angiotensinogen, meanwhile, is being produced in the liver and is converted by renin into angiotensin I, which then is further converted in the lung capillary beds into angiotensin II under the influence of angiotensin converting enzyme (ACE). This has two main effects:

1 To stimulate the adrenal cortex to secrete aldosterone. This increases tubular reabsorption of Na^+ and thus increases water reabsorption, leading to a restoration of blood volume.

2 To act on the smooth muscle in arteriolar walls, leading to the vasoconstriction of arterioles, which in turn leads to an increase in blood pressure.

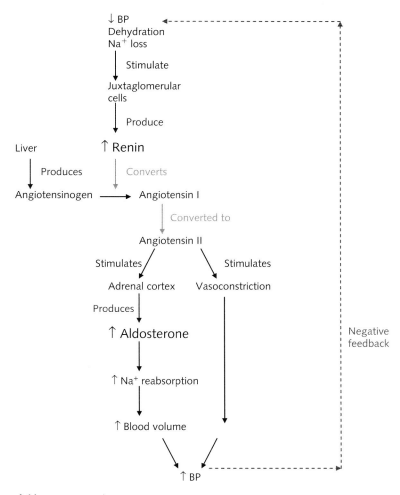

Figure 4.4 Regulation of aldosterone secretion.

Aldosterone levels are known to increase rapidly post-surgery and an impairment in Na^+ excretion has been shown to last for up to a week [11].

Atrial natriuretic peptide (ANP) has also been implicated in the regulation of sodium. It is a hormone that is secreted in both cardiac atria in response to atrial stretching (i.e. on "overfilling" or overcompensation of a low blood volume) and it promotes excretion of both water and sodium. It also suppresses the secretion of antidiuretic hormone (ADH; see below), renin, and aldosterone.

Water balance

ADH is a neuropeptide which is synthesized in the hypothalamus and stored in the posterior pituitary. Its main function is to retain body water and prevent water losses both in the urine and as sweat. Its production is regulated by osmoreceptors in the hypothalamus, which detect dehydration or hypotension. An increase in the plasma level of ADH has three main actions, all of which serve to increase body water:
• Renal tubules retain more water
• Sweat glands decrease output and sweating is diminished
• Arterioles constrict.

Levels of ADH increase following surgery, and administration of morphine, acetylcholine, and nicotine have all been shown to increase ADH production, leading to fluid retention and increased tissue perfusion. This brings with it the potential risk of fluid overload and edema, necessitating careful postoperative fluid monitoring.

Protein metabolism

After trauma of any kind in adults, there is an increase in the basal metabolic rate, breakdown of body protein, and increased nitrogen excretion. The result is a net loss of protein. In the latter stage of the metabolic response to trauma, however, protein anabolism takes over and new protein is synthesized for repair and tissue growth. There is, however, some debate over whether children show the same response as adults; some studies have shown that children and infants show a lack of catabolism following surgery and no increase in protein turnover [12]. Others have shown an increase in protein turnover specifically in neonates on life support [13]. Surgery and its complications, along with sepsis, are the most common causes of protein loss in hospital, otherwise known as protein-energy malnutrition. This term is used to describe the weight loss that occurs as a consequence of either:
• Poor enteral intake secondary to anorexia secondary to the underlying condition
• Increased catabolism, e.g. due to sepsis
• Tumor necrosis factor (TNF) in patients with cancer
• Malabsorption [14].
Nitrogen balance is used as a measure of net protein metabolism. Simplified, this is nitrogen input minus total urinary nitrogen excretion, although the actual results can be rather more difficult to calculate. An increase in urinary urea and ammonia excretion occurs following surgery and negative nitrogen balances are usually seen as a result [2]. This increase in urinary excretion is the effect of protein breakdown in:
• Muscle
• Breakdown of dead and damaged cells
• Hematoma and blood cells.
Of these, muscle breakdown accounts for the majority of the protein loss.

In the starvation state, the small amount of glycogen that is stored in the liver is utilized usually in the first 24 h. Gluconeogenesis is therefore necessary to maintain a supply of glucose for energy. Pyruvate, lactate, glycerol, and amino acids (mainly alanine and glutamine) are the main sources of gluconeogenesis. The majority of protein breakdown occurs in muscle which leads to the inevitable loss of muscle bulk in chronic starvation [14]. Stored triglycerides are also hydrolyzed to glycerol (used for gluconeogenesis as above) and to fatty acids that may be oxidized further to form ketone bodies.

In starvation, adaptation occurs and the basal metabolic rate decreases in an attempt to conserve fuel stores. The brain's choice of substrate changes from glucose to ketone bodies and hepatic gluconeogenesis decreases. Following surgery or trauma, however, that adaptation does not take place; and, coupled with the increase in catecholamines and glucocorticoids, gluconeogenesis and protein breakdown continue in an attempt to provide enough energy to overcome the stress. An enzymatic pathway called the ubiquitin–proteasome pathway (which is a selective degrader of intracellular proteins) is stimulated by these glucocorticoids and cytokines and is responsible for accelerating protein breakdown in muscle in many disease processes [14].

The immune response

There is an immune component to the postsurgery response that is still being understood. It has long been known that cytokines are mediators of the acute phase stress response and it is now known that interleukins and TNF play an additional role in the regulation of the metabolic response.

Interleukins, especially IL-1 and IL-6, stimulate hepatic lipogenesis and IL-1 has an additional role in hepatic gluconeogenesis and in promoting muscle proteolysis [15]. IL-6 is a marker of the stress response in neonates and increases in proportion to the magnitude of the operative insult [16].

TNF increases glucose transport and also promotes hepatic lipogenesis and muscle proteolysis along with IL-1. It also inhibits lipoprotein lipase and has been shown to be the main cause of cachexia in patients with cancer. It has also been postulated that the interleukins and TNF may show a synergistic effect in regulating the metabolic response to trauma [17].

Thermoregulation

Neonates and infants have much more difficulty in regulating and maintaining their own body temperature than older children and adults. This is partly due to an increased surface area/body mass ratio, and partly to do with the make up of their fuel stores. Adults adapt to cold by shivering and vasoconstriction, and conversely to heat by sweating and vasodilation. Newborn babies are unable to mount a shivering response to cold, although they do demonstrate an intact vasoconstriction response [18]. Infants have a particular way of generating heat in the absence of shivering, by way of a specific type of adipose tissue called brown fat which dissipates energy in the form of heat and generates so-called nonshivering thermogenesis. This doubles the normal metabolic rate of the infant, and is accompanied by a threefold rise in the plasma concentration of noradrenaline [19]. During environmental cooling, blood supply to the brown fat increases and heat is generated by the mitochondria within the fat cells [15]. Several studies have shown that under anesthesia (particularly fentanyl), infants are unable to mount a nonshivering thermogenic response which can lead to a sudden increase in their metabolic rate when anesthetic administration is terminated [19]. This reinforces the importance of maintaining a warm environmental temperature both in theater and postoperatively, and of making sure that the stresses on the child are as low as possible in terms of maintaining body temperature.

Laparoscopy versus open surgery

Laparoscopic surgery is increasingly used for a wide variety of operations, associated as it is with reportedly shorter hospital stays, less analgesic requirements postoperatively, and a more rapid postoperative recovery [20–22].

Several studies have investigated whether the body's normal metabolic response to surgery alters in cases where laparoscopy is used as opposed to open surgery. Adult studies have demonstrated that laparoscopy is associated with a small decrease in the inflammatory response with little or no difference in the metabolic response [22, 23]. Conversely, McHoney et al. in 2006 found that laparoscopy in children is associated with an intraoperative hypermetabolic response, where open surgery has no corresponding rise in metabolic rate [24]. The oxygen consumption (VO_2) in children during surgery was used as a marker of metabolic rate and it was found to rise steadily throughout the duration of the laparoscopic surgery. There was also a corresponding rise in core temperature, despite using unwarmed CO_2 for insufflation.

On reviewing the literature for laparoscopic surgery in adults, Vittimberga et al. stated that the body's response to laparoscopy is one of "lesser immune activation" rather than immunosuppression [25]. They also discussed how laparoscopic surgery has been shown to:
• Decrease C-reactive protein (CRP) in cases of cholecystectomy
• Decrease IL-6 concentrations after laparoscopic procedures.
This has also been demonstrated in a study looking specifically at cases of laparoscopy in newborn infants. The operations studied included nephrectomies and

salpingo-oophorectomies, and corroborated the evidence for a significant decrease in the acute phase response in laparoscopic surgery in infants
• Increase histamine response
• Decrease T-cell function
• Decrease postoperative immunosuppression.
There appears to be, however, ongoing debate regarding the changes listed above. Bozkurt et al. [26] studied IL-6 concentrations during emergency laparoscopy and laparotomy in children and found no difference between the two groups. They also undertook measurements of blood prolactin, cortisol, glucose, insulin, lactate, and adrenaline and found that the rise in these substances was equal in both groups [26].

A further study looking at open versus laparoscopic Nissen's fundoplication in children also did not show any difference in concentrations of TNF or IL-1 between the two groups. There was, however, a slight increase in postoperative immune suppression in the open group [27].

This does suggest that the metabolic response is highly variable. The fact that so many studies have been undertaken and yet show differing results does seem to imply that the metabolic response to surgery, while following a similar pathway each time, is not necessarily predictable or quantifiable in different children undergoing different operations.

References

1 Barton RN, Cocks RA, Doyle MO, Chambers H. Time course of the early pituitary-adrenal and metabolic responses to accidental injury. *J Trauma* 1995;39:888–94.
2 Burnand KG, Young AE. *The new Aird's companion in surgical studies.* Churchill Livingstone: London, 1992.
3 Moore FD. *Metabolic Care of the Surgical Patient.* WB Saunders: Philadelphia, 1959.
4 Tortora GJ, Grabowski SR. *Principles of Anatomy and Physiology.* Harper Collins, Newyork, 1996.
5 Cooper CE, Nelson DH. ACTH levels in plasma in preoperative and surgically stressed patients. *J Clin Invest* 1962; 41:1599–1605.
6 Barton RN. Neuroendocrine mobilization of body fuels after injury. *Brit Med Bull* 1985;41:218–25.
7 Walker WF, Johnston IDA. *The Metabolic Basis for Surgical Care.* Heinemann: London, 1971.
8 Traynor C, Hall GM. Endocrine and metabolic changes during surgery: anaesthetic implications. *Brit J Anaesth* 1981;53:153–60.
9 Stoner HB, Frayn KN, Barton RN, Threlfall CJ, Little RA. The relationships between plasma substrates and hormones and the severity of injury in 277 recently injured patients. *Clin Sci* 1979;56:563–73.

10 Frayn KN, Price DA, Maycock PF, Carroll SM. Plasma somatomedin activity after injury in man and its relationship to other hormonal and metabolic changes. *Clin Endocrinol* 1984;20:179–87.

11 Cochrane JPS. The aldosterone response to surgery and the relationship of this response to postopertive sodium retention. *Brit J Surg* 1978;65:744–7.

12 Powis M, Smith K, Rennie M, Halliday D, Pierro A. Effect of major abdominal operations on energy and protein metabolism in infants and children. *J Paediatr Surg* 1998;33:49–53.

13 Keshen TH, Miller RG, Jahoor F, Jaksic T. Stable isotope quantification of protein metabolism and energy expenditure in neonates on pre- and post-extracorporeal life support. *J Paediatr Surg* 1997;32:958–63.

14 Kumar P, Clark M (Editors). *Clinical Medicine.* WB Saunders, London, 1998.

15 Pierro A. Metabolic response to neonatal surgery. *Curr Opin Paediatr* 1999;11:230–6.

16 Jones MO, Pierro A, Hashim IA, Shenkin A, Lloyd DA. Postoperative changes in resting energy expenditure and interleukin-6 in infants. *Brit J Surg* 1994;81:536–8.

17 Hill AG, Hill GL. Metabolic response to severe injury. *Brit J Surg* 1998;85:884–90.

18 Plattner O, Semsroth M, Sessler D, Papousek A, Klasen C, Wagner O. Lack of nonshivering thermogenesis in infants anesthetized with fentanyl and propofol. *Anesthesiology* 1997;86:772–7.

19 Dawkins MJR, Scopes JW. Non-shivering thermogenesis and brown adipose tissue in the human new-born infant. *Nature* 1965;206:201–2.

20 Berggren U, Gordh T, Grama D, Haglund U, Rastad J, Arvidsson D. Laparoscopic versus open cholecystectomy: Hospitalisation, sick leave, analgesia and trauma responses. *Brit J Surg* 1994; 81:1362–5.

21 Joris J, Cigarini I, Legrand M, Jacquet N, De Groote D, Franchimont P *et al.* Metabolic and respiratory changes after cholecystectomy performed via laparotomy or laparoscopy. *Brit J Anaesth* 1992;69:341–5.

22 Kehlet H. Surgical stress response: Does endoscopic surgery confer an advantage? *World J Surg* 1999;23:801–7.

23 Gupta A, Watson DI. Effect of laparoscopy on immune function. *Brit J Surg* 2001;88:1296–1306.

24 McHoney MC, Corizia L, Eaton S, Wade A, Spitz L, Drake DP *et al.* Laparoscopic surgery in children is associated with an intraoperative hypermetabolic response. *Surg Endosc* 2006;20:452–7.

25 Vittimberga FJ, Foley DP, Meyers WC, Callery MP. Laparoscopic surgery and the systemic immune response. *Ann Surg* 1998;227:326–4.

26 Bozkurt P, Kaya G, Altintas F, Yeker Y, Hacibekiroglu M, Emir H *et al.* Systemic stress response during operations for acute abdominal pain performed via laparoscopy or laparotomy in children. *Anaesthesia* 2000;55:5–9.

27 McHoney M, Eaton S, Wade A, Klein N, Stefanutti G, Booth C *et al.* Inflammatory response in children after laparoscopic vs open Nissen fundoplication: Randomised controlled trial. *J Paediatr Surg* 2005;40:908–13.

The Metabolic and Endocrine Response to Surgery II: Management

Benjamin P. Wisner, Douglas Ford and Martin A. Koyle

Key points

- The neonatal kidney has lower glomerular filtration rate and impaired concentrating ability and electrolyte handling.

- Hypotonic fluid administration as well as increased circulating antidiuretic hormone is common cause of postoperative hyponatremia.

- Most postobstructive diuresis is physiologic.

- Bowel segments in continuity with the urinary tract predispose to a number of short- and long-term metabolic consequences.

Introduction

The previous chapter has described the various metabolic and endocrine responses to surgical trauma. This chapter will focus on diagnosis and management of metabolic and endocrine derangements in the pediatric urologic patient.

Developmental changes in renal function

Compared with the mature kidney, the neonatal kidney has impaired concentrating ability as well as lessened abilities for tubular reabsorption of sodium and secretion of potassium and hydrogen. The neonatal kidney also receives a lesser proportion of the cardiac output, which contributes to lower glomerular filtration rate (GFR) [1]. GFR increases markedly over the first 3 months of life, with the transition to adult levels by 2 years of age [2]. Due to impaired countercurrent exchange, maximal neonatal urine concentration is 500–700 mOsm/kg.

Pediatric Urology: Surgical Complications and Management. Edited by Duncan T. Wilcox, Prasad P. Godbole and Martin A. Koyle.
© 2008 Blackwell Publishing, ISBN: 978-1-4051-6268-5.

Routine fluid and electrolyte therapy

The daily water requirements of infants and children are based on estimated caloric expenditures [3]. In a 24-h period, approximately 100 ml water is needed per 100 kcal/kg of energy expended. Sodium and chloride replacement is required at 2–3 mEq/100 ml water per day, and potassium replacement is required at 1–2 mEq/100 ml water per day. Urine is the main source of electrolyte loss; however, in the postsurgical patient, losses from GI sources (e.g. NG suction) may be substantial [4]. Traditional fluid replacement in infants and children with hypotonic fluid has been based on the above-calculated requirements [5].

Disorders of sodium and water balance

Total body water (TBW) consists of both intracellular and extracellular fluid (ECF). ECF makes up approximately 45% of TBW in neonates, this percentage decreases rapidly in the first year of life and then gradually throughout childhood [7]. Renal sodium reabsorption occurs primarily in the proximal tubule via the Na^+–H^+ antiporter on a gradient generated by Na^+–K^+–ATPase. In the collecting duct, sodium resorbtion is regulated mainly by aldosterone and sodium intake, and water handling by ADH [8].

Hyponatremia

Postoperative hyponatremia is a relatively common phenomenon, occurring in approximately 4–20% of patients [5,6,9]. Overall, hyponatremia is the most common electrolyte abnormality observed in hospitalized children [10]. There are many etiologies of postoperative hyponatremia; however, the most common is administration of hypotonic fluid [9]. The hyponatremic effect of free water excess is compounded by an excess of ADH in the first 72 h postoperatively [11–13]. Drugs given in the postoperative period may also contribute to sodium disturbance. Common medications given in children include opioids, NSAIDs, and acetaminophen. Opioids enhance ADH action via mu-receptors [14]. NSAIDs and acetaminophen are known to potentiate water retention by inhibiting prostaglandin synthesis [8]. Vomiting or nasogastric suction can also contribute to hyponatremia.

In a retrospective study of hyponatremia in hospitalized children age 1 month to 18 years, Wattad et al. found that 97.5% of cases fell into the categories of mild or moderate hyponatremia (Serum Na^+ 121–129), and only 2.5% of patients had severe hyponatremia (Serum Na^+ <120). Nine percent of patients with mild and 48% of patients with moderate hyponatremia were symptomatic, most commonly with lethargy and irritability. Two percent of children with mild hyponatremia, 3% with moderate hyponatremia, and 100% with severe hyponatremia had demonstrable neurologic deficits, and, although these children had severe comorbid illness, most had persistence of deficits on discharge from the hospital [15]. In a retrospective series and review of the literature, Medani determined that the average serum sodium in children presenting with seizures was 118 ± 4.3 mEq/l [16]. Hyponatremia has been variably linked to poor outcomes in children, with mortality rates ranging from 8.4% [17] to 12% [15]. It appears that symptomatic hyponatremia is more likely to result in symptoms attributable directly to hyponatremia (e.g. seizures), whereas sequelae such as demyelination are related to rapid correction (>2 mEq/l/h or >20 mEq/l/24 h) and are more likely to occur in patients with chronic hyponatremia [18–20].

The most feared complication of correction of hyponatremia is central pontine myelinolysis (CPM) [21], also termed osmotic demyelination syndrome [22].

In children, CPM has been described in hyponatremic patients; however, these children typically have additional comorbid factors such as liver disease. In a single institution series, only 9/17 cases of CPM occurred in hyponatremic patients, whereas 5/17 had normal sodium and 3/17 had hypernatremia [10]. Most hyponatremia in infants and children is acute in nature, and the benefits of rapid correction to alleviate seizures typically outweighs the risks of demyelination [16, 23, 24].

The first step in the evaluation of hyponatremia is a clinical assessment of volume status. This can be done by evaluation of mucous membranes, urine output, body weight, orthostatic blood pressure, and skin turgor. Next, the urinary sodium concentration allows for determination of whether or not the renal response to hyponatremia is appropriate. This is especially useful in the setting of hypovolemic hyponatremia, in which the normal kidney avidly retains sodium, therefore leading to a low urinary sodium concentration (U[Na] <20 mEq/l). Based on clinical assessment and urinary sodium concentration, the patient can be classified according to the diagram in Figure 5.1. When treating hyponatremia, the importance of serial sodium monitoring cannot be overemphasized.

Hypovolemic hyponatremia

In the pediatric urologic patient, most postoperative hypovolemic hyponatremia is secondary to extrarenal losses. Replacement of sodium and water is required, and isotonic saline is generally appropriate for initial replacement. Once the ECF has been repleted, the stimulus for AVP decreases and rapid correction of hyponatremia occurs via excretion of dilute urine. For this reason, use of hypotonic fluid may be appropriate after repletion of the extracellular fluid volume [24–26]. The sodium deficit calculation may be a useful adjunct to therapy; however, this formula will underestimate the anticipated correction in patients with extrarenal sodium losses such as NG suction or high fever. It should therefore be used only as a guide and is not a substitute for monitoring plasma sodium during deficit replacement.

Sodium deficit = TBW (kg) × (desired [Na] mEq/l – actual [Na] mEq/l) where TBW is estimated as lean body weight (kg) times $0.5 kg^{-1}$ for women, $0.6 kg^{-1}$ for men, and $0.6 kg^{-1}$ for children [24]. The result of this formula is the number of mEq of sodium needed to replace the deficit. This can be given over an appropriate time course to prevent overly rapid correction.

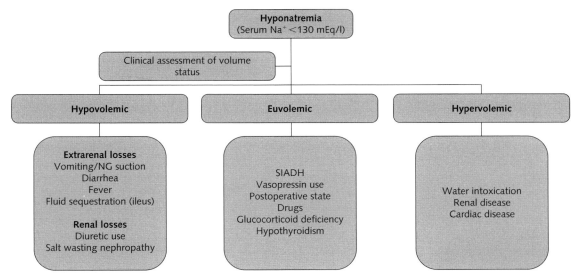

Figure 5.1 Classification of hyponatremia and causes.

Euvolemic hyponatremia

Euvolemic hyponatremia in the pediatric patient can be due to stress, vasopressin administration (for von Willebrand's disease), drugs, glucocorticoid deficiency, hypothyroidism, or SIADH. Should a child have acute (<48 h duration) severely symptomatic euvolemic hyponatremia, correction with hypertonic saline (3%) at 1–2 ml/kg/h plus lasix administration can be undertaken [23]. The goal of therapy in adolescents and adults is to raise serum sodium at 1–2 mEq/l/h until seizures subside [24]. Additional correction should take place at a rate not to exceed 0.33–0.5 mEq/l/h or 8–12 mEq/l in a 24-h period [22,24,27]. In infants and children with seizures, however, more rapid correction may be appropriate if the clinician is confident of an acute symptomatic disturbance in sodium [23].

Asymptomatic euvolemic hyponatremia is treated with fluid restriction to produce a negative free water balance. Restriction to 50% of normal daily goals may be required in some instances [24]. Once again, gradual correction is the goal unless the patient is acutely symptomatic.

Hypervolemic hyponatremia

Hypervolemic hyponatremia is common in infants in children due to water intoxication. It may also be caused by chronic renal or cardiac disease, but these are much less common. Treatment consists of fluid restriction in the asymptomatic patient. In the child with CNS symptoms such as lethargy or seizures, acute correction with 3% saline 5 ml/kg over 10–30 min is an effective strategy, and would tend to raise serum sodium by approximately 5 mEq/l [10,23] (Figure 5.2).

Hypernatremia

Hypernatremia in the pediatric patient arises from excess sodium intake, free water deficit (diabetes insipidus, fever, radiant warmers, phototherapy), or combined sodium and water deficit (postobstructive diuresis, emesis, NG suction, diarrhea) [28]. Hypernatremia can lead to cerebral hemorrhage, and the sodium level should be corrected gradually at a rate not >12 mEq/l/24 h. Water deficit can be calculated by the following formula:

$$\text{Water deficit} = 0.6 \, (\text{body weight (kg)}) \times (1 - (145/\text{current [Na]}))$$

Replacement can be undertaken with normal saline, ½, or ¼ normal saline, depending upon the degree of water deficit. Correction should be monitored with serial plasma sodium measurements.

Disorders of potassium balance

The vast majority of the body's potassium stores are intracellular. The kidney is responsible for secretion of

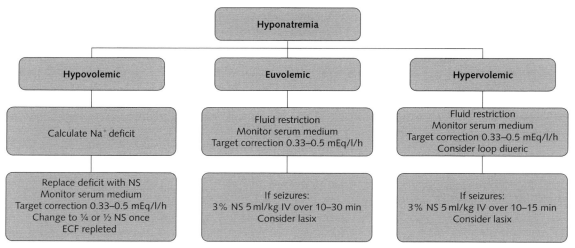

Figure 5.2 Treatment of hyponatremia.
NS, normal saline; ECF, extracellular fluid.

90% of the daily potassium intake [29]. Potassium is absorbed in the proximal tubule and secreted in the distal nephron under the influence of mineralocorticoid. The immature kidney appears to be less efficient in the secretion of potassium load, making the infant more susceptible to hyperkalemia in the setting of handling a potassium load [30].

Hypokalemia

Hypokalemia in the postoperative patient is commonly iatrogenic and is frequently related to nasogastric suction or loop diuretic use. Additional causes are vomiting, diarrhea, insulin administration, and inadequate potassium replacement or intake. Hyperaldosteronism and renal tubular acidosis are also potential causes of hypokalemia. In hyperaldosteronism, hypokalemia is also accompanied by hypertension and alkalosis, and in renal tubular acidosis, a hyperchloremic metabolic acidosis is also present. Symptoms of hypokalemia typically consist of muscle cramps and weakness, but can also include gastrointestinal symptoms with ileus and paresthesias. Treatment of hypokalemia can be accomplished with either intravenous or oral potassium chloride. Should an underlying metabolic abnormality such as renal tubular acidosis be suspected, appropriate evaluation should follow.

Hyperkalemia

Hyperkalemia is a potentially life-threatening condition. Mild hyperkalemia may be asymptomatic; however, symptoms of severe hyperkalemia include characteristic ECG changes, muscle cramps, arrhythmia, and cardiac arrest. Hyperkalemia in infants and children is frequently due to hemolysis, and secondary to the high prevalence of capillary phlebotomy. Another source of fictitious hyperkalemia is usage of IV sites running potassium-containing fluids. Causes of true hyperkalemia include renal failure, bilateral high-grade obstruction, and release of intracellular potassium from destroyed cells, such as crush injury, tumor lysis, or extensive hemolysis. Extracellular shift of potassium due to extreme acidosis, insulin deficiency, or impaired renal secretion such as adrenal insufficiency can also lead to hyperkalemia.

If hemolysis is suspected as the cause of hyperkalemia, repeating the potassium level from a separate venipuncture site is helpful. Potassium should be removed from IV fluids. ECG is helpful in evaluating for cardiac toxicity. Calcium administration may help to stabilize the myocardium from the arrhythmogenic effects of potassium. Excess potassium can be temporarily shifted to an intracellular location by administration of insulin with glucose or by $\beta 2$-agonist inhalers. These agents increase the Na–K–ATPase activity. Loop diuretics enhance potassium secretion and may be useful in therapy. Oral binding solutions such as sodium polystyrene sulfonate

Table 5.1 Bowel segments and associated metabolic derangements.

Bowel segment	Metabolic derangement	Mechanism
Stomach	Hypokalemic, hypochloremic metabolic alkalosis	H^+ and Cl^- loss
Jejunum	Hyperkalemic, hyponatremic metabolic acidosis	Na^+ and Cl^- loss
		K^+ reabsorption
Ileum	Hyperchloremic metabolic acidosis	Ammonium reabsorption
Colon	Hyperchloremic metabolic acidosis	Ammonium reabsorption

(Kayexalate) require a functional GI tract but can be a useful adjunct in therapy. Sodium polystyrene sulfonate should not be given orally in neonates due to the risk of gastrointestinal hemorrhage or colonic necrosis.

Postobstructive diuresis

Postobstructive diuresis can be encountered by the pediatric urologist in a variety of settings. These range from posterior urethral valves to stones to postoperative mishaps such as catheter occlusion, urinary retention after reimplantation, obstruction of a catheterizable stoma, or, rarely, obstructing malignancy such as rhabdomyosarcoma. Postobstructive diuresis can even be encountered in the setting of unilateral obstruction, such as an obstructing ureteral calculus [31,32]. Postobstructive diuresis is caused by many factors. Acutely, there is an early increase in GFR followed by subsequent decrease due to afferent arteriolar constriction [33]. Urinary obstruction also leads to an impairment of sodium and free water reabsorption [34–36]. Altered tubuloglomerular feedback, impaired ADH response, and ANP accumulation have also been implicated [37–39].

The diuresis observed after relief of obstruction is mainly due to the excretion of retained water and solutes [40]. For this reason, aggressive fluid resuscitation is not typically necessary. Due to the impaired concentrating ability and obligatory natriuresis seen as a result of obstruction, some replacement of salt wand water is warranted. In unilateral obstruction, the presence of a normal contralateral kidney typically mitigates natriuresis [41]. Most postobstructive diuresis is benign and corrects within 24–48 h. Approximately 10–20% of these patients, however, will have continued natiuresis that can lead to profound dehydration [42–44]. Patients with signs of volume overload and severe renal impairment may be at higher risk of developing prolonged natiuresis

[45–46]. Gradual decompression does not appear to alter the course of postobstructive diuresis [47].

Interposed bowel segments

The interposition of bowel segments into the urinary tract, such as with bladder augmentation, can create a unique milleu of metabolic derangements. These problems include diarrhea, vitamin malabsorption, and electrolyte abnormalities. Ileal or colonic interposition can result in hyperchloremic metabolic acidosis due to ammonium and chloride absorption [48]. Gastrocystoplasty, which is used much less commonly than other methods of augmentation, can result in development of hypochloremic, hypokalemic metabolic alkalosis (Table 5.1).

Hyperchloremic metabolic acidosis is the most common abnormality encountered with interposed bowel segments in children. Nurse and Mundy [49] found that the incidence of hyperchloremic metabolic acidosis in ileocecal substitution, ileal augmentation, and ileal conduit was 50%, 26%, and 12.5%, respectively. Whitmore and Gittes [50] found a similar overall incidence in intestinocystoplasty, with a hyperchloremic metabolic acidosis occurring in 19% of patients. The risk of developing electrolyte abnormality has been reported to be higher in children with preoperative renal insufficiency, but may also occur in the setting of normal renal function [48–50]. Acidosis can result in bone demineralization as calcium is mobilized to buffer the systemic acid load. Some authors have found a decrease in linear growth after intestinocystoplasty [51–53]; however, this finding is not universal. Mingin *et al.* [54] compared augmented *spina bifida* and exstrophy patients to matched nonaugmented controls. They found that children with intestinocystoplasty had a subclinical hyperchloremic metabolic acidosis, but there were no differences in forearm bone densiometry, height percentile, calcium metabolism, or calcium loss on 24 h urine collection.

Children with interposed bowel segments should be periodically monitored for metabolic and electrolyte abnormalities. Correction of metabolic acidosis can be undertaken with bicarbonate therapy. Severe hyperchloremia can be treated with chlorpromazine or nicotinic acid [4]. Treatment of metabolic acidosis typically requires 0.5–1.0 mEq/kg/d. The amount of bicarbonate needed can be calculated using the following formula:

$$\text{Biocarbonate deficit} = \text{Weight (kg)} \times \text{base deficit} \times 0.3\,\text{mEq/kg/d}$$

Conclusion

Immature renal function in infancy and early childhood, in conjunction with postoperative medications and physiologic changes in ADH and other circulating hormones, makes pediatric patients especially susceptible to water and electrolyte abnormalities. Hyponatremia is by far the most common postoperative electrolyte abnormality, and, when present, appropriate diagnosis is necessary for effective treatment. Care must be taken to provide appropriate postoperative fluids, as well as to monitor patients at risk for electrolyte anomalies.

References

1 Seikaly MG, Arant BS, Jr. Development of renal hemodynamics: Glomerular filtration and renal blood flow. *Clin Perinatol* 1992;19:1–13.

2 Grosfeld JL (Ed). *Pediatric Surgery*, 6th edn. Mosby, Philadelphia, 2006.

3 Hellerstein S. Fluid and electrolytes: Clinical aspects. *Pediatr Rev* 1993;14:103–15.

4 Filston HC, Edwards 3rd, CH, Chitwood R, Jr. *et al.* Estimation of postoperative fluid requirements in infants and children. *Ann Surg* 1982;196:76–81.

5 Duke T, Molyneux EM. Intravenous fluids for seriously ill children: Time to reconsider. *Lancet* 2003;362:1320–23.

6 Burrows FA, Shutack JG, Crone RK. Inappropriate secretion of antidiuretic hormone in a postsurgical pediatric population. *Crit Care Med* 1983;11:527–31.

7 Friis-Hansen B. Body water compartments in children: Changes during growth and related changes in body composition. *Pediatrics* 1961;28:169–81.

8 Barratt MT, Avner ED, Harmon WE (Eds). *Pediatric Nephrology*, 4th edn. Lippincott: Williams & Wilkins, 1999.

9 Chung HM, Kluge R, Schrier RW, Anderson RJ. Postoperative hyponatremia: A prospective study. *Arch Int Med* 1986;146:333–6.

10 Gruskin AB, Sarnaik A. Hyponatremia: Pathophysiology and treatment, a pediatric perspective. *Ped Nephr* 1992;6:280–6.

11 Moran WH, Jr, Miltenberger FW, Shuayb WA *et al.* The relationship of antidiuretic hormone secretion to surgical stress. *Surgery* 1964;56:99–107.

12 Irvin TT, Modgill VK, Hayter CJ *et al.* Plasma-volume deficits and salt and water excretion after surgery. *Lancet* 1972;1159–62.

13 LeQuesne LP, Lewis AAG. Postoperative water and sodium retention. *Lancet* 1953;153–8.

14 Brenner BM, Rector FC, Jr (Eds). *The Kidney*, 5th edn. Philadelphia: WB Saunders, 2008.

15 Wattad A, Chiang ML, Hill LL. Hyponatremia in hospitalized children. *Clin Pediatr (Phila)* 1992;31:153–157.

16 Medani CR. Seizures and hypothermia due to dietary water intoxication in infants. *South Med J* 1987;80:421–5.

17 Arieff AI, Ayus JC, Fraser CL. Hyponatremia and death or permanent brain damage in healthy children. *BMJ* 1992;304:1218–22.

18 Verbalis JG, Martinez AJ. Neurological and neuropathological sequelae of correction of chronic hyponatremia. *Kidney Int* 1991;39:1274–82.

19 Berl T. Treating hyponatremia. Are we Damned if we do and Damned if we don't? *Kidney Int* 1990;37:1008–18.

20 Laureno R, Karp BI. Myelinolysis after correction of hyponatremia. *Ann Intern Med* 1997;126:57–62.

21 Adams RD, Victor M, Mancall EL. Central pontine myelinolysis: A hitherto undescribed disease occurring in alcoholic and malnourished patients. *Arch Neurol Psychiatry* 1959;81:154–72.

22 Sterns RH, Riggs JE, Schochet SS. Osmotic demyelination syndrome following correction of hyponatremia. *NEJM* 1986;314:1535–42.

23 Sarniak AP, Meert KM, Hackbarth R, Fleischmann L. Management of hyponatremic seizures in children with hypertonic saline: A safe and effective strategy. *Crit Care Med* 1991;19:758–62.

24 Adrogue HJ, Madias NE. Hyponatremia. *NEJM* 2000;341:1581–89.

25 Oh MS, Kim HJ, Carroll HJ. Recommendations for treatment of symptomatic hyponatremia. *Nephron* 1995;70:143–50.

26 Kamel KS, Bear RA. Treatment of hyponatremia: A quantitative analysis. *Am J Kidney Dis* 1993;21:439–43.

27 Gross P, Treatment of severe hyponatremia. *Kidney Int* 2001;60:2417–27.

28 Kleigman RM (Ed). *Nelson Textbook of Pediatrics*, 18th edn. Saunders, Philadelphia, 2007.

29 Giebish G, Malnic G, Berliner RW. Control of renal potassium excretion. In *The Kidney*, 5th edn. Edited by BM Brenner, FC Rector, Jr. Philadelphia: WB Saunders, 1996, pp. 371–407.

30 Lorenz JM, Kleinman LI, Disney TA. Renal response of newborn dog to potassium loading. *Am J Physiol* 1986;251: F513–19.

31 Schlossberg SM, Vaughan ED. The mechanism of unilateral post-obstructive diuresis. *J Urol* 1984;131:534–6.

32 Better OS, Arieff AI, Massry SG *et al*. Studies on renal function after relief of complete unilateral ureteral obstruction of three months' duration in man. *Am J Med* 1973;54:234–40.

33 Moody TE, Vaughan ED, Jr., Gillenwater JY. Comparison of the renal hemodynamic response to unilateral and bilateral ureteral occlusion. *Invest Urol* 1977;14:455–9.

34 Buerkert J, Martin D, Head M *et al*. Deep nephron function after release of acute unilateral ureteral obstruction in the young rat. *J Clin Invest* 1978;62:1228–39.

35 Sonnenberg H, Wilson DR. The role of medullary collecting ducts in post-obstructive diuresis. *J Clin Invest* 1976;57:1564–74.

36 Li C, Wang W, Kwon TH *et al*. Altered expression of major Na transporters in rats with bilateral ureteral obstruction and release of obstruction. *Am J Physiol Renal Physiol* 2003;285:F889–901.

37 Wahlberg J, Stenberg A, Wilson DR *et al*. Tubuloglomerular feedback and interstitial pressure in obstructive nephropathy. *Kidney Int* 1984;26:294–302.

38 Frokiaer J, Marples D, Knepper MA *et al*. Bilateral ureteral obstruction downregulates expression of vasopressin-sensitive AQP-2 water channel in rat kidney. *Am J Physiol* 1996:270:F657–68.

39 Ryndin I, Gulmi FA, Chou SY, Mooppan UMM, Kim H. Renal responses to atrial natiuretic peptide are preserved in bilateral ureteral obstruction and augmented by neutral endopeptidase inhibition. *J Urol* 2005;173:651–6.

40 Howards SS, Post-obstructive diuresis: A misunderstood phenomenon. *J Urol* 1973;110:537–40.

41 Wilson DR. Micropuncture study of chronic obstructive nephropathy before and after release of obstruction. *Kidney Int* 1972;2:119–30.

42 Baum N, Anhalt M, Carlton CE, Jr., Scott R, Jr. Post-obstructive diuresis. *J Urol* 1975;114:53–6.

43 Bishop MC. Diuresis and renal functional recovery in chronic retention. *Br J Urol* 1985;57:1–5.

44 O'Reilly PH, Brooman PJC, Farah NB *et al*. High pressure chronic retention. Incidence, aetiology and sinister implications. *Br J Urol* 1986;58:644–6.

45 Jones DA, George NJR, O'Reilly PH. Postobstructive renal function. *Semin Urol* 1987;5:176–90.

46 Vaughan ED, Jr., Gillenwater JY. Diagnosis, characterization and management of post-obstructive diruesis. *J Urol* 1973;109:286–92.

47 Nyman MA, Schwenk NM, Silverstein MD. Management of urinary retention: Rapid versus gradual decompression and risk of complications. *Mayo Clin Proc* 1997;72:951–6.

48 Hall MC, Koch MO, Mc Dougal WS. Metabolic consequences of urinary diversion through intestinal segments. *Urol Clin North Am* 1991;18:725–35.

49 Nurse DE, Mundy AR. Metabolic complications of cystoplasty. *Br J Urol* 1989;63:165–70.

50 Whitmore WF, Gittes RF. Reconstruction of the urinary tract by cecal and ileocecal cystoplasty: Review of a 15 year experience. *J Urol* 1983;129:494–8.

51 Mundy AR, Nurse DE. Calcium balance, growth and skeletal mineralization in patients with cystoplasties. *Br J Urol* 1992;69:257–9.

52 Wagstaff KE, Woodhouse CR, Duffy PG *et al*. Delayed linear growth in children with enterocystoplasties. *Br J Urol* 1992;69:314.

53 Gross DA, Lopatin UA, Gearhart JP *et al*. Decreased linear growth associated with intestinal bladder augmentation in children with bladder exstrophy. *J Urol* 2000;164:917–20.

54 Mingin GC, Nguyen HT, Mathais RS *et al*. Growth and metabolic consequences of bladder augmentation in children with myelomeningocele and bladder exstrophy. *Pediatrics* 2002;110:1193–8.

6

Perioperative Anesthetic and Analgesic Risks and Complications

Philippa Evans and Mark Thomas

Key points

- The mortality associated with anesthesia is low, but is higher at the extremes of age.

- The risks associated with anesthesia have been greatly reduced by improvements in equipment and monitoring techniques.

- Respiratory adverse events are the most common perioperative problems.

- There are side effects or risks associated with all modalities of analgesia. Recent data show epidural analgesia to be associated with fewer complications in children compared with adults.

- Intravenous fluids and blood products should be prescribed with the same caution and consideration as any other medication.

Introduction

Modern anesthesia is extremely safe. In fact the risk of serious injury or death is so small that it makes it difficult to measure accurately. National Confidential Enquiry into Peri-operative Deaths (NCEPOD) data in the UK [1], the Australian Incident Monitoring System (AIMS) project in Australia [2], and the closed claims process in the United States [3] are the best sources of recent data. However, while these sources provide details of death or serious injury they do rely on accurate reporting. Furthermore, they give no indication of the numbers of total anesthetics administered and without this denominator it is not possible to quote accurate rates of risk.

What is clear from the literature is that the mortality associated with anesthesia has decreased dramatically from 6 per 10,000 in the 1950s to 0.36 per 10,000 by the start of this millennium [4–6].

There are several reasons for this. Firstly, we have become much more aware of the need for accurate audit over this time and have used audit as a powerful tool to develop safer practice. Secondly, we have become more subspecialized. There is good evidence that a trained pediatric anesthetist can decrease the incidence of perioperative events [7,8]. Thirdly, we have seen great advances in equipment and monitoring over recent years and have developed minimum monitoring standards to ensure the highest quality of patient care.

Of course, figures quoted for risk are very much dependent on individual patient factors. It is abundantly clear from the studies quoted above that children in the younger age group, specifically below one year of age, have a greater incidence of anesthetic mortality. American Society of Anesthesiologists (ASA) status and comorbidities such as prematurity, obstructive sleep apnea, and congenital abnormalities will all adversely impact upon the risk. However human error and equipment failure account for the majority of negative outcomes and, if they could be eliminated, would make approximately 90% of critical incidents preventable. So, while medical optimization preoperatively remains important the ability to reduce risk further lies squarely with the anesthetist and his or her team and with systems designed to minimize the scope for human error.

Pediatric Urology: Surgical Complications and Management. Edited by Duncan T. Wilcox, Prasad P. Godbole and Martin A. Koyle. © 2008 Blackwell Publishing, ISBN: 978-1-4051-6268-5.

Specific complications of general anesthesia, their prevention and management

Respiratory complications

Respiratory adverse events are the most common perioperative problems faced by the anesthetist [9,10]. The incidence of adverse events is higher in younger children due to the relatively narrow infant airway coupled with the high incidence of respiratory tract infections in this population. The most common events are periods of arterial desaturation, laryngospasm, and bronchospasm [11].

Laryngospasm is the reflex closure of the glottis by adduction of the true or false vocal cords. It can persist after cessation of the stimulus. Common causes include local stimulation of the larynx, e.g. by saliva, blood, or foreign body including a laryngoscope or endotracheal tube. It can also occur in response to other stimulation, e.g. surgery, movement, or stimulation of the anus or cervix. The reflex is abolished in deeper planes of anesthesia. Laryngospasm leads to partial or complete airway obstruction, which presents with stridor and causes hypoxemia and hypoventilation and in the most severe cases negative pressure pulmonary edema. Treatment consists of removing the stimulus, giving 100% oxygen and providing positive end expiratory pressure (PEEP) via the breathing circuit. If the spasm does not resolve with these maneuvres then a small dose of intravenous induction agent or muscle relaxant can be used to break the spasm.

Children with upper respiratory tract infections (URIs) have a sevenfold increase in respiratory complications compared to asymptomatic children [12]. Additional risk factors for developing adverse respiratory events in children with URIs include: the use of an endotracheal tube, age less than five years or a history of prematurity (less than 37 weeks gestation), a history of reactive airway disease or nasal congestion, parental smoking, and surgery on the airway [13].

Airway complications

Control of a patient's airway is the most important aspect of any general anesthetic. Difficulties can arise due to inability to control a patient's airway and provide adequate ventilation by bag-mask ventilation – a "can't ventilate" situation – or when the airway can be managed but intubation is difficult – a "can't intubate" situation. The incidence of difficult laryngoscopy/intubation varies between 1.5% and 13% and failed intubation has been identified as one of the anesthesia-related causes of

death or permanent brain damage [14]. This happens when a "can't intubate can't ventilate" situation arises. There are certain childhood syndromes that are associated with difficult airways and these should be highlighted during preoperative assessment in order that the anesthetic can be planned accordingly. These syndromes include the Pierre Robin Sequence, Crouzon syndrome, Apert syndrome, Pfeiffer syndrome, Treacher-Collins syndrome, craniofacial microsomia, and Goldenhar syndrome [15].

More minor adverse events associated with the airway include dental damage and postoperative sore throat. Oral tissue and dental damage are common complications of general anesthesia and account for a significant proportion of medicolegal claims against anesthetists in adult practice [16]. These injuries tend to occur during laryngoscopy and intubation. A dental history should be obtained during the preoperative visit and children with wobbly teeth (peak ages 6–8 years) should be warned of potential loss! Postoperative sore throat has a reported incidence of 12.1% 24 h after surgery in daycase adult patients. The incidence is higher after intubation than following insertion of a laryngeal mask airway, and interestingly still occurs in some patients who have had no instrumentation of their airway but merely received airway support via a facemask [17].

Cardiovascular complications

Adverse cardiac events are only a quarter as common as respiratory complications during anesthesia. Common events include arrhythmias and bradycardias, and hypertension or hypotension [11]. The results of the Paediatric Perioperative Cardiac Arrest Registry (POCA) found an estimated incidence of anesthesia-related cardiac arrest of 1.4 per 10,000 with a mortality rate of 26% in those affected [6]. Pharmacological (overdose) and underlying cardiac disease were the most common causes; 55% of events occurred in children under the age of one year.

Gastrointestinal complications

Vomiting is the most common postoperative adverse effect associated with anesthesia. Incidence ranges from 9% to 43% [18]. Incidence increases with age, and peaks at 11–14 years corresponding with puberty. The incidence of vomiting is also related to the site of surgery and is highest following strabismus surgery, appendicectomy, ENT surgery, and orchidopexy. High-risk patients include those with a previous history of postoperative nausea and vomiting and/or a history of motion sickness [19]. Anesthetic technique can influence the risk of postoperative vomiting. Techniques should be adjusted and preemptive antiemetics given to those considered to be high risk.

The incidence of perioperative aspiration is low and generally has a good outcome. It is reported as between 1 and 10 per 10,000 with a very low incidence of pneumonitis or need for admission to intensive care [20].

Neurological complications

Peripheral nerve injury has a reported incidence of 1 per 1000 anesthetics in adults. The most commonly affected are ulnar nerve 30%, brachial plexus 23%, and the lumbosacral nerves 16% [21]. Poor positioning intraoperatively is a common underlying factor. The usual mechanism of injury to superficial nerves is secondary to ischemia due to compression of the vasa vasorum by surgical retractors, leg stirrups, or contact with other equipment. Injury is more likely to occur during periods of poor peripheral perfusion due to hypotension and hypothermia. Injury may be less likely in children because of the protection afforded by their increased subcutaneous tissue compared with adults and their lighter weight. The mechanism of injury to the brachial plexus is usually traction caused by excess shoulder abduction. Damage can be avoided by taking meticulous care with patient positioning, using padding to protect pressure points, and avoiding extreme joint positions. Most nerve injuries recover over a period of months; all need to be reviewed by a neurologist.

The commonest type of ocular complication is corneal abrasion. This presents with blurring of vision and usually resolves over 1–2 months [16]. Protective reflexes are lost during anesthesia and eyes need to be taped shut to protect the cornea. Care must be taken to avoid pressure to the eyes and extra padding and protection is needed if the patient is in the prone position for surgery.

Awareness during anesthesia is a state of consciousness that is revealed by explicit or implicit memory of intraoperative events. From adult data, the incidence of conscious awareness with explicit recall and severe pain is estimated to be <1 per 3000 general anesthetics. Conscious awareness with explicit recall but without pain is more common with an incidence between 0.1% and 0.7% [22]. The incidence of awareness is higher in cases where neuromuscular blocking agents are used. Patients who experience awareness are at risk of developing post-traumatic stress disorder. The commonest cause of awareness is drug error: either inadvertent paralysis of an awake patient or failure of delivery of volatile anesthetic agents.

Maladaptive postoperative behaviors have been reported to occur in up to 65% of children undergoing anesthesia and surgery. Changes include anxiety, sleep disturbance, night terrors, and a return to bed wetting. Variables such as young age, degree of patient and parent preoperative anxiety, child's anxiety at induction, type of surgery, and level of postoperative pain have been reported to predict the occurrence of behavioral changes [23]. Prolonged upset occurs even after daycase surgery and anesthesia. Up to 32% of children exhibit negative behavioral changes one month after their operation [24]. Sevoflurane is the volatile anesthetic agent that is most widely used for inhalational induction. Patients who have received sevoflurane are often agitated on their emergence from anesthesia. A short-lived post-anesthetic delirium is well described. However, this emergence delirium associated with sevoflurane is still the subject of some debate and does not seem to develop into prolonged neurocognitive changes. The incidence of maladaptive behaviors seems to be similar with sevoflurane, halothane, and isoflurane [25,26].

Rare but serious complications

Anaphylactic and anaphylactoid reactions during anesthesia are rare but potentially life-threatening allergic events. The two types of reaction are clinically indistinguishable and in their most severe manifestations present with cardiovascular collapse, bronchospasm, and laryngeal edema. Serum histamine and mast cell tryptase levels help confirm the diagnosis [27]. Patients require follow-up with skin-prick test and Radio Allergy Sorbent Test (RASTs) for specific IgE antibodies to identify the triggering agent. The incidence of anaphylaxis is approximately 1 per 6000 anesthetics [28]. The most commonly incriminated agents are the neuromuscular blocking agents (58% of reactions), latex (16.7%), and antibiotics (15%). A history of atopy, asthma, and food allergy are more frequent in cases of latex allergy [29].

Malignant hyperthermia (MH) is a rare autosomal dominant condition that is triggered by volatile anesthetic agent and suxamethonium. It has an incidence of 1 in 15,000 in children and 1 in 50–100,000 in adults [30]. It still has a mortality of 10% and requires prompt and efficient recognition and management [31]. Diagnosis is made by muscle biopsy and relatives of the index case must also be investigated. Anesthesia in susceptible individuals requires careful planning and avoidance of potential trigger agents.

Suxamethonium is a short acting depolarizing muscle relaxant. It is metabolized by plasma cholinesterase. Suxamethonium apnea occurs in patients with reduced cholinesterase activity. This reduced activity arises either as a result of genetic variability in cholinesterase type or secondary to acquired conditions, such as liver disease and cancer. It presents as prolonged nonreversible paralysis at the end of the anesthetic. Management involves continued sedation and ventilation until the drug has been metabolized. This may involve several hours of mechanical ventilation.

Specific complications of pain management

There are very few, if any, urological procedures that are not potentially painful to a greater or lesser extent. Many are easily ameliorated with simple analgesic regime while other require more sophisticated regional techniques in addition.

Systemic analgesia

Of course, when any drug is administered to any patient the potential for error exists. It is always possible to give the wrong drug (in the case of an allergic history for instance), the wrong dose, or to give a drug by the wrong route. Assuming that we are talking about giving appropriate drugs to appropriate patients, it is worth considering the range of agents at our disposal.

Paracetamol

This drug's pharmacokinetics are better known than those of any other drug in the pediatric pharmacopoeia. The main risks in its use relate to the potential for overdose. Suggested maxima are 25 mg\kg per 24 hours at under 30 weeks postconceptional age, 45 mg\kg at less than 34 weeks, 60 mg/kg in term neonates and infants and 90 mg/kg thereafter [32]. Paracetamol is metabolized in the liver mainly by glucuronidation and sulfation but if these pathways become saturated the hepatotoxic oxidative metabolite N-acetyl-p-benzoquinoneimine may accumulate. Risk factors for this include dehydration and sepsis.

Nonsteroidal anti-inflammatory drugs (NSAIDs)

In a large study, the risk of administering a short-term course of ibuprofen was low and similar to paracetamol [33]. Childhood asthma does not seem to be affected by NSAIDs in the way as adult asthma [34]. Impaired renal function and bleeding tendency remain contraindications, however. The use of NSAIDs below six months of age is ill advised because of the risk of pulmonary hypertension and alterations in cerebral and renal regional blood flow that is so dependent on prostaglandins in this age range. A growing body of literature describing the use of NSAIDs for the closure of patent ductus arteriosus in neonates has led to the reappraisal of the lower age limit, and the current United Kingdom national formulary now contains dose-guidance for analgesic use down to one month of age if >5 kg [35].

Opioids

The main side effects of this group are respiratory depression, nausea and vomiting, constipation, urinary retention, itching, and sedation. From a safety perspective clearly the most important of these is respiratory depression.

Since we have moved away from intermittent intravenous bolus and intramuscular injections, the risk has diminished because with infusions and bedside-controlled analgesia pumps the potential for high-peak plasma concentrations is less.

The addition of high background infusion rates to patient–controlled regimes increases the risk of sedation, hypoxia, nausea, and vomiting [36]. However a low rate of 4 mcg/kg/h has advantages in analgesia without this untoward side effect profile [37].

Respiratory depression is readily treatable with naloxone but due to its relatively short duration of action this may need to be repeated or infused. Urinary retention and itching have been successfully treated with lower doses of naloxone while itching often responds to chlorpheniramine.

Nausea and vomiting occurs in 30–45% of children on patient–controlled analgesia pumps and can be reduced by prophylactic anti-emetic administration [38,39]. Adding an anti-emetic to the morphine pump is not effective [40].

Nurse controlled analgesia pumps for children <5 years of age or so is effective [41] but is recommended for use by trained nurses rather than parents [42].

Regional analgesia and local anesthesia
Epidural

A recent national audit of pediatric epidural complications has just been completed in the United Kingdom. Birmingham Children's Hospital painstakingly gathered information from 21 pediatric centers over a 5-year period resulting in data from more than 10,000 epidurals. Ninety-six serious clinical incidents were reported giving an overall incidence of 0.9% [43].

Out of these 96 clinical incidents, 40 were judged by an expert panel to be coincidental to the epidural. These included complications such as pressure sores and compartment syndrome. Of the remaining 56 incidents the

Table 6.1 The incidences of serious complications following pediatric epidurals (United Kingdom National Audit).

Complication	Incidence (out of 10,633 epidurals)
Infection	28
Drug error	14
Nerve injury	6
Postdural puncture headache	6
Local anesthetic toxicity	1
Inadvertent spinal anesthetic	1

commonest was local infection. The relative incidences in this group are given in Table 6.1.

It is clear from the above that epidurals are extremely safe. However, there is still considerable debate within anesthesia as to the merits of epidural analgesia over and above systemic modalities of pain relief. This is not the least because the consequences of a serious complication following an epidural are so great.

Having said that only one patient from the United Kingdom audit had persistent neurological problems more than 12 months postepidural insertion. This compares very favorably with adult epidural data in which the quoted risk of permanent neurological injury is 2–7:10,000 [44]. Furthermore, systemic analgesic techniques are not without complications themselves.

If we were to analyze why there has been a decline in the administration of epidurals, we would most likely attribute it at least in part to the rise of a risk-averse culture. Complications arising from opioids are more likely to be attributed to patient and drug characteristics. Complications arising from the epidural can more readily be apportioned, fairly or not, to poor technique or operator error.

Caudal analgesia

Caudals are the commonest regional technique used in pediatric anesthetic practice. They are relatively easy to perform, especially in children <8 years or so, and are effective. They provide analgesia for 3–10 h depending on the drug combinations used [45]. There are reports on large series of caudals with very few side effects [46,47]. Transient leg weakness and urinary retention should always be anticipated.

The most common additives in the United Kingdom are clonidine and ketamine. The former approximately doubles the duration of a plain local caudal to 5–6 h and

with ketamine a further 4 h or so may be expected [45]. Clearly such prolonged block needs to be anticipated and warned for if inadvertent injury is to be avoided.

Peripheral blocks

As with all blocks, the potential for local anesthetic toxicity exists. The risk is greatest when the solution is injected into vascular tissue or injected inadvertently intravascularly. Most texts recommend an upper limit of 2 mg/kg for bupivacaine (0.8 ml/kg of 0.25%). The recent introduction of levorotatory bupivacaine has been widely embraced into clinical practice since this form has been shown to be equally effective yet less cardio toxic in the event of inadvertent intravascular injection. If cardiotoxicity does occur it may manifest it as ventricular extrasystoles, which can progress to a particularly shock-resistant ventricular fibrillation.

Adrenaline-containing solutions should be avoided near end arteries such as dorsal nerve block or ring block to help avoid the risk of penile necrosis. Ilioinguinal blocks are commonly performed for groin surgery and are extremely safe and effective. The main local risk for these is tracking of the local anesthetic next to the femoral nerve with resultant leg weakness and possible delayed discharge as a result. The increasing use of ultrasound guidance in the accurate placement of blocks may reduce this complication.

Complications associated with intravenous fluids

Recent publications have highlighted the risks of administering infusions of hypotonic solutions to both medical and surgical pediatric patients [48]. The infusion of hypotonic solutions (such as 0.18% sodium chloride with 4% glucose or 5% glucose) is associated with the development of acute hyponatremia. The most serious complication of hyponatremia is hyponatremic encephalopathy, which can lead to permanent neurological damage and death. Over 50% of children with a serum sodium of <125 mmol/l will develop hyponatremic encephalopathy [49]. Hyponatremia is associated with the movement of water into brain tissue, which can lead to cerebral edema. The resultant increase in brain volume can lead to brain herniation and death. Children are at particular risk as they have a higher number of brain cells and a larger brain to intracranial volume ratio compared with adults [50]. In a recent review of 50 cases of hospital-acquired hyponatremic encephalopathy mortality was as high as 50%. More than half the cases occurred in the postoperative setting in previously healthy children undergoing minor surgery [51].

For half a century, fluid therapy in children has been based on Holliday and Segar's formula, which proposed to match children's water and electrolyte requirements on a weight-based calculation using hypotonic solutions [52]. The formula was derived following studies of metabolism in active children. It has been argued that the requirements of hospitalized relatively inactive children are less.

Surgical patients are at particular risk of developing hyponatremia. The postoperative period is associated with a nonosmotic secretion of antidiuretic hormone (ADH). ADH reduces the ability of the kidneys to excrete free water leading to hyponatremia and oliguria. Infusion of hypotonic solutions further exacerbates the situation. Excess ADH secretion can be encountered even after minor surgery [49]. Pain, stress, anxiety, nausea, and vomiting, and morphine can all act stimuli for its release.

Studies have shown that while infusions of hypotonic solutions in the perioperative period are associated with falls in plasma sodium, infusion of isotonic solutions are associated with stable plasma sodium levels [53]. Holliday and Segar have recently changed their recommendations. They suggest halving the average maintenance volume, i.e. 50 ml/kg/day for the first day of the infusion and monitoring serum sodium if the need for intravenous fluids continues [54].

Fluid therapy in surgical patients should be designed to provide for different requirements: fluid deficits, maintenance fluid requirements, and volume of fluid needed to maintain an adequate tissues perfusion (and counteract the effects of anesthetics). Fluid deficits consist of preoperative deficits (fasting, gastrointestinal, renal, or cutaneous losses), hemorrhage and third space losses. The National Patient Safety Agency in the United Kingdom has recently produced a Patient Safety Alert with regard to intravenous fluid therapy in children [55]. They recommend the immediate removal of sodium chloride 0.18% with glucose 4% from use. In units where this has occurred, there have been no further cases of iatrogenic hyponatremia [56]. They emphasize that the prescribing of fluids should be afforded the same considerations as the prescription of other drugs with reference to indications, contraindications, and dose [57] and that prescriptions should be individualized [58]. They recommend that intravascular volume depletion should be managed using bolus doses of sodium chloride 0.9%

(isotonic), and that ongoing losses should be replaced with a similar biochemical solution. In most cases this would be an isotonic solution such as sodium chloride 0.9%, sodium chloride with glucose 5% or Hartman's solution (or Ringer's lactate). They state that sodium chloride 0.45% with glucose 5% or 2.5% can safely be prescribed for the majority of children as maintenance fluid. They urge closer patient monitoring with regular weights and measurement of plasma sodium. They also call for a review of drug prescription charts so that maintenance fluids can be prescribed separately to other intravenous fluids [55].

Complications associated with blood transfusion

Children are more susceptible than adults to the harmful effects of hypovolemia. Volume correction is therefore of paramount importance and can be achieved with crystalloids and artificial colloids. In general children tolerate hemodilution well and perioperative levels of 6 g/dl are acceptable in a hemodynamically stable child. There are of course many potential complications of transfusion namely hypocalcemia, hyperkalemia, hypomagnesemia, metabolic acidosis, and hypothermia. However, all of these are generally correctable [59]. What is of greater concern to parents and children is the infective risk of blood transfusion.

Infectious disease transmission risk

Infectious risks of transfusion have decreased dramatically secondary to improved screening, detection of infected agents, and advances in pathogen inactivation. Nonetheless the risk of infection, especially of human immunodeficiency virus and hepatitis C, is often of great concern to the parents of children who may need blood transfusion. The incidence varies between countries and is dependent upon the prevalence of these infections within the donor community and the resources used to screen the blood products. Tables 6.2 and 6.3 illustrate the current situation in the United States.

Besides viral pathogens, bacterial contamination can occur. This is most commonly seen with platelets [60]. Standards for testing platelets for bacterial growth are being developed. Other infectious diseases that can potentially be transmitted by transfusion include Chagas disease, Lyme disease, malaria, and Creutzfeldt-Jakob disease (CJD). Although no specific nucleic acid or antigen testing for these diseases exist, donor screening and

Table 6.2 Current blood screening tests used on donated blood in the United States.

Screening tests
Hepatitis B surface antigen (HBsAg)
Hepatitis B core antibody (anti-HBc)
Hepatitis C virus antibody (anti-HCV)
HIV-1 antibody (anti-HIV-1)
HIV-2 antibody (anti-HIV-2)
HTLV-I antibody (anti-HTLV-I)
HTLV-II antibody (anti-HTLV-II)
Nucleic acid amplification testing (NAT) for HIV-1 and HCV
Serologic test for syphilis
Nucleic acid amplification for West Nile virus

Source: Data from www.aabb.org.

Table 6.3 Risk of transfusion-related viral transmission and viral window for negative screening test.

Virus	Risk	Days possible to transmit disease, i.e. false negative screen
Hepatitis A	–	'Occasional cases'
Hepatitis B	1 per 137,000	59
Hepatitis C	1 per 1,000,000	82
Human T-lymphotrophic virus I and II	1 per 641,000 or less	51
HIV	1 per 1,900,000	22

Source: Data from www.aabb.org.

the deferral of those with potential symptoms helps prevent transfusion-related transmission. In the United Kingdom all blood products are leukocyte-depleted and clotting products are sourced from the United States to reduce the risk of transmission of new variant CJD.

Incompatibility and other immunologic considerations

Clerical error is the most common cause of mismatched transfusion. Severe acute hemolytic reactions most often result from immunologic destruction of red cells because of ABO incompatibility. Less frequently,

serologic incompatibilities not detected by standard antibody screens can cause an acute hemolytic reaction. Anaphylactoid reactions with bronchospasm, laryngeal edema, and urticaria are dangerous but rare and typically occur in IgA-deficient individuals. The mandatory use of leukocyte-depleted products in the United Kingdom has significantly reduced transfusion reactions and immune modulation caused by cytokines and leukocyte-degradation products. Formation of antihuman leukocyte antigen (HLA)-antibodies and febrile transfusion reactions have also been virtually eliminated [61].

References

1 An acute problem? The first of two reports published in 2005 by the National Confidential Enquiry into patient Outcome and Death (1 June 2003 to 31 June 2003) CD Version. London, 2005.

2 Van der Walt JH, Sweeney DB, Webb RK. Pediatric incidents in anesthesia: An analysis of 2000 incident reports. *Anaesth Intens Care* 1993;21:655–8.

3 Mooray JP, Geiduschek JM, Caplan RA *et al*. A comparison of pediatric and adult anesthesia closed malpractice claims. *Anesthesiology* 1993;78:461–7.

4 Short TG, O'Regan A, Jayasuriya JP *et al*. Improvements in anaesthetic care resulting from a critical incident reporting programme. *Anaesthesia* 1996;51:615–21.

5 Rackow H, Salnitre E, Green LT. Frequency of cardiac arrest associated with anaesthesia in infants and children. *Pediatrics* 1961;28:697.

6 Morray JP, Geiduschek JM, Ramamoorthy C *et al*. Anesthesia-related cardiac arrest in children. Initial findings of the Pediatric Perioperative Cardiac Arrest (POCA) Registry. *Anesthesiology* 2000;93:66–71.

7 Keenan RL, Shapiro JH, Kane FR *et al*. Bradycardia during anesthesia in infants. *Anesthesiology* 1994;80:976–81.

8 Auroy Y, Ecoffey C. The relationship between complications of pediatric anestheisa and volume of pediatric anesthetics. *Anesth Analg* 1997;84:234.

9 Tay C, Tan G, Ng S. Critical incidents in paediatric anaesthesia: An audit of 10,000 anaesthetics in Singapore. *Paediatr Anaesth* 2001;11:711–18.

10 Cohen MM, Cameron CB, Duncan PG. Pediatric anesthesia morbidity and mortality in the perioperative period. *Anesth Analg* 1990;70:160–67.

11 Murat I, Constant I, Maud'Huy H. Perioperative morbidity in children: A database of 24 165 anaesthetics in France over a 30-month period. *Paediatr Anaesth* 2004; 14:158–64.

12 Cohen MM, Cameron CB. Should you cancel the operation when a child has an upper respiratory tract infection?. *Anesth Analg* 1991;72:282–8.

13 Tait AR, Malviya S, Voepel-Lewis T *et al*. Risk factors for perioperative adverse respiratory events in children with

upper respiratory tract infections. *Anesthesiology* 2001; 95:299–306.

14 Randell T. Prediction of difficult intubation. *Acta Anaesthesiol Scand* 1998;42:136–7.

15 Dinwiddie R. Congenital upper airway obstruction. *Paediatric Resp Reviews* 2004;5:17–24.

16 Jenkins K, Baker AB. Consent and anaesthetic risk. *Anaesthesia* 2003;58:962–84.

17 Higgins PP, Chung F, Mezei G. Postoperative sore throat after ambulatory surgery. *BJA* 2002;88:582–4.

18 Kermode J, Walker S, Webb I. Postoperative vomiting in children. *Anaesth Intensive Care* 1995;23:196–9.

19 Cohen MM, Duncan PG, DeBoer *et al.* The post operative interview: assessing risk factors for nausea and vomiting. *Anesth Analg* 1994;78:7–16.

20 Borland CM, Sereika SM, Woelfel SK *et al.* Pulmonary aspiration in pediatric patients during general anesthesia: incidence and outcome. *J Clinical Anesth* 1998;19:95–102.

21 Kroll DA, Caplan RA, Posner K *et al.* Nerve injury associated with anesthesia. *Anesthesiology* 1990;73:202–7.

22 Schwender D, Klasing S, Davinderer M *et al.* Awareness during general anaesthesia. Definition, incidence, clinical relevance, causes, avoidance and medicolegal aspects. *Anaesthetist* 1995;44:743–54.

23 Kain Z. Postoperative maladaptive behavioural changed in children: Incidence, risk factors and interventions. *Acta Anaesthesiol Scand* 2000;51:217–26.

24 Kontincerni LH, Ryhanen PT, Moilanen IK. Behavioural changes following routine ENT operations in two-to-ten year old children. *Paediat Anaesth* 1996;6:45–9.

25 Kain Z, Caldwell-Andrews A, Weinberg M *et al.* Sevoflurane versus halothane: postoperative maladaptive behavioural changes. *Anesthesiology* 2005;102:720–6.

26 Meyer RR, Munster P, Werner C, Brambrink AM. Isoflurane is associated with a similar incidence of emergence agitation/delirium as sevoflurane in young children-a randomised controlled study. *Paediatr Anaesth* 2007;17:56–60.

27 Suspected anaphylactic reactions associated with anaesthesia. Revised Edition 2003. The Association of Anaesthetists of Great Britain and Ireland and the British Society for Allergy and Clinical Immunology, August 2003.

28 Laxenaire MC, Mertes PM. Anaphylaxis during anaesthesia. Results of a 2 year study in France. *BJA* 2001;87:549–58.

29 Mertes PM, Laxenaire MC, Alla F. Anaphylactic and anaphylactoid reactions occurring during anesthesia in France in 1999–2000. *Anesthesiology* 2003;99:536–45.

30 Nelson TE, Flewellen EH. Current concepts. The malignant hyperthermia syndrome. *N Engl J Med* 1983;309:416–18.

31 Guidelines for the management of a malignant hyperthermia crisis. The Association of Anaesthetists of Great Britain and Ireland. A4 laminated sheet 2007.

32 Anderson BJ, van Lingen RA, Hansen TG *et al.* Acetaminophen developmental pharmacokinetics in premature neonates and infants: A pooled population analysis. *Anesthesiology* 2002;96:1336–45.

33 Lesko SM, Mitchell AA. The safety of acetaminophen and ibuprofen among children younger than two years old. *Pediatrics* 1999;104:E39.

34 Lesko SM, Louik C, Vezina RM *et al.* Asthma morbidity after short-term use of Ibuprofen in children. *Pediatrics* 2002;109:E20.

35 British National Formulary for Children 2006. BMJ Publishing Group. RPS Publishing & RCPCH Publications 2006.

36 Doyle E, Harper I, Morton NS *et al.* Comparison of patient-controlled analgesia with and without a background infusion after lower abdominal surgery in children. *Br J Anaesth* 1993;71:670–73.

37 Doyle E, Harper I, Morton NS *et al.* Patient-controlled analgesia with low dose background infusions after lower abdominal surgery in children. *Br J Anaesth* 1993;72:818–22.

38 Doyle E, Byers G, McNicol LR *et al.* Prevention of postoperative nausea and vomiting with transdermal hyoscine in children using patient-controlled analgesia. *Br J Anaesth* 1994;72:72–6.

39 Allen DC, Jorgensen C, Sims C. Effect of tropisetron on vomiting during patient-controlled analgesia in children. *Br J Anaesth* 1999;83:608–10.

40 Munro FJ, Fisher S, Dickson U *et al.* The addition of antiemetics to the morphine solution in patient-controlled analgesia syringes used by children after an appendicectomy does not reduce the incidence of postoperative nausea and vomiting. *Paediatr Anaesth* 2002;12:600–603.

41 Monitto CL, Greenberg RS, Kost-Byerly S *et al.* The safety and efficacy of parent-/nurse-conrolled analgesia in patients less than six years of age. *Anaesth Analg* 2000;91:573–9.

42 Howard RF. Current status of pain management in children. *JAMA* 2003;290:2464–9.

43 Llewellyn N, Moriarty A. The UK National Paediatric Epidural Audit. *Paediatr Anaesth* 2007; in press.

44 Faccenda KA, Finucane BT. Complications of regional anaesthesia. Incidence and prevention. *Drug Saf* 2001;24:413–42.

45 de Beer DA, Thomas ML. Caudal additives in children… solutions or problems?. *Br J Anaesth* 2003;90:487–98.

46 Veyckemans F, Vanobbergh LJ, Gouverneur JM. Lessons from 1100 pediatric caudal blocks in a teaching hospital. *Reg Anaesth* 1992;17:119–23.

47 Dalens B, Hasnaoui A. Caudal anaesthesia in pediatric surgery: Success rate and adverse effects in 750 consecutive patients. *Anesth Analg* 1989;68:83–9.

48 Choong K, Kho ME, Menon K, Bohn D. Hypotonic versus isotonic saline in children: A systematic review. *Arch Dis Child* 2006;91:528–35.

49 Mortiz M, Ayus JC. Preventing neurological complications from dysnatraemias in children. *Pediatr Nephrol* 2005;20:1687–700.

50 Paut O, Lacroix F. Recent developments in the perioperative fluid management for the paediatric patient. *Curr Opin Anaesthesiol* 2006;19:268–77.

51 Moritz M, Ayus J. Prevention of hospital-acquired hyponatraemia: A case for using isotonic saline. *Pediatrics* 2003;111:227–30.

52 Holliday M, Segar W. The maintenance need for water in parental fluid therapy. *Pediatrics* 1957;19:823–32.

53 Brazel PW, McPhee IB. Inappropriate secretion of antidiuretic hormone in postoperative scoliosis patients: The role of fluid management. *Spine* 1996;21:724–7.

54 Holliday M, Segar W. Reducing errors in fluid therapy management. *Pediatrics* 2003;111:424–5.

55 NPSA 2006 Patient Safety Alert. Reducing the risk of harm when administering intravenous fluids to children. National Patient Safety Agency United Kingdom, 2006.

56 Cosgrove M, Wardhaugh A. Iatrogenic hyponatraemia. *Arch Dis Child* 2003;88:646–7.

57 Stern RH, Silver SM. Salt and water: Read the packet insert. *QJMed* 2003;96:549–52.

58 Shafiee MAS, Bohn D, Hoorn EJ, Halperin ML. How to select optimal maintenance intravenous fluid therapy. *QJMed* 2003;96:601–10.

59 Barcelona SL, Thompson AA, Cote C. Intraoperative pediatric blood transfusion therapy: A review of common issues. Part I: hematologic and physiologic differences from adults; metabolic and infectious risks. *Pediatr Anesth* 2005;15:716–26.

60 Smith LA, Wright-Kanuth MS. Bacterial contamination of blood components. *Clin Lab Sci* 2003;16:230–8.

61 Solheim BG, Wesenberg F. Rational use of blood products. Paediatric Update. *Eur J Cancer* 2001;37:2421–7.

Open Surgery of the Upper Urinary Tract

7

Nephrectomy

Paul Crow and Mark Woodward

Key points

- With the advent of laparoscopic surgery, open simple nephrectomy is rarely performed.

- The retroperitoneal approach is preferable to the transabdominal approach as it does not lead to the formation of intraperitoneal adhesions.

- Conversion of laparoscopic to open nephrectomy is usually achieved by joining or extending port site incisions.

- Preoperative imaging provides valuable anatomical information useful in planning nephrectomy, particularly when the kidney is ectopic.

- Careful preoperative planning and surgical technique can minimize the morbidity associated with hemorrhage or damage to perirenal structures.

Introduction

The advent of laparoscopic surgery has made open nephrectomy an infrequent undertaking in pediatric urology. The most common indications for open nephrectomy are now malignant disease (see Chapter 33) and trauma (see Chapter 38).

Contraindications to elective, simple laparoscopic nephrectomy are increasingly rare, with some centers now reporting successful laparoscopic surgery for xanthogranulomatous pyelonephritis [1]. These facts, together with the absence of contemporary publications on elective open simple nephrectomy, would seem to confirm that laparoscopic surgery has now taken over as the gold standard approach.

Although infrequently applied, a good working knowledge of open approaches to the kidney remains important to the pediatric urological surgeon. In particular, the ability to convert rapidly from laparoscopic to open nephrectomy, whether it is to control hemorrhage or for nonprogression, remains an essential surgical skill. In addition, familiarity with the choice of open approaches

to both normally positioned and ectopic kidneys is vital on the rare occasion that laparoscopy is contraindicated.

This chapter will cover open approaches to the kidney, concentrating on the anatomical basis, advantages, and potential complications of each approach.

Surgical approaches to the kidney

The first intentional nephrectomy was performed by Gustav Simon in 1869 in the treatment of an ureterovaginal fistula. The first pediatric nephrectomy for a Wilms tumor was performed in Leeds, by Richard Jessop in 1877. Retroperitoneal flank approaches had a lower incidence of postoperative peritonitis and were the approach of choice in the first half of the 20th century. Advancements in the surgical technique led to a revival of transabdominal approaches in the 1950s. The modern surgeon has numerous choices of approach, which can be tailored to the needs of each individual case.

Retroperitoneal approaches

The majority of surgeons prefer a retroperitoneal approach to simple nephrectomy, the principal advantage being avoidance of the peritoneal cavity and the associated risk of forming intraperitoneal adhesions. Open access to the retroperitoneum can be achieved through loin, lumbotomy, and anterior approaches. Readers are referred

---

Pediatric Urology: Surgical Complications and Management. Edited by Duncan T. Wilcox, Prasad P. Godbole and Martin A. Koyle.
© 2008 Blackwell Publishing, ISBN: 978-1-4051-6268-5.

to excellent operative texts of the various approaches while the advantages and disadvantages of the various approaches are described here.

Loin (flank) approach

Advantages   Good access to renal parenchyma and collecting system [2].
Good access in obese patients.

Disadvantages Exposure of renal pedicle inferior to anterior approaches.
Relatively large incision with higher incidence of wound pain and muscle bulge.

Dorsal lumbotomy

Advantages   Rapid access without cutting muscle [3].
Useful for bilateral procedures without patient repositioning.
Less postoperative pain and bulge.
Fresh approach in those with previous loin or abdominal surgery.

Disadvantages Exposure may be limited and access to the kidney and pedicle inferior, so more suitable for low, small, or cystic kidneys.

Anterior subcostal/transverse

Advantages   Good access to the renal pedicle.
Disadvantages Retraction of peritoneal cavity can limit access.

Transabdominal approaches

The increased postoperative recovery time and risk of intraperitoneal adhesion formation means that these approaches are generally reserved for malignant or traumatic cases (see Chapters 33 and 38). The advantage of these approaches is that they allow excellent access to the renal pedicle and great vessels. Transverse/subcostal or midline incisions are most frequently employed, although occasionally a thoracoabdominal incision may be used.

The advantages/disadvantages of the transverse/subcostal approach have been discussed; converting it to a transabdominal procedure simply involves opening rather than retracting the peritoneum. This approach allows excellent access to the lateral and superior portion of the kidney. If required the incision can be extended across the midline, although this involves further muscle division.

A midline incision is generally preferred in traumatic cases or when the patient has a narrow subcostal angle.

It allows for rapid access without muscle cutting via incision of the linea alba and provides good access to the entire peritoneal cavity. The incision is made from the xiphoid to the caudal aspect of the umbilicus but is easily extended inferiorly. Mass closure is performed.

A thoracoabdominal approach tends to be reserved for large upper pole tumors [4] and has the obvious disadvantage of entering the thoracic cavity and cutting costal cartilage.

Independent of incision choice, once the peritoneal cavity has been entered, the colon can be reflected medially by incising its lateral peritoneal attachment. On the left side this is facilitated by dividing the splenocolic ligaments, which also prevents undue traction on the spleen. On the right side the duodenum is reflected along with the colon. Exposure may be maintained with the use of a ring retractor. Vascular anatomy is variable, but on the right side the renal vein normally receives no tributaries, but is short and care must be taken not to damage the vena cava. If retraction of the right renal vein is difficult, the renal artery can be taken between the vena cava and aorta as opposed to lateral to the cava. On the left, the renal vein is long and typically receives gonadal, adrenal, and lumbar tributaries. These are ligated and divided to facilitate retraction of the renal vein and ligation of the renal artery. The kidney is mobilized by sharp dissection starting laterally to provide better access to posterior hilar area where friable veins may be present.

Surgical approaches in specific situations

Conversion from laparoscopic to open nephrectomy

The choice of conversion technique depends on the reason for conversion and the laparoscopic approach employed. Emergency conversion for severe hemorrhage should be via whichever route the surgeon feels will allow fastest vascular control. If possible, pressure should be applied to the bleeding point with a pledget or open swab pushed through a port site. If the reason for conversion is less precipitous, then the surgeon can be more circumspect about the incision. In retroperitonoscopy, conversion is usually achieved by joining the port sites in the form of a subcostal loin incision. In transabdominal laparoscopy, the port site best placed to give access to the area of difficulty is extended.

Approaches to ectopic kidneys [5]

Ectopic kidney position can be a result of abnormal migration (e.g. pelvic kidney) or abnormal fusion (e.g. horseshoe kidney and crossed fused renal ectopia). The choice of incision will depend on the position, size, and vascular supply of the renal unit to be removed, as determined by the preoperative imaging. An extraperitoneal iliac fossa approach is often the best for a pelvic kidney. An oblique skin incision is deepened by dividing the external oblique aponeurosis inline with its fibers. The internal oblique and transversus abdominis muscles are divided by muscle splitting. The peritoneum is bluntly mobilized and retracted medially to give access to the retroperitoneal space and the kidney. The ectopic renal vessels can derive from the lower aorta or iliac vessels and the anatomy must be carefully defined before the vessels are taken and kidney removed.

An anterior subcostal extraperitoneal incision is usually the favored approach for a horseshoe kidney heminephrectomy, although a transverse supraumbilical transabdominal approach is better if access to both sides of the kidney is required. A midline incision is often preferred in older children and adolescents. The vascular supply varies considerably between individuals and preoperative CT reconstruction can provide valuable information. The lower poles and isthmus frequently receive blood from the common iliac vessels, which can be intimately related to the gonadal vessels and ureters. Again, careful dissection is required to define the vascular anatomy. The isthmus can be thin and fibrous, and if so can be divided between clamps and the edges oversewn. In a thicker isthmus the renal capsule is incised and the arcuate vessels are ligated individually, with any calyceal breaches repaired.

Complications

Complications are uncommon in simple open nephrectomy in children. While there are numerous contemporary publications outlining complication rates following laparoscopic nephrectomy, there are no recent series with outcome data from open nephrectomy. In this section, the more frequently encountered and the potentially more serious complications are discussed together with the methods by which they can be avoided and treated.

Intraoperative complications
Hemorrhage
Intraoperative hemorrhage is very unusual in open nephrectomy in children, and blood is usually only cross-matched if the surgeon anticipates difficulties, e.g. XGP nephrectomy. Preoperative contrast CT is rarely required.

If hemorrhage is encountered, it is vital that the anesthetist is immediately made aware of the problem. As a general rule, brisk hemorrhage is best initially dealt with by applying pressure while ensuring that suction and vascular equipment is available. Proper exposure of the area allows for precise vascular control and is more reliable than blind diathermy or clip application. Venous hemorrhage tends to be more troublesome and difficult to locate than arterial bleeding. The sites of venous bleeding are to some extent predictable, with four areas most commonly encountered:

1 Lumbar veins entering the posterolateral aspect of the vena cava at each vertebral level. They may be damaged by traction on the cava and should be identified and ligated if the cava needs to be mobilized. If a lumbar vein is avulsed, compression should be applied to the cava above and below. The cava is then rolled medially and the ostium clamped with Allis clamps. The defect is then closed with a vascular suture. The proximal end of the lumbar vein can retract back into the psoas muscle leading to troublesome hemorrhage. If the vein cannot be grasped with a clip, the area of hemorrhage is oversewn.

2 Right gonadal vein entering anterolateral surface of the vena cava. Similarly, this thin-walled vein is at risk during mobilization or traction of the cava and avulsion can be repaired as described above.

3 Lumbar veins drain into the left renal vein just lateral to the aorta and into the vena cava close to the entry of the right renal vein.

4 Right adrenal vein draining into the vena cava.

Venous injury is less commonly encountered if dissection is undertaken in the relatively bloodless plane immediately adjacent to the cava's wall. If the cava itself is damaged, repair is best effected with pressure above and below the tear, using Allis or Satinsky clamps to facilitate the placement of a vascular suture.

Hemorrhage can also rarely be encountered as a result of splenic or hepatic injury. Traction is the most common mechanism of injury to the spleen and this can be prevented by taking down the lienorenal and splenocolic ligaments early in the procedure. Small, superficial tears in either organ can be controlled with pressure and application of hemostatic gauze (Surgicel). Deeper lacerations may require repair with mattress sutures, over Surgicel bolsters, if necessary. More extensive damage to the spleen can be managed by placing it in a bag or mesh to apply external pressure. Splenectomy is rarely necessary and only used as a last resort.

Bowel injury
The duodenum is particularly at risk in right nephrectomy and colon can be damaged on either side. Careful mobilization (Kocherization) of the duodenum reduces

the risk of unwitting injury from retraction or diathermy. If the duodenum is breached, it should be sutured directly, after debriding the area in the case of diathermy injury. The same holds for colonic injury, with a defunctioning stoma reserved for large or severely contaminated injury.

Pancreatic injury

If recognized intraoperatively, injury to the tail of pancreas is best managed with partial amputation to avoid pancreatic fistula.

Pneumothorax

The pleura is not infrequently breached, both deliberately and inadvertently, during nephrectomy. Small defects can be closed with running sutures taking care to avoid the lung. Once the sutures are loosely in place, the lung is inflated to push out the fluid and air that has accumulated in the pleural space, before tightening the suture line. This process can be facilitated by placing a tube in the pleural space, which is removed when the lung is fully inflated. Larger defects are closed as fully as possible, leaving chest drain *in situ*. A postoperative chest radiograph should be taken to confirm resolution of the pneumothorax.

Early postoperative complications (<30 days)
Pancreatic fistula

This presents in a similar fashion to acute pancreatitis and with fluid discharge from the wound. US or CT scan reveals a retroperitoneal collection and fluid analysis shows high pH and amylase. Treatment is done by percutaneous drainage to prevent pseudocyst formation. The majority of fistulae close but extended periods of drainage and dietary support may be required.

Ileus

More commonly encountered following transabdominal incisions, most cases will resolve with nasogastric drainage and careful fluid and electrolyte replacement. Although the majority are due to bowel handling, care must be taken not to miss a more serious etiology such as bowel injury, hemorrhage, or pancreatic fistula. Ileus lasting more than a few days or accompanied by systemic sepsis should be treated with suspicion.

Wound infection and dehiscence

Superficial wound infections are managed by opening superficial layers and appropriate dressings. Unless accompanied by systemic infection or spreading cellulitis, many do not require use of antibiotics. Wound dehiscence is rarely encountered with modern suture materials and wound closure techniques and generally reflects poor surgical technique. Deep wound dehiscence, particularly in transabdominal incisions, requires early surgical intervention but most can simply be resutured.

Chest infection

Atelectasis is common after nephrectomy, particularly with flank incisions. Both the operative and nonoperative sides can be affected by the surgery itself and the flexed intraoperative position. The risk of chest infection is increased by inadequate postoperative analgesia, leading to poor chest expansion, expectoration, and mobilization.

Secondary hemorrhage and hematoma

The presentation depends on the briskness of the bleed. Severe hemorrhage is usually obvious, presenting with signs of shock and abdominal distension. Dry wound drains do not rule out the diagnosis and the hemoglobin does not necessarily fall in the acute phase of bleeding. Immediate surgical intervention is required in conjunction with resuscitation with intravenous fluid and blood. Slower hemorrhage may be less obvious and lead to hematoma formation, particularly in retroperitoneal incisions. Abdominal distension, abdominal wall bruising, and fall in hemoglobin are common findings. Treatment can be conservative or by radiological or surgical drainage depending on the extent of the collection.

Renal insufficiency

Preoperative renograms are always obtained to give differential function, so unpredicted postoperative renal impairment is exceptionally rare following nephrectomy for unilateral renal disease. If nephrectomy is contemplated in bilateral renal disease, a pediatric nephrologist is usually involved, and it may be necessary to assess GFR formally prior to surgery. Where unexpected renal insufficiency is encountered postoperatively, acute reversible causes need to be actively ruled out and again, a nephrology opinion sought.

Late postoperative complications (>30 days)
Pain

Chronic wound pain can be encountered after any incision but is more common after loin approaches. In the majority of cases the wound appears well healed and there is no readily appreciable cause for the pain. In many individuals the pain is due to local nerve injury. If simple analgesia is not effective, input from the pain team should be sought.

Wound bulge

Loin incisions are frequently accompanied by postoperative wound bulge, especially in infants. This does not usually represent a hernia but rather a localized muscle weakness secondary to muscle stretching or subcostal nerve neurapraxia which tends to resolve spontaneously. Incisional hernia can complicate any of the approaches and when encountered, surgical repair should be considered. Mesh can be used depending on the site and size of the defect.

Conclusion

Most pediatric urologists will increasingly rarely perform open simple nephrectomy. A good understanding of the surgical technique and the issues that surround the procedure remains important, particularly to laparoscopic surgeons who may have to convert to an open approach as a matter of urgency.

References

1 Kapoor R, Vijjan V, Singh K *et al.* Is laparoscopic nephrectomy the preferred approach in xanthogranulomatous pyelonephritis? *Urology* 2006;68:952–5.
2 Woodruff LM. Eleventh rib, extrapleural approach to the kidney. *J Urol* 1955;73:183.
3 Gardiner RA, Naunton-Morgan TC, Whitefield HN *et al.* The modified lumbotomy versus the oblique loin incision for renal surgery. *Br J Urol* 1979;51:256.
4 Clarke BG, Rudy HA, Leadbetter WF. Thoracoabdominal incision for surgery of renal, adrenal and testicular neoplasms. *Surg Gynecol Obstet* 1958;106:363.
5 Hinman F. *Atlas of Paediatric Urologic Surgery*. Hinman text book: published by Saunders (W.B.) Co Ltd (Sep 1994), pp. 135–40.

Partial Nephrectomy

Marc-David Leclair and Yves Héloury

Key points

- Partial nephrectomy in children has a low complication rate.
- Most important complications are urinary leak and functional impairment of the remaining moiety.

- Very few patients will require further surgery for treatment of a symptomatic ureteric stump.

Introduction

Partial nephrectomy may be performed in children with either duplex kidney or single system. Indications of partial nephrectomy in a normal nonduplicated urinary tract are merely represented by renal tumors in very selected cases, like Wilms tumor arising in a solitary kidney, in bilateral kidneys, or in a context of predisposing syndrome. Oncological results and complications of nephron sparing surgery in these cases will not be detailed in this chapter.

Duplication of the ureter and the renal pelvis is one of the most common malformations of the upper urinary tract. Ureteral duplication occurs with an incidence of 0.8%, predominantly in females, and may be bilateral in 20–40% of the cases [1]. Although most duplicated systems remain asymptomatic, there is an increased incidence of childhood urinary tract infections, as might be expected with the associated increased incidence of reflux and obstruction. Duplex kidney may also be associated with renal hypoplasia or dysplasia, in correlation with the abnormal location of the ureteral orifice [2]. Partial nephrectomy is a well-established treatment of nonfunctioning moieties in duplicated renal collecting systems. The most frequent indications for upper pole

heminephrectomy include nonfunctional upper moiety with ectopic ureter or ureterocele. Indications for lower pole heminephrectomy are mainly represented by damaged lower-moieties with massive vesicoureteric reflux (VUR), or rarely pyeloureteric junction (PUJ) obstruction of the lower collecting system.

Outcomes from operation

Upper pole partial nephrectomy for ectopic ureterocele

The primary treatment of ectopic ureterocele may involve initial endoscopic decompression by intravesical puncture, and subsequent total reconstruction with ureterocele excision, reconstruction of the detrusor, and reimplantation of the ureter (usually the ipsilateral lower pole ureter) combined with partial nephrectomy of the dysplastic upper moiety. Such trigonal reconstructions can be challenging, especially when performed early in infancy; therefore, a simplified approach based on a primary upper pole heminephrectomy was developed, considering that in most of duplex kidneys with ectopic ureterocele, the dysplastic upper pole unit usually does not have sufficient function to warrant salvage.

The "simplified approach" with primary upper pole heminephrectomy was deemed to allow ureterocele decompression, and to facilitate later staged approach to bladder-level surgery. In some cases, it could be expected that ureterocele decompression would obviate the need

Pediatric Urology: Surgical Complications and Management. Edited by Duncan T. Wilcox, Prasad P. Godbole and Martin A. Koyle. © 2008 Blackwell Publishing, ISBN: 978-1-4051-6268-5.

for subsequent bladder procedure. Experience with the simplified approach suggests that the overall need for eventual bladder surgery is very much related to the presence of VUR at diagnosis. Partial nephrectomy alone can be the definitive treatment in 85% of children with ectopic ureterocele with no associated VUR [3,4]. However, it is rare that extravesical ureterocele on duplex kidneys show no reflux. In addition, new onset VUR may be observed in 25–40% of cases after upper tract surgery [4–6]. Conversely, preoperative contralateral or ipsilateral lower pole VUR, particularly when high-grade, appears to increase the likelihood of subsequent bladder-level surgery. Husmann *et al.* reported a reoperation rate of 96% with high-grade VUR or involving more than one renal moiety [3,4]. Overall, after upper pole partial nephrectomy, a significant proportion of children will require subsequent ureterocelectomy and ureteral reimplantation for definitive treatment of persistent or new onset reflux and recurrent urinary tract infections. The overall reoperation rate may vary between series with ureterocele type, age at surgery, or degree and number of renal moieties with VUR. Shekarriz and coworkers showed that almost half of patients treated with upper pole heminephrectomy eventually require further surgery after long-term follow-up [5].

Partial nephroureterectomy alone may result in urinary incontinence in a small subset of patients [3]. In these rare occasions, a large distended ureterocele may have created an intrinsic muscular defect in the bladder neck to cause incontinence after decompression. Exceptionally, a ureterocele may prolapse to the perineum after upper pole partial nephrectomy [7].

Upper pole partial nephrectomy for ectopic ureter

Most ectopic ureters are associated with duplex kidneys and poorly functioning upper moieties. Their surgical management usually involves upper pole partial nephrectomy. Rarely, the upper moiety shows enough function to warrant conservation of the parenchyma, and a ureteropyelostomy or ureteroureterostomy to drain the ectopic upper collecting system into the lower system may be appropriate [8,9].

Most duplex ectopic ureters occur in females, and those ending distal to the external sphincter may cause incontinence. The outcome of upper pole partial nephrectomy performed in this context is usually straightforward, with immediate relief of the symptom. Rarely, reflux of voided urine into the residual ureteral stump may lead to a small amount of dribbling incontinence after micturition or recurrent infection [10].

Lower pole partial nephrectomy

Most of lower pole heminephrectomies are carried out for nonfunctioning lower moieties due to renal scarring by reflux nephropathy or associated dysplasia. Outcome and risk of subsequent surgery usually depends on the outcome of contralateral reflux.

Management of the retained ureteral stump

It is generally accepted that in the absence of reflux, the stump of the excised upper pole ureter can be left opened, occasionally with a small feeding tube in the lumen to ensure that the ureterocele effectively decompresses [10]. When there is associated reflux in the excised ureter (as it is often the case after primary ureterocele endoscopic incision), the stump should be ligated [11].

There has been much debate about the natural history of the remaining ureteral stump after heminephrectomy and the necessity of removing the lower part. Removal of the defunctionalized ureter requires additional lower abdominal incision and possible dissection into the bladder neck and the urethra, particularly in ectopic ureters. Moreover, despite separation of the two orifices in the bladder, distal ureters in complete duplication are in a common sheath and share common vasculature, and close dissection of one of the ureters may lead to ischemic injury of the other. On the other hand, stasis of infected urine in the remaining stump is suspected to increase the risk of recurrent urinary infections, although documentation of isolated stump infection is difficult to prove. Persad *et al.* showed that the ureteral stump may behave like a bladder diverticulum and cause symptoms mimicking pyelonephritis, and therefore recommended that the whole ureter be excised [12]. In the Great Ormond Street series of upper pole partial nephrectomies performed on children detected prenatally, the reoperation rate to deal with ureteric stump was 8%, and the authors concluded that the risk of injury to the good ureter might outweigh the benefits of a complete ureterectomy [13].

After partial nephrectomy for ureterocele, it is likely that the risk for recurrent urinary tract infections related to the stump is higher in incompletely drained ureteroceles and refluxing ureteral stumps [6]. However, the risk for a secondary surgery in ectopic ureteroceles does not only depend on the fate of the ureteral stump, but also relies on the outcome of bladder function and reflux in the remaining lower renal unit.

After partial nephrectomy for duplex ectopic ureter, Plaire *et al.* [14] reported a 12% rate of ectopic ureteric stump excision, although most indications of secondary procedure were related to VUR in either upper or lower moiety. In this series, none of the ectopic ureters presenting with incontinence required repeat surgery [14]. Contradictory results from a study of 15 renal units with ectopic ureter treated with partial nephrectomy suggested that ectopic retained ureter, with or without reflux, rarely necessitated stump removal [6]. The removal of the lower segment of an ectopic ureter can be technically difficult and may cause injury to bladder continence mechanisms. Modern techniques of laparoscopic or retroperitoneoscopic heminephrectomy offers a unique exposition of the whole urinary tract, and allow to carry out the dissection lower down to the bladder level with excellent visualization. These minimally invasive techniques should provide an excellent way to minimize further stump-related complications without the need for additional flank incision in ectopic ureters.

The natural history of the refluxing ureteral stump remains to be investigated. Despite recommendations that refluxing distal ureteric stumps should be removed at nephrectomy [12], there is little evidence that it is responsible for significant morbidity. In large published series, secondary procedures to remove refluxing ureteral stump are necessary in <5% of the cases [11,15–17]. It is possible that the distal ureteral stump retain some peristaltic activity that prevents urinary stasis [17].

Complications

There is very little data in pediatric urology literature on complications of partial nephrectomies in duplex kidneys. The postoperative course of this procedure is usually uneventful, and its morbidity is probably much lower than in adult surgery. Complications are rare, represented mainly by urinary leaks and ischemic complications of the remaining moiety.

Main published experience in the field comes from the adult urological practice, where partial nephrectomies are performed for renal tumor excision. The complications observed in this context in adults are mainly urinary fistula, infections, bleeding, and acute renal failure when performed in solitary kidney. Up to 30% of nephron sparing procedures can be associated with technical- or renal-related complications, but most of them can be satisfactorily managed nonoperatively or endourologically and only few will require further open surgery [18].

Heminephrectomy in duplicated collected system is obviously facilitated by the fact that there is usually distinct segmental vascular supply with separate branches to the lower and upper halves of the kidney. In addition, the transected renal surface between the two moieties is ideally a plane where no entry into the collecting system should be necessary, hence minimizing the risk of urinary leakage.

Urinoma

Urinoma or urinary leak is reported on very few occasions in most published series. In our personal series of 75 heminephrectomies (30 open and 45 retroperitoneoscopic partial nephrectomies), a calyceal breach was recognized and sutured intraoperatively in four cases (three open partial nephrectomies, and one laparoscopic partial nephrectomy converted to open for suturing).

Urinoma represents an accumulation of urine around the remaining moiety, and may be explained either by some residual functioning parenchyma or a contained urine leak from a small calyceal breach in the collecting system of the remaining moiety [19] not recognized intraoperatively. Urinary leak diagnosed postoperatively usually remains asymptomatic and requires no treatment as it usually resolves spontaneously [20].

There is little evidence that minimally invasive surgery actually modifies the incidence of postoperative urinoma. Classic principles of open partial nephrectomy recommended preserving a strip of renal capsule, sutured for covering of the remaining moiety. This maneuvre, which is not routinely performed in endosurgical procedures, was deemed to decrease the risk of urine leak. One series reported a 20% rate of postoperative urinoma with laparoscopy [21], but subsequent comparative studies failed to demonstrate a clear difference with open surgery [22]. Even if the risk of postoperative urine leakage is slightly higher with endosurgical procedures, this difference may not be clinically relevant as this complication usually resolves by itself.

Cysts

Ultrasound postoperative follow-up often shows asymptomatic residual cysts in contact with the transected parenchyma [13,16,20,21,23,24]. This very well known event is usually asymptomatic. In a series of 60 open heminephrectomies, Gundeti et al. reported that such cysts could be observed in up to 18% of the cases [25], and half of them were still present more than 2 years after surgery. Percutaneous aspiration, although unnecessary in most of the cases have been reported. Results of fluid analysis are consistent with the diagnosis of seroma, likely secondary to disruption of lymphatics during dissection [20]. Other explanations could be a collection of fluid under the renal capsule, or some retained glomeruli with no drainage system [25]. It seems that this complication is being observed more frequently with laparoscopic or retroperitoneoscopic approach [23] although the reason for that remains unclear.

Ischemia/atrophy/functional loss of the remaining pole

Basic surgical principles of heminephrectomy focus on careful identification of both moieties vessels to prevent unintended injury. This involves initial dissection of the renal hilum to clearly identify the blood supply to the moiety that needs to be kept. This dissection carries an inherent risk of injury to the remaining pole vasculature, leading to subsequent atrophy of the remaining renal unit [26,27].

Even in the absence of erroneous division of vascular branches and when no ischemic changes are noted intraoperatively, progressive atrophy of the remaining moiety may be observed on postoperative follow-up in up to 5% of the cases [26,28]. Excessive traction on the kidney and its pedicle may also be responsible for intimal injury and subsequent thrombosis [29]. Precautions during open surgery, with minimal traction on a kidney left *in situ* could help to prevent this outcome [29]. However, this complication is still being observed with laparoscopic or retroperitoneoscopic approach, where mobilization of the kidney is usually limited. In their series of 23 retroperitoneal laparoscopic partial nephrectomies, Wallis *et al.* observed a functional loss of the remaining moiety in two patients, aged 7 and 9 months [20]. This finding underlined that laparoscopic heminephrectomy remains technically challenging, especially in young infants. We had a similar experience, with one case of functional loss of a nonrefluxing lower moiety in the postoperative follow-up of an upper pole partial nephrectomy in a series of 45 retroperitoneoscopic heminephrectomies [30]. This complication occurred among the first cases of our experience, and led us to a strict policy of conversion to open surgery when clear identification of renal vasculature cannot be ascertained.

Renal function outcome of the remaining moiety after partial nephrectomy has been previously reported [25]. This important study assessed changes in differential renal function on MAG 3 or DMSA nuclear renograms pre- and postoperatively, and showed an overall significant decrease of 7% in renal function of the remaining moiety, including 5/60 cases in whom decrease of renal function was more than 10%. Possible explanations included removal of healthy renal parenchyma, small function attributed to the removed moiety, and intraoperative ischemic injury to the remnant kidney.

Injury of the remaining collecting system

Clear identification of the collecting system anatomy should be ascertained before proceeding to section of the ureter. This is usually facilitated by an important difference in size between the two ureters. Indeed, indications for partial nephrectomy are mainly represented by gross uretero-hydronephrosis of obstructive origin (upper pole partial nephrectomy) or high-grade reflux (lower pole partial nephrectomy). However, erroneous section of the wrong ureter may happen and needs to be recognized and repaired intraoperatively.

Torsion of the remaining moiety

Torsion of the remaining renal unit may occur, after complete dissection of peritoneal attaches contributes to abnormal mobility of the kidney in the renal bed. This exceptional complication is similar to the torsion sometimes occurring on renal transplants [31]. Some authors have advocated routine nephropexy of the renal remnant, with a suture fixing the capsule to the adjacent musculature [16]. To our knowledge, this complication has never been reported after laparoscopic heminephrectomy, where freeing of the remaining pole is probably more limited.

Hemorrhage

Intraoperative bleeding is obviously an important issue in adult renal surgery without duplication of the collecting system. Conversely, blood loss is usually minimal in pediatric partial nephrectomy, with most series showing intraoperative bleeding <50 ml [23]. Usually, most blood losses come from the transected parenchymal surface. Bleeding originating from a nonligated ureteral stump (ureterocele) has also been reported [32]. No difference in blood loss has been shown between open or minimally invasive partial nephrectomy. With the widespread use of modern section and coagulation devices such as Harmonic Scalpel®, it is likely that the amount of blood loss will become insignificant in the outcome of these children.

Preventing and managing complications

Urinary leak, cysts

Postoperative urinoma is common and usually requires no treatment. The majority of urinary leak documented by increased drain output will resolve spontaneously if there is no obstruction of urinary drainage from the involved renal unit [33]. Persistent urinary leak can benefit from bladder drainage with a transurethral Foley catheter [20]. In the rare event of a symptomatic urinary fistula not resolving spontaneously, the collecting system of the remaining moiety should be drained, ideally with an internal ureteral JJ stent. When an internal drainage fails to address the problem, it may be necessary to place a percutaneous drain [32], or even to close surgically the calyceal breach.

Some authors advocate systematic placement of a drain in contact with the transected parenchyma at the end of the procedure although there is no clear evidence that it would really decrease the incidence of urinoma formation [32] or postoperative cysts.

Injury to the collecting system

Although clear identification of ureters is usually easy in the context of partial nephrectomy, there are few situations where understanding of collecting systems anatomy will be more challenging, like small ectopic nonobstructed ureter draining a tiny upper moiety, or lower pole low-grade reflux. In these situations, it may be necessary to start the procedure with a cystoscopy to insert endoscopically a ureteral stent. This stent can be inserted either in the ureter that will need to be kept, or in the one to be removed, with the plan to inject methylene blue intraoperatively to facilitate identification of an open calyx.

Inadvertent opening of the pelvis or ureter of the remaining moiety will need to be carefully closed, and can be drained with bladder drainage, internal JJ stent, and/or direct suction drain.

Ischemia and atrophy of the remaining moiety

Direct observation of ischemic changes on the remaining moiety during heminephrectomy is a rare event, and intraoperative decision will be difficult to make. If further dissection shows evidence of definitive section of the remaining pole vessels, it is likely there is no other option than total nephrectomy. In every other situation, the remaining moiety should be left in place and monitored carefully.

Localized ischemia is probably relatively frequent at the level of the transection in the parenchyma, as the section may not be exactly performed between the two moieties and is preferably done on the side that is removed. Indeed, mild fever is very frequently observed

in our experience after partial nephrectomy one or two days postoperatively and may be related to the phenomenon of local ischemia.

Renal atrophy and functional loss of the remaining moiety diagnosed on long-term ultrasound or functional follow-up should not need reoperation in most of the cases, unless a complication like arterial hypertension occurs. Therefore, follow-up of an atrophied renal remnant should be limited to annual monitoring of arterial blood pressure.

Partial nephrectomy is an important procedure in the surgical armamentarium of pediatric surgeons dealing with complete ureteral duplication. This technique may be technically demanding, especially with the onset of modern minimally invasive approaches. However, there are remarkably few complications following this procedure, apart from the risk of injury to the remaining moiety. The outcome of this procedure in the pediatric population is mainly determined by the underlying condition and the relevance of the indication.

References

1 Campbell MF. Anomalies of the ureter. In *Urology*, 3rd edn. Edited by MF Campbell, JH Harrison. Philadelphia: WB Saunders, 1970: Vol. 2, Chapter 37, pp. 1487–542.

2 Mackie GG, Stephens FD. Duplex kidneys: A correlation of renal dysplasia with position of the ureteral orifice. *J Urol* 1975;114:274–80.

3 Husmann DA, Ewalt DH, Glenski WJ, Bernier PA. Ureterocele associated with ureteral duplication and a non functioning upper pole segment: Management by partial nephrectomy alone. *J Urol* 1995;154:723–6.

4 Husmann D, Strand B, Ewalt D, Clement M, Kramer S, Allen T. Management of ectopic ureterocele associated with renal duplication: A comparison of partial nephrectomy and endoscopic decompression. *J Urol* 1999;162:1406–9.

5 Shekarriz B, Upadhyay J, Fleming P, Gonzales R, Spencer-Barthold J. Long-term outcome based on the initial surgical approach to ureterocele. *J Urol* 1999;162:1072–6.

6 De Caluwé D, Chertin B, Puri P. Fate of the retained ureteral stump after upper pole heminephrectomy in duplex kidneys. *J Urol* 2002;168:679–80.

7 Ben Meir D, Livne PM. Prolapsed ureterocele after upper pole heminephrectomy. *Urology* 2002;60:1111.

8 Mandell J, Bauer SB, Colodny AH, Lebowitz RL, Retik AB. Ureteral ectopia in infants and children. *J Urol* 1981;126:219–22.

9 El Ghoneimi A, Miranda J, Truong T, Monfort G. Ectopic ureter with complete ureteric duplication: Conservative surgical management. *J Pediatr Surg* 1996;31:467–72.

10 Cooper CS, Snyder HM. Ureteral duplication, ectopy, and ureteroceles. In *Pediatric Urology*, Edited by JP Gearhart,

RC Rink, PDE Mouriquand. WB Saunders, Philadelphia 2001: Chapter 28, pp. 430–49.

11 Adroulakakis PA, Stephanidis A, Antoniou A, Christophoridis C. Outcome of the distal ureteric stump after heminephrectomy and subtotal ureterectomy for reflux or obstruction. *BJU Int* 2001;88:586–9.

12 Persad R, Kamineni S, Mouriquand PDE. Recurrent symptoms of urinary tract infection in eight patients with refluxing ureteric stumps. *Br J Urol* 1994;74:720–2.

13 Ade-Ajayi N, Wilcox DT, Duffy PG, Ransley PG. Upper pole heminephrectomy: Is complete ureterectomy necessary? *BJU Int* 2001;88:77–9.

14 Plaire JC, Pope JC, Kropp BP, Adams MC, Keating MA, Rink RC, Casale AJ. Management of ectopic ureters: Experience with the upper tract approach. *J Urol* 1997;158:1245–7.

15 De Caluwé D, Chertin B, Puri P. Long-term outcome of the retained ureteral stump after lower-pole heminephrectomy in duplex kidneys. *Eur Urol* 2002;42:63–6.

16 Mor Y, Mouriquand PDE, Quimby GF, Soonawalla PF, Zaidi SZ, Duffy PG, Ransley PG. Lower pole heminephrectomy: Its role in treating non-functioning lower pole segments. *J Urol* 1996;156:683–5.

17 Cain MP, Pope JC, Casale AJ, Adams MC, Keating MA, Rink RC. Natural history of refluxing distal ureteral stump after nephrectomy and partial ureterectomy for vesicoureteral reflux. *J Urol* 1998;160:1026–8.

18 Campbell SC, Novick AC, Streem SB, Klein E, Licht M. Complications of nephron sparing surgery for renal tumors. *J Urol* 1994;151:1177–80.

19 Lee RS, Retik AB, Borer JG, Diamond DA, Peters CA. Pediatric retroperitoneal laparoscopic partial nephrectomy: Comparison with an age matched cohort of open surgery. *J Urol* 2005;174:708–12.

20 Wallis MC, Khoury AE, Lorenzo AJ, Pippi-Salle JL, Bägli DJ, Farhat WA. Outcome analysis of retroperitoneal laparoscopic heminephrectomy in children. *J Urol* 2006;175:2277–82.

21 Valla JS, Breaud J, Carfagna L, Tursini S, Steyaert H. Treatment of ureterocele on duplex ureter: Upper pole nephrectomy by retroperitoneoscopy in children based on a series of 24 cases. *Eur Urol* 2003;43:426–9.

22 El Ghoneimi A, Farhat W, Bolduc S, Bagli D, McLorie G, Khoury A. Retroperitoneal laparoscoic vs open partial nephroureterectomy in children. *BJU Int* 2003;91:532–5.

23 Robinson BC, Snow BW, Cartwright PC, de Vries CR, Hamilton BD, Anderson JB. Comparison of laparoscopic versus open partial nephrectomy in a pediatric series. *J Urol* 2003;169:638–40.

24 Borzi PA, Yeung CK. Selective approach for transperitoneal and extraperitoneal endoscopic nephrectomy in children. *J Urol* 2004;171:814–16.

25 Gundeti MS, Ransley PG, Duffy PG, Cuckow PM, Wilcox DT. Renal outcome following heminephrectomy for duplex kidney. *J Urol* 2005;173:1743–4.

26 Decter RM, Roth DR, Gonzales ET. Individualized treatment of ureteroceles. *J Urol* 1989;142:535–7.

27 Jednak R, Kryger JV, Barthold JS, Gonzales R. A simplified technique of upper pole heminephrectomy for duplex kidney. *J Urol* 2000;164:1326–8.

28 Belman AB, Filmer RB, King LR. Surgical management of duplication of the collecting system. *J Urol* 1974;112:316–21.

29 Mor Y, Ramon J, Raviv G, Jonas P, Goldwasser B. A 20-year experience with treatment of ectopic ureteroceles. *J Urol* 1992;147:1592–4.

30 Leclair MD, Supply E, Vidal I, Heloury Y. Laparoscopic partial nephrectomy in infants and children. How difficult is it? XVIIIth ESPU annual congress, April. Brugge, Belgium, 2007.

31 Roza AM, Johnson CP, Adams M. Acute torsion of the renal transplant after combined kidney-pancreas transplant. *Transplantation* 1999;67:486–8.

32 Piaggio L, Franc-Guimond J, Figueroa TE, Barthold JS, Gonzales R. Comparison of laparoscopic and open partial nephrectomy for duplication anomalies in children. *J Urol* 2006;175:2269–73.

33 Novick AC, Streem SB. Surgery of the kidney. In *Campbell's Urology,* 6th edn. Edited by PC Walsh, AB Retik, TA Stamey. Elsevier Science, Philadelphia 1992: Chapter 97, p. 2973.

9

Ureteropelvic Junction Obstruction

Jenny Yiee and Duncan T. Wilcox

Key points

- Gold-standard Anderson–Hynes success rate >95%.

- Age, presentation, and preoperative criteria do not affect outcome.

- Most common complications are urinary leak and urinary infection.

- Use of stents and/or nephrostomy tubes may decrease complications and improve outcomes.

- Urine leaks and obstruction should be managed with immediate diversion with stent preferred.

- Failures can be treated with endopyelotomy, but repeat pyeloplasty remains the gold standard.

Introduction

Ureteropelvic junction obstruction is a common diagnosis within pediatric urology, which has been increasing with the introduction of prenatal ultrasound. Treatment options for ureteropelvic junction obstruction encompass the urologic spectrum. Watchful waiting, balloon dilation, endopyelotomy, laparoscopic pyeloplasty, robotic pyeloplasty, and open pyeloplasty are all current approaches. Controversies in the management of ureteropelvic junction obstruction include indication for surgical intervention versus watchful waiting, timing of operations, surgical approach, the use of drains, and management of complications. This chapter will attempt to elucidate factors affecting patient outcomes and provide an approach in the management of complications.

Surgical techniques

Kuster first described a "uretero-pyeloneostomy" as a direct anastomosis of the ureter to the renal pelvis in 1891. In 1892 Fenger adapted for urology the Heineke–Mikulicz, a general surgical technique for pyloric stenosis.

The Fenger technique splits a stenosed Ureteropelvic junction (UPJ) longitudinally to close transversely. In an attempt to achieve a smooth pelvic-ureteral transition with minimal excess tissue, the Foley Y-plasty evolved. This procedure advances a Y-shaped incision to close as a V [1]. A variety of flaps then ensued such as the spiral flap by Culp–DeWeerd [2,3], the vertical flap by Prince–Scardino [4], the advancing V-flap by Devine [5], and the dismembered V-flap by Diamond–Nguyen [6].

The now common Anderson–Hynes dismembered pyeloplasty was first described in 1949 by British plastic and urologic surgeons J.C. Anderson and Wilfred Hynes [7]. As evidenced by the myriad of other techniques described above, its elevation to gold-standard status was not immediate. In its original description, an L-shaped wedge of redundant renal pelvis was excised. The vertical arm of the L was closed primarily while the lower arm was anastomosed to a spatulated ureter. The original description did not include a stent, an issue under much current debate. In older studies, the Davis intubated ureterotomy, Anderson–Hynes, and Prince–Scardino reported success rates >80% [4,8] (Figure 9.1).

Outcomes

As the indication to perform a pyeloplasty is varied, so is the definition of outcome. These can include improved

Pediatric Urology: Surgical Complications and Management. Edited by Duncan T. Wilcox, Prasad P. Godbole and Martin A. Koyle. © 2008 Blackwell Publishing, ISBN: 978-1-4051-6268-5.

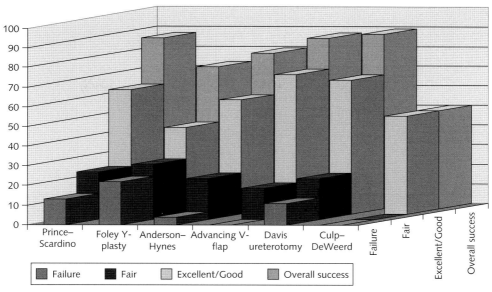

Figure 9.1 Historic success rates from 1961 and 1982. (Adapted from Prince and Scardino [4] and Tynes *et al.* [8].)

symptoms (e.g. flank pain or urinary tract infection), improved hydronephrosis on ultrasound, stabilization of renal function on radionuclide scan, and improved T1/2 by radionuclide scan. Large historic series consisting mostly, but not exclusively, of dismembered repairs have reported successful repairs in as high as 210/214 (98%) [9] and 152/153 (99%) [10].

In a more recent and large series of dismembered repairs, Sheu *et al.* [11] retrospectively reviewed 102 patients with 109 kidneys. Their average age at operation was 21.7 months with a mean follow-up of 44 months (Table 9.1). All patients received a perinephric Penrose drain, but no collecting system drains were used. Four patients (3%) required reoperation. These consisted of repeat pyeloplasties and one nephrectomy. Renal function improved or remained stable in 99 (97%) patients. Preoperatively 92.5% of patients had T1/2 > 20 min. This decreased to 7.5% postoperatively.

Another large series, by Tal *et al.* [12], retrospectively reviewed 103 patients. The mean age at operation was 12 months with mean follow-up of 32 months. The use of collecting system drains were left to the discretion of the surgeon. This series reported no incidences of reoperation, sepsis, or mortality. Decreased hydronephrosis was seen in 83 (80.6%) patients, improved drainage by renal scan seen in 90 (87.4%) patients, and improved or preserved renal function by renal scan seen in 92 (89.3%) patients (Table 9.1).

Outcomes by preoperative criteria

Whether one can predict functional improvement, i.e. who are the best operative candidates, remains a subject of active investigation. Zaccara *et al.* [13] retrospectively reviewed 69 patients who underwent stented Anderson–Hynes repairs. In attempting to correlate age, anterior–posterior diameter, parenchymal thickness, glomerular filtration rate, and differential renal function with post-operative improvement in differential renal function, no association could be found. The authors concluded that improvement based on renal scan criteria was a random event.

Outcomes by presentation

It has been shown that the manner of presentation, whether prenatal hydronephrosis, urinary infection, or pain, has no affect on initial differential renal function [14]. In assessing whether the mode of presentation affects outcome, most series agree that initial presentation has little effect.

In the series by Sutherland *et al.* [15], 108 patients <1 year old presented with a prenatal ultrasound in 86 (80%) patients and urinary infection in 9 (8.3%). Conversely the presentation of children >1 year old was dominated by pain in 47 (48%), urinary infection in

Table 9.1 Modern presentations and outcomes of Anderson–Hynes dismembered pyeloplasty.

		Sheu et al. [11]	Tal et al. [12]
	No. patients	109	103
	Mean age (months)	21.7	12
	Mean follow-up (months)	44	32.4
Presentation (Tal) or Surgical indication (Sheu)	Prenatal ultrasound	31%	77.5%
	Differential function <40%	60%	N/A
	T1/2 > 20 min	22%	N/A
	Urinary infection	3%	7.8%
	Flank pain	14%	4.9%
Postoperative imaging	Decreased/stable hydronephrosis	98%	80.6%
	Improved/stable renal function	97%	89.3%
	T1/2 improved	76%	87.4%
Complications	Fever	N/A	31.1%
	Urinary infection	3.7%	12.6%
	Leakage	3.7%	7.8%
Outcome	Repeat pyeloplasty	3%	0
	Nephrectomy	1%	0

Source: Adapted from Sheu *et al.* [11] and Tal *et al.* [12].

29 (24%), incidental in 13 (11%), and hematuria in 12 (10%). Outcomes did not differ between the two groups.

Tal *et al.* [12] noted that patients presenting with a urinary tract infection versus prenatal detection were more likely to be females and older. This was associated with an increased complication rate, but did not affect overall outcomes as measured by ultrasound or renal scan.

Salem *et al.* [16] in their series of 95 patients observed that symptomatic patients (e.g. urinary infection, abdominal pain, or palpable mass) showed a significantly greater improvement than asymptomatic patients presenting with ultrasound findings alone. This significance, however, did not persist on logistic regression analysis. The lack of association between outcomes and age or presentation supports that of a prior study by Macneily *et al.* [14].

A significant difference that did persist on logistic regression analysis was renal function improvement as predicted by preoperative differential renal scan. Salem *et al.* found that patients with preoperative differential functions of <40% were significantly more likely to improve at least 5% than those with >40% function. This finding is likely influenced by the fact that well-functioning kidneys have little room to improve.

Outcomes by age

A consequence of increasing diagnoses by prenatal ultrasound is the evolution of patient age. Most series prior to the 1980s consisted exclusively of symptomatic older toddlers and children whereas most series from the turn of the century are now populated by asymptomatic infants. While early studies reported higher infection and complication rates in those <1 year old [17], more recent studies support successful outcomes in infants.

Sutherland *et al.* [15] reviewed their series of pyeloplasties from 1974 to 1994. This yielded 234 renal units who underwent Anderson–Hynes repairs via a flank incision. The use of stents or nephrostomy tubes depended on surgeon preference and did not correlate to age. One hundred and eight of these patients were <1 year old and 119 were >1 year old. Decreased dilation on postoperative intravenous pyelogram or ultrasound was seen in 95% in those <1 year old and 96% in those >1 year old. They concluded that pyeloplasties were effective regardless of age.

Woo and Farnsworth [18] reported a series of 51 patients all <1 year old with a mean operative age of 3.7 months. All underwent dismembered pyeloplasties with variable drainage tubes employed. Their success rate was 94% as defined by improved renal scan.

Salem *et al.* [16] reported a series of 95 patients who received renal scans pre- and postoperatively. They found no difference in functional improvement in age groups ranging from <3 months to >5 years old. As a group about one-third of patients showed improved function and two-thirds showed stability.

If age does not affect outcome, two conclusions can be made. One is that surgical anatomy and technique is unhindered in the young infant and the other is whether prompt surgery on young infants is indicated given equivalent outcomes at a later age.

Outcomes by delayed repair

Surgical versus nonsurgical management of ureteropelvic junction obstruction remains controversial. Immediate surgical repair was favored in the past; however, a study by Ransley *et al.* [19] revealed the possibility of conservative management. In this nonrandomized study, only 23% of children with an initial differential renal function, >40% function, managed nonsurgically eventually deteriorated to require surgical correction. Not all patients regained or improved their renal function after pyeloplasty. This prompts the question whether waiting until the development of deterioration affects overall outcomes.

In a study by Apocalypse *et al.* [20], 77 children were managed surgically or with watchful waiting. Of 38 children initially conservatively managed, 12 (32%) eventually required surgical intervention due to deterioration on imaging or urinary tract infections. Though this group experienced a transient decrease in renal function, after repair there was no difference in renal function by DMSA scan between the conservative, early surgery, and delayed surgery groups.

Another study by Chertin *et al.* [21] retrospectively reviewed 44 patients who underwent delayed pyeloplasty for a >5% worsening of renal function by renal scan. All patients (100%) showed improvement in hydronephrosis by ultrasound. Forty-two patients (95%) showed improvement of their renal function with 36 (82%) regaining initial levels of renal function. They found no correlation between age, degree of hydronephrosis, or initial renal function and subsequent improvement of renal function.

Outcomes by surgical technique

Laparoscopic, robotic, and endoscopic techniques are discussed in other chapters of this book. In open repairs,

the Anderson–Hynes is now used almost universally. One variable to the dismembered pyeloplasty is the choice of flank versus dorsal lumbar incision. Though the flank incision is more common in modern days, the dorsal lumbar incision has historic roots, being described as early as 1870 [22]. The dorsal lumber approach offers exposure of the renal pelvis and hilum at the expense of the upper pole and distal ureter.

Wiener and Roth [23] described 33 consecutive children undergoing an Anderson–Hynes pyeloplasty. The first 17 patients received a flank incision with the next 16 patients all receiving a dorsal lumber incision. Overall success rates were similar. One patient in the flank incision required reoperation while none required reoperation in the dorsal lumbotomy group. Overall complication rate in the flank incision group was 22% with 2 stent placements and 2 urinary tract infections. The complication rate for the dorsal lumbar incision group was 12% with stents required for an urinoma and worsening hydronephrosis. One statistically significant finding was the decrease in operative time in those older than 12 months by dorsal lumbotomy.

A similar study by Kumar and Smith [22] retrospectively examined 91 infants. The choice of incision was surgeon dependent. The authors concluded that the dorsal lumbotomy was superior given the significantly decreased hospital stay (3 versus 7 days), faster time to oral intake (48 versus 83 h), perceived superiority of exposure, and minimal learning curve.

Both groups support the dorsal lumbar incision based on its excellent operative time, time to recovery and decreased hospital stay. Both groups also note that operative and recovery time are similar to those of endopyelotomy while providing an improved success rate. More recent studies show even shorter hospital stays between 2 and 3 days [24].

Complications

Prevention of complications during surgery starts with gentle tissue handling, preserving blood supply, and providing an adequate, tension-free anastomosis. Other factors such as identification of a crossing vessel, drainage tubes, and surgical approach can also affect postoperative recovery.

Most complications are present in the immediate postoperative period. Failures usually present within 2 years, however failures have been described as distantly as 8 years postoperatively in the pediatric population

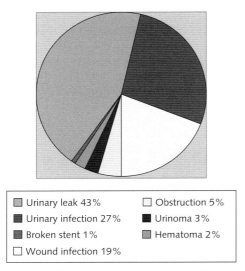

Urinary leak 43%   □ Obstruction 5%
Urinary infection 27%   ■ Urinoma 3%
Broken stent 1%   ■ Hematoma 2%
□ Wound infection 19%

Figure 9.2 Distribution of complications by type. Total infection rate 108/833 (13%) patients. (Adapted from Smith *et al.* [24], with permission from Elsevier.)

[25–27]. A review of literature by Smith *et al.* [24] compiled 833 patients from prior studies with an overall complication rate of 13%. Urinary leakage, urinary tract infection, and wound infection make up almost 90% of these complications (Figure 9.2).

Complications by use of drains

The use of indwelling stents, externalized stents, or nephrostomy tubes is heterogenous. This practice is largely dependent on surgeon preference. In most studies, a perinephric Penrose drain is ubiquitous. The theoretical advantages to collecting system drains include decreased urinary extravasation, decreased urinoma formation, decreased obstruction secondary to postoperative edema, ability to assess radiographically via a nephrostomy, and optimization of alignment of the anastamosis. Those who do not use drains cite possible higher infection rates, dislodgement of tubes, continued possibility of obstruction or extravasation, need for further anesthesia in tube removal, and the questionable quality of a dry anastomosis.

Woo and Farnsworth [18] presented 54 patients, 13 of whom received no tubed drainage, 6 of whom received nephrostomy only drainage, and 34 of whom received stent only drainage. Results regarding need for repeat pyeloplasty and incidence of urinary infection and leakage favored the stent only group.

Repeat pyeloplasties were required in 2 (15%) of the tubeless drainage group, 1 (17%) of the nephrostomy group, and 0 of the stented group. Similarly there were no incidents of urinary leakage among the stented group, but occurred in 31–50% of the other two groups. The authors noted that while there was one stented patient (3%) with a urinary infection, this patient did not need further surgical intervention. Conversely, of the 4 (31%) patients in the tubeless group who developed a urinary infection, 50% later went on to require a repeat pyeloplasty. This observation led to the conclusion that an infection in the face of leakage could have devastating consequences on anastomotic scarring. Therefore these authors advocated a stent in all patients.

In assessing the utility of both a stent and a nephrostomy, Smith *et al.* [24] presented a retrospective, non-randomized series of patients. Fifty-two patients had an externalized stent and nephrostomy tube while 65 patients were tubeless.

This series found a similar overall complication rate between stent + nephrostomy versus tubeless (13% and 17%, respectively). There was a trend toward a higher urinary tract infection rate with tubes (6%) than without (1.5%). While no patients with tubed drainage required repeat pyeloplasty compared to three patients in the tubeless group, this finding did not reach statistical significance. A review of literature presented in this chapter demonstrated significantly more follow-up procedures needed in the tubeless group (9%) versus the tubed repairs (4%).

In support of the routine use of nephrostomy tubes, Austin *et al.* [28] presented findings on 132 patients. All patients underwent postoperative nephrostograms prior to nephrostomy removal. Notably, nephrostomy tubes were capped early in the postoperative course on postoperative day 0 or 1. Average length of follow-up was 2.1 years. Though 9% of nephrostograms initially showed extravasation, all nephrostograms later showed patent anastomoses with no subsequent obstruction. Their rate of urinary infection was 1.5%, comparable to other series. These authors concluded that their low rate of complications warranted the use of a nephrostomy tube as a means to achieve temporary diversion, perform radiographic assessment, and reduce extravasation.

In a randomized prospective trial, Arda *et al.* [29] divided patients into externalized stent versus no stent groups. Stents were removed on postoperative day 3 and Penrose drains on postoperative day 4, unless urine leakage

Table 9.2 Combined rates of complications in tubed drainage versus no tubed drainage.

	Tubed drainage	No tubed drainage
No. patients	244	94
Repeat pyeloplasties (%)	1 (0.4)	5 (5)
Overall complications (%)	17 (7)	19 (20)
Urinary tract infections (%)	6 (2)	6 (6)
Urine leak/Obstruction/ Urinoma (%)	21 (9)	13 (14)

Source: Adapted from Smith *et al.* [24], Austin *et al.* [28], Ransley *et al.* [19], and Woo and Farnsworth [18].

was observed. In patients with Penrose drains only, drains were removed on postoperative day 3, unless urine leakage was observed.

Arda *et al.* found no difference in hospital stay, urine leakage, or favorable results between those with an externalized stent and those without. A persistent urinary tract infection was present in one patient in the nonstented arm of the study. Based on this investigation, the authors recommend the use of a stent only in selected patients such as those with poor renal function, severe hydronephrosis, a solitary kidney, or a revision pyeloplasty.

Table 9.2 shows combined data from the above studies. There exists a trend toward decreased complications of all types and a decreased need for repeat pyeloplasties in those with any type of tubed drainage. Though these data are not definitive, it does suggest that tubes do not increase complications and may even improve outcomes.

Managing complications

As described above, the most common complications of pyeloplasties include urinary leakage, infection, and obstruction. The ultimate goals in managing complications are to preserve renal function and to prevent repeat surgery. Management of certain complications is a part of general medical knowledge. For example, most physicians would manage urinary tract infections with cultures and tailored antibiotic care. Management of other complications is not as straightforward. Specifically, how should leakage, obstruction, or malfunctioning drainage tubes be treated in order to minimize distress to the patient while maximizing function?

Initial management

Initial management of urinary leakage, obstruction, urinoma, or infection focusses on relieving symptoms and trying to prevent scar formation. Urinary extravasation, especially in the setting of infection, is thought to promote scar and subsequent long-term failure. Therefore all infections should be treated promptly, especially in the setting of extravasation.

It is also agreed upon that urine should be diverted to limit anastomotic scarring. Nephrostomies and stents are thought by some to be equally adequate modes of drainage, however several authors [15,18] believe a stent is superior in maintaining a patent anastomosis. Sutherland *et al.* noted that of their patients who developed urinary leakage or obstruction, 3 of 4 (75%) patients treated with a nephrostomy eventually needed a repeat pyeloplasty whereas 0 of 5 patients treated with a stent eventually needed a repeat pyeloplasty.

After diversion and sterile urine are achieved, the patient may be reassessed in 6–8 weeks after an adequate period of recovery (Figure 9.3).

Definitive management

If obstruction persists after a trial of urinary diversion, definitive management should be attempted. Options include balloon dilation, endopyelotomy, repeat pyeloplasty, or ultimately nephrectomy.

Anatomic factors contributing to failure include scar tissue, a redundant pelvis, and crossing vessels that had been missed or are new since the prior surgery. Methods used to maximize success in reoperation vary. Some advocate antegrade or retrograde pyelograms prior to any reoperation [30] to define the anatomy. Others believe CT scans before the primary or salvage surgery are warranted to evaluate for crossing vessels. Rohrmann *et al.* utilize a transperitoneal approach to gain access to virgin tissue planes. In the cases of an ureterocalicostomy, employment of an omental wrap can decrease leakage and enhance blood supply. Ironically, though the use of stents and nephrostomy tubes is variable during primary repairs, their role in salvage repairs is more widely accepted.

The collective results of five case series show all 37 (100%) attempted repeat pyeloplasties were successful (Table 9.3). An additional six patients underwent successful ureterocalicostomy. Three patients underwent nephrectomy as the primary salvage technique due to

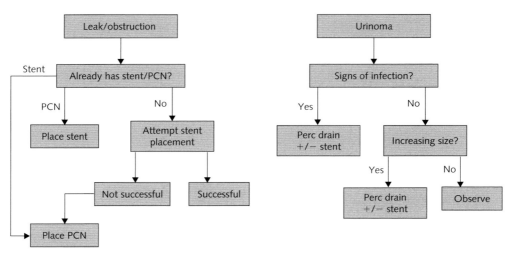

Figure 9.3 Initial treatment algorithm for urinary leak, obstruction, or urinoma.

Table 9.3 Presenting symptoms and outcomes of recurrent ureteropelvic junction obstruction.

		Thomas *et al.* [35]	Lim *et al.* [27]	Rohrmann *et al.* [30]	Persky *et al.* [26]	Sutherland *et al.* [15]
	No. patients	103	127	336	N/A	227
	No. failed (%)	7 (93)	3 (98) + 9 referrals	10 (97) + 6 referrals	8 (N/A)	9 (96)
Presenting symptom	Pain/obstruction	6 (86)	2 (17)	4 (25)	1 (13)	5 (56)
	Abnormal imaging	1 (14)	6 (50)	2 (13)	7 (88)	N/A
	Prolonged leak	0	3 (25)	5 (31)	1 (13)	4 (44)
Initial treatment	Stent	4	4	0	0	4
	Nephrostomy	1	2	10	0	5
	Balloon dilation (No. successful)	5 (1)	0	3	0	0
	Endopyelotomy (No. successful)	1 (0)	0	0	0	0
	Success with initial treatment (%)	1 (14)	0	0	0	6 (67)
Definitive treatment	Repeat pyeloplasty	3	10	13	8	3
	Ureterocalicostomy	3	0	3	0	0
	Nephrectomy	0	3	0	0	0
	Crossing vessel found (%)	2 (33)	2 (17)	0	0	0
	Percentage of successful kidney salvage	100	75	100	100	100

renal function, intraoperative findings, and family preference. Therefore, in 42 attempted salvage repairs of recurrent ureteropelvic junction obstruction, all were successful.

Though open surgery is the most definitive approach, the use of endopyelotomy or balloon dilation is attractive given decreased morbidity. Jabbour *et al.* [31] reported a series of patients undergoing endopyelotomy after failed pyeloplasty. Though children were a part of this group, the mean age was 35 years old. The interval between pyeloplasty and endopyelotomy averaged 57 months. Mean follow-up at 88.5 months revealed that 63 of 72 patients (87.5%) had success as defined by resolution of symptoms and improved intravenous pyelogram findings. All patients who failed presented within 1 year. Failures were subsequently treated with nephrectomy (44%), repeat pyeloplasty (33%), endopyelotomy (11%), and ileal interposition (11%). The authors did not advocate preoperative CT scan to assess for existing vessels, but Clayman reports that doing so has decreased his postoperative bleed rate from 6.9% to 0% [32]. This technique provides an acceptable success rate while obviating the need to re-explore a scarred system. Unfortunately, this technique has yet to be well studied in the pediatric population.

Balloon dilation in the treatment of primary pediatric ureteropelvic junction obstruction has reported success rates from 47–70% [33,34]. No studies dedicated to balloon dilation for recurrent ureteropelvic junction obstruction exist. Combined data from Thomas *et al.* and Rohrmann *et al.* (Figure 9.3) suggest that balloon dilation as a treatment for recurrent ureteropelvic junction obstruction has only a 1/8 (12.5%) success rate. Though morbidity is minimal with this intervention, its low success rate does not make it a definitive treatment.

Conclusion

The Anderson–Hynes dismembered pyeloplasty offers a >95% success rate for a common diagnosis in pediatric urology. The criteria for and timing of operation are often surgeon dependent; however, age preoperative factors, delayed surgery, and mode of presentation do not affect outcomes. Outcomes are affected by choice of incision with a lumbar dorsal incision providing a shorter hospital stay and time to gastrointestinal recovery over the more common flank incision. The use of stents and nephrostomy tubes is also largely surgeon dependent, though data may suggest that complication rates decrease with tubed urinary drainage. When complications do occur, any urinary extravasation or obstruction should be managed with diversion. A stent is preferred when possible over a nephrostomy tube. Pyeloplasty failures are definitively treated with a repeat pyeloplasty, though adult literature suggests endopyelotomy may be an option.

References

1 Foley F. A new plastic operation for stricture at the ureteropelvic junction. *J Urol* 1937;38:643–72.

2 Culp OS, DeWerd J. A pelvic flap operation for certain types of ureteropelvic obstruction: Observations after two years' experience. *J Urol* 1954;71:523–9.

3 Culp OS, DeWerd J. A pelvic flap operation for certain types of ureteropelvic obstruction: Preliminary report. *Proc Staff Meet Mayo Clin* 1951;26:483–8.

4 Prince CL, Scardino P. Results of various procedures used for correction of congenital ureteropelvic obstruction. *J Urol* 1962;87:315–18.

5 Devine CJ, Devine PC, Prizzi AR. Advancing V-flap modification for the dismembered pyeloplasty. *J Urol* 1970;104:810.

6 Diamond DA, Nguyen H. Dismembered V-flap pyeloplasty. *J Urol* 2001;166:233–5.

7 Anderson JC, Hynes W. Retrocaval ureter. *Br J Urol* 1949;21:209.

8 Tynes WV, Warden SS, Devine CJ. Advancing V-flap dismembered pyeloplasty. *Urology* 1981;18:235–7.

9 Johnston JH, Evans JP, Glassberg KI, Shapiro SR. Pelvic hydronephrosis in children: A review of 219 personal cases. *J Urol* 1977;117:97–101.

10 Henren WH, Radhakrishnan J, Middleton AW. Pediatric pyeloplasty. *J Pediatr Surg* 1980;15:133–43.

11 Sheu JC, Koh CC, Chang PY, Wang NL, Tsai JD, Tsai TC. Ureteropelvic junction obstruction in children: 10 years' experience in one institution. *Pediatr Surg Int* 2006;22:519–23.

12 Tal R, Bar-Sever Z, Livne PM. Dismembered pyeloplasty in children: A review of 5 years single center experience. *Int J Urol* 2005;12:1028–31.

13 Zaccara A, Marchetti P, La Sala E, Caione P, De Gennaro M. Are preoperative parameters of unilateral pyelo-ureteric junction obstruction in children predictive of postoperative function improvement. *Scand J Urol Nephrol* 2000;34:165–8.

14 Macneily AE, Maizels M, Kaplan WE, Firlit CF, Conway JJ. Does early pyeloplasty really avert loss of renal function? A retrospective review. *J Urol* 1993;150:769–73.

15 Sutherland RW, Chung SK, Roth DR, Gonzales ET. Pediatric pyeloplasty: Outcome analysis based on patient age and surgical technique. *Urology* 1997;50:963–6.

16 Salem YH, Majd M, Rushton HG, Belman AB. Outcome analysis of pediatric pyeloplasty as a function of patient age, presentation, and differential renal function. *J Urol* 1995;154:1889–93.

17 Snyder HM, Lebowitz RL, Colodny AH, Bauer SB, Retik AB. Ureteropelvic junction obstruction in children. *Urol Clin North Am* 1980;7:273.

18 Woo HH, Farnsworth R. Dismembered pyeloplasty in infants under the age of 12 months. *Br J Urol* 1996;77:449–51.

19 Ransley PG, Dhillon HK, Gordon I, Duffy PG, Dillon MJ, Barratt TM. The postnatal management of hydronephrosis diagnosed by prenatal ultrasound. *J Urol* 1990;144:584–7.

20 Apocalypse GT, Oliveira EA, Rabelo EAS, Diniz JSS, Marino VSP, Pereira AK *et al.* Outcome of apparent ureteropelvic junction obstruction identified by investigation of fetal hydronephrosis. *Int Urol Nephrol* 2003;35:441–8.

21 Chertin B, Rolle U, Farkas A, Puri P. Does delaying pyeloplasty affect renal function in children with a prenatal diagnosis of pelvi-ureteric junction obstruction? *Br J Urol Int* 2002;90:72–5.

22 Kumar R, Smith G. Dorsal lumbotomy incision for pediatric pyeloplasty-a good alternative. *Pediatr Surg Int* 1999;15:562–4.

23 Wiener JS, Roth D. Outcome based comparison of surgical approaches for pediatric pyeloplasty: Dorsal lumbar versus flank incision. *J Urol* 1998;159:2116–19.

24 Smith KE, HN, Lieb JI, Mandell J, Baskin LS, Kogan BA. Stented versus nonstented pediatric pyeloplasty: A modern series and review of the literature. *J Urol* 2002;168:1127–30.

25 Psooy K, PJ, Leonard MP. Long-term followup of pediatric dismembered pyeloplasty: How long is long enough? *J Urol* 2003;169:1809–12.

26 Persky L, MW, Kedia K. Management of initial pyeloplasty failure. *J Urol* 1981;125:695–7.

27 Lim DJ, WR. Management of failed pyeloplasty. *J Urol* 1996;156:738–40.

28 Austin PF, CM, Rink RC. Nephrostomy tube drainage with pyeloplasty: Is it necessarily a bad choice. *J Urol* 2000;163:1528–30.

29 Arda IS, OP, Sevmis S. Transanastomotic stents for dismembered pyeloplasty in children. *Pediatr Surg Int* 2002;18:115–18.

30 Rohrmann D, SH, Duckett JW, Canning DA, Zderic SA. The operative management of recurrent ureteropelvic junction obstruction. *J Urol* 1997;158:1257–9.

31 Jabbour ME, GE, Klima WJ, Stravodimos KG, Smith AD. Endopyelotomy after failed pyeloplasty: The long-term results. *J Urol* 1998;160:690–2.

32 Clayman R. Endopyelotomy after failed pyeloplasty: The long-term results (editorial comment). *J Urol* 1998;160:692.

33 Mackenzie RK, YG, Hussey JK, Mahomed AA. Is there a role for balloon dilatation of pelvi-ureteric obstruction in children? *J Pediatr Surg* 2002;37:893–6.

34 Sugita Y, CT, Hutson JM. Retrograde balloon dilatation for primary pelvi-ureteric junction stenosis in children. *Br J Urol* 1996;77:587–9.

35 Thomas JC, DeMarco RT, Donohoe JM, Adams MC, Pope JC 4th, Brock JW 3rd. Management of the failed pyeloplasty: a contemporary review. *J Urol* 2005 Dec; 174(6):2363–6.

10

Ureteral Reimplant Surgery

Laurence S. Baskin and Gerald Mingin

Key points

- Open ureteral reimplantation has a success rate of 98%.
- Outcome is affected by a failure to recognize underlying voiding dysfunction or neurogenic bladder.
- Most complications are transient; ureteral obstruction is the most serious complication and should be managed with renal drainage.
- Persistent reflux can be treated endoscopically or with repeat open surgery.

Introduction

Vesicoureteral reflux (VUR) is among the most common problems encountered in pediatric urologic practice. Controversies in the management of reflux include observation versus medical therapy, versus the need for surgical intervention. Among the latter, there is disagreement as to the timing and type of intervention, i.e. either endoscopic or open. This chapter will focus on the surgical treatment of reflux including open, laparoscopic, and robotic ureteral reimplantation. Those factors affecting the success of the surgery as well as the potential complications and their management will be discussed.

Who needs surgical intervention and in what form

Observation of VUR with and without antibiotic prophylaxis is still the most common option in the initial treatment scheme of children with VUR. With the advent of safe endoscopic therapy it could be argued that reflux should be corrected, or at least that option be offered at the time of diagnosis. This would eliminate the need

Pediatric Urology: Surgical Complications and Management. Edited by Duncan T. Wilcox, Prasad P. Godbole and Martin A. Koyle. © 2008 Blackwell Publishing, ISBN: 978-1-4051-6268-5.

for antibacterial prophylaxis with its concomitant poor patient compliance and potential resistance issues. We still advocate the more traditional approach of medical management since endoscopic intervention still requires a general anesthetic. In addition, Benoit *et al.* [1] have recently supported medical management as being more cost effective than endoscopic treatment. A complete discussion of the merits of open versus endoscopic correction is beyond the scope of this chapter. It appears that both techniques have a role in the surgical armamentarium; however, surgeon preference and bias is also an important factor.

Surgical techniques

Surgical treatment of reflux has evolved rapidly over the last decade and ranges from transvesical to extravesical, laparoscopic, robotic, and endoscopic treatments. Regardless of the treatment options, all procedures aim to create a flap valve mechanism where the ureter lies in a submucosal bladder tunnel where the ratio of the tunnel length to ureteral diameter is 5:1 or greater. The most widely used open technique is the Cohen cross-trigonal reimplant [2]. The ureters are mobilized transvesically and submucosal tunnels are created so that the new hiatus is on the opposite side. Other often-used open techniques include the Glenn–Anderson ureteral advancement [3] and the Politano–Leadbetter ureteroneocystostomy [4].

In the former the ureter is mobilized and a submucosal tunnel is developed toward the bladder neck. The latter technique utilizes the creation of a new hiatus cranial to the original one.

The technique utilized for extravesicle reimplantation is the Lich–Gregoir or one of its modifications [5,6]. Here an incision is made in the serosal and muscular layers of the bladder sufficient for the ureter to be placed into the trough and the muscle reapproximated over the ureter. When ureteral reimplantation is performed laparoscopically or with robotic assistance, the technique is often a variation on the Lich–Gregoir, however, the laparoscopic cross-trigonal transvesical technique has been performed successfully in some centers [7]. The techniques used for laparoscopic or robotic laparoscopic-assisted ureteral reimplantation are similar. Transurethral cystoscopy is performed and the bladder is distended with saline. The camera port is placed in the dome of the bladder using an open technique or under direct vision after percutaneous placement of a traction suture. The saline is removed and the bladder is insufflated with CO_2 to 10–12 mmHg. Ureteral stents are placed and a cross-trigonal reimplant is performed as described in the open procedure.

Outcomes of surgical technique

In open transvesicle repairs the Cohen cross-trigonal procedure is the most widely utilized with a success rate of 98% in primary reflux [8]. For secondary reflux, the success rates range from 89% to 95% [9,10]. The results are similar for the Politano–Leadbetter repair [11]. With regard to the extravesicle Lich–Gregoir the overall success rates are 96% for both unilateral and duplicated systems [12]. Success with laparoscopic transvesicle repair approaches 96% [7]. Robotic ureteral reimplantation is still in its infancy with no large series reported to date. However, anecdotally there appears to be approximately 80% successful correction rate for unilateral reflux.

Factors affecting the outcome of surgical correction

Persistence of VUR is the most common complication after reimplant surgery. Although this occurrence may be due to technical error, more often than not it is due to overt bladder pathology or failure to recognize underlying bladder pathology. Pathology can be in the form of neurogenic bladder, anatomic pathology, or voiding dysfunction. It also may be due to a large ureteral diameter where an adequate tunnel length is not achieved.

In most cases the cause of a neurogenic bladder will be obvious such as a myelomeningocele or spinal cord injury. A more subtle presentation would be an older child with an occult presentation of tethered cord. In most cases reflux will resolve or improve by directly decreasing bladder pressure via intermittent catheterization, anticholinergic therapy, or bladder augmentation. In the rare infant experiencing recurrent infection especially with ongoing renal scarring or progressive hydronephrosis despite adequate medical management, vesicostomy is a temporary option that assures bladder drainage. Anatomical causes of bladder dysfunction that may worsen the results of reimplantation include the presence of a ureterocele, or posterior urethral valves.

Voiding dysfunction or dysfunctional elimination by far accounts for the majority of treatment failures. These patients can be identified based on a history that elicits symptoms such as infection, incontinence, urgency, frequency, and constipation. Aggressive treatment, including strict adherence to voiding and bowel regiments will lead to resolution of reflux as well as associated lower urinary tract infection. If these children have failed reimplantation surgery, correction of the underlying voiding dysfunction will often eliminate the need for further intervention.

Megaureter

The management of megaureter is dependent on whether the dilation is associated with primary obstruction or reflux. Management also takes into account whether the patient is asymptomatic or not.

In the absence of infection, increasing hydroureteronephrosis or failure to demonstrate obstruction on a nuclear scan conservative management is the rule. Conservative management also applies to the refluxing megaureter. If the patient is symptomatic the type of intervention is age dependent. In children 6 months of age or older, ureteral tailoring either excisional [13] or tapered with intravesicle or extravesicle reimplant may be considered [14]. The decision to tapper is based on whether a 5:1 ratio of tunnel length to ureteral diameter can be obtained. In younger children ureteral reimplantation with excessive tailoring can potentially jeopardize the vascularity of the distal ureter. The success rates vary depending on associated obstruction versus reflux and the approach utilized for reimplantation. Correction of obstructed megaureters had a higher success rate than refluxing ureters: 90% versus 74%. Ureters reimplanted using an intravesicle technique had a higher success rate when compared to the extravesicle technique: 86% versus 76% [15]. This difference may be attributed to differences in collagen to smooth muscle ratios at the ureterovesicle junction.

If the child is not a candidate for definitive correction due to age/size, nephrostomy tube placement or cutanous ureterostomy are possible options. Nephrostomy tubes are not well tolerated in children and placement has lead to a significant complication rate (4–8%) [16] including hemorrhage, septicemia, and puncture of the pleura or peritoneum and for this reason cutanous ureterostomy often is a better option. In this procedure the distal ureter can be dissected off of the bladder and brought out to the skin through a small Pfannenstiel incision. This allows for decompression of the ureter. Infection and stomal stenosis are associated complications [17]. Recently, the use of a refluxing ureteral reimplant in children with megaureter has been described. In this procedure, the ureter is implanted as to allow free reflux of urine. The advantage is that obstruction is traded for reflux [18].

Preventative measures to avoid complications

There are a number of technical precepts, which if followed will help to ensure a successful result. Chief among these is adequate detrusor muscle backing. Whether an open, laparoscopic, or robotic approach is used in the submucosal tunnel or trough length should be at least 4–5 times the ureteral diameter. It is important that the chosen technique be done in such a fashion that avoids excessive trauma to the tissue in order to prevent secondary obstruction.

Thus, gentle tissue handling cannot be overemphasized. This includes careful dissection of the ureter from the bladder so as to avoid devascularization of the distal ureter. The mucosa of the orifice should not be touched thereby preventing edema. The judicious use of retraction sutures facilitates minimal touch techniques. These sutures will also allow the surgeon to maintain proper orientation and avoid torsion of the ureter.

Importance is placed on a tension-free anastomosis, while avoiding placement of the new hiatus laterally in order to prevent kinking of the ureter. The anastomosis should be fixed securely. We advocate placement of a suture through bladder mucosa and muscle taking

ureteral serosa and mucosa to ensure that the ureter does not retract into the submucosal tunnel. Finally, the original hiatus is closed to avoid a bladder diverticulum, taking care not to occlude the ureter.

Two additional technical points are controversial, the need for routine ureteral stenting, and the placement of a penrose drain in the space of Retzius. Stenting should at least be considered when the distal ureter has been transected or excessive handling has occurred and in infants and those with a thickened and scarred bladder. Stenting the ureter may be advantageous in a laparoscopic/ robotic approach were the stiffness could help with easy identification of the ureter. The placement of a penrose drain has been advocated for the prevention of urinary extravasation [19] but equally good results have been reported calling into question the necessity of drain placement [20]. We do not advocate routine perivesicle drains. In the rare event of leakage from the suture line a urethral catheter can be placed and re-exploration therefore is rarely necessary.

Complications

Operative complications are divided into two groups, those that occur in the immediate postoperative period and those that can occur up to several years out.

Early complications

Early complications occur in the first few days postsurgery and are usually transient. They include low urine output, hematuria, bladder spasm, retention, voiding dysfunction, and infection. Preoperative dehydration, obstruction at the level of the ureter (edema) or bladder outlet (clot or catheter balloon) cause decreased urine output. Initially, the position of the catheter and absence of clots should be assured with gentle bladder irrigation. Inadequate hydration usually is then uncovered as the culprit. Prevention of this problem is paramount by assuring vigorous hydration during the intraoperative period followed by 12 h of fluid replacement at 1.5 times maintenance. Often despite such aggressive fluid replacement, a fluid bolus of 10 ml/kg of isotonic saline may need to be administered. If anuria or oliguria persists beyond 24–48 h despite the above interventions, a renal bladder ultrasound should be performed to look for urinary extravasation or obstruction. Extravasation may be treated initially with prolonged Foley catheter drainage, whereas complete obstruction requires placement of ureteral stents or nephrostomy tube drainage. Placement of ureteral stents such as feeding tubes in the newly positioned ureteral orifices often will require reopening the incision and bladder with open ureteral catheterization especially if the cross-trigonal technique has been used. Since this is typically within 48–72 h of the original surgery, little wound healing has taken place and the skin, fascia, and bladder incision can be retraced with little effort. The new orifices are typically edematous but will always accept a stent initiating a brisk postobstructive diuresis. Nevertheless, placement of nephrostomy tubes avoids a fresh incision but has its own disadvantages. Nephrostomy tubes may require more intensive postoperative care to prevent dislodging and can be more uncomfortable for the child. They do offer an option for antegrade stent placement in the rare occasions where this may be necessary.

Hematuria and bladder spasms are seen with open surgery and usually resolve within a week of surgery. These symptoms can be distressing; however, reassurance and selective use of anticholinergics are all that is necessary.

Transient voiding dysfunction has been reported in open surgery, whether this will hold true for robotic and endoscopic treatment remains to be seen. Symptoms include urge incontinence and nocturnal enuresis due to inflammation, which resolves over several weeks. Patients who have a bilateral extravesicle repair are at an increased risk for postoperative voiding dysfunction. Inefficient bladder emptying, requiring intermittent catheterization was seen in 26% of patients after bilateral reimplantation [21]. However, spontaneous voiding resumed in all of these patients within 1 month. Patients with a previous history of voiding dysfunction must be encouraged to continue their voiding regiment.

It is not uncommon for patients to develop a febrile urinary tract infection after surgery. This can be avoided by obtaining a preoperative urine culture. Since a preoperative urine culture is not always practical a urinalysis or urine dip the morning of surgery will alert the physician to the possibility of infection. Regardless, perioperative antibiotic prophylaxis should be administered and at discharge prior suppressive antibiotic regimens resumed.

Late complications

Ureteral obstruction is the most common late complication. As mentioned previously, anuria or oliguria persisting beyond 48 h mandates imaging to rule out obstruction. Obstruction in open surgery is caused by kinking due to excessive angulation or devascularization of the distal ureter and occurs in 2–8% of cases, 8% of European cases in IRS [22].

Avoidance of placing the new hiatus to laterally on the bladder wall and care in closing the old hiatus should avoid this problem. There are two additional circumstances were obstruction is prone to occur. During an extravesicle reimplant if a ureteral advancement suture is placed, care must be taken to avoid excessive angulation (Personal communication of Gerald Mingin). In the case where the Politano–Leadbetter procedure is utilized the ureter must be freely mobilized off the peritoneal reflection to a distance of 6–8 cm. Failure to adequately mobilize the ureter can also lead to excessive angulation. It is recommended that this part of the procedure be done under direct vision to avoid perforating the peritoneum, ileum, or colon [23].

Complete obstruction necessitates nephrostomy tube and/or ureteral stent drainage. Although there is the occasional anecdotal report of resolution up to a year, most patients will require reoperation. It is not unusual to see temporary resolution with continuous Foley catheter drainage. Angulation may not occur in the decompressed bladder and is seen only with filling. However, this treatment should not be a replacement for surgical revision.

Table 10.1 Treatment of anuria/oliguria.

Anuria/Oliguria	Flush urethral catheter
	Fluid bolus of 0.45 normal saline
Persistence beyond 48 h	Renal bladder ultrasound
Urine extravasation	Continued urethral catheterization
Hydroureteral nephrosis	Obstruction mandates placement of ureteral stents or a percutanous nephrostomy tube
Long-term obstruction	Redo-reimplantation

Postoperative reflux

Postoperative reflux may be due to persistent reflux in the reimplanted ureter(s) or new onset contralateral reflux. For open bladder surgery the reported incidence is up to 1.5% [24]. For unilateral extravesicle reimplantation this number is reported to be as high as 5.5% [12]. In almost all cases observation is the preferred treatment as spontaneous resolution occurs over time. Rarely in the case of ureterovesical fistula continued reflux warrants reoperation with excision of the ureter distal to the fistula.

New onset contralateral reflux is observed in 19% of open unilateral reimplants [25] and with Deflux injections as well. Resolved contralateral reflux is a risk factor for new onset occurrence and is seen in 45% of patients where only a single side is surgically corrected [26]. The majority of these patients will resolve over time and observation is recommended. Most recommend that at the time of the procedure bilateral treatment can be performed even if one side has resolved spontaneously. In a recent study of patients undergoing unilateral extravesicle reimplantation contralateral reflux developed in 5.6% of patients with complete resolution in all patients by 31 months [27]. Redo surgery after observation has a high success rate.

However, great care must be exercised to avoid ischemic ureteral injury. The surgeon must be prepared to deal with a paucity of ureteral length. In these cases a psoas hitch may prove useful if further length is needed, a Boari flap can provide up to 14 cm in patients with adequate bladder capacity [28]. In almost all situations where length is compromised a transureterostomy can be performed avoiding the need for bowel interposition with the exception of history of stone disease. Transureteroureterostomy has proved highly successful in patients with failed ureteral reimplant surgery [29]. In the case of a persistently dilated ureter, ureteral tapering should be performed.

Finally, subureteral injection of dextranomer/hyaluronic acid has been proposed as an alternative to open surgery for failed ureteroneocystotomy. The success rate is 70% with a single injection, but has been reported to ultimately reach 100% after the second injection [30]. Endoscopic treatment of VUR is discussed in Chapter 15.

Suggested follow-up postreimplantation

Patients should be kept on prophylactic antibiotics until postoperative studies have been verified. A standard protocol would include obtaining a renal ultrasound 4–6 weeks postsurgery to ensure the absence of obstruction. Mild dilation is expected due to transient edema. Moderate hydronephrosis may be a sign of significant obstruction and would require further testing. It is important that preoperative cystogram be checked as we have often seen *de novo* severe hydronephrosis in those with massive dilatation of the collecting system with a preoperative normal ultrasound. In case where obstruction must be excluded, we prefer a nuclear lasix renogram to confirm these findings. If standard open or extravesicle reimplantation is performed especially for nondilating reflux, we do not obtain a postoperative cystogram in light of the

Table 10.2 Suggested follow-up after ureteral reimplantation surgery.

4–6 weeks	Renal bladder ultrasound
3–4 months	Voiding cystourethrogram, only in the case of laparoscopic/robotic procedures
Yearly	Blood pressure measurement/urinalysis

success rate of these techniques. If the surgery is performed robotically or endoscopically, the success rate is not as yet predictable in most surgeons' hands and hence a voiding urethral cystogram 3–4 months postsurgery is recommended until results approaching those of open surgery are achieved.

Decades long prospective studies on the outcome of patients treated for VUR in childhood are lacking. A recent retrospective study with an average follow-up time of 35 years looked at the outcomes in kidneys with no scaring, unilateral scarring, and bilateral scarring. Information on renal function was available on 55% of patients. Mild renal damage (GFR 60–89 ml/min/1.73 m^2) was found in 64% of patients. This was true of patients with either unilateral scarring or no scarring. There was also an increased tendency for hypertension in those patients with scarring. Finally, a total of 83% of patients with bilateral scarring had lowered kidney function, a quarter presented with proteinuria and half with hypertension [31].

Screening for late occurring complications of VUR is performed yearly and includes measurement of blood pressure and a urinalysis to look for hypertension and infection. Normal values for spot urine protein are inconsistent. Based on the above measurement of urine, protein is more likely to be of benefit in those individuals with bilateral scarring.

References

1 Benoit RM, Peele PB, Cannon GM, Jr., Docimo SG. The cost-effectiveness of dextranomer/hyaluronic acid copolymer for the management of vesicoureteral reflux. *J Urol* 2006;176:2649–53.

2 Cohen SJ. Ureterozystoneostomie: Eine neue antireflux Technik. *Aktuelle Urol* 1975;6:1.

3 Glenn JF, Anderson EE. Distal tunnel ureteral reimplantation. *J Urol* 1967;97:623–6.

4 Politano VA, Leadbetter WF. An operative technique for the correction of vesicoureteral reflux. *J Urol* 1958;79:932–41.

5 Lich R, Jr., Howerton LW, Davis LA. Recurrent urosepsis in children. *J Urol* 1961;86:554–8.

6 Gregoir W, Van Regemorter G. Le reflux vesicoureteral congenital. *Urol Int* 1964;18:122–36.

7 Yeung CK, Sihoe JD, Borzi PA. Endoscopic cross-trigonal ureteral reimplantation under carbon dioxide bladder insufflation: A novel technique. *J Endourol* 2005;19:295–9.

8 Ehrlich RM. Success of the transvesicle advancement technique for vesicoureteral reflux. *J Urol* 1982;128:554–7.

9 Kondo A, Ontani T. Correction of reflux with the ureteric crossover method: Clinical experience in 50 patients. *Br J Urol* 1987;60:36–8.

10 Ehrlich RM. Success of transvesicle advancement technique for vesicoureteral reflux. *J urol* 1982;128:554–7.

11 Burbige KA. Ureteral reimplantation: A comparison of results with the cross-trigonal and Politano–Leadbetter techniques in 120 patients. *J Urol* 1991;146:1352–3.

12 Lapointe SP, Barrieras D, Leblanc B, Williot P. Modified Lich–Gregoir ureteral reimplantation: Experience of a Canadian center. *J Urol* 1998;159:1662–4.

13 Hendren WH. Operative repair of megaureter in children. *J Urol* 1965;101:491.

14 Perdzynski W, Kalicinski ZH. Long-term results after megaureter folding in children. *J Pediatr Surg* 1996;31:1211.

15 Defoor W, Minevich E, Reddy P, Polsky E, McGregor A, Wacksman J, Sheldon C. Results of tapered ureteral reimplantation for primary megaureter: Extravesicle vs intravesicle approach. *J Urol* 2004;17:164.

16 Wah TM, Weston MJ, Irving HC. Percutanous nephrostomy insertion: Outcome data from a prospective multi-operator study at a UK training centre. *Clin Radiol* 2004;59:255.

17 MacGregor PS, Kay R, Straffpm RA. Cutanous ureterostomy in children: Long-term followup. *J Urol.* 1985;34:518.

18 Lee DL, Lee SD, Akbal C, Kaefer M. Refluxing ureteral reimplant as temporary treatment of obstructing megaureter in neonate and infant. *J Urol* 2005;173:1357.

19 Cain MP, Rink, RC. *Complications of Ureteral Reimplantation, Megaureter Repair and Ureteroceles: Complications of Urologic Surgery.* Philadelphia: W.B. Saunders, 2001.

20 Park J, Retik AB. Surgery for vesicoureteral reflux. In *Pediatric Urology.* Edited by Gearhart J, Rink R and Mouriquand P. Philadelphia: W.B. Saunders, 2001.

21 Houle AM, Mclorie GA, Heritz DM, McKenna PH, Churchill BM, Khoury AE. Extravesical nondismembered ureteroplasty; a renewed technique to correct vesicoureteral reflux in children. *J Urol* 1992;148:704.

22 Mesrobain HGJ, Kramer SA, Kelalis PP. Reoperative ureteroneocystostomy; a review of 69 patients. *J Urol* 1985;133:388–90.

23 Tocci PE, Politano VA, Lynne, CM, Carrion HM. Unusual complications of transvesicle ureteral reimplantation. *J Urol* 1976;115:731–5.

24 The American Urological Association pediatric vesicoureteral reflux clinical guidelines panel. *The Management of Primary Vesicoureteral Reflux in Children.* Baltimore, MD: American Urological Association, 1997.

25 Hoenig DM, Diamond DA, Rabinowitz R, Caldamone AA. Contralateral reflux after unilateral ureteral reimplantation. *J Urol* 1996;156:196–7.

26 Ross JH, Kay R, Nasrallah P. Contralateral after unilateral reimplantation in patients with a history of resolved contralateral reflux. *J Urol* 1995;154:1171–2.

27 Minevich E, Wacksman J, Lewis AG, Sheldon C. Incidence of contralateral reflux following unilateral extravesical detrusorrhaphy (ureteroneocystotomy). *J Urol* 1998;159:2126–8.

28 Aronson W. *Complications of Ureteral Surgery: Management and Prevention in Complications of Urologic Surgery.* Philadelphia: W.B. Saunders, 2001.

29 Hendren WH, Hensle TW. Transureteroureterostomy: Experience with 75 cases. *J Urol* 1980;123:826.

30 Jung C, DeMarco RT, Lowrance WT, Pope JC, Adams MC, Dietrich MS *et al.* Suberteral injection of dextranomer/hyaluronic acid copolymer for persistent vesicoureteral reflux following urteroneocystotomy. *J Urol* 2007;177:312–15.

31 Lahdes-Vasama T, Niskanen K, Ronnholm K. Outcome of kidneys in patients treated for vesicoureteral reflux during childhood. *Nephrol Dial Transplant* 2006;21:2491–7.

11 Ureteroureterostomy

Job K. Chacko and Martin A. Koyle

Key points

- Ureteroureterostomy is a safe, effective procedure for managing ureteral duplication anomalies.
- Urinary drainage with stents and/or drains is crucial for preventing postoperative complications.
- VUR can develop or persist after surgical intervention and usually can be managed conservatively.

- Problems with anastomosis patency are uncommon.
- Transureteroureterostomy can be a viable option for salvage procedures and diversion/undiversion.

Introduction

Ureteral duplication anomalies with complete ureteral duplications can present in many different ways. Vesicoureteral reflux (VUR) often associated with the lower pole can be seen in conjunction with an upper pole ureterocele and/or ectopic upper pole ureter. There are a number of ways to surgically approach this including incision/excision of the ureterocele, upper/lower pole heminephrectomy, pyelopyelostomy, or common sheath reimplant. One potentially underutilized technique is the ipsilateral ureteroureterostomy (U-U). Evidence in the literature suggests that U-U can be used with high success with minimal morbidity and complication.

Another use of U-U is transureteroureterostomy (TUU) for salvage procedures as well as diversion/undiversion.

This chapter will address these surgical techniques and attempt to troubleshoot complications and provide steps for management.

Pediatric Urology: Surgical Complications and Management. Edited by Duncan T. Wilcox, Prasad P. Godbole and Martin A. Koyle. © 2008 Blackwell Publishing, ISBN: 978-1-4051-6268-5.

Surgical techniques

Ipsilateral ureteroureterostomy

The initial use of U-U was first described by Buchtel in 1965 [1]. The patient is placed supine on the operating table. Most cases can be performed through a modified Gibson incision or Pfannenstiel incision. If cystoscopy is necessary for stent placement into recipient ureter, this can be done with dorsal lithotomy and fluoroscopy. The ureteral complex is located as it passes below the obliterated umbilical artery and the ureters are separated above the common distal blood supply. The donor ureter is then transected and ligated distally if necessary. The recipient ureter is then opened lengthwise to match the diameter of the donor ureter. The ureteral anastomosis is performed end-to-side with 7:0 polydioxane (PDS) absorbable suture. An indwelling stent can be placed prior to the anastomosis. Ureterocele excision and recipient ureter reimplant can be performed through this same incision. After the surgery is finished, the incision is closed and a Penrose drain can be brought through the incision.

Transureteroureterostomy

The technique for TUU involves greater exposure because of the need to mobilize the donor ureter to the recipient ureter for the anastomosis. This usually involves a larger, midline transperitoneal incision. The posterior peritoneum is incised to expose the retroperitoneum and access to the ureters. The bowel is mobilized cephalad to provide maximum exposure. The donor ureter is then mobilized and ligated as distal as possible, taking care to preserve the adventitia. The gonadal vessels often have to be ligated for mobilization. The donor ureter is then brought across to the recipient ureter above or below the inferior mesenteric artery – this decision is based intraoperatively on which will bring the donor ureter to the recipient ureter off tension for a good anastomosis. An end-to-side anastomosis is performed similar to the ipsilateral U-U. An indwelling stent is placed prior to completion of the anastomosis. External drainage with Penrose or Jackson-Pratt drains can be placed to monitor urinary leak from the anastomosis.

Outcomes from operations

Outcomes from ipsilateral U-U have historically been very good. The largest series by Lashley *et al.* [2] of 100 ureteroureterostomies had an average patient age of 28 months with a hospital stay of 4.6 days. The anastomoses patency was 94% and they found that the most common complication was prolonged Penrose drain output. Of 13 patients with prolonged drain output, one required percutaneous drainage of the kidney, and one required percutaneous drainage of urinoma. Other complications included fever of unknown origin (2) and blood transfusions (2). In addition, one patient each had ileus, retained drain, gastroenteritis, febrile urinary tract infection (UTI), and pneumonia. Six patients were considered failures. Three patients had U-Us requiring revision secondary to obstruction. Two patients had VUR that subsequently underwent ureteral reimplants, and one patient had a nondraining ureteral stump that required excision. None of the complications were seen in these six patients with a failed procedure.

Another series from Chacko *et al.* [3] of 41 U-Us had an average age of 31 months and hospital stay average of 1 day. The patency rate was 100%. Complications seen were *de novo* VUR in two patients that had U-U alone. One patient underwent ureteral reimplant, and the other underwent subureteric injection. Two patients with U-U and concomitant common sheath reimplant had persistent VUR that was treated with observation in one patient and subureteric injection in the other. In children having concomitant U-U and reimplant, two patients without indwelling stents developed transient postoperative urinomas that required subsequent drainage. Another patient presented with transient ipsilateral urinary obstruction that required percutaneous drainage that resolved spontaneously.

Bieri *et al.* [4] reported on 24 U-Us with an average age of 4 years and a hospital stay of 3 days. Complications noted were UTI in one patient and U-U revision for prolonged drain output. Long-term patency rates were 100%.

Jelloul and Valayer [5] performed 19 U-Us on patients with a mean age of 3.5 years that averaged 6 hospital day stays. They did not note any complications at an average follow up of 38 months.

U-U can be used as a primary and a salvage procedure. Choi and Oh [6] reviewed their management of ureteral duplication pathology. Eighteen U-Us were performed of which 13 were primary U-Us. Five U-Us were performed as salvage procedures for prior failed approaches in which all succeeded. They noted that U-U had the lowest failure rate of the different techniques they used. Overall they observed an 89% success rate for U-U. Two patients with primary U-Us required intervention. One patient underwent remnant ureterocele excision, while another had a ureterocele excision with ureteral reimplant for VUR with infection.

Bochrath *et al.* [7] reported on 13 U-Us on patients ranging from 2 to 14 years. The hospital stay ranged from 2 to 10 days with a median of 3 days. Complications noted were VUR into three ureteral stumps, and persistent VUR in one patient. The three patients with ureteral stumps needed no further intervention as well as the patient with persistent VUR.

Outcomes for ipsilateral U-Us are displayed in Table 11.1.

Outcomes for TUUs in pediatrics have been reported by a number of groups. An early study reviewing TUU in children was performed by Halpern *et al.* [8]. They performed TUU in 38 children – 14 TUUs alone and 24 TUUs with cutaneous ureterostomy. The majority of patients had underlying bladder pathology. Complications included avulsion of the TUU resulting in eventual death, two patients with ureteral necrosis resulting in ileal conduit diversions.

Hodges *et al.* [9] reviewed their 25 year experience with 100 patients. The age ranges were 1–83 years. Two cases resulted in postoperative death from other sources of pathology. Complications included prolonged urinary drainage (2), inferior mesenteric syndrome (2), anastomotic disruption (1), VUR (1), acute pyelonephritis (5).

Hendren and Hensle [10] described experience with 75 cases of TUUs. The main indications were for failed

Table 11.1 Outcomes of ipsilateral ureteroureterostomies.

Study	Number	Age	Hospital stay	Follow-up	Success rate (U-U patency) (%)	Complications
Chacko et al. [3]	41	31 months	1 day	3–34 months (average 12 months)	100	VUR (4); urinoma (2); transient obstruction (1)
Lashley et al. [2]	100	28 months	4.6 days	2.5–24 months	94	Prolonged Penrose output (13) – one required percutaneous nephrostomy tube, one required percutaneous drain; U-U obstruction (3); non-draining stump with UTI (1); fever (2); ileus (2); VUR (2); retained drain (1); gastro-enteritis (1); pneumonia (1); no yo-yo reflux
Choi et al. [6]	18	0–12 years	–	Median 7.6 years	89	VUR (1) required reimplant; excision ureterocele for UTI (1)
Bieri et al. [4]	24	4 years	3 days	41.4 months	100	UTI (1); U-U revision (1); no yo-yo reflux
Jelloul et al. [5]	19	3.5 years	6 days	38 months	100	UTI (1); VUR (2); no yo-yo reflux
Bochrath et al. [7]	13	2–14 years	3 days	55 months	100	VUR stump (3); VUR (1); no yo-yo reflux

VUR, vesicoureteral reflux.

ureteral reimplants or urinary undiversion. They noted no deaths, anastomotic leaks, or nephrectomies. Three patients developed reoperative complications. One patient required a revision for an anastomosis that was too anterior on the recipient ureter, causing excessive angulation. Another patient had a kink in the recipient ureter distal to the anastomosis that required resection. The last patient needed revision of a bowel segment used to drain a donor renal pelvis into a recipient ureter, which was subsequently moved to drain into the opposite recipient renal pelvis.

Rushton et al. [11] used TUU for 31 patients for urinary diversions/undiversions and failed ureteral reimplants. They noted neurogenic bladders in 26 patients and 4 others with bladder pathology. Complications included two stent placements for transient obstruction and ureterocutaneous drainage. Another patient developed obstruction after tapered reimplant requiring cutaneous

ureterostomy. Lastly, one patient developed a large urinoma due to ischemic necrosis of the upper ureter that resulted in nephrectomy. Two complications including partial small bowel obstruction and vesicocutaneous fistula both resolved without intervention. There were no complications with any of the TUU anastomoses.

A review of 69 TUUs by Mure et al. [12] for multiple indications, for salvage and reconstruction, for diversion/undiversion noted a low complication rate. Three patients required reoperation – one for postoperative urinoma and the other for common ureteral trunk ischemia that required separate ureteral reimplantation into the existing sigmoid conduit. The last patient required donor nephrectomy for deterioration and infection. No complications with the TUU anastomoses were noted.

Lastly, Pesce et al. [13] had 70 patients requiring TUUs with the majority (97%) for salvage procedures for failed ureteral reimplants. Complications included

Table 11.2 Outcomes of transureteroureterosotomies.

Study	Number	Age	Salvage/ diversion-undiversion	Follow-up	Success rate (U-U patency) (%)	Complications
Pesce *et al.* [13]	70	2–13 years	68/2	4–21 years (average 10.8 years)	100	Temporary obstruction requiring PNT (1); distal obstruction requiring dilation (1); 4 patients with neurogenic bladder: progression of pre-exisitng renal disease (2); Renal stones donor pelvis (1); distal ureteral stenosis requiring reimplant (1)
Mure *et al.* [12]	69	1 month to 21 years (mean 8.6 years)	22/47	Median 6 years	100	Urinoma (1); ureteral trunk ischemia (1); nephrectomy donor kidney (1)
Rushton *et al.* [11]	31	5 weeks to 17 years	8/23	>1 year	100	Transient obstruction requiring stent (1); obstruction tapered reimplant (1); ureterocutaneous fistula requiring stent (1); nephrectomy (1); partial small bowel obstruction (1); vesicocutaneous fistula (1); 30 patients with neurogenic bladder or bladder pathology
Hendren and Hensle [10]	75	Newborn to 36 years	35/40	–	98.6	Angulation at U-U (1); common stem obstruction (1); dilated bowel to ureter problem (1)
Hodges *et al.* [9]	100	1–83 years	22/78	>1 year	99	Prolonged urinary drainage (2); inferior mesenteric syndrome (2); U-U disruption (1); VUR (1); pyelonephritis (5)
Halpern *et al.* [8]	38	4 months to 10 years	7/31 –	–	97	U-U avulsion resulting in death (1); ureteral necrosis requiring ileal conduit (2)

one temporary obstruction requiring stent placement and one distal obstruction of the recipient ureteral reimplant treated with balloon dilation. Four patients with neurogenic bladders developed complications unrelated to the TUUs. There were no complications related to the TUU anastomoses. Results are shown in Table 11.2.

Complications

Reported complications with ipsilateral U-U are depicted in Figure 11.1. The most common problems were prolonged drain output and VUR, whether *de novo* or persistent versus VUR into the stump. Few of the patients that had prolonged drain output required intervention and were managed conservatively until it resolved.

VUR after surgery invariably is lower grade and often can be managed with conservative measures including subureteric injection and observation. Kaplan *et al.* [14] reported on conservative management of patients with complete duplication and VUR and of the observed group, 48% had resolution of VUR. In addition, the high success rates of subureteric injection with lower grade VUR can and has been applied to VUR seen after U-U.

Complications

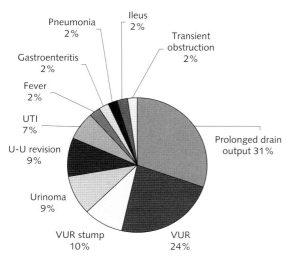

Figure 11.1 Complications of ipsilateral ureteroureterostomies.

Lastly, VUR into the remaining stump after U-U can be minimized by dissecting the stump to the level of the bladder, which can be easily accomplished with the low incision used for U-U.

Obstruction of the U-U anastomosis was uncommon and in cases where revision was necessary, it was easily accomplished with 100% success after the revision. Urinoma formation was relatively uncommon and the chance for leakage from the anastomosis can be minimized with drainage. All studies advocated using some form of urinary drainage, whether it was urinary stent, drain, or both.

One concern many have with U-U is potentially leaving behind a dysplastic upper pole. Smith *et al.* [15] compared U-U versus upper pole nephrectomy. They found that 9.5% of patients on pathology of the upper pole had evidence of marked dysplasia and half of the patients had no dysplasia or insignificant evidence of pyelonephritis. The decision for U-U was based on the appearance of the upper pole intraoperatively, and if it appeared healthy and U-U was technically feasible, it was performed. Husmann [16] reviewed consequences of leaving tissue behind in multicystic dysplastic kidneys and duplicated dysplastic segments and found them very rarely associated with urinary infection, hypertension, and renal tumors.

Another concern is ureteral disparity during U-U anastomosis and the potential for yo-yo reflux between the two ureters. This appears to be an academic concern and no investigators have reported any problems with ureteral disparity from donor to recipient ureter and no instances of yo-yo reflux have occurred.

Ureteral anastomosis complications with TUU are uncommon and all studies have shown excellent success. Since the TUU is mainly used for salvage and more complex reconstructive and creative surgeries, the chance for complications invariably increases. Many cases are reoperative procedures from the beginning and often the patients have other comorbidities that can increase the risk for complications. The most important point is to anticipate problems and have a higher suspicion for complications postoperatively.

Preventing complications

Preoperative

Preoperative evaluation is crucial because of the variety of anomalies seen in complete ureteral duplication. Information that is necessary consists of presence or absence of ureterocele, location of the insertion of the upper pole moiety and is it ectopic, obstructed, or refluxing. In addition, lower pole VUR and contralateral VUR need to be evaluated. Also, the character of the upper pole parenchyma is important as well. Most of these answers can be elucidated by a renal/bladder ultrasound (RBUS) and voiding cystourethrogram (VCUG). Anatomical definition not seen on VCUG can be evaluated by intravenous pyelogram (IVP). Further evaluation of upper pole function can be performed using nuclear medicine imaging. An upper pole function of >10% should be considered for U-U. Often times, the less invasive RBUS can give an idea of the quality and amount of upper pole parenchyma.

Intraoperative

Prior to making the incision in the lower abdomen, cystoscopy with retrograde ureteropyelography can be performed if preoperative imaging does not provide an accurate map of the duplicated anatomy. It may be helpful to identify ectopic ureteral orifices. If cystoscopy is not warranted, ureteral stenting can be performed at the time of the U-U anastomosis.

At the time of identifying the ureteral complex, care must be taken when exposing the ureters to preserve the blood supply. Minimal tissue handling is important to prevent postoperative urine leak and stricture, in addition to stenting/drain. Ureteral luminal disparity from donor to recipient ureter has not been a problem, but it is crucial to make an appropriate length incision on the recipient ureter to match the dilated donor ureter. The anastomosis should be performed with a 6-0 or 7-0 monofilament absorbable suture in a running stitch. Using a lower abdominal incision allows for concurrent procedures to be performed including ureterocele excision, low resection of donor ureter stump in addition to U-U with reimplant if VUR exists in the lower pole ureter. If VUR exists on the contralateral side, reimplants are best done intravesically to avoid potential bladder neuropraxia from bilateral extravesical manipulation.

In patients with TUUs, the same principles of tissue handling and urinary drainage apply. Other key points are to create a tension-free anastomosis, as well as making sure the donor ureter crosses the abdomen without interference from the inferior mesenteric artery.

Postoperative

Patients postoperatively generally do well. It is important to monitor drain output and remove it when it is dry to prevent urinoma formation. Patients generally do well, but if they present with UTI, pain, or fever, they warrant urinalysis and culture and possible imaging with CT scan or RBUS.

Normal routine follow-up should include RBUS at 6 weeks postoperatively. In addition, patients with other renal and bladder comorbidities should have routine creatinine and blood pressure monitoring.

Managing complications

Initial

Management of initial complications consists of evaluation of symptoms. Early signs of problems can manifest as fever, malaise, or urinary symptoms. All patients with a documented, febrile UTI need evaluation for VUR with a VCUG. Evaluation for urinoma or obstruction is best evaluated by CT scan with contrast to assess size and location of urine leak as well as hydronephrosis.

Definitive

Problems at the U-U can manifest in two forms: obstruction or leak. Obstruction at the U-U site will manifest as dilation in the donor renal segment. Management consists of percutaneous nephrostomy drainage and empiric antibiotics until infection is proven. After the acute period resolves, antegrade nephrostogram should be performed to assess patency of the anastomosis. If the U-U is not open and draining, surgical intervention may be necessary.

Urinary leak at the U-U site can occur and the risk increases if stent and/or drains are not left in place postoperatively. If urinoma does occur, percutaneous drainage or open drainage is necessary. After resolution of the urine leak, most studies show no problems with patency with the U-U anastomosis. Of patients that did need redo of the anastomosis, all of them resulted in patency postoperatively.

VUR after surgery was a common complication. The most definitive treatment historically performed was ureteral reimplant. However, other management strategies that have been successful, specifically observation or subureteric injection, offer less morbidity. Yo-yo reflux in all studies has not been an observed phenomenon and is more of an academic concern.

Conclusion

Ipsilateral U-U is a safe and effective technique for managing ureteral duplication anomalies. Postoperative complications can be minimized based on patient selection and recognizing pitfalls early and treating them appropriately as they arise. For the right patient, it offers good cosmesis, short recovery, and excellent success rates.

TUU is also a safe and effective procedure for both salvage procedures after failed ureteral reimplants and urinary diversion/undiversion procedures in more complex patients. Although postoperative problems are uncommon, when they occur, they can be challenging to manage. However, this should not deter the pediatric urologist from using TUU as one of many methods for managing these difficult cases.

References

1 Buchtel HA. Uretero-ureterostomy. *J Urol* 1965;93:153–7.

2 Lashley DB, McAleer IM, Kaplan GW. Ipsilateral ureteroureterostomy for the treatment of vesicoureteral reflux or obstruction associated with complete ureteral duplication. *J Urol* 2001;165:552.

3 Chacko JK, Koyle MA, Mingin GC, Furness III PD: Ipsilateral ureteroureterostomy in the surgical management of the severely dilated ureter in ureteral duplication. *J Urol* 2007; 178 (4 pt 2): 1689–92.

4 Bieri M, Smith CK, Smith AY, Borden TA. Ipsilateral ureteroureterostomy for single ureteral reflux or obstruction in a duplicate system. *J Urol* 1998;159:1016.

5   Jelloul L, Valayer J. Ureteroureteral anastomosis in the treatment of reflux associated with ureteral duplication. *J Urol* 1997;157:1863.

6   Choi H, Oh SJ. The management of children with complete ureteric duplication: The use of ureterouretrostomy as a primary and salvage procedure. *BJU Int* 2000;86:508.

7   Bochrath JM, Maizels M, Firlit CF. The use of ipsilateral ureterouretrostomy to treat vesicoureteral reflux or obstruction in children with duplex ureters. *J Urol* 1983;129:543.

8   Halpern GN, King LR, Belman AB. Transureteroureterostomy in children. *J Urol* 1973;109:504.

9   Hodges CV, Barry JM, Fuchs EF, Pearse HD, Tank ES. Trans ureteroureterostomy: 25-year experience with 100 patients. *J Urol* 1980;123:834.

10 Hendren WH, Hensle TW. Transureteroureterostomy: Experience with 75 cases. *J Urol* 1980;123:826.

11 Rushton HG, Parrott TS, Woodard JR. The expanded role of transureteroureterostomy in pediatric urology. *J Urol* 1987;134:357.

12 Mure P, Mollard P, Mouriquand P. Transureteroureterostomy in childhood and adolescence: Long-term results in 69 cases. *J Urol* 2000;163:946.

13 Pesce C, Costa L, Campobasso P, Fabbro MA, Musi L. Successful use of transureteroureterostomy in children: A clinical study. *Eur J Pediatr Surg* 2001;11:395.

14 Kaplan WE, Nasrallah P, King LR. Reflux in complete duplication in children. *J Urol* 1978;120:220.

15 Smith FL, Ritchie EL, Maizels M, Zaontz MR, Hseuh W, Kaplan WE *et al.* Surgery for duplex kidneys with ectopic ureters: Ipsilateral uretero-ureterostomy versus polar nephrectomy. *J Urol* 1989;142:532.

16 Husmann DA. Renal dysplasia: The risks and consequences of leaving dysplastic tissue in situ. *Urology* 1998;52:533.

IV Surgery of the Bladder

12

Epispadias–Exstrophy Complex

Ahmad A. Elderwy and Richard Grady

Key points

- Epispadias–Exstrophy Complex (EEC) is a rare, challenging birth defect.
- Preservation of kidney function and external genitalia is a major concern.
- Complications associated with this condition are common and can be severe.
- Familiarity and experience in the care of these patients are essential for proper management.

Introduction

With Epispadias–Exstrophy Complex (EEC), the anterior portion of the bladder and/or urethra and abdominal wall structures are deficient and the pubis symphysis is widely separated. Interestingly, classic bladder exstrophy and epispadias often occur in isolation, while cloacal exstrophy or exstrophy variants are usually associated with anomalies of intestines, neurological system, upper urinary tract, and skeletal system [1]. The complications associated with this condition include those of the untreated state as well as those that occur as a consequence of surgical intervention. In this chapter, we will discuss bladder exstrophy and epispadias.

Overview

Options to approach bladder exstrophy are discussed in Table 12.1.

No treatment

Although bladder exstrophy is not a lethal anomaly in infancy, these patients are often social pariahs because

Table 12.1 Options to approach bladder exstrophy.

1 No treatment
2 Anatomical reconstruction:
   - Complete primary repair
   - Staged repair
   - Repair using radical mobilization of soft tissues
   - Radical single-stage reconstruction
3 Urinary diversion (incontinent, anal sphincter-based continence or continent reservoir) and genital reconstruction with or without excision of bladder plate

of associated odor and hygiene problems. In addition, 66–75% of affected patients die by age 20 due to pyelonephritis and renal failure [2]. The untreated exstrophic patient has a 17.5% risk of bladder neoplasia after age of 20 years, with high mortality rate. Early cystectomy is not protective (Figure 12.1) [3].

Surgical intervention

Surgeon preference, patient anatomy, and availability of tertiary care facilities all play a role in which operative procedures are chosen.

Anatomical reconstruction of EEC
Bladder exstrophy repair

Early attempts (up to the 1970s) at bladder exstrophy closure were dogged by high morbidity and poor long-term

Pediatric Urology: Surgical Complications and Management. Edited by Duncan T. Wilcox, Prasad P. Godbole and Martin A. Koyle. © 2008 Blackwell Publishing, ISBN: 978-1-4051-6268-5.

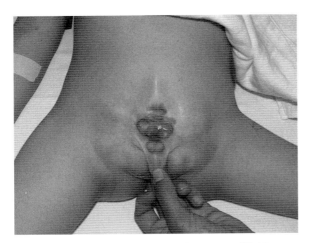

Figure 12.1 Untreated bladder exstrophy (8 years old). Note chronic changes of the bladder plate.

outcomes for continence and renal function [4,5], and many surgeons favored the use of primary urinary diversion. However, the advent of the staged repair approach demonstrated that anatomic reconstruction of the exstrophic bladder was feasible and safe [6]. This approach led to significant improvements in continence, renal preservation as well as excellent cosmetic results [7,8]. In literature, the rate of continence has varied. Some patients require clean intermittent catheterization (CIC) and bladder augmentation or diversion to achieve dryness [9,10].

More recently, newer techniques of single-stage exstrophy repair (including complete primary repair of bladder exstrophy, CPRE) have been developed [11–14] in addition to modifications of the staged repair (modern staged repair of bladder exstrophy, MSRE) [15]. Neonatal exstrophy closure is recommended but salvage single-stage reconstruction in delayed cases (>6 months of age) is associated with lower continence rate [16,17]. These new techniques of single-stage reconstruction appear to be safer than that used in the past, and enhance bladder capacity, stability, and compliance more than staged approach [18].

Epispadias repair

Early efforts were associated with high rate of complications [19]. Current methods (Cantwell-Ransley, and Mitchell penile disassembly techniques) use dissection of the corporal bodies and transposition of the tubularized urethral plate to the ventral aspect of the penis with satisfactory cosmesis and lower overall complications [19,20].

Urinary diversion

This approach may achieve some of the primary goals of surgical intervention for EEC with fewer operations. It is useful for patients who may not have reliable access to health care facilities, and the patients who have not achieved urinary dryness despite attempts at functional reconstruction.

Ureterosigmoidostomy (USO) is associated with high daytime urinary dryness rates of 92–97% without reliance on catheters or external appliances. Despite the reduction of complications for USO after improvements in ureteral reimplantation, chronic metabolic acidosis (up to 100%), chronic pyelonephritis (22%), ureteral obstruction or reflux (up to 29%), significant upper tract scarring and calculi (18%), and nighttime incontinence (42%) necessitate secondary interventions [21,22]. Furthermore, on longer-term follow-up, daily fecal-urinary incontinence (26% and 48%, respectively) with pelvic organ prolapse (48%), and delayed development of neoplasms in the colon or the bladder remnant (overall risk is 38%) have dampened enthusiasm for this procedure [3,23]. Recently, low-pressure rectal reservoirs have been proposed again as a treatment for bladder exstrophy with acceptable day and night urinary dryness (100% and 91%, respectively), and less complications. Alkali supplementation and a regular follow-up surveillance colonoscopy are still needed for these patients [24].

Incontinent urinary diversions were popular in the past but had the significant disadvantage of an incontinent abdominal stoma. Urinary conduits, especially ileal loops, are not free of complications (renal deterioration up to 41%). So, if necessary, colonic conduits with non-refluxing ureterocolic anastmosis are preferred [25,26].

The popularization of CIC has led to the development over the past 15–20 years of *continent urinary diversions* such as the Indiana pouch, which was developed for the exstrophy population. Preservation of the native bladder and bladder augmentation [27] allows the native bladder to act as a convenient substrate for ureteral and Mitrofanoff reimplantation.

Complications of anatomical reconstruction of EEC

It is sometimes difficult to differentiate the failure to reconstruct the primary pathophysiological defects of

Table 12.2 Complications following surgery for EEC.

Problem	Early	Late
Urinary	Bladder dehiscence, urinary fistulae, catheters malfunction, HUN	BOO, UTI, urinary calculi, renal scarring, incontinence, stress incontinence, NE, CIC, bladder augmentation/diversion, renal failure, bladder malignancy
Genital (male)	Loss of glans or corpora, loss of penile skin	Inadequate phallus, psychosexual delay, retrograde or difficult ejaculation, subfertility, erectile dysfunction, sexual reassignment[*]
Genital (female)	Loss of urethra-vaginal septum, loss of clitoris, vaginal deficiency	Genital cosmesis defects, vaginal stenosis, uterine prolapse, miscarriage, elective cesarean section
Fascial	Hematoma, wound infection, fascial dehiscence	Hernias, cosmesis defects in suprapubic area/umbilicus
Orthopedic	Transient femoral nerve palsy	Gait problems, abnormal hip dynamics, back pain
Others	Latex allergy, abdominal distension, abdominal compartment syndrome,[*] death	Rectal prolapse, fecal incontinence, short bowel syndrome,[*] fecal stoma/ACE,[*] multiple anesthesia, anxiety disorders, recurrence of exstrophy, death

HUN, hydroureteronephrosis; BOO, bladder outlet obstruction; UTI, urinary tract infection; NE, nocturnal enuresis; CIC, clean intermittent catheterization.
[*]Specific complications with cloacal exstrophy.

EEC from complications associated with treatment. The different approaches (CPER, MSRE, staged repair, etc.) are designed to improve the long-term outcome, and all rely on the same surgical principles, successful initial closure, surgeon experience, and proper postoperative management.

In most discussions of EEC, the subject of urinary incontinence dominates the whole topic, to an extent that the other disabilities resulting from the disorder receive little attention [28]. Bladder exstrophy requires a median of five operations per patient [29]. Successful closure of isolated epispadias is achieved by single operation in 80–91% [19,20] (Table 12.2).

Urinary complications

Bladder dehiscence has decreased from up to 13% to up to 3% with recent techniques. It may be precipitated by many factors including postoperative abdominal distention, bladder prolapse, and the loss of ureteral stents before postoperative day 7. Dehiscence necessitates about a 6-month recovery period before a second attempt at closure can be made. Tension-free reclosure with osteotomy, preoperative testosterone, and combine epispadias and bladder repair are important factors in subsequent closures but up to a 40% failure rate at reclosure is reported. Failure of the primary closure

markedly decreases the chance and onset for eventual continence with volitional voiding from 30% if a patient underwent two closures to less than 20% for who had undergone more than two closure attempts. Primary use of osteotomy may be protective against bladder dehiscence [14,15,30,31].

Catheter malfunction is uncommon; catheter patency should be confirmed at initial closure. Early loss of the suprapubic catheter is a particular cause for concern. We recommend replacing this with another tube or urethral catheter as soon as possible if this happens within the first 2 weeks following closure. Ureteric catheters malfunction may necessitate early repositioning with open surgery [12] or with fluoroscopy [32].

Urethrocutaneous fistula formation at the penopubic junction is the most common surgical complication of CPRE. In the setting of newborn exstrophy closure, fistulas may occur in 14–35% of cases [14,29]. This fistula rate is increased to 26–52% in delayed or redo cases [16,17]. Two-layer closure covered with a single layer small intestinal submucosa onlay help to prevent fistulae [33]. With the staged exstrophy repair, postoperative fistula develops in 21% of patients with intact plate versus 25% if para-exstrophy flaps are used [34].

Spontaneous fistula closure rate is expected in 25–100% within 7.5 months. If not, surgical closure is indicated with urethrocystoscopy to evaluate the repair. Implications of bladder neck (BN) fistula in reference to urinary continence remain to be seen [17,33].

Urinary outlet obstruction is one of the potentially dangerous failed outcomes of bladder closure because it can cause renal deterioration, increase the risk for chronic urinary tract infection (UTI), and may decrease the chance to achieve urinary continence. This may be somewhat subtle; however, routine ultrasonography of the bladder and upper urinary tracts also should be performed frequently after closure to detect hydronephrosis (especially in combination with high postvoid residual) that may indicate outlet obstruction and cystoscopy may also be needed [35].

Neourethral stricture or tortuosity is often associated with para-exstrophy skin flap use, one stage urethroplasty by flap/graft interposition, meatal stenosis, or pubic suture erosion. A stricture develops at the proximal anastomotic site in 10–67% of patients with exstrophy who have para-exstrophy skin flaps used at the initial closure [36]. We prefer to convert exstrophy cases with the inherently short urethral plate (50–77%) into hypospadias to avoid complications of flap/graft interposition [14]. Combined bladder and epispadias repair for delayed or redo cases is associated with up to 10.5% stricture rate [16,17].

Interim management of bladder outlet obstruction (BOO) usually includes urethral dilation, internal urethrotomy, CIC, surgical revision, or diversion. Long-term urinary diversion (e.g. suprapubic catheter) increases the likehood of bladder augmentation [36]. The popularization of the Mitrofanoff principle has significantly improved the management of those patients with tortuous neourethra following urethral reconstruction.

Bladder and kidney infections. Patients are routinely maintained on suppressive antibiotic therapy as vesicoureteral reflux (VUR) occurs almost universally after exstrophy closure. This is continued until VUR is corrected or resolves spontaneously (up to 16%) [14,29]. Febrile UTIs occur in up to 22% of patients while 70% experience one or more episodes of asymptomatic bacteriuria. These patients should be appropriately evaluated (to ensure that they have no evidence of outlet obstruction) and aggressively treated [29]. Early ureteral reimplantation or deflux injection is indicated if recurrent febrile infections occur in the setting of adequate prophylaxis. Cephalotrigonal technique is preferred for ureteral reimplantation as a cross-trigone technique may complicate future bladder neck reconstruction (BNR) [37].

Renal damage is related to outlet obstruction and febrile UTIs. With improvement of techniques and

follow-up, it is decreased from 25% to up to 7.5% [10,13,14,38].

Transient hydroureteronephrosis (HUN) occurs in up to 23% of children following their initial surgery, which may be related to gradual accommodation of the bladder as it cycles urine in the presence of VUR. About half of children with HUN may require CIC even though there is no evidence of BOO. Spontaneous improvement is expected in most, but this is unpredictable [14,38]. If HUN persists, ureteral reimplantation, bladder augmentation, or diversion may be indicated to provide a low-pressure urine storage reservoir. Long-term study of EEC patients following staged reconstruction has found that about 24% had significant upper tract damage in the form of renal scarring and/or moderate or severe hydronephrosis. Serum creatinine remained normal in 97%, mild renal insufficiency developed in 1.5%, and renal transplantation was performed in 1.5% [10]. The storage of urine in intestinal reservoirs did not change renal function for at least 10 years in 80% of the patients. The remaining (20%) had some deterioration in renal function, usually from identifiable and remediable causes [39].

Incontinence. Universally accepted definitions for continence remain a topic for discussion. For the purpose of this chapter, we define urinary continence as 2- to 3-h dry intervals with volitional voiding without bladder augment or diversion.

Successful CPRE may be associated with primary daytime continence (bladder emptying volitionally of with the use of clean CIC) at age of toilet training [14,17]. However, many exstrophy patients are partially continent after initial closure and show on urodynamics a low leak point, wide BN and reasonable bladder compliance and capacity (>60–85 ml). For these patients, formal BNR or endoscopic injection of the BN is indicated and continence is achieved in up to 60–87%. Most surgeons use for BNR either Young-Dees-Leadbetter or Mitchell BNR (which also moves fibrotic tissue at the level of the original BN away from the new BN) [14,15]. At the time of BNR, we typically perform ureteral reimplantation (if not done before) and construct a Mitrofanoff channel [14]. The mean time to daytime continence after BNR is 14 months (range 4–21) and the mean time to nighttime continence is 22 months (range 11–33) [40]. These children void volitionally and may catheterize one to two times a day to ensure bladder emptying.

In some patients (5–52%), the bladder does not grow to an adequate capacity (<50–60 ml) and/or has impaired compliance with upper tract deterioration. This may be due to postoperative complications (e.g. bladder prolapse or dehiscence, BOO, recurrent UTIs, bladder calculi, and long-term diversion), or can occur despite technically successful reconstruction efforts (especially if delayed or redo closure, delayed epispadias repair, very small bladder plate at initial closure, or neuropathic bladder). In this situation, concomitant BNR, bladder augmentation with or without Mitrofanoff channel is recommended [8,27,30].

Many adjuvant measures may be helpful to achieve continence, control stress incontinence, and enuresis. Again, urodynamics help to decide the needed maneuver.

• Endourethral injection (1–3 sessions) of dextranomer based implants (Deflux®) remained beneficial in 40% of patients with 7-years follow-up [41]. A history of previous surgery and gender had no significant effect on the outcome. A maximum of three injections is predictive with reasonable certainty of any benefit from the procedure [42].

• Anticholinergic agents, low-dose desmopressin [43], or imipramine [44] may also be helpful.

Despite near or total subjective continence and "good" voiding in children who had undergone staged reconstruction for exstrophy, of these patients 72% have clinical problems related to emptying, which include recurrent UTIs, epididymitis, and bladder calculi. Objective urodynamic parameters confirm poor voiding in most patients. One must question the normalcy of the voiding pattern and price to achieve continence among patients with exstrophy [45].

If urinary continence is not achieved within 2 years following formal BNR and the above measures, future success is elusive [40]. Treatment choice depends on the results of urodynamic studies and other clinical and social factors.

• Rarely, the urodynamic evaluation reveals a bladder with adequate capacity and compliance with wide BN and low detrusor leak point pressure. In these cases BNR, artificial urinary sphincter, or other BN procedures (wrap/sling/closure) can be performed. BNR revision rarely achieves continence with volitional voiding [46]. The creation of a Mitrofanoff channel in this situation is invaluable.

• Most of the patients demonstrate an inadequate bladder capacity and a low detrusor leak point pressure and usually require bladder augmentation or diversion. Often, bladder augmentation is combined with a BN procedure and Mitrofanoff channel to optimize the chance for urinary dryness.

In long-term follow-up, about 60% of patients with initially successful bladder closures and BNR have required further surgery (augment/diversion) in their second decade of life because of the gradual development of poorly compliant, low-capacity bladders that cause urinary incontinence [47]. This may be due to fixed outlet resistance with multiple BN procedures. It remains to be seen if CPRE will experience late continence failures as these children age.

Bladder malignancy. Early reconstruction decreases the risk of malignancy in the exstrophic bladder from 17.5% to 3.3% at a median age of 42 years [3]. Moreover, patients who have undergone augmentation cystoplasty using intestinal segments are at increased risk for malignant degeneration [48]. Life-long surveillance with cystoscopy and urine cytology is recommended. In the event of malignancy, treatment options include radical cystectomy with urinary diversion [49]. Four cases have been reported with severe perineal pain after bladder augmentation that was probably secondary to the abnormal retained bladder remnants. Cystectomy cured the pain and may also have removed a potential site of future malignant tumor [50].

The male genital complications

Atrophy of the corporal bodies, glans, and/or urethra. In experienced hands, these complications are unusual. It has been described after the initial stage of a staged reconstruction [51,52] as well as CPRE (up to 5%) [53,54]. These catastrophic complications can arise from violation of tissue planes. Overly aggressive attempts at mobilizing the corporal bodies from the pubis symphysis and penile lengthening may result in corporal denervation and/or devascularization [13] without additional lengthening of the congenitally deficient exstrophic penis [55]. Efforts to avoid this complication include assessment of the glans penis for ischemia after pubic rami reapproximation; if there is any color change, apply papaverine, and replace the sutures higher in the pubis, and/or consider osteotomy if not done.

With loss of the urethral plate and significant amounts of penile skin, other sources of replacement tissues (grafts/flaps) can be used for later reconstruction [56]. Ischemia of the glans and penile skin within 24–48 h after closure is reversible in more than half of the cases by observation. The use of vasodilators may be helpful. Reoperation with higher replacement of pubic sutures appears to be of no value in the setting of prolonged ischemia [54]. Acute postoperative penile ischemia should prompt immediate reoperation to release tight sutures, restore circulation, and salvage the penis [13].

A short phallus and/or persistent chordee. Complete penile disassembly provides satisfactory cosmetic and functional penile outcome [14]. In the Cantwell-Ransley repair, up to 7% of patients require early penile straightening surgery [34]. Revision rate for genitoplasty is 29% after puberty [57]. In another study, erections were curved in 34% with no curvature so severe as to prevent sexual intercourse [58].

Penile degloving and division of suspensory ligament can maximize the available penile length. A dorsal dermal corporal graft, ventral corporal plication, or rotation may additionally help lengthen as well as correct any chordee/asymmetry. Scar excision can be closed in a plastic fashion (Z-plasty) if enough penile skin is available. Otherwise, rotational flaps, tissue expanders, or full-thickness skin grafts can be used [52,59].

Sexual dysfunction. Adolescent males with exstrophy are psychosexually delayed 2–4 years compared with their peers [60]. Libido, erection, and orgasm are usually intact. About 50–70% of men described intimate relationships as serious and long-term [58,61,62].

Subfertility. Ejaculation is often present in up to 63–90% of men despite the extensive reconstructive procedures done for these patients. Sperm quality and quantity is impaired (at least in 40%) despite testes that are believed to be intrinsically normal. This may be due to partial obstruction, retrograde ejaculation, slow seminal emission, or recurrent infections. Despite this, about half of men do not require assisted reproductive techniques to father children [58,61,62].

The female genital complications

Loss of urethrovaginal septum occurs in rare situations. This usually occurs during dissection of urethral plate from the underlying vagina or transaction and lengthening of urethral plate with para-exstrophy flaps [56,63]. Mobilization of the BN, urethra, and vagina as a unit helps prevention of this complication [14].

Further reconstruction of the female genitalia, if needed, can be done during adolescent years. Mons-plasty with hair-bearing skin and fat should be used to cover the midline defect. Most patients required vaginal dilatation or a cut-back/Y-V vaginoplasty to allow satisfactory intercourse in the mature female. Initiation of sexual activity tends to be delayed until early adulthood. All of the female patients described intimate relationships as serious and long term [63,64].

Uterine and vaginal prolapse occur in up to 50% of patients. Early primary bladder reconstruction may decrease this risk. Fixation of the uterus to the anterior abdominal wall in childhood may be helpful to prevent prolapse while allowing normal pregnancy [65]. Uterine suspension procedures such as sacrocolpopexy can correct uterine prolapse in the exstrophy patient and may preserve fertility in young patients [66].

Obstetric implications. Fecundity is unimpaired in female patients with exstrophy, but maintenance of a pregnancy is significantly more difficult and requires interdisciplinary cooperation. Successful pregnancy is reported in 10–25% of patients [67]. Complications in the past have included maternal deaths [2]. Nowadays, these pregnancies are more often complicated by:
• *Obstetric complications* that include uterine or vaginal prolapse (>50%), preterm labor (40%), miscarriages (28%), and malpresentation (25%). Bed rest is necessary in the later stages of pregnancy for most of these patients [68–70].
• *Urinary complications* that include transient secondary urinary incontinence, recurrent UTIs (17–52%), hydronephrosis requiring drainage (10%), Mitrofanoff difficulties, and ileal prolapse (in those with ileal conduit). Antibiotic prophylaxis is recommended and patients may require indwelling catheters. The usual voiding pattern can be resumed after delivery. Pregnancy has no long-term effect on renal function and does not compromise reconstruction [68–70].

Spontaneous vaginal deliveries (if not precluded by malpresentation) are done in those women who had undergone prior permanent urinary diversions. Vaginal delivery may carry the risk of obstructed labor (due to vaginal stenosis) and later prolapse. Most recommend elective cesarean sections before term for women with functional bladder closures to eliminate stress on the pelvic floor and the urinary sphincter mechanism [2,71].

Fascial abnormalities

• *Fascial dehiscence* may occur within 1 week after repair in up to 3% of patients and require immediate repair. This complication does not affect the integrity of the bladder or urethral reconstruction [14] (Figure 12.2).
• *Inguinal hernias* have been reported in 56–82% of boys and 11–15% of girls with bladder exstrophy, and 33% in boys with complete epispadias. Incarcerated hernias affect up to 50% of boys during the first year following their initial procedure. The incidence of synchronous or asynchronous bilaterality is about 80%. At the time of bladder exstrophy closure, these hernias should be bilaterally repaired using a preperitoneal approach to the internal ring. The overall recurrence rate is 8–17% [72–74].

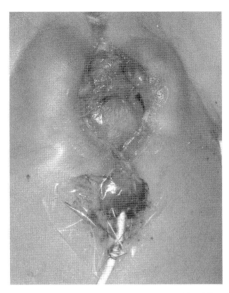

Figure 12.2 Fascial dehiscence following initial bladder closure.

Orthopedic complications

These are associated with the orthopedic management of exstrophy in about 4% of patients [75]. These include transient femoral nerve palsy, delayed union of osteotomy, and osteomyelitis.

• *Complications of traction.* Pressure sores and compartment syndrome with permanent muscle weakness can occur with tight wrapping of legs [75]. Significant transient hypertension was reported with inappropriately applied traction [76]. We use a spica cast for 3 weeks for postoperative immobilization of neonates, which facilitates early discharge and nursing care with excellent results [14].

• *Gait abnormalities* in these children arise as a consequence of underlying bone abnormalities. Many of these children initially learn to ambulate with a wide waddling gait that resolves as the children grow. Few develop gait problems, hip dysplasia, or back pain [77]. A recent study showed that early pelvic osteotomy has long-term effects on patients' instinctive walking patterns and neutralizes some of the effects of bladder exstrophy [78].

Other complications

• *Latex allergy.* One-third of patients with bladder exstrophy developed latex symptoms and another third have latex sensitization. Multiple surgical procedures and atopy play a major role in the development of latex hypersensitivity [79].

• *Psychosocial concerns and long-term adjustment.* Children with exstrophy undergo multiple surgeries and have potential problems with respect to urinary continence, sexual function, and self-esteem problems. Children who achieved continence after the age of 5 years are more likely to have problems with acting-out behavior. They do not have clinical psychopathology and improving outcomes may be achieved through a focus on normal adaptation [80]. Current recommendations include early psychiatric intervention and advised to continue with long-term psychiatric support into adult life [61]. There are a number of websites that can prove very helpful to parents and patients (http://www.bladderexstrophy.com/support.htm).

• *Mortality.* Currently, exstrophy repair carries a low risk of mortality (up to 1.5% in the United States, all of whom had been born prematurely) [81]. Late mortality may be related to development of malignancy [3].

Conclusion

Although results of therapy are far from perfect, they reflect remarkable accomplishments from many physicians. There is great potential for further improvement such that 1 day children born with exstrophy will be treated early and completely and never know that they had a major problem.

References

1 Diamond DA, Jeffs RD. Cloacal exstrophy: A 22-year experience. *J Urol* 1985;133:779–82.

2 Clemston C. Ectopia vesicae and split pelvis. *J Obstet Gynaecol Br Commonw* 1958;65:973–81.

3 Smeulders N, Woodhouse CR. Neoplasia in adult exstrophy patients. *BJU Int* 2001;87:623–8.

4 Trendelenburg F. The treatment of ectopia vesicae. *Ann Surg* 1906;44:281–9.

5 Johnston JH, Kogan SJ. The exstrophic anomalies and their surgical reconstruction. *Curr Probl Surg* 1974(Aug);1–39.

6 Fisher JH, Retik AB. Exstrophy of the bladder. *J Pediatr Surg* 1969;4:620–6.

7 Oesterling JE, Jeffs RD. The importance of a successful initial bladder closure in the surgical management of classical bladder exstrophy: Analysis of 144 patients treated at the Johns Hopkins Hospital between 1975 and 1985. *J Urol* 1987;137:258–62.

8 Husmann DA, Vandersteen DR, McLorie GA *et al.* Urinary continence after staged bladder reconstruction for cloacal exstrophy: The effect of coexisting neurological abnormalities on urinary continence. *J Urol* 1999;161:1598–602.

9 Hollowell JG, Ransley PG. Surgical management of incontinence in bladder exstrophy. *Br J Urol* 1991; 68:543–48.

10 Bolduc S, Capolicchio G, Upadhyay J *et al.* The fate of the upper urinary tract in exstrophy. *J Urol* 2002;168:2579–82.

11 Grady RW, Mitchell ME. Complete primary repair of exstrophy. *J Urol* 1999;162:1415–20.

12 Fuchs J, Gluer S, Mildenberger H. One-stage reconstruction of bladder exstrophy. *Eur J Pediatr Surg* 1996;6:212–15.

13 Kelly JH. Radical soft tissue mobilisation in the repair of classic bladder exstrophy: An alternative to pelvic osteotomy. *Prog Paediatr Urol* 2000;3:119–46.

14 Grady RW, Joyner BD, Mitchell ME. The CPRE technique for the repair of bladder exstrophy and epispadias: Long-term follow-up. *Abstract presented in AAP* 2003.

15 Gearhart JP, Baird AD. The modern staged repair (MSRE) of bladder exstrophy: A contemporary series. *Abstract presented in XVIIth Annual Congress of the ESPU* 2006.

16 Baird AD, Mathews RI, Gearhart JP. The use of combined bladder and epispadias repair in boys with classic bladder exstrophy: Outcomes, complications and consequences. *J Urol* 2005;174:1421–4.

17 Hafez AT, El-Sherbiny MT, Shorrab AA *et al.* Complete primary repair of bladder exstrophy in children presenting late and those with failed initial closure: Single center experience. *J Urol* 2005;174:1549–52.

18 Borer JG, Gargollo PC, Kinnamon DD *et al.* Bladder growth and development after complete primary repair of bladder exstrophy in the newborn with comparison to staged approach. *J Urol* 2005;174:1553–7.

19 Kajbafzadeh AM, Duffy PG, Ransley PG. The evolution of penile reconstruction in epispadias repair: A report of 180 cases. *J Urol* 1995;154:858–61.

20 Mitchell ME, Bagli DJ. Complete penile disassembly for epispadias repair: The Mitchell technique. *J Urol* 1996;155:300–04.

21 Stein R, Fisch M, Stockle M *et al.* Urinary diversion in bladder exstrophy and incontinent epispadias: 25 years of experience. *J Urol* 1995;154:1177–81.

22 Koo HP, Avolio L, Duckett JW, Jr. Long-term results of ureterosigmoidostomy in children with bladder exstrophy. *J Urol* 1996;156:2037–40.

23 Miles-Thomas J, Gearhart JP, Gearhart SL. An initial evaluation of pelvic floor function and quality of life of bladder exstrophy patients after ureterosigmoidostomy. *J Gastrointest Surg* 2006;10:473–7.

24 Pahernik S, Beetz R, Schede J *et al.* Rectosigmoid pouch (Mainz Pouch II) in children. *J Urol* 2006;175:284–7.

25 Middleton AW, Jr., Hendren WH. Ileal conduits in children at the Massachusetts General Hospital from 1955 to 1970. *J Urol* 1976;115:591–5.

26 Stein R, Fisch M, Stockle M *et al.* Colonic conduit in children: Protection of the upper urinary tract 16 years later? *J Urol* 1996;156:1146–50.

27 Kajbafzadeh AM, Quinn FM, Ransley PG. Radical single stage reconstruction in failed exstrophy. *J Urol* 1995; 154:868–70.

28 Williams DI. Exstrophy. *Ann Chir Infant* 1971;12:483–92.

29 Borer JG, Gargollo PC, Hendren WH *et al.* Early outcome following complete primary repair of bladder exstrophy in the newborn. *J Urol* 2005;174:1674–8.

30 Gearhart JP, Ben-Chaim J, Sciortino C *et al.* The multiple reoperative bladder exstrophy closure: What affects the potential of the bladder? *Urology* 1996;47:240–3.

31 Husmann DA, McLorie GA, Churchill BM. Closure of the exstrophic bladder: An evaluation of the factors leading to its success and its importance on urinary continence. *J Urol* 1989;142:522–4.

32 Binsaleh S, Jednak R, Pippi-Salle JL. Case report: Azotemia secondary to bilateral ureteral kinking from ureteral stents placed at the time of bladder exstrophy closure. *Can J Urol* 2005;12:2724–5.

33 Alpert SA, Cheng EY, Kaplan WE *et al.* Bladder neck fistula after the complete primary repair of exstrophy: A multi-institutional experience. *J Urol* 2005;174:1687–9.

34 Surer I, Baker LA, Jeffs RD *et al.* The modified Cantwell-Ransley repair for exstrophy and epispadias: 10-year experience. *J Urol* 2000;164:1040–2.

35 Baker LA, Jeffs RD, Gearhart JP. Urethral obstruction after primary exstrophy closure: What is the fate of the genitourinary tract? *J Urol* 1999;161:618–21.

36 Gearhart JP, Peppas DS, Jeffs RD. Complications of paraexstrophy skin flaps in the reconstruction of classical bladder exstrophy. *J Urol* 1993;150:627–30.

37 Canning DA, Gearhart JP, Peppas DS *et al.* The cephalotrigonal reimplant in bladder neck reconstruction for patients with exstrophy or epispadias. *J Urol* 1993;150:156–8.

38 Husmann DA, McLorie GA, Churchill BM. Factors predisposing to renal scarring: Following staged reconstruction of classical bladder exstrophy. *J Pediatr Surg* 1990;25:500–4.

39 Fontaine E, Leaver R, Woodhouse CR. The effect of intestinal urinary reservoirs on renal function: A 10-year follow-up. *BJU Int* 2000;86:195–8.

40 Chan DY, Jeffs RD, Gearhart JP. Determinants of continence in the bladder exstrophy population: Predictors of success? *Urology* 2001;57:774–7.

41 Lottmann HB, Margaryan M, Lortat-Jacob S *et al.* Long-term effects of dextranomer endoscopic injections for the treatment of urinary incontinence: An update of a prospective study of 61 patients. *J Urol* 2006;176:1762–6.

42 Burki T, Hamid R, Ransley PG *et al.* Injectable polydimethylsiloxane for treating incontinence in children with the exstrophy-epispadias complex: Long-term results. *BJU Int* 2006;98:849–53.

43 Caione P, Nappo S, De Castro R *et al.* Low-dose desmopressin in the treatment of nocturnal urinary incontinence in the exstrophy-epispadias complex. *BJU Int* 1999;84:329–34.

44 Dave S, Grover VP, Agarwala S, Mitra DK, Bhatnagar V. The role of imipramine therapy in bladder exstrophy after bladder neck reconstruction. *BJU Int* 2002;89:557–60.

45 Yerkes EB, Adams MC, Rink RC, Pope JC IV, Brock JW, 3rd. How well do patients with exstrophy actually void? *J Urol* 2000;164:1044–7.

46 Burki T, Hamid R, Duffy P *et al.* Long-term followup of patients after redo bladder neck reconstruction for bladder exstrophy complex. *J Urol* 2006;176:1138–41.

47 Woodhouse CR, Redgrave NG. Late failure of the reconstructed exstrophy bladder. *Br J Urol* 1996;77:590–2.

48 Fernandez-Arjona M, Herrero L, Romero JC *et al.* Synchronous signet ring cell carcinoma and squamous cell carcinoma arising in an augmented ileocystoplasty. Case report and review of the literature. *Eur Urol* 1996;29:125–8.

49 Paulhac P, Maisonnette F, Bourg S *et al.* Adenocarcinoma in the exstrophic bladder. *Urology* 1999;54:744.

50 Phelps SR, Malone PS. Severe perineal pain after enterocystoplasty in bladder exstrophy. *BJU Int* 2004;93:835–7.

51 Woodhouse CR, Kellett MJ. Anatomy of the penis and its deformities in exstrophy and epispadias. *J Urol* 1984;132:1122–4.

52 Amukele SA, Lee GW, Stock JA *et al.* 20-year experience with iatrogenic penile injury. *J Urol* 2003;170:1691–4.

53 Hammouda HM. Results of complete penile disassembly for epispadias repair in 42 patients. *J Urol* 2003;170:1963–5.

54 Husmann DA, Gearhart JP. Loss of the penile glans and/or corpora following primary repair of bladder exstrophy using the complete penile disassembly technique. *J Urol* 2004;172:1696–700.

55 Silver RI, Yang A, Ben-Chaim J *et al.* Penile length in adulthood after exstrophy reconstruction. *J Urol* 1997;157:999–1003.

56 Gearhart JP, Baird AD. The failed complete repair of bladder exstrophy: Insights and outcomes. *J Urol* 2005;174:1669–72.

57 VanderBrink BA, Stock JA, Hanna MK. Aesthetic aspects of abdominal wall and external genital reconstructive surgery in bladder exstrophy-epispadias complex. *Curr Urol Rep* 2006;7:149–58.

58 Avolio L, Koo HP, Bescript AC *et al.* The long-term outcome in men with exstrophy/epispadias: Sexual function and social integration. *J Urol* 1996;156:822–5.

59 Woodhouse CR. The management of erectile deformity in adults with exstrophy and epispadias. *J Urol* 1986;135:932–5.

60 Reiner WG, Gearhart JP, Jeffs R. Psychosexual dysfunction in males with genital anomalies: Late adolescence, Tanner stages IV to VI. *J Am Acad Child Adolesc Psychiatry* 1999;38:865–72.

61 Ben-Chaim J, Jeffs RD, Reiner WG *et al.* The outcome of patients with classic exstrophy in adult life. *J Urol* 1996;155:1251–2.

62 Woodhouse CR. Sexual function in boys born with exstrophy, myelomeningocele, and micropenis. *Urology* 1998;52:3–11.

63 Ben-Chaim J, Jeffs RD, Gearhart JP. Loss of urethrovaginal septum as a complication of exstrophy closure in girls. *Eur Urol* 1998;33:206–8.

64 Woodhouse CR. The gynaecology of exstrophy. *BJU Int* 1999;83:34–8.

65 Stein R, Fisch M, Bauer H *et al.* Operative reconstruction of the external and internal genitalia in female patients with bladder exstrophy or incontinent epispadias. *J Urol* 1995;154:1002–7.

66 Rose CH, Rowe TF, Cox SM *et al.* Uterine prolapse associated with bladder exstrophy: Surgical management and subsequent pregnancy. *J Matern Fetal Med* 2000;9:150–2.

67 Mathews RI, Gan M, Gearhart JP. Urogynaecological and obstetric issues in women with the exstrophy–epispadias complex. *BJU Int* 2003;91:845–9.

68 Peneau M, Body G, Lansac J *et al.* Bladder exstrophy and pregnancy. Apropos of 2 cases. *Ann Urol (Paris)* 1985;19:47–52.

69 Hensle TW, Bingham JB, Reiley EA *et al.* The urological care and outcome of pregnancy after urinary tract reconstruction. *BJU Int* 2004;93:588–90.

70 Greenwell TJ, Venn SN, Creighton S *et al.* Pregnancy after lower urinary tract reconstruction for congenital abnormalities. *BJU Int* 2003;92:773–7.

71 Krisiloff M, Puchner PJ, Tretter W *et al.* Pregnancy in women with bladder exstrophy. *J Urol* 1978;119:478–9.

72 Husmann DA, McLorie GA, Churchill BM *et al.* Inguinal pathology and its association with classical bladder exstrophy. *J Pediatr Surg* 1990;25:332–4.

73 Stringer MD, Duffy PG, Ransley PG. Inguinal hernias associated with bladder exstrophy. *Br J Urol* 1994;73:308–9.

74 Connolly JA, Peppas DS, Jeffs RD *et al.* Prevalence and repair of inguinal hernias in children with bladder exstrophy. *J Urol* 1995;154:1900–1.

75 Okubadejo GO, Sponseller PD, Gearhart JP. Complications in orthopedic management of exstrophy. *J Pediatr Orthop* 2003;23:522–8.

76 Husmann DA, McLorie GA, Churchill BM. Hypertension following primary bladder closure for vesical exstrophy. *J Pediatr Surg* 1993;28:239–41.

77 Jani MM, Sponseller PD, Gearhart JP *et al.* The hip in adults with classic bladder exstrophy: A biomechanical analysis. *J Pediatr Orthop* 2000;20:296–301.

78 Svenningsson A, Gutierrez-farewik E, Svensson J *et al.* Gait analysis in children with bladder exstrophy: Effects of an early pelvic osteotomy. *Abstract presented in ESPU/AAP section on urology – 2nd joint meeting, 2005.*

79 Ricci G, Gentili A, Di Lorenzo F *et al.* Latex allergy in subjects who had undergone multiple surgical procedures for bladder exstrophy: Relationship with clinical intervention and atopic diseases. *BJU Int* 1999;84:1058–62.

80 Montagnino B, Czyzewski DI, Runyan RD *et al.* Long-term adjustment issues in patients with exstrophy. *J Urol* 1998;160:1471–4.

81 Nelson CP, Dunn RL, Wei JT, Gearhart JP. Surgical repair of bladder exstrophy in the modern era: Contemporary practice patterns and the role of hospital case volume. *J Urol* 2005;174:1099–1102.

13 Umbilical and Urachal Anomalies

Paul F. Austin

Key points

- The urachus is an embryonic remnant of the allantois.
- The urachal anomaly subtypes are reflective of the location of the incomplete involution of the urachus.
- The medial umbilical ligaments are vestigial urachal structures and useful landmarks for identifying the ureters.
- Ultrasound and/or sinography are useful diagnostic modalities for the majority of urachal anomalies.

The urachus, or median umbilical ligament, is a cordlike structure that is continuous with the anterior dome of the bladder inferiorly and extends in an extraperitoneal fashion to the umbilicus superiorly. The urachus is a normal embryonic remnant of the primitive bladder dome and may be affected by disorders related to the arrest of its normal involution. There are four clinical entities relating to the incomplete involution of the urachus during embryogenesis. These urachal anomalies include a patent urachus, urachal cyst, urachal sinus, and vesicourachal diverticulum (Figure 13.1).

Prevalence

Urachal anomalies are rare. In a large pediatric autopsy series, the historical incidence of a patent urachus is 1 in 7610 cases and the incidence of a urachal cyst is 1 in 5000 [1]. Another example of the infrequency of urachal anomalies includes a report of 315 cases accumulated

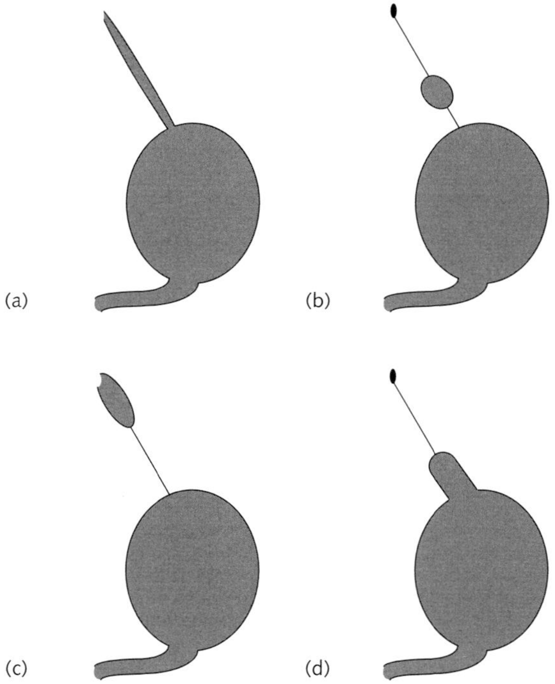

Figure 13.1 Urachal anomalies: (a) patent urachus, (b) urachal cyst, (c) urachal sinus, and (d) vesicourachal diverticulum.

Pediatric Urology: Surgical Complications and Management. Edited by Duncan T. Wilcox, Prasad P. Godbole and Martin A. Koyle. © 2008 Blackwell Publishing, ISBN: 978-1-4051-6268-5.

over a 40-year period [2]. The most frequent urachal abnormalities that typically present are either an urachal sinus or an urachal cyst [3–5]. There is generally a 2:1 incidence of urachal anomalies in males compared to females and urachal anomalies, usually present in early childhood, may be clinically silent and remain unrecognized until adulthood.

Embryology

The urachus is an embryonic remnant of the allantois [6]. The allantois in embryos of reptiles, birds, and some mammals has a respiratory function and may act as a reservoir for urine during embryonic life. The allantois remains very small in human embryos but is involved with early blood formation and associated with development of the urinary bladder [6]. As the bladder enlarges, the allantois becomes the urachus and is represented in adults as the median umbilical ligament. The blood vessels of the allantois become the umbilical arteries and veins. The obliterated umbilical arteries or medial umbilical ligaments are important landmarks to help locate the underlying ureters when performing surgery on the bladder and ureter (e.g. extravesical ureteroneocystomy).

The allantois arises from the yolk sac and extends to the cloaca – the precursor to the bladder (urogenital sinus) and the rectum (hindgut). With further development and division of the urogenital sinus and hindgut by the urorectal septum, the allantois is initially continuous with the bladder but soon constricts and becomes a thick, fibrous cord called the urachus. During the 4th and 5th months of development, the urachus narrows to a small caliber tube lined by transitional epithelium [7].

Anatomy

The urachus lies within the space between the peritoneum posteriorly and the transversalis fascia anteriorly that is known as the space of Retzius [8]. The urachus is bounded by the umbilicovesical fascia, which extends laterally to each umbilical artery. Inferiorly, the fascial layers spread out over the dome of the bladder to the hypogastric artery posteriorly and to the pelvic diaphragm anteriorly. Thus, a potential pyramidal shaped space is created that is completely self-contained and separate from the peritoneal cavity. These fascial planes act to limit the spread of an urachal infection or neoplasm. Knowledge of this anatomy becomes important in the diagnosis and treatment of urachal diseases [9].

Clinical urachal anomalies

Urachal anomalies result from a failure of fibrosis and involution of the urachus during embryonic development. A variety of clinical urachal anomalies exist and are dependent on where the failure of involution occurs in the urachal tract between the bladder and the umbilicus (Figure 13.1).

Diagnosis

The diagnosis of an urachal anomaly is made from a combination of presenting history, physical exam, and imaging. Periumbilical discharge suggests either a patent urachus or an urachal sinus while a palpable umbilical mass suggests an umbilical cyst. Patients may present with abdominal, suprapubic, or periumbilical pain. Periumbilical erythema and tenderness suggest an underlying infection and patients with urachal anomalies may present with dysuria, fever, and a urinary tract infection.

A variety of imaging may be used to make the diagnosis of an urachal anomaly. The appearance of a fixed, midline, cystic, extraperitoneal swelling between the umbilicus and the bladder on ultrasonography (US) is suggestive of an urachal anomaly [10]. During a work-up of abdominal or pelvic pain, computed tomography (CT) may allow the diagnosis of an urachal anomaly [11] Figure 13.3b. Several studies have advocated that US is the test of choice if an urachal cyst is suspected with a periumbilical mass and sinography is the best modality to identify a patent urachus or urachal sinus [3,4,12]. Other imaging modalities may diagnose urachal anomalies including a voiding cystourethrogram (VCUG) may demonstrate an urachal diverticulum commonly seen in patients with prune belly syndrome.

Analysis of the umbilical fluids may provide another means of diagnosing an urachal anomaly. Fluid analysis would include measuring the umbilical fluid for content of urea and creatinine. Injecting methylene blue transurethrally or indigo carmine intravenously and observing a color change in the draining fluid; or conversely, injecting indigo carmine into the fistulous tract and looking for a color change in the urine may also provide the diagnosis [9]. Finally, cystoscopy has also been reported to assist in the characterization of urachal anomalies [7].

Outcomes and complications of urachal anomalies

Congenital anomalies of the urachus represent an arrest of the normal process of involution of the urachus and may not present until adulthood. Common presenting symptoms are periumbilical discharge, umbilical mass, periumbilical pain, and dysuria [13]. Bladder prolapse or eversion has been reported in a patent urachus [14,15] mimicking an omphalocoele on antenatal scans. Sepsis secondary to a patent urachus has also been reported [16,17]. Urachal cysts may become infected. Usually the infection is restricted to the space of Retzius but occasionally the cyst may rupture intraperitoneally with resultant bowel fistula formation [18]. A urachal sinus usually presents with symptoms and signs of localized sepsis. Occasionally, intra-abdominal contents may be densely adherent to the inflammatory mass and may be injured during resection. A vesicourachal diverticulum rarely requires treatment unless it is large with poor emptying due to a narrow neck or paradoxical contraction.

In a report by Ueno and associates, the authors advocate that patients with asymptomatic urachal remnants do not require follow-up, and urachal remnants, especially those under 1 year of age, do not require surgical resection unless the patient has multiple symptomatic episodes [19]. Their conclusions were based upon the finding of only 1 patient out of 44 patients that developed recurrent symptoms during follow-up (maximum follow-up was 32 months). The authors also cite the spontaneous involution rate of the normal urachus during infancy [20] and found that nearly one-third of their asymptomatic patients had disappearance of their urachal remnant.

One of the concerns of leaving an urachal remnant is if untreated, urachal carcinoma may develop within these anomalies. Urachal carcinoma is rare in children (0.01%) [21] and accounts for 0.34% of all bladder cancers [22,23]. The most common type is adenocarcinoma although other histological types have been reported [21,23–26]. The patients usually have a poor prognosis due to late presentation with local invasion. In a histologic review of 23 urachal remnants removed over a 10-year period, Upadhyay and Kukkady found normal urothelial lining in 17 urachal remnants, whereas 6 (25%) showed abnormal epithelium. This abnormal epithelium included colonic epithelium, small intestinal epithelium, and squamous epithelium which suggest concern for malignant degeneration. Given this potential risk of malignancy along with the minimal invasiveness of laparoscopy, a case may be made for laparoscopy as a treatment modality for asymptomatic urachal remnants [27].

Diagnosis and management of urachal anomalies

Patent urachus

A patent urachus usually presents itself at or soon after birth when the umbilical cord is ligated and urine drains from the umbilicus. Historically, lower urinary tract obstruction has been considered a contributing factor in its pathogenesis [28], but this is not seen in the majority of cases. In fact, urethral tubularization occurs after the urachal lumen obliterates during fetal development [29]. Subsequently, it suggests that infravesical obstruction has little influence on urachal development.

As previously mentioned, the diagnosis is frequently confirmed after injecting the patent urachal opening with contrast during a sinogram or by analyzing the umbilical fluid. Other conditions that may present with a wet umbilicus include anomalies of the omphalomesenteric duct (completely patent omphalomesenteric duct, omphalomesenteric duct sinus, vitelline cyst, Meckel's diverticulum) or an umbilical granuloma [30].

In the management of a patent urachus, observation may be indicated in young infants without symptoms because the involution of the urachus is not complete at birth and spontaneous closure can occur in the first few months of life [31]. If there is an associated bladder outlet obstruction, management of the bladder outlet obstruction is often adequate to cause involution of the patent urachus.

When drainage is persistent, complete excision of the urachus with a small cuff of bladder by an extraperitoneal approach is recommended [32] (Figure 13.2).

Urachal cyst

The majority of urachal cysts develop in the lower third of the urachus. Most urachal cysts go undetected unless they become infected or enlarge to a size causing mechanical symptoms [33]. Following enlargement

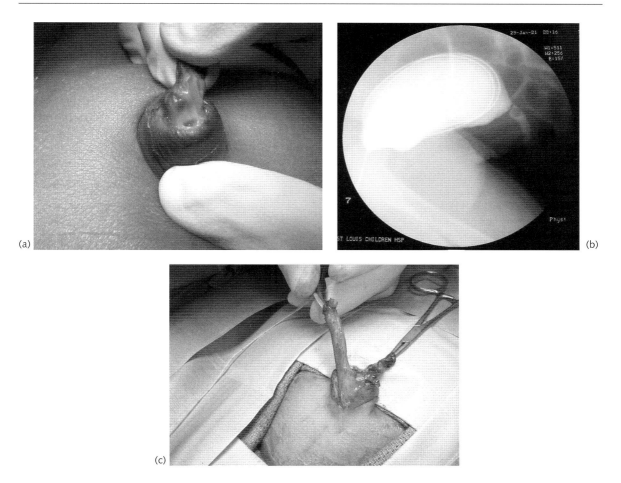

Figure 13.2 Patent urachus: (a) patent opening inferior to umbilical cord, (b) patent urachus visualized on cystogram and sinogram, and (c) operative dissection of patent urachus.

of the cyst, symptoms include lower abdominal pain, a feeling of heaviness, and urinary frequency. Urachal cysts may become infected and develop into an urachal abscess. The majority of these are infected with *Staphylococcus aureus* [3,4] and these generally manifest in adulthood. US is the most common diagnostic modality to identify urachal cysts [4] (Figure 13.3a). CT scan is beneficial when there is a large cystic abscess or there is severe periumbilical cellulitis which may cause misinterpretation on ultrasound [12] (Figure 13.3b).

Treatment of urachal cysts involves complete excision. However, when infection is present, management by perioperative drainage and antibiotics followed by subsequent elective excision may represent the most effective surgical option [34–36]. Excision of the urachal cyst

may be done openly or may be performed laparoscopically [37,38].

Urachal sinus

An urachal sinus most likely represents an urachal cyst that becomes infected and dissects to the umbilicus (Figure 13.4). Additionally, an urachal sinus may drain into the bladder or it may drain into either the umbilicus or the bladder and is termed an alternating sinus. These patients typically present in childhood with periumbilical pain and tenderness and may have umbilical erythema, excoriation, or reactive granulation tissue. A fistulogram is usually diagnostic and will help delineate the extent of the sinus tract [4,12]. After treatment of the acute infection, surgical excision of the sinus tract is recommended.

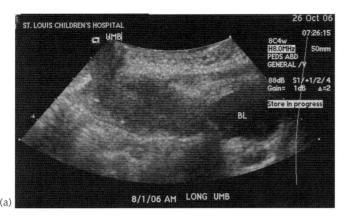

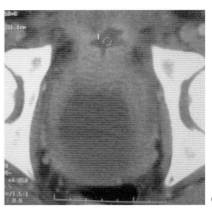

Figure 13.3 Urachal cyst: (a) ultrasound image of urachal cyst, note proximity to bladder (BL) and (b) CT scan evaluation of abdominal pain revealing infected urachal cyst.

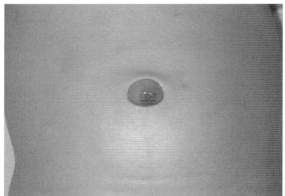

(a)

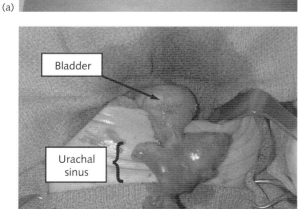

(b)

Figure 13.4 Urachal sinus: (a) urachal sinus presenting as a protuberant umbilical mass with drainage and (b) operative dissection of alternating urachal sinus. Note connection to bladder and umbilicus.

Vesicourachal diverticulum

A vesicourachal diverticulum is frequently seen in a child with prune belly syndrome. A vesicourachal diverticulum may be seen in the setting of lower urinary tract obstruction (e.g. posterior urethral valves) but may also be discovered incidentally during an imaging work-up (e.g. VCUG for evaluation of vesicoureteral reflux). Patients who have this urachal anomaly are usually asymptomatic. A vesicourachal diverticulum is thought to occur when there is incomplete obliteration and closure of the lower portion of the urachus and the bladder apex. No treatment is usually necessary since this anomaly is primarily morphological and bears no functional consequences.

References

1 Rubin A. *Handbook of Congenital Malformations*. Philadelphia: Saunders, 1967.
2 Blichert-Toft M, Nielsen OV. Congenital patient urachus and acquired variants: Diagnosis and treatment. Review of the literature and report of five cases. *Acta Chir Scand* 1971;137:807–14.
3 Mesrobian HG, Zacharias A, Balcom AH, Cohen RD. Ten years of experience with isolated urachal anomalies in children. *J Urol* 1997;158:1316–8.
4 Cilento BG, Jr., Bauer SB, Retik AB, Peters CA, Atala A. Urachal anomalies: Defining the best diagnostic modality. *Urology* 1998;52:120–2.
5 Choi YJ, Kim JM, Ahn SY, Oh JT, Han SW, Lee JS. Urachal anomalies in children: A single center experience. *Yonsei Med J* 2006;47:782–6.
6 Moore KL, Persaud TVN. *The Developing Human: Clinically Oriented Embryology*, 5th edn. Philadelphia: Saunders, 1993.
7 Nix JT, Menville JG, Albert M, Wendt DL. Congenital patent urachus. *J Urol* 1958;79:264–73.

8 Hammond G, Yglesias L, Davis JE. The urachus, its anatomy and associate fasciae. *Anat Rec* 1941;80:271–87.

9 Bauer SB, Retik AB. Urachal anomalies and related umbilical disorders. *Urol Clin North Am* 1978;5:195–211.

10 Holten I, Lomas F, Mouratidis B, Malecky G, Simpson E. The ultrasonic diagnosis of urachal anomalies. *Australas Radiol* 1996;40:2–5.

11 Yu JS, Kim KW, Lee HJ, Lee YJ, Yoon CS, Kim MJ. Urachal remnant diseases: Spectrum of CT and US findings. *Radiographics* 2001;21:451–61.

12 Nagasaki A, Handa N, Kawanami T. Diagnosis of urachal anomalies in infancy and childhood by contrast fistulography, ultrasound and CT. *Pediatr Radiol* 1991;21:321–3.

13 Cilento BG, Jr., Bauer SB, Retik AB *et al.* Urachal anomalies: Defining the best diagnostic modality. *Urology* 1998;52:120.

14 Lugo B, McNulty J, Emil S. Bladder prolapse through a patent urachus: Fetal and neonatal features. *J Pediatr Surg* 2006;41:e5–7.

15 Yeats M, Pinch L. Patent urachus with bladder eversioin. *J Pediatr Surg* 2003;38:e12–13.

16 Takamura C, Ikegami M, Han YS *et al.* Patent urachus associated with abdominal abscess: Report of a case. *Hinyokika Kiyo* 1991;37:87–90.

17 Buckspan MB. Patent urachus and infected urachal cyst in an adult: A case report. *Can J Surg* 1984;27:496.

18 Nunn LL. Urachal cysts and their complications. *Am J Surg* 1952;84:252.

19 Ueno T, Hashimoto H, Yokoyama H, Ito M, Kouda K, Kanamaru H. Urachal anomalies: Ultrasonography and management. *J Pediatr Surg* 2003;38:1203–7.

20 Zieger B, Sokol B, Rohrschneider WK, Darge K, Troger J. Sonomorphology and involution of the normal urachus in asymptomatic newborns. *Pediatr Radiol* 1998;28:156–61.

21 Clapuyt P, Saint-Martin C, De Batselier P *et al.* Urachal neuroblastoma: First case report. *Pediatr Radiol* 1999;29:320.

22 Henly DR, Farrow GM, Zincke H. Urachal cancer: Role of conservative surgery. *Urology* 1993;42:635.

23 Sheldon CA, Clayman RV, Gonzalez R *et al.* Malignant urachal lesions. *J Urol* 1984;131:1.

24 Yokoyama S, Hayashida Y, Nagahama J *et al.* Rhabdomyosarcoma of the urachus: A case report. *Acta Cytol* 1997;41:1293.

25 Defabiani N, Iselin CE, Khan HG *et al.* Benign teratoma of the urachus. *Br J Urol* 1998;81:760.

26 D'Alessio A, Verdelli G, Bernardi M *et al.* Endodermal sinus (yolk sac) tumor of the urachus. *Eur J Pediatr Surg* 1994;4:180.

27 Navarrete S, Sanchez Ismayel A, Sanchez Salas R, Sanchez R, Navarrete Llopis S. Treatment of urachal anomalies: A minimally invasive surgery technique. *JSLS* 2005;9:422–5.

28 Hinman F, Jr. Surgical disorders of the bladder and umbilicus of urachal origin. *Surg Gynecol Obstet* 1961;113:605–14.

29 Schreck WR, Campbell WA, 3rd. The relation of bladder outlet obstruction to urinary-umbilical fistula. *J Urol* 1972;108:641–3.

30 Homsy YL. Bladder and urachus. In *Pediatric Urology*, 3rd edn. Edited by B O'Donnell, SA Koff. Oxford/Boston: Butterworth-Heinemann, 1997: pp. 483–93.

31 Zieger B, Sokol B, Rohrschneider WK *et al.* Sonomorphology and involution of the normal urachus in asymptomatic newborns. *Pediatr Radiol* 1998;28:156.

32 Nix JT, Menville JG, Albert M. Congenital patent urachus. *J Urol* 1958;79:264.

33 MacNeily AE, Koleilat N, Kiruluta HG, Homsy YL. Urachal abscesses: Protean manifestations, their recognition, and management. *Urology* 1992;40:530–5.

34 McCollum MO, Macneily AE, Blair GK. Surgical implications of urachal remnants: Presentation and management. *J Pediatr Surg* 2003;38:798–803.

35 Pesce C, Costa L, Musi L, Campobasso P, Zimbardo L. Relevance of infection in children with urachal cysts. *Eur Urol* 2000;38:457–60.

36 Minevich E, Wacksman J, Lewis AG, Bukowski TP, Sheldon CA. The infected urachal cyst: Primary excision versus a staged approach. *J Urol* 1997;157:1869–72.

37 Khurana S, Borzi PA. Laparoscopic management of complicated urachal disease in children. *J Urol* 2002;168:1526–8.

38 Cadeddu JA, Boyle KE, Fabrizio MD, Schulam PG, Kavoussi LR. Laparoscopic management of urachal cysts in adulthood. *J Urol* 2000;164:1526–8.

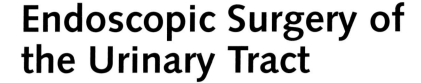

V

Endoscopic Surgery of the Urinary Tract

14

Cystoscopy and Cystoscopic Interventions

Divyesh Y. Desai

Key points

- Primary endoscopic resection of both anterior and posterior urethral valves is the preferred treatment option in majority of cases.
- Routine second look procedures ensure completeness of resection and de-obstruction.
- With modern instrumentation and good surgical technique, complications directly related to endoscopic manipulation are rare, e.g. iatrogenic urethral strictures.
- Endoscopic treatment of pediatric urethral strictures is associated with a cure rate of 50%,

with best results achieved for the short segment idiopathic bulbar strictures.

- Endoscopic ureterocele puncture is an effective method of producing upper tract decompression and can be curative for the single system intravesical ureteroceles.
- JJ stenting as the initial treatment for primary obstructive megaureter is curative in up to 50% of cases but is associated with a high morbidity (up to 70%).

Introduction

Pediatric endoscopy has come a long way in the past two decades, and advances and refinements in fiber optic technology, along with miniaturization of equipment, allow endoscopic visualization of almost the entire urinary tract. Miniaturization has allowed the endoscopic appraisal of most neonatal urethras including those of preterm babies weighing 2000 g or more. There are a wide array of instruments available today which allow for safe assessment and intervention with minimal complications provided one remains within the limitations of the available equipment.

Posterior urethral valves

Introduction

Posterior urethral valves remain the most common cause of lower urinary tract outflow obstruction in

male infants with an estimated incidence of 1:5000 live births. The majority are suspected on antenatal ultrasound screening and referred to specialist centers at birth. Modern endoscopic equipment along with long-term outcome data has dramatically changed the surgical approach to valve treatment. In the past, many newborns were treated with a vesicostomy primarily because of the relatively large instrumentation available. Supravesical diversions were in vogue due to their undisputed short-term benefits on renal function; however, the long-term outcome of these diversions show no benefit for renal function and raise concern regarding the effect on outcome on bladder function. This chapter will cover the various approaches to the endoscopic ablation of posterior urethral valves, their complications, and an approach to avoiding these complications in the 21st century.

Surgical techniques and outcomes

In 1972, Whitaker et al. [1] reported the results of 112 patients in whom valves were ablated endoscopically with an infant McCarthy panendoscope, using either a bugbee (30) or a loop electrode (82) to destroy the valve

Pediatric Urology: Surgical Complications and Management. Edited by Duncan T. Wilcox, Prasad P. Godbole and Martin A. Koyle. © 2008 Blackwell Publishing, ISBN: 978-1-4051-6268-5.

membrane. In situations where the urethra (meatus and submeatal region) would not accommodate the instrument, a small perineal urethrostomy was made by cutting down upon the tip of a small sound placed in the urethra, and the panendoscope was introduced via the perineum just distal to the external sphincter. The valve membrane was ablated using coagulating diathermy current. Many authors have expressed concern about iatrogenic stricture disease with this technique. Whitaker does not report on the incidence in his series; however, Myers and Walker [2] reported a 50% incidence of strictures in his series of valves ablated in infancy with a 25% incidence in the group as a whole.

Whitaker and colleagues [1] reported a 33% incidence of continuous incontinence with a further 55% stress incontinence in their series of 112 patients. It is difficult to attribute a cause to incontinence as some of their patients had additional bladder neck surgery, and the noncompliant valve bladder had not been ruled out. An addendum to that publication reported a dramatic improvement in daytime incontinence in five boys following treatment with imipramine.

In 1973, Williams and associates [3] advocated ablating the valves with a diathermy hook electrode under radiological control. This technique avoided a perineal urethrostomy and was successful in several cases, but complications arose when the hook engaged adjacent tissue like the bladder neck or verumontanum. Whitaker and Sherwood [4] subsequently modified the hook, which minimized the risk of adjacent tissue injury but did not completely eliminate it.

Hendren [5] was a proponent of valve ablation under direct vision and in the narrower urethra passed the insulated wire electrode (3F) alongside an 8F endoscope, a technique he described as "a little awkward." He ablated the valves using cutting diathermy current and reported no strictures with this technique. Several boys in his series required further resection of the valves, and once again the continence outcome was muddied by synchronous or metachronous bladder neck surgery.

In 1986, Diamond and Ransley [6] described the Fogarty balloon catheter ablation technique and noted that while not universally successful, they achieved satisfactory results in nine of ten carefully selected patients. The bladder is filled with contrast material via a small feeding tube, which is then removed. A no. 4 Fogarty balloon catheter is passed and the balloon inflated within the bladder. The catheter is then slowly withdrawn under fluoroscopic control until the balloon engages the valve. A sharp tug causes rupture of the anterior membrane. The balloon is then deflated and the catheter is removed. Cromie and associates [7] describe a similar procedure using a modified venous valvulotome in which under fluoroscopic control the valvulotome is used to engage and cut the obstructing membrane. They reported completeness of ablation in 13 of 15 patients treated. Both reports describe a 0% stricture incidence with their respective techniques.

Other described techniques include Mohan's [8] urethral valvotome in which the valves are engaged and destroyed without any fluoroscopy control and under local analgesia, relying on the instrument design to "catch" the valves. Mohan reports good results in eight boys treated using his instrument based on symptoms and improved radiologically findings on repeat voiding cystourethrogram (VCUG).

Percutaneous, endoscopic, antegrade diathermy valve ablation has been popularized by Zaontz and Firlit [9] with a subsequent description by Gibbons and associates [10] of endoscopic antegrade diathermy valve ablation through a vesicostomy.

A bugbee or insulated wire electrode passed through an infant (5–7.5F) cystourethroscope is a useful technique in very small infants. Similarly, laser ablation using the pottasium titanyl phosphate (KTP) (or Nd-YAG) laser via a small fiber passed through the working channel of the infant cystoscope has been reported as a safe technique in newborn infants with no stricture formation up to 3 years follow-up. This technique relies on coagulative necrosis of the membranous tissue and the tip of the electrode or fiber is placed in direct contact with the valve tissue and the current is applied. The process is repeated at multiple sites.

Videoendoscopy using a 8.5F (5° lens) to 10F (0° lens) resectoscope and a cold knife hook working element allow safe and effective ablation of urethral lesions without risk of thermal injury or significant bleeding and can be employed in infants as small as 2000 g. At the present time, this is the safest and most effective technique for ablation of membranous lesions of the infant urethra and is the gold standard against which other techniques will be compared. The membrane is cut at the 5 and 7 o'clock positions until its connection with the verumontanum is lost. Some surgeons advocate additional routine incision at the 12 o'clock position. The bladder is drained via a 6–8F feeding tube for 24–48 h and subsequently removed.

A review of the last 100 valve resections at the author's institution using a bugbee/insulated wire or the cold knife resection technique shows a 21% incidence of re-resection at planned follow-up check cystoscopy and a 0% incidence of urethral stricture disease.

The instrumentation available for valve ablation at the author's institution includes:
1 6–7.5F graduated Wolff cystourethroscope with a 3F working channel
2 10, 11, or 13.5F resectoscopes with cold knife hook working element
3 Bugbee electrodes, Colling's Knife, and resectoscope loops.

In situations where the available instrumentation was too large to be safely accommodated in the infant urethra, valve ablation was deferred to a later date. In the interim, the urethra was serially and passively dilated using increasing calibre urethral catheters changed on a weekly basis.

Complications
Urethral stricture

Table 14.1 Incidence of urethral stricture following ablation of posterior urethral valves.

Author valve	Age at (n) ablation (year)	Number (year)	Follow-up (%)	Stricture
Myers [2]	<1	14	1–10	50
Myers [2]	>1	14	1–10	0
Nijman [11]	< and >1	85	5–19	0
Mitra [12]	0–15	82	1–21	3.6
Crooks [13]	1.5–?	36	4–?	08
Churchill [14]	<1 to >1	173	?	12

Dense strictures following diathermy ablation are on the decline and most recent series report a <5% incidence of strictures. Diagnosed early they may be amenable to dilatation or visual internal urethrotomy. Recurrent strictures or long segment strictures will require definitive anastomotic or augmented urethroplasty.

Incomplete valve ablation

Completeness of valve ablation must be confirmed on follow-up VCUG and or cystourethroscopy. Incidence of incomplete ablation varies and in our review was seen in 21% of cases. It is more likely following bugbee or insulated wire ablation through a small cystoscope, as the vision is limited due to relatively poor flow of irrigation fluid.

It is prudent to rescope the urethra within 6–12 weeks of the initial ablation to check completeness of resection, as the consequences of persistent obstruction are potentially disastrous.

Obstructive oliguria or anuria

True uretero–vesical junction obstruction is rare in boys with posterior urethral valves (PUV). Temporary UVJ obstruction, presumed to be due to entrapment of the UVJ by the thickened detrusor following decompression of the bladder, is seen not uncommonly in clinical practice. The oliguria or in severe cases anuria typically lasts for 24–48 h and resolves spontaneously. There may be associated perirenal urinary extravasation and nephrostomy drainage of one or both kidneys may occasionally become necessary, however most cases can be managed with a policy of watchful waiting.

Sarkis *et al.* [15], Noe and Jenkins, and Jordan and Hoover have all reported individual cases and Sarkis recommends use of non-self-retaining tubes to drain the bladder to minimize the risk.

Urinary tract infection

It is not uncommon for these children to have impaired renal function, making these neonates particularly vulnerable to developing urine infection following urethral instrumentation, VCUG, and valve ablation. In addition they may acquire drug resistant organisms and with prolonged antibiotic treatment, secondary fungal infections which are extremely difficult to treat.

Renal impairment

The condition is associated with considerable morbidity and accounts for 16% of children with end-stage renal failure and for 25% of all children with end-stage renal disease (ESRD) who undergo renal transplantation, according to the UK Transplant Registry 2005. Early renal failure is attributed to inherent renal dysplasia. The etiology of late onset renal impairment is more complex, and dysplasia, bladder dysfunction, and urinary tract infections are all implicated.

The fragile renal function in the neonatal period is exquisitely sensitive and vulnerable to fluid imbalance and urinary infection. Adequate precautions along with input from nephrological colleagues help to maintain optimum function and nadir creatinine levels along with a formal glomerular filteration rate (GFR) value at 1 year of age helps predict long-term outcome in these children.

Urinary incontinence

At the present time, urinary incontinence as a consequence of valve ablation and associated sphincter damage is rare. In the past, a high incidence was reported: 33% continuous and an additional 55% stress incontinence in a series of 34 patients who had both valve ablation and bladder neck surgery [1]. The subsequent description of the valve bladder and the abnormal urodynamic patterns observed in these children clarified the etiopathogenesis of incontinence in majority of these patients.

Parkhouse and associates [16] reported daytime urinary incontinence at 5 years of age to associate with poor long-term renal outcome. A further compounding factor, which may be responsible, is polyuria, secondary to impaired renal function.

Recent studies, which have prospectively looked at the development of bladder function in these children, have shown a high incidence of bladder dysfunction (up to 70% [17]). Serial invasive urodynamic studies have documented a changing pattern over time with a different etiology for incontinence at varying time points [18].

Preventing complications
Urethral stricture
The neonatal urethra is extremely delicate and forced or over sized instrumentation will inevitably result in narrowing. It is good practice to prophylactically dilate the meatus and submeatal region prior to introduction of the endoscopes. Generous lubrication and gentle manipulation will minimize trauma. It is essential to have an array of instruments available, which will allow safe and satisfactory valve ablation.

The new pediatric resectoscopes have a blunt metal rounded tip compared to the Bakelite sharp beaks found on older instruments. This design feature helps to minimize injury during introduction.

Cold knife incision is neat, specific, and not associated with surrounding tissue damage. Diathermy ablation has the potential to injure adjacent structures, and the current can penetrate to the deeper tissues, which has the potential to promote scarring. A pure cut setting on the diathermy is less damaging than coagulating current and the smaller surface area of the Colling's knife is more precise compared to the resectoscope loop.

Limiting operative time to a minimum, ensuring adequate visualization of the important landmarks during resection, and minimizing postoperative bladder drainage all contribute toward lowering the risk of stricture formation.

It was felt that a "dry urethra" following valve ablation promotes stricturing; however, Mitra found no evidence to support this hypothesis in his study.

In the uncommon situation where the available instrumentation is found to be too large, deferring valve ablation or a temporary vesicostomy further reduce the risk of complications and improve outcomes.

Obstructive oliguria or anuria
Decompressing the bladder via suprapubic or urethral catheter usually results in a period of postobstructive diuresis. Paradoxically, draining the bladder can sometimes result in a temporary obstruction at one or both vesicoureteric (VU) junctions producing obstructive oliguria, anuria with or without calyceal rupture and urinomas. Sarkis et al. [15] have attributed this to the balloon of the urethral catheter obstructing the ureteric orifices in a small thick-walled bladder.

An alternative explanation is that the hypertrophied detrusor clamps down on the intramural part of the lower ureter, temporarily kinking of the lumen to occlude the flow of urine. We have observed this phenomenon both pre and post valve ablation and we do not use balloon catheters to drain the bladder.

Avoiding balloon catheters, minimizing the length of tubing within the bladder when using feeding tubes, and avoiding repeated insertions by draining the bladder suprapubically (5F Cystofix® Minipaed) are measures that may minimize the risk. Slow decompression of the chronically distended bladder is recommended in adults, however this is difficult to achieve in the neonate.

Incomplete valve ablation and sphincteric incontinence
Adequate visualization during valve ablation is the key to successful and complete resection. A selection of instrumentation should be available to allow safe and satisfactory ablation in majority of cases. Routine second look appraisal of the urethra within 6–12 weeks will minimize complications as a consequence of incomplete resection. Avoid concomitant bladder neck surgery as proposed recently [19] because in the past this approach has been shown to be associated with high morbidity.

Urinary tract infections and renal impairment
Routine prophylactic antibiotic and antifungal cover around the VCUG, and valve ablation minimizes the incidence of infections in the neonatal period. Antibiotic prophylaxis in infancy and ensuring a good fluid intake along with elective circumcision offered at the time of second look check cystoscopy are measures that will reduce the risk of urinary infections in infancy.

Conclusions
Video endoscopic valve ablation using the hook cold knife offers a safe and effective way to ablate the valves in the neonatal period. A lesser number will require ablation using bugbee or insulated wire electrodes.

Prophylactic dilatation of the urethra, generous lubrication, avoiding forcible use of over sized instruments, and gentle manipulation minimize complications.

Routine second look procedures ensure completeness of resection.

Careful monitoring and recruiting nephrological colleagues in the care of these children optimizes outcome. Routine periodic follow-up with appropriately timed investigations to address aberrations in urinary continence and renal function ensure optimal long-term outcome in these children.

Anterior urethral valves or syringocele

Introduction
Anterior urethral valves (AUV) were first described by Watts in 1906 as a cause of urethral obstruction in boys. The origin is attributed to a cystic dilatation (syringocele) of the main bulbourethral glands described by Cowper in 1705. The paired Cowper's glands lie dorsal to and on either side of the membranous urethra. The ducts from these glands are 2–3 cm long and enter the urethra individually or fuse proximally to enter as a single orifice. These mucus secreting glands begin to function by 4 months, gestation and their secretion acts as a lubricant and transport medium for sperm during ejaculation.

The common location of the lesion, approximately 1 cm proximal to the fossa navicularis, suggests a faulty union between the glanular and penile urethra as the cause. Other plausible explanations suggested include, congenital urethral stricture, abortive urethral duplication, and transient urethral obstruction in utero.

Rupture of the syringocele causes the distal lip to lift up and abut against the anterior wall of the urethra during voiding, acting as a flap valve resulting in urinary outflow impairment. The diagnosis is made on an VCUG.

Clinical presentation is variable and includes prenatal hydronephrosis, penile swelling, urinary tract infections, and voiding symptoms like poor urinary stream and dribbling.

Surgical techniques and outcomes
Transurethral incision or fulgration of the valve is the proedure of choice in the majority. Provided a significant defect in the corpus spongiosum has been eliminated on clinical exam and VCUG, no further intervention is necessary.

Bauer and associates [20], in a series of 9 cases over 40 years, found incision to be successful in three-quarters of cases, with one child requiring a subsequent urethroplasty.

Bagli et al. [21] in their series of 17 cases found this technique successful in all 6 cases treated with a transurethral incision of the valve leaflet.

A urethroplasty or diverticulectomy is recommended in cases where the spongiosal defect is large resulting in poor urethral support. The urethroplasty may be performed as either a one- or two-stage procedure and the published results of two of the series mentioned earlier show a success rate approaching 100%.

A vesicostomy as the primary treatment has been recommended in neonates and infants with associated high-grade bilateral vesicoureteral reflux (VUR). Subsequent management will depend on the degree of the spongiosal defect and may include correction of VUR.

In general, the effects of intravesical obstruction due to AUV are less severe than those due to posterior urethral valves (PUV). AUV cause few long lasting upper tract radiographic changes and are associated with a chronic renal failure incidence of 0–5% compared to up to 60% in children with posterior urethral valves (PUV). Similarly, bilateral VUR is not associated with a poor prognosis in children with AUV suggesting majority of reflux is secondary and resolves after treatment of the AUV.

In Bagli et al.'s [21] series, patients with anterior urethral valves were found to be continent of urine and free of urinary tract infections and obstructive symptoms at long-term follow-up.

Complications and management
Urinary extravasation
Urinary extravasation has been described in isolated cases following transurethral incision. In these patients, the subcutaneous tissue and corpus spongiosum is attenuated and allows for urinary extravasation. On removal of the catheter and subsequent voiding, urine leaks to track along the penile shaft and scrotum producing a boggy swelling. Reintroduction of a urethral catheter and a further period of drainage usually resolve the problem. Aspiration or drainage may be indicated if the urinoma is infected and in rare cases a subsequent urethroplasty may be necessary.

Urethral fistula
Urethral fistulae may occur following one- or two-stage urethroplasty and are managed in the same way as those occurring following a hypospadias repair.

VUR
Persistent VUR following successful relief of obstruction due to AUV may require intervention if symptomatic. Treatment options include endoscopic correction and surgery. Bladder dysfunction is rare in children with AUV.

Conclusions

AUV is a rare cause of male urethral obstruction; the majority can be treated endoscopically and the condition is associated with good long-term outcome for both renal and bladder functions.

Urethral strictures

Introduction

Pediatric urethral strictures are uncommon and their etiology can be divided into "inflammatory," traumatic, and idiopathic. The inflammatory category includes nonspecific urethritis, lichen sclerosis balanitis xerotica obliterans (BXO), and urethralgia posterior. Trauma is commonly iatrogenic and attributed to instrumentation or surgery but also includes the more dramatic fall astride and road traffic accident (RTA) injuries. The majority of the idiopathic strictures occur at the junction of the proximal and middle sections of the bulbar urethra in adolescents or young adults with no previous history, suggesting a "congenital" etiology.

In the pediatric population, the most common cause of strictures is previous hypospadias repair and in one series [22] was responsible for 40% of cases. Other etiologies include idiopathic in 18%, postinstrumentation in 12%, traumatic in 10%, and the remaining following surgery for ano rectal malformation (ARM), pelvic radiation, balanitis xerotica obliterans (BXO), and posterior urethral valves (PUV) ablation.

Surgical techniques and outcomes

The time-honored method of treatment is urethral dilatation, which stretches the stricture and more commonly disrupts it. An alternative treatment with an equally long history is a urethrotomy. Initially this was performed blindly but with the development of endoscopic instrumentation is now carried out under vision. It is now widely accepted that both dilatation and urethrotomy are equally effective and can cure up to 50% of short bulbar strictures when first used. Alternatives such as laser urethrotomy, indwelling urethral stents, or intermittent self-catheterization are not curative and of these only self-catheterization is occasionally helpful.

If instrumentation is required more frequently or is complicated then a urethroplasty is the only curative option.

Excision and end-to-end anastomosis or anastomotic urethroplasty is the best option for short strictures, 1–2 cm long of traumatic or idiopathic origin in the bulbar or membranous urethra. For all other locations or recurrent strictures >2 cm in length, a substitution urethroplasty is the procedure of choice. A stricturotomy and patch graft (foreskin, posterior auricular Wolfe graft, or buccal mucosa) is more successful than excision and circumferential repair, and in situations where excision of the stricture becomes necessary, a two-stage repair is a more successful and reliable option [23].

Outcome of visual internal urethrotomy

Table 14.2 Outcomes of visual internal urethrotomy for urethral stricture.

Author	Number (n)	Success (%)	Follow-up (month)
Kirsch et al. [22]	40	50	24
Stormont et al. [24]	199	68	42
Pansadoro and Emiliozzi [25]	224	32	60
Heyns et al. [26]	163	39	24
Gonzalez et al. [27]	37	21	?

Complications of visual internal urethrotomy

Well-recognized complications of internal urethrotomy include:
1 Bleeding
2 Fever
3 Epididymitis
4 Incontinence

Table 14.3 Incidence of complications of visual internal urethrotomy.

Author	Number (n)	Complication rate (%)
Kirsch et al. [22]	40	04
Stormont et al. [24]	199	18
Smith et al. [28]	?	27
Muller et al. [29]	937	6.7

In the adult literature, serious complications like erectile dysfunction, rectal perforation, and chordee have been described [30,31].

Conclusion

Visual internal urethrotomy is a minimally invasive procedure associated with a cure rate of approximately 50% in carefully selected cases.

The best results are achieved in short-segment idiopathic bulbar strictures with a low-associated complication rate.

If a patient develops a recurrent stricture following a urethrotomy, however long the interval, further instrumentation is rarely curative. Similarly, penile or long-segment strictures are rarely cured by urethrotomy. In these situations it is best to proceed to a urethroplasty early.

Endoscopic management of ureteroceles

Introduction

The aim in ureterocele management is prevention of renal damage secondary to obstruction (with or without the associated comorbidity of VUR and urinary infections). The treatment should at the same time maintain continence and minimize surgical morbidity. Endoscopic puncture is minimally invasive, can achieve definitive decompression or act as a temporizing procedure that reduces the risk of infection and has the potential to allow recovery of renal function.

It is generally accepted that endoscopic puncture of the ureterocele is a definitive procedure in children with a single nonrefluxing system with an intravesical ureterocele.

The management of children with ectopic ureteroceles and ureteroceles associated with duplex systems is controversial, with management strategies ranging from periodic follow-up to open ablative and reconstructive surgery.

Surgical techniques and outcomes

Montfort and associates [32] described endoscopic ureterocele incision in 1985 and found that a small incision was less likely to cause reflux compared to the previous practice of deroofing the ureteroceles.

In 1994, ureterocele puncture was described which has supplanted incision to become the mainstay in the endoscopic management of ureteroceles.

The success rate of endoscopic management when assessed by the rate of decompression and subsequent urinary tract infections has been shown to be high although outcomes from some groups suggest that it is ineffective in preventing urinary infections. Endoscopic management is most successful in patients with intravesical single system ureteroceles. In children with ectopic ureteroceles associated with duplex systems, endoscopic puncture does not appear to be definitive, but it is successful in achieving decompression and minimizing the risk of urinary tract infections.

A recent meta-analysis of surgical practice in the endoscopic management of ureteroceles by Byun and Merguerian [33], where the outcome measure was secondary operation concluded:

1 Reoperation rate was significantly greater in patients with ectopic compared to intravesical ureteroceles.
2 A greater rate of reoperation in patients with duplex versus single system ureteroceles.
3 Presence of reflux preoperatively was associated with a significantly greater risk of reoperation.

The drawback of this meta-analysis is that the outcome measure of reoperation includes surgery for persistent reflux and a residual nonfunctioning decompressed upper moiety of a duplex system. The management of these clinical situations is varied and does not necessarily mandate further surgery.

Complications and their management

Inadequate decompression

Ureterocele management has moved from the extensive deroofing to the current precise puncture of the lesion in a dependent position. This approach can result in an inadequate opening, particularly in thick-walled ureteroceles, causing persistent obstruction. Antibiotic prophylaxis and a repeat ultrasound assessment 4–6 weeks following the procedure will minimize the risk and will help determine the need for further puncture.

VUR

Ipsilateral or contralateral VUR into the lower moiety may persist following ureterocele decompression and occasionally VUR into the decompressed moiety may develop following endoscopic intervention.

Asymptomatic VUR is not in itself an indication for further intervention and may be a reflection of the developmentally distorted anatomy at the trigone. Persistent VUR in association with recurrent breakthrough urinary tract infections or voiding dysfunction will determine the need for further surgery.

Voiding dysfunction

Voiding dysfunction occasionally develops following ureterocele puncture, particularly in association with large thin-walled ureteroceles. The distal lip can act as a flap valve to obstruct the bladder outlet during voiding. Treatment usually involves excision of the ureterocele, repair of any defect in the bladder wall with or without ureteric reimplantation.

With the more complex caecoureteroceles there may be associated bladder neck deficiency which results in urinary incontinence. They tend to occur in females and the trigone is grossly abnormal. Surgical intervention in such cases is indicated for continence and in addition to ureterocele excision and repair some form of bladder neck surgery is necessary in order to improve continence.

Conclusions

Endoscopic ureterocele puncture is an effective treatment modality for producing upper tract decompression and minimizing the risk of urinary tract infections. It is curative in the majority of single system intravesical ureteroceles and effectively decompresses a significant proportion of obstructed upper moieties of duplex systems so that no further interventions are necessary in carefully selected cases.

JJ stenting for primary obstructive megaureter

Introduction

The majority (up to 80%) of perinatally detected primary obstructive megaureters resolve spontaneously, hence conservative management with watchful waiting is considered a safe initial approach for this condition. An increasing number of these cases are detected on routine antenatal screening and can result in a clinical dilemma when associated with ipsilateral reduced renal function. The need to temporize bladder/trigone surgery before 1 year of age because of the fear of jeopardizing evolving bladder function further compounds the problem. External urinary diversion is a well-established temporizing measure but is not without problems. Stenosis, inadequate drainage, and the need for further surgery suggest the need to look for alternative treatment modalities. JJ stenting of the vesicoureteric junction (VUJ) is one such minimally invasive alternative to achieve temporary internal drainage.

Surgical techniques and outcomes

JJ stenting for symptomatic VUJ obstruction in infancy was reported in 1999. The limitation to endoscopic insertion in infancy is the calibre of the urethra and available instrumentation. 3F/12 cm length ureteric JJ stents are available (Rusch International, Germany) which are suitable for endoscopic insertion.

Indications for stenting include distal ureteric dilatation >10 mm, reduced differential renal function (≤40%), a drop in differential function, and an obstructive curve on diuretic renography.

The ureteric orifice and distal end of the ureter can be difficult to negotiate and conversion rates to open cystotomy, dilatation, and open insertion (of a larger 5F or 6F) of the stent are high.

In cases of bilateral megaureter, a single longer length (20–24 cm) stent can be used, with the looped ends up

the ureter and a short length of the straight segment forming a bridge between the ureteral orifices. Open insertion was necessary in 50% of cases in Grazia *et al.*'s [34] series and can be higher.

The stents are left in position for 6 (recommended) to 9 months and the urinary tract is periodically assessed with ultrasonography and isotope renography during this period. Antibiotic prophylaxis is recommended. Fifty percent of cases treated in this manner require no further intervention [34]. Morbidity associated with this approach has been reported as high as 70% due to stent-related complications.

Complications
- Breakthrough urinary infections
- Stent blockage/encrustations
- Bladder spasms
- Hematuria
- Fungal urinary tract infection

Management of complications

Careful monitoring with monthly ultrasonography for the first 3 months following stent insertion is prudent. Consideration must be given to synchronous circumcision with stent insertion in male patients. Ensuring a minimum amount of free tubing within the bladder will minimize bladder spasms. A high index of suspicion must be maintained when interpreting findings on ultrasound of debris within the collecting system, and urine must be examined for hyphae to rule out fungal infections. In the event of stent-related complications, early removal followed by either a diversion or reimplantation is warranted in the presence of ongoing obstruction.

Conclusions

JJ stent insertion across the VUJ can allow effective drainage in primary obstructive megaureters and in a proportion (up to 50% [34]) is curative.

There is some evidence to suggest that in those requiring subsequent reimplantation of the ureter, the need for ureteral tapering is obviated but the numbers are small.

The technique is associated with a high morbidity rate (up to 70% [34]) and a high rate of conversion to an open insertion method.

Given the high spontaneous resolution rate in primary obstructive megaureter and the high complication rate associated with stenting, its use should be restricted to carefully selected cases that are very critically monitored following placement of the stent.

The technique's potential to decrease the need for ureteral tapering needs further evaluation.

Botox® injections for neurogenic bladder dysfunction

Introduction
Neurogenic bladder and bowel dysfunction is present in a large proportion of children with neural tube defects and caudal regression syndrome. Detrusor overactivity, impaired bladder compliance, and detrusor sphincter dysynergia are responsible for deterioration in renal function and early management in these patients remains controversial. It is generally agreed that aim of urological management in these children is preservation of the upper tracts in infancy and early childhood and the subsequent attainment of urinary continence in later life. The management of the hostile bladder is varied, ranging from anticholinergic medication with or without clean intermittent catheterisation (CIC), urinary diversion (vesicostomy), to bladder augmentation with a catheterisable channel to aid bladder emptying. Of these, anticholinergic medication is the least invasive and reversible of the options and is the preferred first choice by both patients and physicians.

However, problems arise when nonsurgical treatment fails. Approximately 10% of patients are nonresponders to anticholinergic medications and a further proportion develop side effects to these drugs even when administered intravesically. Restoring safe bladder dynamics in these patients has thus far been achieved by bladder enlargement surgery until the publication of encouraging reports describing the beneficial effects of Botulinum-A toxin into the hyper-reflexive detrusor in adults with spinal cord injuries.

Surgical techniques and outcomes
Botox® in the dose of 10 IU/kg (maximum 300 IU) or Dysport® in the dose of 40 IU/kg (maximum 1200 IU) is injected submucosally into the detrusor muscle, at multiple sites sparing the trigone. The effect usually lasts for 9–12 months and can be repeated if necessary.

Evaluation of outcomes in the limited studies published in children so far suggests significant subjective and objective benefits as evidenced by:
- Decrease in detrusor overactivity
- Increase in bladder compliance

- Increase bladder capacity
- Reduction in detrusor voiding pressures

In addition one study has noted a significant improvement in bowel symptoms in 66% of the patients treated [35].

Complications
Early reports suggest that this is a safe treatment with a small risk of hematuria and urinary infection. Urinary retention is a theoretical possibility and patients are counselled regarding the need for intermittent catheterization.

Conclusions
Preliminary results suggest Botulinum-A toxin to be a safe alternative in the management of neurogenic bladder dysfunction and the improvements demonstrated in urodynamic parameters and continence are encouraging [36]. There is some suggestion that this may have beneficial effects on bowel function and needs further validation.

The unanswered question is whether or not repeat injections provide long-term relief without the development of an antibody response to repeated exposure, and if so this treatment holds promise in carefully selected cases. If shown to be safe in the long-term, an extended application will be in the treatment of resistant nonneurogenic bladder dysfunction.

References

1 Whitaker RH, Keeton JE, Williams DI. Posterior urethral valves: A study of urinary control after operation. *J Urol* 1972;108:167–71.
2 Myers DA, Walker RD. Prevention of urethral strictures in the management of posterior urethral valves. *J Urol* 1981;126:655–7.
3 Williams DI, Whitaker RH, Barratt TM, Keeton JE. Urethral valves. *Br J Urol* 1973;45:200–10.
4 Whitaker RH, Sherwood T. An improved hook for destroying posterior urethral valves. *J Urol* 1986;135:531–2.
5 Hendren WH. A new approach to infants with severe obstructive uropathy: Early complete reconstruction. *J Peditar Surg* 1970;5:184–99.
6 Diamond DA, Ransley PG. Fogarty balloon catheter ablation of neonatal posterior urethral valves. *J Urol* 1987;137:1209–11.
7 Cromie WJ, Cain MP, Bellinger MF, Betti JA, Scott J. Urethral valve incision using a modified venous valvulotome. *J Urol* 1994;151:1053–5.
8 Abraham MK. Mohan's urethral valvotome: A new instrument. *J Urol* 1990;144:1196–8.

9 Zaontz MR, Firlit CF. Percutaneous antegrade ablation of posterior urethral valves in premature or underweight term neonates: An alternative to primary vesicostomy. *J Urol* 1985;134:139.

10 Gibbons MD, Koontz WW, Smith MJV. Urethral strictures in boys. *J Urol* 1979;121:217.

11 Nijman RJM, Scholtmeijer RJ. Complications of transurethral electro-incision of posterior urethral valves. *Br J Urol* 1991;67:324–6.

12 Lal R, Bhatnagar V, Mitra DK. Urethral strictures after fulguration of posterior urethral valves. *J Ped Surg* 1998;33:518–9.

13 Crooks KK. Urethral strictures following transurethral resection of posterior urethral valves. *J Urol* 1982;127:1153–4.

14 Churchill BM, Krueger RP, Fleisher MH, Hardy BE. Complications of posterior urethral valve surgery and their prevention. *Urol Clin North Am* 1983;10:519–30.

15 Sarkis P, Robert M, Lopez C, Veyrec C, Guiter J, Averous M. Obstructive anuria following fulguration of posterior urethral valves and foley catheter drainage of the bladder. *Br J Urol* 1995;76:664–5.

16 Parkhouse HF, Barratt TM, Dillon MJ, Duffy PG, Fay J, Ransley PG, Woodhouse CR, Williams DI. Long term outcome of boys with posterior urethral valves. *Br J Urol* 1988;62:59–62.

17 De Gennaro M, Capitanucci ML, Silveri M, Morini FA, Mosiello G. Detrusor hypocontractility evolution in boys with posterior urethral valves detected by pressure flow analysis. *J Urol* 2001;165:2248–52.

18 Holmdahl G, Sillen U, Bachelard M, Hansson E, Hermansson G, Hjälmås K. Bladder dysfunction in boys with posterior urethral valves before and after puberty. *J Urol* 1996;155:694–8.

19 Payabvash S, Kajbafzadeh AM. Results of prospective clinical trial comparing concurrent valve ablation/bladder neck incision (BNI) with simple valve ablation in children with posterior urethral valve posterior urethral valves (PUV). J Pediatr Urol 2007;3:S36–S37.

20 McLellan DL, Gaston MV, Diamond DA, Lebowitz RL, Mandell J, Atala A, Bauer SB. Anterior urethral valves and diverticula in children: A result of ruptured Cowper's duct cyst? *BJU Int* 2004;94:375–8.

21 Van savage JG, Khoury AE, McLorie GA, Bägli DJ. An algorithm for the management of anterior urethral valves. *J Urol* 1997;158:1030–2.

22 Hsiao KC, Baez-Trinidad L, *et al.* Direct vision internal urethrotomy for the treatment of pediatric urethral strictures: Analysis of 50 patients. *J Urol* 2003;170:952–5.

23 Mundy AR. Management of urethral strictures. *Postgrad Med J* 2006;82:489–93.

24 Stormont TJ, Suman VJ, Osterling JE. Newly diagnosed bulbar urethral strictures: Etiology and outcome of various treatments. *J Urol* 1993;150:1725.

25 Pansadoro V, Emiliozzi P. Internal urethrotomy in the management of anterior urethral strictures: Long term follow up. *J Urol* 1996;156:73.

26 Heyns CF, Steenkamp JW *et al.* Treatment of male urethral strictures: Is repeated dilatation or internal urethrotomy useful? *J Urol* 1998;160:356.

27 Duel BP, Barthold JS, Gonzalez R. Management of urethral strictures after hypospadias repair. *J Urol* 1998;160:170–1.

28 Smith PJ, Robert JB, Ball AJ, Kaisary AV. Long term results of optical urethrotomy. *Br J Urol* 1983;55:698.

29 Albers P, Fichtner J *et al.* Long term results of internal urethrotomy. *J Urol* 1996;156:1611–4.

30 Inversen Hansen R, Guldberg O, Moller I. Internal urethrotomy with the Sachse urethrotome. *Scand J Urol Nephrol* 1981;15:189.

31 McDermott DW, Bates RJ, Heney NM, Althausen A. Erectile impotence as complication of direct vision cold knife urethrotomy. *Urology* 1981;18:467.

32 Montfort G, Morisson-Lacombe G *et al.* Simplified treatment of ureterocoeles. *Chir Pediatr* 1985;26:26.

33 Byun E, Merguerian PA. A meta-analysis of surgical practice patterns in the endoscopic management of ureterocoeles. *J Urol* 2006;176:1871–7.

34 Castagnetti M, Cimador M, Sergio M, De Grazia E. Double-J stent insertion across vesicoureteral junction – Is it a valuable initial approach in neonates and infants with severe primary nonrefluxing megaureter? *Urology* 2006;68:870–5.

35 Kajbafzadeh AM, Moosavi S, Tajik P, Arshadi H, Payabvash S, Salmasi AH, Akbari HR, Nejat F. Intravesical injection of Botulinum Toxin type A: Management of neuropathic bladder and bowel dysfunction in children with myelomeningocoele. *Urology* 2006;68:1091–6.

36 Riccabona M, Koen M, Schindler M, Goedele B, Pycha A, Lusuardi L, Bauer SB. Botulinum-A Toxin injection into the detrusor: A safe alternative in the treatment of children with myelomeningocoele with detrusor hyperreflexia. *J Urol* 2004;171:845–8.

15

Vesicoureteric Reflux

Christian Radmayr

Key points

- Endoscopic treatment is an option when dealing with vesicoureteric reflux.
- Endoscopic treatment has an excellent safety profile and is a simple outpatient procedure.
- Success rates of 79% after single use are achievable depending on different substances and injection techniques.
- Success rates decrease with increasing reflux grade.

- For higher reflux grades multiple treatments may be necessary.
- Long-term follow-up data up to 7.5 years after successful injection prove the durability of therapy.
- Endoscopic treatment is an option for duplex systems, neuropathic bladders, after initial treatment failure, or even after failed open reimplantation.

Introduction

For more than two decades, subureteric injection for treating vesicoureteric reflux (VUR) has been used as an alternative to conventional open surgical therapy [1]. A variety of agents have been used to correct VUR; these include: *polytetrafluoroethylene, cross-linked bovine collagen, synthetic calcium hydroxyapatite ceramic, autologous chondrocytes,* and *polydimethylsiloxane.* But following the approval of dextranomer/hyaluronic acid copolymer (Dx/HA) as a bulking agent by the Food and Drug Administration (FDA) in 2001, the interest in the endoscopic management of VUR has become increasingly popular. The minimally invasive nature of the procedure and the encouraging results make it a very attractive alternative to either prolonged antibiotic prophylaxis or open surgery [2].

Surgical techniques

Transurethral subureteric injection

The standard method for endoscopic treatment of VUR was originally developed and described in by Matouschek

more than 25 years ago [3]. Following this initial experience tetrafluoroethylene paste was introduced by O'Donnell and Puri and clinically popularized [4]. However, concerns regarding particle migration [4] arose and this substance never gained FDA approval. In this procedure the implant is placed underneath the ureteric orifice in the bladder creating a bolus, which lengthens the submucosal tunnel of the ureter and may additionally serve as a fixation point as well [5]. This procedure is carried out with the child in lithotomy position under general anesthesia. A routine 9.5 french pediatric cystoscope with a working channel is mandatory. Under direct vision the needle enters the submucosal space approximately 2–3 mm distal to the refluxing orifice at the 6 o'clock position and the needle is moved forward approximately 4–5 mm while injecting the bolus.

After successful injection a bulge appears in the floor of the ureter and the orifice looks volcano shaped with the ureteral entering in a sickle-shaped contour. No postoperative urine drainage is necessary and the child can be discharged the same day after voiding spontaneously.

Hydrodistension implantation technique

Using the hydrodistension technique the bulking agent is placed differently using the flow of water from the cystoscope to distend the very distal part of the ureter. The substance is placed submucosally but within the

Pediatric Urology: Surgical Complications and Management. Edited by Duncan T. Wilcox, Prasad P. Godbole and Martin A. Koyle. © 2008 Blackwell Publishing, ISBN: 978-1-4051-6268-5.

ureteric tunnel. With this modification the whole floor of the intravesical ureter is lifted up and subsequently the injected bolus leads to a complete cooptation of the intravesical ureter [6, 9]. With this sort of intraureteral injection combined with hydrodistension, a success rate of 90% or even higher for each reflux grade is reported in the short term, which is only slightly lower than the results for ureteral reimplantation. But this series represents a single center's experience only and it still has to be proven by other institutions as well as in the long term.

A study comparing the hydrodistension technique with the original subureteric injection method revealed a success rate of 89% versus 71% 3 months postoperatively as proven by standard voiding cystourethrogram. This difference in outcome is statistically significant with a p-value of less than 0.05 [10].

Outcome after subureteral injection in single systems

A meta-analysis [3] on reflux resolution after endoscopic therapy revealed a resolution rate following a single injection in children without ureteral duplication or neuropathic bladder of 67.1%, irrespective of grade or bulking agent. In these studies with a total population of 882 patients, polytetrafluoroethylene, collagen, dextranomer, polydimethylsiloxane, and chondrocytes were used as bulking agents. When calculating success rates by ureters (total number of ureters was 2450), the resolution rate was higher at 75.7%. When analyzed by reflux grade success of endoscopic therapy was highest at 78.5% for grades I and II, intermediate for grade III reflux (72%), and progressively lower for grades IV (63%) and V reflux (51%), respectively (Figure 15.1).

The long-term results are available for polytetrafluoroethylene with a published follow-up period of 10–16 years [7] with a total of 258 children (205 girls, 53 boys) with a total of 393 ureters treated and an age range from 3 months to 14 years (mean age 5.1 years). All children had high-grade reflux (grades III–V). One hundred and twenty-nine were bilateral, 92 unilateral, and 37 refluxing duplex systems with 6 of these bilateral, respectively. Complete reflux resolution after the first injection comprised a total of 76.8% with a further cessation of VUR after the second injection in additional 13.5% (Figure 15.2).

Multicenter studies of subureteral teflon injections in a large series of 8332 children (12,251 refluxing ureters) with 41 centers worldwide involved a reflux cessation rate of 75.3% (according to affected ureters) after single injection and an additional 12% after second injection and a supplementary 2% after three or four injections [8].

A series using synthetic calcium hydroxyapatite reported a resolution rate of 24 out of 74 patients at 1 and 2 years (32%). Ureteral resolutions were 46% and 40% at 1 and 2 years, respectively. But with 35 patients treated and 85% compliance with the required 2-year voiding cystourethrogram, the primary center achieved 2-year cure rates of 66% of patients and 72% of ureters [6].

Concerning outcome after single injection using the modified technique with intraureteral injection combined with hydrodistension, a success rate of 90% or even higher for each grade (I–V) is reported, which is indeed only slightly lower than the results for open reimplantation procedures [10]. The question is whether these outstanding results can be proven at other centers as well in a prospective multicenter setting and whether these results are durable.

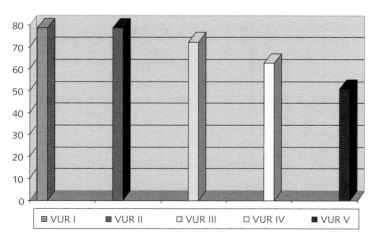

Figure 15.1 Reflux resolution after single injection for different reflux grades based on a meta-analysis. (Adapted from Elder [2].)

Altogether the published series are lacking important information in case of failure after first injection. Neither grades during the second injection are reported, nor intraoperative findings such as shifting or vanishing of the bulking agent. A possible assumption might be that there would be a tendency toward downstaging reflux grade during the second treatment course. The success with the second procedure was only 54.4%, compared to 67.1% for the first injection when patient resolution was assessed. In case the first two injections were unsuccessful, the published studies account a fairly low success rate for a third attempt at only 33.9% [3]. Of course according to that meta-analysis the aggregate success rate following 1, 2, or even 3 procedures was 85–87% when ureters and patients were analyzed. This outcome is certainly comparable to the favorable success rates of open reimplantation techniques with the disparity that it may take two or even three events under general anesthesia to achieve this outcome.

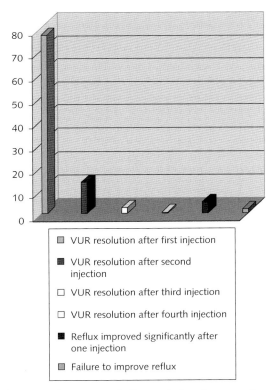

Figure 15.2 Percentages of reflux resolution after one and additional injections in a total of 393 ureters treated with polytetrafluoroethylene. (Adapted from Puri [8].)

Outcome in duplicated systems

The entity of complete ureteral duplication and associated high-grade VUR (IV and V) is related to a definitively lower spontaneous resolution rate than compared to those with a single collecting system [9], whereas in children with low-grade reflux and a duplicated collecting system the available published data are contradictory [10]. A meta-analysis clearly pointed out a significantly lower success rate for a duplicated system following a single injection compared to a single system [3]. Perhaps the altered ureteral anatomy in patients with a duplicated system can cause technical difficulties that may lead to shifting or malpositioning of the bulking agent [11].

A published series, using Teflon, investigated 43 patients with duplex systems. All patients had lower pole reflux and 29 also had upper pole reflux. After 2–8 years' follow-up they reported a success rate of 87% with a single injection [12]. Other series with the use of that bulking agent showed similar results with over two-thirds of complete resolution rate and almost 90% downstaging of reflux grade after one injection with a follow-up of 2 years [13].

Outcome in neuropathic bladders

Reflux in children with neuropathic bladder is unlikely to resolve spontaneously, with significantly lower resolution rates than in normal bladders [3]. Such bladders are often noncompliant with a thickened bladder wall and a high detrusor pressure. Of course reflux can be partially controlled by various bladder decompression procedures, but despite that it rarely resolves spontaneously. Endoscopic treatment has also become popular in these cases although significant detrusor fibrosis may sometimes cause difficulties in achieving proper placement of the bulking material. Some authors report that subureteral placement of the material has not been possible because the orifices could not be identified due to severe trabeculation [14]. Moreover, continuing high detrusor pressure might add to displacement of the injected material. Therefore, it is recommended to maintain a low intravesical pressure generally by using anticholinergics and clean intermittent catheterization. Another important aspect is that neuropathic bladders are potentially infected. Consequently antibiotic prophylaxis is another tool to achieve a proper outcome. Unfortunately in a meta-analysis, the attempt to analyze the results of endoscopic treatment in this particular patient population was ineffective due to insufficient data [3]. Only single center experiences with the use of Teflon are available reporting success rates of 55% and above after a single injection. However, recurrence has been as high as 30% in some series [15,16].

Outcome after initial treatment failure

Failures of endoscopic treatment are still seen in many patients; a repeat injection is considered before opting for an alternative treatment modality. A recently published single center series of 42 children with 37 girls and 5 boys and an age range from 18 months to 14 years reported a successful outcome in 35 of these children (83%) and in 47 of the total of 53 ureters (89%) treated, respectively using the hydrodistension implantation technique and dextranomer/hyaluronic acid as bulking agent. Ureteral success as categorized by preoperative VUR grade was 88% for grade I, 92% for grade II, and 85% for grade III [17] (Figure 15.3). Interestingly in this series the most common finding noted on repeat cystoscopy was caudal migration of the implant. The authors concluded that material migration might be secondary to bladder contractions or, more likely, ureteral peristalsis

although the real causes might be multifactoral and are still not clearly understood.

Outcome of endoscopic treatment for persisting reflux after ureteral reimplantation

Patients with previously failed open ureteral reimplantation usually have the same treatment options as for newly diagnosed children with VUR including observation with antibiotic prophylaxis, open redo procedures, and suburethral injection of bulking agents. The recurrence rate of VUR after open ureteroneocystostomy is approximately 2–4% [18]. Reoperation in failed reimplanted ureters is a major undertaking associated with a significant morbidity [19]. A meta-analysis exposed a success rate of 65% in these cases of persisting postoperative reflux with only one injection [3]. Unfortunately, the reviewed articles lacked the information on the different reimplantation techniques used.

A recently published single center experience using dextranomer/hyaluronic acid in 12 patients with 14 refluxing ureters stratified their heterogeneous patient population [20]. Before open ureteroneocystostomy three ureters had a grade V reflux, three had an associated ureterocele, one had prior open ureteroneocystostomy, and one had an associated neurogenic bladder secondary to caudal regression syndrome. Nine of these ureters were implanted using the Politano-Leadbetter technique, two using the Glenn-Anderson technique, and one using the Cohen crosstrigonal technique. Additionally, ureteral tapering was necessary for two ureters and common sheath reimplantation for a total of four ureters. Only nine patients with a total of 10 ureters were available for adequate follow-up. Ureteral success was reported in 7 out of 10 ureters after the initial injection. Of the three failed ureters reflux grade was unchanged in one, downgraded in another one, and resolved ipsilateral but new contralateral reflux in the remaining one. The authors conclude that considering the difficulties inherent in repeat surgery and the high success rate of dextranomer/hyaluronic acid injection, this alternative treatment is an appealing and reasonable option for patients failing open surgery.

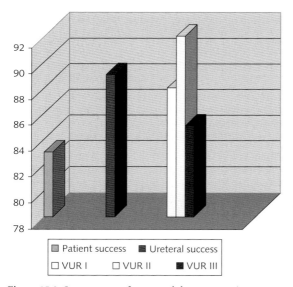

Figure 15.3 Success rates after second dextranomer/hyaluronic acid injection in percentages for patients, ureters, and according to preoperative reflux grades. (Adapted from Elmore [17].)

Complications

So far there have been no product-related serious adverse events encountered independent of the injected material.

Polytetrafluoroethylene as well as polydimethylsiloxane have possible migration potentials as described in several animal studies [4,5]. But so far no clinical data are available on children treated with these substances.

Urinary tract infections

In a long-term survey of 228 treated children, the frequency of a urinary tract infection was as low as 8% (19/228) after the injection of dextranomer/hyaluronic acid. But only one case of urinary tract infection was directly related to the treatment itself, whereas the remaining happened more than 3 months after the procedure till the end of the follow-up period of a total of 6 years [21].

Ureteral obstruction

Postoperative obstruction is a concern since occlusion of the orifice is a major goal in the treatment procedure. This may lead to postoperative flank pain in the affected children. With the use of dextranomer/hyaluronic acid an incidence of 4% was reported, but all of them were self-limiting without any need for intervention [9,10,25]. So far only a single case of a ureteral stenosis after injection of dextranomer/hyaluronic acid has been reported in the literature. In this particular case, it remained unclear whether this was due to the injected material itself since the treated refluxing ureter was a dysmorphic ureter anyway [22].

In the long-term follow-up in a series of 258 children with high-grade (grades III–V) reflux treated with subureteral polytetrafluoroethylene injections, only one obstruction occurred [11]. This patient was readmitted to hospital because of severe unilateral ureteral obstruction the day after bilateral subureteric injection of polytetrafluoroethylene for grade IV reflux. A ureteral stent had to be placed for 5 consecutive days till the edema at the ureterovesical junction subsided. A long-term follow-up voiding cystourethrogram of this patient 9 years later revealed no reflux and no obstruction.

De novo contralateral reflux

Contralateral *de novo* reflux after endoscopic treatment occurs in about 10–32% [23]. It has been suggested that surgical distortion of the contralateral trigone during the procedure or the elimination of a low-pressure pop-off mechanism from the bladder may result in contralateral neoreflux. In a series of 495 children treated with polytetrafluoroethylene with unilateral grades III–V reflux, 37 (7%) developed neocontralateral VUR after previous successful correction of VUR, with 40% of these occurring within the first 3 months [11]. Another study of 134 children treated unilaterally with dextranomer/hyaluronic acid revealed a *de novo* contralateral reflux incidence of 4.5% (6/134), 3 months after the injection [9,10]. These two studies suggest that if this phenomenon of new onset contralateral reflux is due to a pop-off mechanism, then the incidence would be similar in both open surgical and endoscopic techniques; however, the lower incidence with injection procedures suggests that trigonal distortion during open surgery is the more likely mechanism [24].

Concerning technical skills the learning curve with either injection technique (conventional subureteral injection or modified intraureteral injection combined with hydrodistension) has to be taken into account. Available date clearly demonstrate that improvement in success to 70% with a single-treatment course is achievable after the first 20 cases. But to reach an improved outcome of 80% or even more a total of 100 cases is necessary [9]. This study clearly points out that any endoscopic intervention for treating VUR should be concentrated in centers with appropriate settings and numbers of cases. Especially in rather complicated cases like duplicated system, this is even more mandatory, since a published meta-analysis [3] ruled out a significantly lower success rate for endoscopic treatment of a refluxing duplicated system following a single injection compared to a single system.

Conclusions

Available data demonstrate that reflux resolution rate following endoscopic therapy is favorable, although it is lower compared to current reports of open surgical procedures. The AUA guidelines report and other contemporary reports supported the statistics of an overall success rate of almost 96% in children with VUR grades I–IV, a persistent reflux in 2%, and ureteral obstruction in 2% when treated with conventional open surgery [2,22]. In contrast a recently published meta-analysis of endoscopic therapy revealed resolution of reflux in 79% of ureters with grades I and II, 72% with grade III, and 65% with grade IV reflux following a single injection of a bulking agent [3]. Following one or more injections the ureteral success rate was 85% and 87% for patients, respectively.

With the introduction of a modified implantation technique using intraureteral injection of dextranomer/hyaluronic acid combined with hydrodistension, a success rate of up to 90% or even higher for each grade (I–IV) might be achievable, which is only slightly lower than the results for ureteral reimplantation [9,10].

It can be concluded that endoscopic subureteral injection of tissue augmenting substances has indeed become an established alternative to long-term antibiotic prophylaxis and surgical intervention in the management of children suffering from VUR. It is a simple outpatient procedure with an excellent safety profile, although technical skills as well as a distinct number of cases (learning curve) [9] are necessary to achieve the best possible outcome in terms of effectiveness and long-term successful results for the affected.

References

1 Puri P, Granata C. Multicenter surgery of endoscopic treatment of vesicoureteral reflux using polytetrafluoroethylene. *J Urol* 1998;160:1007.
2 Elder JS, Peters CA, Arant BS *et al.* Pediatric vesicoureteral reflux guidelines panel summary report on the management of primary vesicoureteral reflux in children. *J Urol* 1997;157:1846.
3 Matouschek E. New concept for the treatment of vesicoureteral reflux. Endoscopic application of teflon. *Arch Esp Urol* 1918;34:385.
4 O'Donnell B, Puri P. Treatment of vesicoureteric reflux by endoscopic injection of Teflon. *Br Med J* 1984;289:7.
5 Kirsch AJ, Perez-Brayfield MR, Scherz HC. Minimally invasive treatment of vesicoureteral reflux with endoscopic injection of dextranomer/hyaluronic acid copolymer: the Children's Hospitals of Atlanta experience. *J Urol* 2003;170:211.
6 Kirsch AJ, Perez-Brayfield M, Smith EA. The modified STING procedure to correct vesicoureteral reflux: Improved results with submucosal implantation within the intramural ureter. *J Urol* 2004;171:2413–16.
7 Puri P. Endoscopic treatment of vesicoureteral reflux. In *Pediatric Urology*, Edited by JP Gearhart, RC Rink, PDE Mouriquand. Philadelphia: W. B. Saunders Company, 2001: pp. 411–20.
8 Puri P, Granata C. Multicenter survey of endoscopic treatment of vesicoureteral reflux using polytetrafluoroethylene. *J Urol* 1998;160:1007–1011.
9 Afshar K, Papanikolaou F, Malek R *et al.* Vesicoureteral reflux and complete ureteral duplication. Conservative or surgical management. *J Urol* 2005;173:1725.
10 Lee PH, Diamond DA, Duffy PG *et al.* Duplex reflux: A study of 105 children. *J Urol* 1991;146:657.
11 Perez-Brayfield M, Kirsch AJ, Hensle TW *et al.* Endoscopic treatment with dextranomer/hylauronic acid for complex cases of vesicoureteral reflux. *J Urol* 2004;172:1614.
12 Miyakita H, Ninan GK, Puri P. Endoscopic correction of vesicoureteric reflux in duplex systems. *Eur Urol* 1993;24:111–15.
13 Dewan PA, O'Donnell B. Polytef paste injection of refluxing duplex ureters. *Eur Urol* 1991;19:35–8.
14 Engel JD, Palmer LS, Cheng EY. Surgical versus endoscopic correction of vesicoureteral reflux in children with neurogenic bladder dysfunction. *J Urol* 1997;157:2291–4.
15 Misra D, Potts SR, Brown S *et al.* Endoscopic treatment of vesicoureteric reflux in neurogenic bladder – 8 years experience. *J Pediatr Surg* 1996;31:1262–4.
16 Puri P, Guiney EJ. Endoscopic correction of vesicoureteric reflux secondary to neuropathic bladder. *Br J Urol* 1986;58:504–06.
17 Elmore JM, Scherz HC, Kirsch AJ. Dextranomer/Hyaluronic acid for vesicoureteral reflux: Success rates after initial treatment failure. *J Urol* 2006;175:712–15.
18 Barrieras D, Lapointe S, Reddy PP *et al.* Are postoperative studies justified after extravesical ureteral reimplantation? *J Urol* 2000;164:1064.
19 Mesrobian HGJ, Kramer SA, Kelalis PP. Reoperative ureteroneocystostomy: Review of 69 patients. *J Urol* 1985;133:388.
20 Jung C, DeMarco RT, Lowrance WT *et al.* Subureteral injection of dextranomer/hyaluronic acid copolymer for persistent vesicoureteral reflux following ureteroneocystostomy. *J Urol* 2007;177:312–15.
21 Läckgren G, Wahlin N, Sköldenberg E *et al.* Long-term follow-up of children treated with dextranomer/hyaluronic acid copolymer for vesicoureteral reflux. *J Urol* 2001;166:1887–92.
22 Snodgrass WT. Obstruction of a dysmorphic ureter following dextranomer/hyaluronic acid copolymer. *J Urol* 2004;171:395–6.
23 Diamond DA, Rabinowitz R, Hoenig DM *et al.* The mechanism of new onset contralateral reflux following unilateral ureteroneocystostomy. *J Urol* 1996;156:665–7.
24 Kumar R, Puri P. Newly diagnosed contralateral reflux following successful endoscopic correction. Is it due to a pop off mechanism? *J Urol* 1997;158:1213–15.

Interventional Procedures

Korgun Koral

16

Key points

- Communication between the interventional radiologist and urologist is key to successful procedures.

- General anesthesia is necessary for many of the procedures.

- Percutaneous nephrostomy technique is different in newborns and young infants than it is in older children and adults.

- If an interventional radiologist is involved in gaining access for percutaneous nephrolithotripsy, it usually saves time and decreases the radiation dose to gain access in the angiography suite and move the patient to the operating room.

A pediatric interventional radiologist can play a role in the management of a child before, during, or after a surgical intervention. A good working relationship between the surgeon and radiologist is essential to maximize patient care.

Patient preparation

Prior to the procedures, coagulation parameters and platelet count are assessed to determine the risk of bleeding. Procedures are not performed if the platelet count is <50,000 per milliliter or International Normalized Ratio is greater than 1.5. For procedures that require percutaneous access, if the patient has urosepsis, intravenous (IV) broad spectrum antibiotics may be given. Alternatively, if there is no urosepsis 1 h prior to the procedure, 40–50 mg/kg of IV cefazolin may be administered [1].

Sedation and general anesthesia

Many relatively short pediatric urinary interventional procedures can be performed with IV sedation [2].

Pediatric Urology: Surgical Complications and Management. Edited by Duncan T. Wilcox, Prasad P. Godbole and Martin A. Koyle. © 2008 Blackwell Publishing, ISBN: 978-1-4051-6268-5.

When available, general anesthesia is certainly preferable over sedation, as the radiologist can concentrate solely on the procedure. For longer procedures and for procedures that require absolute immobilization general anesthesia is mandatory.

Procedures

There are many common steps in percutaneous interventional procedures. The percutaneous access will be described in detail in the percutaneous nephrostomy (PN) section.

Percutaneous nephrostomy

PN is an established technique for urinary diversion that is occasionally used in children [3]. The most common indications for PN in children are listed in Table 16.1. Performance of PN procedure presents unique difficulties in the newborns and young children.

The patient is placed prone with the side in interest raised approximately 20–30° from the horizontal plane. The posterior aspect of the kidney has an area of relative avascularity (Broedel's line), which is preferred for placement of needles and catheters [4]. A subcostal approach aimed at puncture of an inferior calyx is preferred. If subsequent placement of a stent is contemplated, a more cranial calyx approach may be performed so that the

Table 16.1 Common indications for percutaneous nephrostomy in children.

Bilateral UPJ obstruction
Unilateral UPJ obstruction of a single functioning kidney
Obstruction after pyeloplasty
Urolithiasis
Ureterovesical junction obstruction
Posterior urethral valves
Primary obstructing megaureter
Pyonephrosis/fungus ball
Pelvic/retroperitoneal tumors
Trauma
Assessment of function in a cystic mass
Decompression of a cystic renal mass to facilitate surgical manipulation

angle from the renal pelvis to the ureter is more favorable. Inadvertent puncture of an anterior calyx may also impede subsequent wire and catheter manipulation [5]. For access prior to the percutaneous nephrolithotomy, the calyx or part of the pelvis harboring the stone is punctured. A direct renal pelvis puncture should be avoided because of increased risk of hemorrhage during manipulation. Ultrasound (US) guidance is preferred for access. The anesthesiologist may suspend respiration to help with immobilization of the kidney during puncture, but this is rarely necessary. Lidocaine or bupivacaine may be used for local anesthesia. Initial access is with a 22-gauge needle Chiba (Cook, Bloomington, Indiana) or Inrad (Inrad, Kentwood, Michigan) needle. It is relatively easy to visualize the echogenic needle in the hypoechoic collecting system. If a small vessel is inadvertently punctured, hyperechoic blood may accumulate in the collecting system. Return of urine ensures that the needle tip is in the collecting system. The remainder of the procedure is performed using fluoroscopy guidance. The entire procedure may be performed with US guidance, but this is not recommended as there is relatively poor control of the wires. Also, performing the procedure using only US guidance requires two very experienced operators. Fluoroscopy must be used as conservatively as possible with minimal exposure rates. A small amount of nonionic contrast material is administered to opacify the renal pelvis. Air should not be introduced during this step, because if access is lost inadvertently, presence of air in the collecting system will make ultrasonographic visualization very difficult. A 0.018-inch stainless steel wire is advanced through the needle into the renal pelvis.

It is desirable to advance the wire into the ureter to facilitate subsequent dilator and catheter manipulations. If ureter cannot be negotiated, the wire is coiled in the renal pelvis. A small skin incision is made at the puncture site. The needle is removed. Generally one must place a working wire (with a diameter equal or greater than 0.035 inch) in order to place a nephrostomy tube. Over the 0.018-inch wire either a micropuncture set (Cook) or a Neffset (Cook) is loaded. Neffset is preferred because it has a metallic stiffener, which has a superior robustness over micropuncture set as it traverses the tissues. Care must be taken not to bend the wire and not to advance the Neffset too much as it is loaded over the wire. The inner metallic dilator of the Neffset and the wire are removed. The outer dilator of Neffset is a 6 French tube, which accepts a 0.035-inch or 0.038-inch working wire. The outer dilator of the Neffset is removed. If an 8 French or larger catheter is going to be placed, the tract is dilated with fascial dilators. One must always be parallel to the path of the initial puncture as the dilators and nephrostomy tube are advanced over the wire to avoid bending the wire. The nephrostomy tube is loaded over the wire and advanced while the wire is held firmly. It is important to release the stiffener from the catheter when the tip of the catheter is in the renal pelvis. When the catheter is in the renal pelvis, the stiffener and the wire are removed. Contrast material is administered to document the position of the catheter and study the ureter. The string of the catheter is pulled and the tip of the catheter is locked. Usage of sutures to secure the catheter to skin is optional. There are special adhesive catheter holders (e.g. Statlock, Venetec, San Diego, California) to secure the catheter. Sterile dressings are applied over the catheter. The catheter is connected to drainage bag.

The described conventional technique works successfully in the great majority of the pediatric patients. However in the newborns and young infants who have very little urine in their dilated collecting systems, it may be difficult to perform a successful PN, because the small amount of urine may drain into the perirenal tissues during manipulation of wires and catheters. This is particularly true for newborns with ureteropelvic junction (UPJ) obstruction in whom placement of a wire into the ureter is problematic (Figure 16.1). The modified 2-step technique addresses this problem [6]. For newborns and young infants, the collecting system is punctured with an 18-gauge vascular needle (Merit, South Jordan, Utah). A 0.035-inch wire is advanced through the needle. Following a small skin incision the needle is removed and a 6 French Navarre (Bard, Covington, California) catheter is loaded over the wire and placed in the collecting

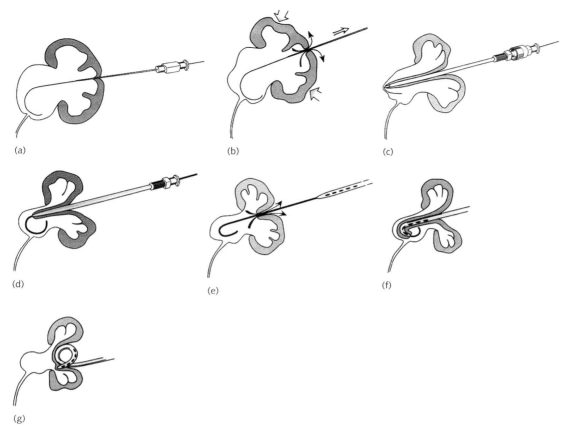

Figure 16.1 Proposed mechanism for failed micropuncture technique in a kidney with UPJ obstruction. (a) The collecting system is punctured with a 22-gauge micropuncture needle. (b) As the 0.018-inch wire is advanced through the micropuncture, needle decompression of the collecting system begins. (c) An attempt is made to place a micropuncture set. The thin renal parenchyma, which is very pliable, offers little resistance. The small collecting system and inability to negotiate the 0.018-inch wire into the ureter, which is usually the case in severe UPJ obstruction, result in incomplete placement of the micropuncture set. (d) As the 0.035-inch wire is advanced through the outer portion of the micropuncture set, the wire may or may not enter the collecting system. The figure shows the soft tip of the wire in the collecting system. (e) There is continuous decompression of the collecting system with each step. An attempt is made to place the nephrostomy tube over the 0.035-inch wire. (f) The catheter cannot be advanced into the collecting system because the wire cannot be negotiated into the ureter. The collecting system has nearly completely decompressed. On fluoroscopy, it is difficult to know whether the catheter is in the collecting system. (g) The wire is removed, leaving the nephrostomy tube outside the decompressed collecting system. There is usually a urinoma outside the kidney at this stage. (Reproduced from Koral *et al.* [6], with permission from the Society of Interventional Radiology.)

system. The tapered and relatively sharp tip of the Navarre catheter allows for penetration of the tissues without necessitating prior dilation.

Percutaneous nephrostomy in transplant kidney
Hydronephrosis can develop early or late following renal transplantation. The technique is the same as described for native kidneys, except for patient position (Figure 16.2).

An ultrasound transducer with greater resolution (i.e. higher MHz) may be used because of the decreased distance from the skin to the collecting system. The renal pelvis should be avoided during puncture.

The PN is not meant to be a definitive means of urinary diversion in children. The PN catheter should be kept in place as briefly as possible. It is generally not advisable to discharge pediatric patients with existing PN catheters.

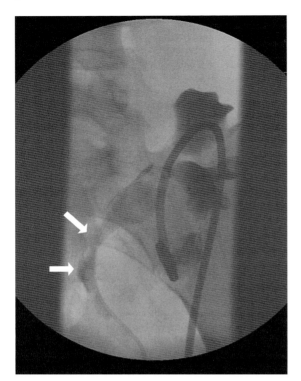

Figure 16.2 PN placement to a left lower quadrant transplant kidney. A calcified ureteric stent (arrows) is present.

Table 16.2 Complications of percutaneous nephrostomy.

Hemorrhage (into the pelvis or perirenal tissues)
Sepsis
Catheter dislodgement
Arteriovenous fistula (very rare)
Pseudoaneurysm (very rare)

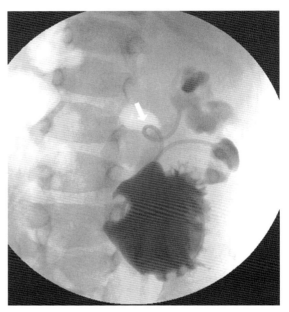

Figure 16.3 Six-year-old patient with solitary left kidney with duplicated collecting system. The patient had cloacal exstrophy and a neobladder. Double-J stents could not be placed cystoscopically. Two stents were placed. The upper stent's cranial coil (arrow) was not perfectly deployed, but it still served the purpose of identifying the ureterovesical junction at a later exploration.

The PN placement is a relatively safe procedure. In the general population the complication rate is reported to be around 4% [5]. Minimal discoloration of the urine due to a small amount of hemorrhage is expected and parents/patients should be informed about this prior to the procedure. The potential complications are listed in Table 16.2.

Ureteric stent placement/balloon ureteroplasty/stent retrieval

The indications for antegrade ureteric stent placement are usually limited to when placement of a retrograde ureteric stent is not possible or contraindicated. The stents are usually required in children following pyeloplasty or ureter resection and/or reimplantation. Ureteric stent placement is one of the most difficult procedures in pediatric interventional radiology. The difficulties stem from relatively small size of the renal pelvis and difficulty to work with small caliber stents. Also, the procedure includes a final step (the advancement of the pelvic loop

of the double-J stent) during which there is relatively little control (Figure 16.3).

The steps to obtain access are identical to those described under the section of PN. It is recommended that a safety wire (usually a 0.018 inch, 40 cm stainless steel wire) be placed, either from the same access site (a sheath has to be used for this) or from another puncture, in case access is lost during the procedure. The safety wire ensures access to the drained collecting system. Having a sheath in place also allows administration of contrast material into the system to study the anatomy. The access must be through a calyx from which the pelvis and ureter can be easily negotiated. A relatively more cranial calyx is preferred, but this is not mandatory if a favorable angle can be used through a lower calyx approach. To negotiate the ureter – if there is difficulty with a regular 0.018 wire – instead of using a glidewire which is relatively difficult to control, a V-18 control wire (Boston Scientific, Natick, Massachusetts) is preferred. V-18 control wire has a hydrophilic soft tip in addition to a relatively stiff body. If there is difficulty in negotiating the ureterovesical junction an angled glide catheter can be placed over the wire and a wire–catheter combination may be used. Through the catheter or through the sheath, the anatomy of the ureter is studied with administration of contrast material. If there is a significant narrowing of the ureterovesical junction, balloon ureteroplasty may be performed. Once the catheter is in the bladder (it is important to communicate with the surgeon and be familiar with the surgery, because a very long ureter tunnel in the bladder wall may generate the false appearance of intravesical position of the catheter tip, Figure 16.4) a 0.035 super stiff working wire (Amplatz, Cook) is exchanged with the V-18 control wire. The wire is coiled in the bladder. If balloon ureteroplasty is performed, a balloon that is at least 4 cm in length is preferred to ensure coverage of the stenotic segment (Figure 16.5). Appearance and resolution of the waist during inflation of the balloon indicate satisfactory coverage of the stenotic area and application of adequate pressure. The balloon is kept inflated for 30–60 s. The inflation may be repeated if necessary. Subsequently, the distance from the ureterovesical junction to the renal pelvis is measured using either the V-18 wire or the Amplatz wire. Placing a radiopaque ruler underneath the patient is also useful. The antegrade stents are identical to retrograde stents. The author's experience is with 4.7, 4.8, and 5 F double-J stents which can be loaded over Amplatz wires. In antegrade placement, the knot of the string is cut but the string is kept in place until final deployment. If a sheath is in place, the sheath is removed and over the Amplatz wire the stent is advanced with a pusher catheter. The bladder coil is formed first and Amplatz wire is withdrawn to ureter. Using the radiopaque marker of the stent, the operator judges the position of the cranial tip of the stent. The wire is pulled further into the renal pelvis as the stent is pushed. If the position of the upper coil is satisfactory, the strings are pulled and the wire is removed while the pusher is kept still. Then the pusher is also removed. It is prudent to place a nephrostomy tube using the safety wire at the end of the procedure because

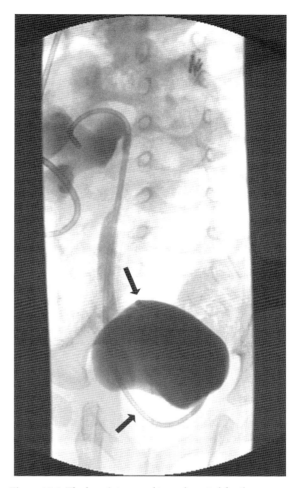

Figure 16.4 The long intramural tunnel created for the reimplanted ureter necessitates placement of a longer double-J stent (arrows).

local edema and hemorrhage may obstruct the ureter. The nephrostomy tube is kept open to bag drainage for 24 h and then closed. The patient is observed for 24 h for pain and fever while the tube is closed to drainage. If there are no complaints, before discharge, the nephrostomy tube is removed under fluoroscopy guidance utilizing a wire, so that the upper coil of the double-J stent remains intact in the renal pelvis. The retrieval of the stent is generally performed by the urologist with cystoscopy.

Very rarely, if removal of a stent is not feasible with cystoscopy, the interventional radiologist may remove the stent from the urethra using a snare catheter.

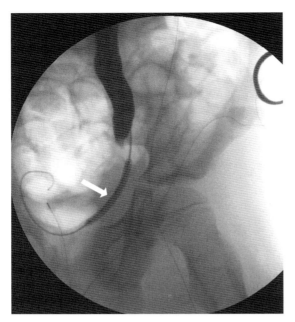

Figure 16.5 Ureteroplasty using 4 mm (caliber), 4 cm (length) angioplasty balloon (arrow) prior to the placement of a double-J stent.

If transurethral removal is not feasible, the collecting system is accessed and the catheter may be retrieved by capturing the cranial tip of the double-J stent. This is, in fact very difficult to achieve in a nondilated system. As a last resort one can advance the snare catheter through the ureter into the bladder and capture the distal end of the double-J stent and retrieve it (Figure 16.6).

Percutaneous fluid collection drainage

Fluid collections that require percutaneous drainage include postoperative urinomas, hematomas, abscesses, and lymphoceles. The diagnosis of the fluid collection is usually made with US or computerized tomography (CT). The author prefers to perform these procedure using US and fluoroscopy guidance, instead of CT guidance for two reasons: first, one can perform needle placement much faster and with greater accuracy using US guidance; second, fluoroscopy allows for real-time visualization of the needles and wires decreasing the likelihood of loss of access. Use of CT-fluoroscopy is controversial in children in whom exposure to ionizing radiation should be kept to a minimum.

Abscess drainage

Perirenal abscesses are rare in children and they rarely need to be drained. It must be kept in mind that not all fluid collections seen on CT are amenable to percutaneous

drainage. Due to lesser spatial resolution of CT compared to US, fine septae within a fluid collection may not be apparent. If multiple, these septa may make a successful drainage impossible. However, if specimen collection is the goal, presence of multiple septa will not impede the procedure. The patient is positioned depending on the location of the collection. For a collection around a native kidney, the patient is positioned prone with the side of the abnormality elevated approximately 20–30° similar to the position for PN. For collections around a transplant kidney the patient is kept supine. One should avoid marking the skin entry site with a pen, as one can inadvertently "tattoo" the skin while going through the mark. Depending on the size and appearance of the fluid collection a 22- or 18-gauge needle may be used. If the fluid collection is small and multiple passes are expected generally a 22-gauge Chiba needle is used for access. After access, the steps are identical to those of PN placement. If a drainage catheter of ≥8 French size is placed, then the tract is dilated with fascial dilators. For children, usually 8–10 French catheters are used for drainage. Drainage tubes larger than 12 French are generally avoided in children. Drainage catheters with metallic stiffeners are preferred. One can administer contrast material to identify the fluid collection, extrarenal position of the catheter, and check for inadvertent puncture of the collecting system of the kidney. US can be used to assess the position of the catheter tip in the fluid collection. One should try to aspirate as much fluid as possible during the procedure by manipulating the catheter. The specimen is sent for Gram stain and cultures. The drainage is intended to be by gravity. It is recommended that the catheter be flushed with 2–3 ml of saline daily to keep it patent. For abscesses and hematomas, it is rarely necessary to keep a drain longer than 3–4 days. If the drainage over 24 h is <2–3 ml, the drain is removed, usually after checking the resolution of the collection with US. Sedation is not necessary for removal of drainage catheters.

Urinoma/lymphocele drainage

Urinoma drainage is usually performed for diagnostic purposes. Using US guidance and a small needle (usually a 22 gauge) a sample is collected and sent for Gram stain, cultures, and creatine level. It is desirable to aspirate as much fluid as possible. To facilitate aspiration, for large collections, a vacuumed drainage container may be used. If the urinoma is large and is expected to reaccumulate, until definitive correction of the cause of the urinoma, a drain may be placed.

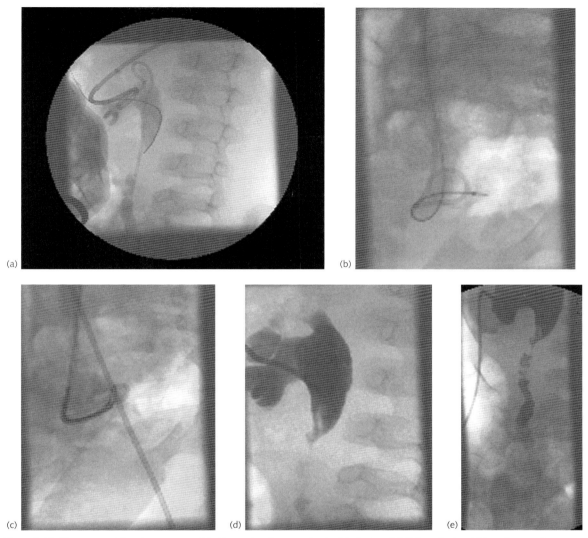

(a)

(b)

(c)

(d)

(e)

Figure 16.6 Three-year-old male status post-bladder exstrophy repair and reimplantation of the right ureter. The indwelling right double-J stent could not be removed cystoscopically. (a) The renal pelvis was accessed. The upper coil of the stent could not be captured with a snare catheter. The collecting system was not dilated enough for adequate deployment of the snare. (b) A PN catheter was placed. Through a different access site a V-18 wire was advanced into the ureter alongside the double-J stent. (c) Using a hydrophilic catheter–wire combination the bladder was catheterized. There was more room in the bladder to deploy the snare catheter. (d) The distal coil of the double-J stent was captured. (e) The double-J catheter was withdrawn into the renal pelvis and removed. The nephrostogram demonstrated no extravasation with passage of contrast material into the bladder.

Lymphoceles generally occur following renal transplantation. The access is generally for diagnostic purposes; if there is mass effect compromising renal function or reaccumulation occurs, a drainage catheter may be used.

Nephrolithotomy

The role of interventional radiology in percutaneous nephrolithotomy is primarily to acquire satisfactory access for the urologist. Percutaneous nephrolithotomy is indicated in children whose therapy with shock wave lithotripsy (SWL) or ureteroscopy (URS) has failed and in those who have anatomic abnormalities that impair urinary drainage and stone clearance [7,8].

The procedure can be performed in the operating room (OR) or in the angiography suite. In nondilated systems and patients with increased body fat, obtaining percutaneous access can be laborious. In the OR, portable C-arm fluoroscopy results in an increased dose of radiation both to the patient and the operator, due to inability to change the source–receptor distance and lack of shielding. Moreover, the image quality is inferior to that of a conventional fluoroscopy unit. Therefore, at the author's institution percutaneous nephrolithotomy procedures are performed in a staged fashion. Understandably, the urologist feels more comfortable in the OR. Access is obtained in the angiography suite by the radiologist by placement of a catheter into the calyx harboring the stone. An access that will facilitate advancement of a wire into the ureter should be obtained. If the nephrolithotomy is done on the same day, a security wire is advanced into the bladder from the same access site. Then the patient is transferred to OR while still under anesthesia. If the nephrolithotomy is not performed on the same day, the nephrostomy tube stays in place until the day of the procedure. Some urologists prefer placement of a nephroureterostomy tube, which is done by advancing the tip of the catheter into the bladder.

Whitaker test

To distinguish between an obstructive dilation of the renal collecting system from nonobstructed dilation, usually following pyeloplasty, Whitaker test is occasionally performed [5]. The procedure is performed under anesthesia because even minimal motion may alter the pressure recordings. The procedure is performed in the angiography suite under fluoroscopy. For access, US guidance and two 22-gauge Chiba needles are used. One needle is connected to contrast material infusion bag, the other to the pressure monitor. A Foley catheter is placed and connected to pressure monitor. This procedure is performed when the referring urologist is present.

If this is not possible, results should be communicated to the referring urologist before terminating the test, because the test may need to be tailored accordingly. To ensure accuracy of the measurements, one can change the tubings of the contrast material injection and pressure monitor without removing the needles. The final interpretation is made by the urologist.

Conclusion

In summary, pediatric interventional radiologist may play an important role in the management of children with urinary problems. A detailed discussion, regarding the indication and treatment plan, with the patient's family and urologist is of utmost importance prior to committing to a procedure.

References

1 Schmidt MB, James CA. Genitourinary intervention in children. *Sem Interv Radiol* 2002;19:51–7.
2 Mason KP, Michna E, DiNardo JA, Zurakowski D, Karian VE, Conner L, Burrows PE. Evolution of a protocol for ketamine-induced sedation as an alternative to general anesthesia for interventional radiologic procedures in pediatric patients. *Radiology* 2002;225:457–65.
3 Stanley P, Diament MJ. Pediatric percutaneous nephrostomy: Experience with 50 patients. *J Urol* 1986;135:1223–6.
4 Scatorchia GM, Berry RF. A review of renal anatomy. *Sem Interv Radiol* 2000;17:323–8.
5 Lee MJ. Percutaneous genitourinary intervention. In *The Requisites: Vascular and Interventional Radiology*. Edited by JA Kaufman, MJ Lee. Philadelphia: Mosby, 2004: pp. 602–35.
6 Koral K, Saker MC, Morello FP, Rigsby CK, Donaldson JS. Conventional versus modified technique for percutaneous nephrostomy in newborns and young infants. *J Vasc Interv Radiol* 2003;14:113–6.
7 Kroovand RL. Pediatric urolithiasis. *Urol Clin North Am* 1997;24:173–84.
8 Jackman SV, Hedican SP, Peters CA, Docimo SG. Percutaneous nephrolithotomy in infants and preschool children: Experience with a new technique. *Urology* 1998;52:697–701.

17

Minimally Invasive Interventions for Stone Disease

H. Serkan Dogan and Serdar Tekgül

Key points

- There are a variety of options to treat children with stone disease, namely extracorporeal shock wave lithotripsy (ESWL), ureteroscopy (URS), percutaneous nephrolithotomy (PCNL), and open surgery.

- Treatment is either by an individual modality or in combination and is tailored to each patient according to the size, location, and type of stone.

- ESWL is the principal treatment for patients with a single renal pelvis stone <20 mm, lower pole stones <10 mm, and upper ureteric stones.

- URS should be the first treatment choice for lower and middle ureteral stones.

- PCNL has reported a success rate of over 90% for any size and composition of renal stones.

- Open stone surgery stands as a reserved option in a very small percentage of patients who are too young with large stones, and have congenital structural urinary system abnormalities which need surgical correction.

- Bladder stones can be managed by transurethral lithotripsy or percutaneous cystolithotripsy depending on stone size with open surgery reserved for very big stones.

Extracorporeal shock wave lithotripsy

Since its introduction in 1980 extracorporeal shock wave lithotripsy (ESWL) has become the most widely used technique to treat stone disease in children [1]. However, the rate of complications is greater in children than adults. Many of these complications arise from inappropriate patient selection, imprudent use of the shock wave energy, and unfamiliarity with secondary endourologic procedures. There are multiple different lithotriptors and they are developed day by day with the advents in the technology. As in adults, success and complication rates in children also are affected by multiple factors such as size, location, composition and visibility of the stone, number and energy of the shock waves.

Pediatric Urology: Surgical Complications and Management. Edited by Duncan T. Wilcox, Prasad P. Godbole and Martin A. Koyle. © 2008 Blackwell Publishing, ISBN: 978-1-4051-6268-5.

The main difference from adult ESWL practice is the need for anesthesia in children. For the children <10 years old general anesthesia is usually needed [2,3]. However, ESWL can be safely used even in infants [4].

Outcomes

ESWL is the principal treatment for patients with a single renal pelvis stone <20 mm, lower pole stones <10 mm, and upper ureteric stones. Increasingly it is being used for larger stones, multiple locations, or lower ureteral with good results.

Stone size

As the stone size increases stone-free rate decreases. Published series on ESWL report stone-free rates as 87.8%, 75.5%, and 56.7% for the sizes <1 cm, 1–2 cm, and >2 cm, respectively [5]. In addition, some authors advocate ESWL even in staghorn cases with a stone-free rate of 80%; however, they state the need for prophylactic stenting to reduce complications [6,7].

Stone location

The location of the stone is a critical factor for success. Because of the effects of gravity lower pole stones are not so successfully treated, with low stone-free rates at 50–62% [5,8,9]. However, others report a success rate >90% regardless of the lower caliceal anatomy [10]. One of the largest studies on ESWL treatment for ureteric stones in children reports an overall stone-free rate of 91% (proximal: 94%, middle: 94%, and distal: 89%) with a 49% retreatment rate [11].

Stone composition

Cystine, brushite (dicalcium phosphate dihydrate), and whewellite (calcium oxalate monohydrate) are known to respond to ESWL poorly, and in patients with larger stones with these compositions alternative treatment options should be preferred. Moreover, "*metabolic*" or "*anatomic abnormalities*" have been shown to have an adverse effect on ESWL results. Patients with metabolic or anatomic problems have significantly lower stone-free rates (31.7% versus 69.4%) following ESWL [12].

Complications

Renal colic is caused by the passage of stone fragments or by the effect of the shock waves passing through tissue and is observed in the majority of patients. In the pediatric literature, renal colic is reported in only 2–19% [5,8,11,13–17]. This is less in adults and may be due to differences in pain perception or because the pediatric ureter is more efficient in transporting the stone fragments [15]. Pain without persistent signs of obstruction can be alleviated by antispasmodic and analgesic medication. Unrelieved pain should be evaluated further and presence of significant obstruction must be excluded.

Fever and *UTI* are described in 0.8–8.5% and 1.2–7.7% of patients, respectively [5,10–14,17–19]. Fever itself can be transient, though association with UTI needs antibiotic treatment. The infectious complications can occur with the fragmentation of the stone that may harbor bacteria even in the presence of preoperative sterile urine. Although routine use of prophylactic antibiotic is not recommended, urine should be sterile preoperatively. In the presence of unresolved bacteriuria, the procedure must be performed under appropriate antibiotic treatment. In those children who developed fever or UTI, close follow-up is mandatory, since progression to sepsis is infrequent, but possible.

Stone-street (steinstrasse) is one of the specific complications of ESWL and occurs mostly in the lower ureter. Its incidence depends on the pretreatment stone size and stenting and reported as 1.1–17.4% [5,10,13,14,17–19]. In staghorn stone cases prophylactic ureteral stenting has been advised to prevent this complication [20]; however, others report lower stone-free rates in patient with pre-ESWL inserted J-stents [10]. Routine stenting before ESWL is not advisable and should be reserved for very large stones in which stone-street formation is suspected or cases with significant hydronephrosis. When stone-street develops, it should be managed conservatively. If spontaneous passage does not occur ureteroscopic intervention is the treatment of choice. However, repeat ESWL might be an option. Accompanying pyelonephritis might need percutaneous drainage. In addition, the inability to pass the stone through the urethra occurs in <1% of patients and may necessitate urethroscopic intervention [12,17].

Dermal ecchymosis or *bruises* are variably reported with a range from 0% to 100% [5,8,19]. The severity depends on the generation of the machine, shock wave energy, and number of shocks. It is transient and does not need medical treatment. However, the effect of shock waves inside the body is more significant. *Perirenal (subcapsular)* and *enteric wall hematoma* is reported in <1% and managed conservatively [13,19]. *Microscopic hematuria* is common and *gross hematuria is* reported in up to 11.3% of patients [12,14]. Other rare complications, so far only reported in adults, include: hepatic injury, pancreatitis, anemia due to red blood cell hemolysis, hypertension, cardiac arrhythmia, and skeletal trauma.

The most serious pulmonary complication is *hemoptysis* secondary to lung contusion, fortunately reported only three times in the literature [21–23]. Shielding the lungs with shock-absorbing material or altering the mode of mechanical ventilation during the procedure may be an option to avoid the pulmonary complications.

The effect of ESWL on the renal functions has been studied in very few studies. These studies revealed renal function returns to baseline values within 15 days and additionally mid- and long-term studies showed an increased renal function after ESWL [24–26].

Ureteroscopy

Since the efficacy of ESWL in lower and middle ureteral stones decreases, ureteroscopy (URS) is often considered the first choice in these patients. URS will provide approximately 90% stone-free rates irrespective of the composition or radioopacity of the stone. These figures increase up to 100% with the adjuvant treatments and with the use of small caliber flexible instruments [27–37]. Although the stone-free rates are similar, it is well-established that the efficacy quotient of URS is significantly higher than ESWL in lower ureteral stones [11,27].

The technique is well-described and similar to adults'. Working under direct vision, the use of guide wires and fluoroscopic guidance are recommended. Routine dilation of the orifice and postoperative stenting is optional and should be decided individually. As the experience increases, active dilation is less required; if necessary, hydrodilation with Perez-Castro irrigation pump should be tried first [38]. Postoperative stenting depends on the invasiveness of the procedure and 1–2 weeks is sufficient in cases with high suspicion of trauma [39].

With the advent of pediatric instruments and increased surgical experience, complications, although still present, have decreased.

Intraoperative complications

Stone migration is undesirable and occurs approximately 6.5% of the time [30]. Cautious use of irrigation fluid and new cone-baskets reduce this problem [40]. When using the lithotripsy, gently squeezing the stone between the probe and the ureteral wall will be helpful and laser energy sources seem to minimize migration. Occasionally the stone migrates to the calyces, with these patients a flexible ureteroscope and laser fiber lithotripter is needed. In the absence of these tools, a stent should be left *in situ* and ESWL or percutaneous nephrolithotomy (PCNL) should be considered.

Ureteral perforation is another serious complication of URS. It might occur due to the loss of direct vision during the procedure or oversqueezing the stone between the probe and the ureteral wall. In the recent literature, the incidence is 0–6% [14,28,31,33,34]. In laser lithotripsy, keeping at least 1 mm from the mucosa and applying the lowest possible power will reduce inevident ureteral trauma. In cases of superficial mucosal trauma, the procedure can be carried on cautiously. However, in cases of significant perforation, the session must be ceased and a stent left. A very infrequent complication seen with perforation is dislodgement of the stone or fragments out of the ureter [33]. In this case, leaving a stent in the ureter and close follow-up of the patient is needed.

Inability to access the stone or *inability to place the guide wires* is reported in 0–12% of patients [32]. It occurs mostly secondary to the edematous reaction at the orifice, impaction of the stone, or due to tortuosity of the ureter. In these patients caution is required as the tissue is easily traumatized and extravasation can occur [36]. If

access to the stone is impossible leaving a double J stent for a period of 2–8 weeks (median 3 weeks) is effective in these patients [41]. Inability to place a safety guide wire before the procedure is another problem, traversing the orifice, and advancing through the ureter might be an option, however, this should be done with maximum care. Conversion to open surgery should be the last option. *Conversion to open surgery* is reported in up to 13.5% of patients [14,28,34]. It can occur secondary to the factors mentioned previously. Although it was not reported in pediatric URS literature, *ureteral avulsion*, which may develop due to application of harsh force with an inappropriate size instrument, also necessitates open surgery. Another point which should be considered is the inadvertent applications of laser energy on endourological tools that may cause breakage within seconds [42].

Early postoperative complications

Hematuria is the most frequent complication of URS in children. Its frequency may be as high as 27% [14,30,34]. Usually it is self-limiting, however, in cases of profuse bleeding it must be evaluated promptly.

Infectious complications are the other important issues. Its severity varies from simple asymptomatic bacteriuria to sepsis. Different series report various frequencies for urinary tract infection (UTI), pyelonephritis, and sepsis. *Pyelonephritis* has been reported to occur in approximately 4% of patients [29,30]. *Sepsis* has not been reported in most of the series, however one study reported 8.1% (3 of 37 cases), which is unexpectedly high [14]. The authors relate this high rate to the high pressures produced by electrohydraulic lithotripter during the disintegration of the infection stones. All these cases have been treated successfully by antibiotic therapy. To prevent these complications, preoperative urine must be sterile. Antibiotic prophylaxis with a broad-spectrum antibiotic (e.g. cephalosporines) during anesthetic induction should routinely be used. If sterile urine cannot be obtained preoperatively because of anatomic abnormalities, obstruction or presence of stones, the surgery must be performed under appropriate antibiotic treatment.

Stent migration is an infrequent complication reported in one series with 4% (1 in 25 cases) [29]. It occurs due to use of inappropriate size of catheter or uncontrolled placement under fluoroscopy. It can be easily corrected with an additional endoscopic session.

Late postoperative complications

Stricture is reported in the literature with an incidence between 0% and 2% and may need open surgical correction [28,35]. Stricture is most commonly thought to relate to active dilation of the orifice. Dilation itself facilitates the introduction of the instruments and lessens the instrument-related trauma. On the other hand, the mucosal tears during the active dilation may heal with fibrosis which can cause secondary fibrosis. Hydrodilation with Perez-Castro irrigation pump can be an alternative [38]. Some authors suggest passive dilation by placing a stent 3–4 weeks prior to the surgery [41]. They state that no dilation during the stone surgery was needed. However, this option carries a disadvantage of two sessions under anesthesia.

Routine stenting is also controversial. Often a stent is not required, however, in cases with suspicion of ureteral trauma the surgeon should not feel any hesitation about stenting. A suture attached to the stent, which exits from the external urethral meatus, will ease the pull of the catheter even under office conditions after the required time period.

Vesicoureteral reflux has been reported in 0–18% of cases [28,29,32,34]. In all cases with detected reflux, reflux grade was low, transient, and no intervention for reflux was needed. Consequently, a cystogram postoperatively is not usually required.

Percutaneous nephrolithotomy

Although practice of PCNL needed 10 years of adult experience before performing it in children [43], recent literature reports stone-free rates between 86.9% and 98.5% in any size and composition of stones [44–52]. These figures include even the staghorn stone series [52]. The stone-free rates reach to 100% with adjunctive treatment modalities (second-look PCNL, URS, ESWL). There is now considerable experience showing that even simultaneous bilateral PCNLs are possible with good success [51].

With the advent of appropriate size instruments, flexible nephroscopes, and laser lithotripters, age and weight are no longer limitations and even outpatient "tubeless" PCNL is begun to be reported with less pain, reduced risk of complications, and shorter hospital stays [53].

The effect of surgery on a developing organ has been questioned and none of the studies reported a significant adverse effect on kidneys by both dynamic and static scintigraphic evaluations [44].

Complications

Bleeding which requires transfusion is the most commonly described complication of PCNL as in adults. It is reported between 0.4% and 23.9% [44–52]. It mostly occurs due to complex manipulation in the kidney. Levering the nephroscope is the most frequent mistake during the operation which causes uncontrolled parenchymal laceration and bleeding. It should be kept in mind that making another access to the kidney may be less invasive than forceful attempts to reach a stone at a difficult location. A flexible instrument may also be helpful. The authors' preferences when deciding on the access to the kidney are:
1 a posterior calyx to an anterior one,
2 a dilated calyx,
3 infundibulum should be long and wide,
4 the selected calyx should offer access to the maximum amount of stone burden and the pelvis with a relatively straight line [46].
Bleeding is associated with operative time, stone burden, width of dilation, and number of tracts. When bleeding starts which disturbs vision, placing the working sheath into the kidney will help to decrease the bleeding as it presses the parenchymal vessels. Fulguration of the vessel – if apparent – is also possible after replacing the irrigation fluid with a nonelectrolyte containing fluid. If these conservative measures are not adequate, operation should be stopped and a nephrostomy left in the kidney. Clamping the nephrostomy catheter for a time approximately 20–30 min in association with forced diuresis is helpful. Conversion to open surgery because of bleeding is very rare and reported to occur in only 3 of 62 and 1 of 55 cases [14,45].

Minor renal pelvis extravasation is reported to occur in 5%, whereas apparent *renal pelvis perforation* is 1% in one series [44]. It can occur as a result of inadvertent manipulation with the nephroscope or during disintegration of the stone. It is managed conservatively by leaving the nephrostomy catheter longer. Renal pelvis perforation can also cause the migration of stone out of the kidney. In this case, no attempts to retrieve the stone from the extrarenal area should be attempted, as it is possible to injure the renal pedicle.

Extrarenal fluid collection is mostly retroperitoneal but in some instances intraperitoneal collection may occur. Small perirenal retroperitoneal collections are common and inconsequential. Large fluid collections are reported to occur in <1% (1 of 138) of cases and easily managed by a percutaneous drainage catheter [48]. No intraperitoneal fluid collection was reported following PCNL in children. However, it was reported in percutaneous cystolithotomy cases and said to be managed in the same way [54].

Neighboring organ injury is a possible complication. However, in the pediatric PCNL literature no organ injury is reported except one which reported only one *hydrothorax* amongst the 62 cases which has been managed with a chest tube [14]. The explanation for this low neighboring organ injury could be that surgeons gain a significant experience before attempting pediatric cases and moreover they behave more cautiously in a pediatric case.

"*Fever*" with or without documented UTI is the most reported postoperative complication. It is reported within a wide range between 2% and 49% [14,44–52]. Preventive measures are similar for all endoscopic stone surgeries, as described previously.

"*Prolonged urinary leakage*" after the removal of nephrostomy catheter is reported to happen in up to 8% of cases [46,48]. It is mostly due to ureteral obstruction, secondary to an unnoticed residual fragment. A double J stent placement will normally resolve this issue.

Open surgery

ESWL and endoscopic techniques are used to treat almost all children with stone disease. However, open stone surgery is still an option in a few patients who are too young with large stones, and have congenital structural urinary system abnormalities which need surgical correction. Also, severe orthopedic deformities may be a limitation for endoscopic procedures and open surgery becomes the only alternative.

Bladder calculi

Bladder stones constitute a separate group of stone disease with a male predominance, early presentation, and high frequency of ammonium acid urate composition [54]. It is mainly the problem of developing countries and endemic areas for stone disease. Different treatment modalities have been used. ESWL with its least invasive nature may be a good option. However, positioning the child and the passage of fragments through the narrow urethra is more difficult. ESWL treatment for bladder calculi in children was shown to be less effective with reported stone-free rates between 47.6% and 83% [14,55,56]. In most of the cases, several ESWL sessions and auxiliary procedures are required for complete clearance. Transurethral lithotripsy and percutaneous cystolithotripsy have equal efficacies approximately 100% [14,54]. Percutaneous route has the advantage of not to traumatize urethra since multiple passages through

narrow pediatric urethra has the risk of future stricture formation. Open surgery for bladder calculi is reserved for very big stones and additional anatomic abnormality necessitating surgical correction.

References

1 Newman DM, Coury T, Lingeman JE *et al*. Extracorporeal shock wave lithotripsy experience in children. *J Urol* 1986;136:238–40.
2 Aldridge RD, Aldridge RC, Aldridge LM. Anesthesia for pediatric lithotripsy. *Paediatr Anaesth* 2006;16:236–41.
3 Ugur G, Erhan E, Kocabas S, Ozyar B. Anaesthetic/analgesic management of extracorporeal shock wave lithotripsy in paediatric patients. *Paediatr Anaesth* 2003;13:85–7.
4 McLorie GA, Pugach J, Pode D *et al*. Safety and efficacy of extracorporeal shock wave lithotripsy in infants. *Can J Urol* 2003;10:2051–5.
5 Muslumanoglu AY, Tefekli A, Sarilar O *et al*. Extracorporeal shock wave lithotripsy as first line treatment alternative for urinary tract stones in children: A large scale retrospective analysis. *J Urol* 2003;170:2405–8.
6 Lottmann HB, Traxer O, Archambaud F, Mercier-Pageyral B. Monotherapy extracorporeal shock wave lithotripsy for the treatment of staghorn calculi in children. *J Urol* 2001;165:2324–7.
7 Al-Busaidy SS, Prem AR, Medhat M. Pediatric staghorn calculi: The role of extracorporeal shock wave lithotripsy monotherapy with special reference to ureteral stenting. *J Urol* 2003;169:629–33.
8 Tan MO, Kirac M, Onaran M *et al*. Factors affecting the success rate of extracorporeal shock wave lithotripsy for renal calculi in children. *Urol Res* 2006; 34: 215–21.
9 Ozgur Tan M, Karaoglan U, Sen I, Deniz N, Bozkirli I. The impact of radiological anatomy in clearance of lower calyceal stones after shock wave lithotripsy in paediatric patients. *Eur Urol* 2003;43:188–93.
10 Ather MH, Noor MA. Does size and site matter for renal stones up to 30-mm in size in children treated by extracorporeal lithotripsy? *Urology* 2003;61:212–5,discussion 215.
11 Muslumanoglu AY, Tefekli AH, Altunrende F, Karadag MA, Baykal M, Akcay M. Efficacy of extracorporeal shock wave lithotripsy for ureteric stones in children. *Int Urol Nephrol* 2006;38:225–9.
12 Tan AH, Al-Omar M, Watterson JD, Nott L, Denstedt JD, Razvi H. Results of shockwave lithotripsy for pediatric urolithiasis. *J Endourol* 2004;18:527–30.
13 Slavkovic A, Radovanovic M, Vlajkovic M, Novakovic D, Djordjevic N, Stefanovic V. Extracorporeal shock wave lithotripsy in the management of pediatric urolithiasis. *Urol Res* 2006;34:315–20,Epub 2006, July 26.
14 Rizvi SA, Naqvi SA, Hussain Z, Hashmi A, Hussain M, Zafar MN *et al*. Management of pediatric urolithiasis in Pakistan: Experience with 1,440 children. *J Urol* 2003;169:634–7.

15 Gofrit ON, Pode D, Meretyk S *et al*. Is the pediatric ureter as efficient as the adult ureter in transporting fragments following extracorporeal shock wave lithotripsy for renal calculi larger than 10 mm? *J Urol* 2001;166:1862–4.

16 Rodrigues Netto N, Jr., Longo JA, Ikonomidis JA, Rodrigues Netto M. Extracorporeal shock wave lithotripsy in children. *J Urol* 2002;167:2164–6.

17 Raza A, Turna B, Smith G, Moussa S, Tolley DA. Pediatric urolithiasis: 15 Years of local experience with minimally invasive endourological management of pediatric calculi. *J Urol* 2005;174:682–5.

18 Demirkesen O, Onal B, Tansu N, Altintas R, Yalcin V, Oner A. Efficacy of extracorporeal shock wave lithotripsy for isolated lower caliceal stones in children compared with stones in other renal locations. *Urology* 2006;67:170–4,discussion 174–5.

19 Aksoy Y, Ozbey I, Atmaca AF, Polat O. Extracorporeal shock wave lithotripsy in children: Experience using a mpl-9000 lithotriptor. *World J Urol* 2004;22:115–19.

20 Al-Busaidy SS, Prem AR, Medhat M. Pediatric staghorn calculi: The role of extracorporeal shock wave lithotripsy monotherapy with special reference to ureteral stenting. *J Urol* 2003;169:629–33.

21 Malhotra V, Gomillion MC, Artusio JF, Jr. Hemoptysis in a child during extracorporeal shock wave lithotripsy. *Anesth Analg* 1989;69:526–8.

22 Sigman M, Laudone VP, Jenkins AD *et al*. Initial experience with extracorporeal shock wave lithotripsy in children. *J Urol* 1987;138:839–41.

23 Tiede JM, Lumpkin EN, Wass CT, Long TR. Hemoptysis following extracorporeal shock wave lithotripsy: A case of lithotripsy-induced pulmonary contusion in a pediatric patient. *J Clin Anesth* 2003;15:530–3.

24 Villanyi KK, Szekely JG, Farkas LM, Javor E, Pusztai C. Short-term changes in renal function after extracorporeal shock wave lithotripsy in children. *J Urol* 2001;166:222–4.

25 Vlajkovic M, Slavkovic A, Radovanovic M, Siric Z *et al*. Long-term functional outcome of kidneys in children with urolithiasis after ESWL treatment. *Eur J Pediatr Surg* 2002;12:118–23.

26 Goel MC, Baserge NS, Babu RV, Sinha S, Kapoor R. Pediatric kidney: Functional outcome after extracorporeal shock wave lithotripsy. *J Urol* 1996;155:2044–6.

27 De Dominicis M, Matarazzo E, Capozza N, Collura G, Caione P. Retrograde ureteroscopy for distal ureteric stone removal in children. *BJU Int* 2005;95:1049–52.

28 A Busaidy SS, Prem AR, Medhat M. Paediatric ureteroscopy for ureteric calculi: A 4-year experience. *Br J Urol* 1997;80:797–801.

29 Schuster TG, Russell KY, Bloom DA, Koo HP, Faerber GJ. Ureteroscopy for the treatment of urolithiasis in children. *J Urol* 2002;167:1813–16,discussion 1815–16.

30 Bassiri A, Ahmadnia H, Darabi MR, Yonessi M. Transureteral lithotripsy in pediatric practice. *J Endourol* 2002;16:257–60.

31 Raza A, Smith G, Moussa S, Tolley D. Ureteroscopy in the management of pediatric urinary tract calculi. *J Endourol* 2005;19:151–8.

32 Satar N, Zeren S, Bayazit Y, Aridogan IA, Soyupak B, Tansug Z. Rigid ureteroscopy for the treatment of ureteral calculi in children. *J Urol* 2004;172:298–300.

33 Dogan HS, Tekgul S, Akdogan B, Keskin MS, Sahin A. Use of the holmium:YAG laser for ureterolithotripsy in children. *BJU Int* 2004;94:131–3.

34 Al-Busaidy SS, Prem AR, Medhat M, Al-Bulushi YH. Ureteric calculi in children: Preliminary experience with holmium:YAG laser lithotripsy. *BJU Int* 2004;93:1318–23.

35 Minevich E, Defoor W, Reddy P, Nishinaka K, Wacksman J, Sheldon C *et al*. Ureteroscopy is safe and effective in prepubertal children. *J Urol* 2005;174:276–9.

36 Thomas JC, DeMarco RT, Donohoe JM, Adams MC, Brock JW, 3rd, Pope JC, 4th. Pediatric ureteroscopic stone management. *J Urol* 2005;174:1072–4.

37 Tan AH, Al-Omar M, Denstedt JD, Razvi H. Ureteroscopy for pediatric urolithiasis: An evolving first-line therapy. *Urology* 2005;65:153–6.

38 Soygur T, Zumrutbas AE, Gulpinar O, Suer E, Arikan N. Hydrodilation of the ureteral orifice in children renders ureteroscopic access possible without any further active dilation. *J Urol* 2006;176:285–7,discussion 287.

39 Wu HY, Docimo SG. Surgical management of children with urolithiasis. *Urol Clin North Am* 2004;31:589–94, 159–94.

40 Desai MR, Patel SB, Desai MM, Kukreja R, Sabnis RB, Desai RM *et al*. The Dretler stone cone: A device to prevent ureteral stone migration – the initial clinical experience. *J Urol* 2002;167:1985–8.

41 Hubert KC, Palmer JS. Passive dilation by ureteral stenting before ureteroscopy: Eliminating the need for active dilation. *J Urol* 2005;174:1079–80,discussion 1080.

42 Honeck P, Wendt-Nordahl G, Hacker A, Alken P, Knoll T. Risk of collateral damage to endourologic tools by holmium:YAG laser energy. *J Endourol* 2006;20:495–7.

43 Woodside JR, Stevens GF, Stark GL, Borden TA, Ball WS. Percutaneous stone removal in children. *J Urol* 1985;134:1166–7.

44 Dwaba MS, Shokeir AA, Hafez AT *et al*. Percutaneous nephrolithotomy in children: Early and late anatomical and functional results. *J Urol* 2004;172:1078–81.

45 Zeren S, Satar N, Bayazit Y, Bayazit AK, Payasli K, Ozkeceli R. Percutaneous nephrolithotomy in the management of pediatric renal calculi. *J Endourol*. 2002;16:75–8.

46 Desai MR, Kukreja RA, Patel SH, Bapat SD. Percutaneous nephrolithotomy for complex pediatric renal calculus disease. *J Endourol* 2004;18:23–7.

47 Badawy H, Salama A, Eissa M *et al*. Percutaneous management of renal calculi: Experience with percutaneous nephrolithotomy in 60 children. *J Urol* 1999;162:1710–13.

48 Holman E, Khan AM, Flasko T, Toth C, Salah MA. Endoscopic management of pediatric urolithiasis in a developing country. *Urology* 2004;63:159–62,discussion 162.

49 Samad L, Aquil S, Zaidi Z. Paediatric percutaneous nephrolithotomy: Setting new frontiers. *BJU Int* 2006;97:359–63.

50 Salah MA, Toth C, Khan AM, Holman E. Percutaneous nephrolithotomy in children: Experience with 138 cases in a developing country. *World J Urol* 2004;22:277–80.

51 Salah MA, Tallai B, Holman E, Khan MA, Toth G, Toth C. Simultaneous bilateral percutaneous nephrolithotomy in children. *BJU Int* 2005;95:137–9.

52 Aron M, Yadav R, Goel R, Hemal AK, Gupta NP. Percutaneous nephrolithotomy for complete staghorn calculi in preschool children. *J Endourol* 2005;19:968–72.

53 Jackman SV, Hedican SP, Peters CA, Docimo SG. Percutaneous nephrolithotomy in infants and preschool age children: Experience with a new technique. *Urology* 1998;52:697–701.

54 Salah MA, Holman E, Khan AM, Toth C. Percutaneous cystolithotomy for pediatric endemic bladder stone: Experience with 155 cases from 2 developing countries. *J Pediatr Surg* 2005;40:1628–31.

55 Kostakopoulos A, Stavropoulos NJ, Makrichoritis C, Picramenos D, Deliveliotis C. Extracorporeal shock wave lithotripsy monotherapy for bladder stones. *Int Urol Nephrol* 1996;28:157–61.

56 Delakas D, Daskalopoulos G, Cranidis A. Experience with the Dornier lithotriptor MPL 9000-X for the treatment of vesical lithiasis. *Int Urol Nephrol* 1998;30:703–12.

18 General Laparoscopy

Chris Kimber and Neil McMullin

Key points

- Laparoscopy is safe in trained surgical hands.
- Attention to equipment setup and ergonomics improves task performance.
- Energy sources must be fully understood and used judiciously.
- Unrecognized bowel perforation is a catastrophic complication and must be considered in the septic postoperative patient.

Introduction

As surgery progresses there is no doubt that the modalities of visualizing target organs are increasing while the trauma related to wound access is decreasing. Laparoscopy is a step in this progression that is likely to be superseded by open MRI intervention and robotic surgery. Caution is required with laparoscopy and a well-trained surgeon is essential. Laparoscopy is now widely used in pediatric surgery and urology for the removal of solid tissue (dysplastic, malignant, or infected), reconstruction (i.e. pyeloplasty, orchidopexy), and diagnosis (i.e. intersex trauma). The following chapter will document basic endoscopic techniques while focusing on the complications of laparoscopy in general.

History

Initial visualization of the abdominal cavity by papyrus was attempted by early Egyptians. Insufflation followed

the introduction of the Veress needle in the 1930s and finally in 1982 Kurt Semm performed the first laparoscopic appendicectomy. Improved equipment and the development of instrumentation enabled widespread introduction of laparoscopy in the 1990s. Laparoscopy and endoscopic surgery are now considered routine in pediatric surgery and urology.

Procedure

Basic laparoscopy involves insertion of a primary optic trocar by open technique, usually in a transumbilical fashion, establishment of a pneumoperitoneum, visualization via a rigid telescope, and the insertion of secondary trocars for instrumentation. The diameter of the ports, telescope size, and instrumentation is extremely variable and based on the availability of equipment at the institution and surgical expertise. It is inappropriate to prescribe a rigid diagnostic laparoscopy formula. Retroperitoneal or lateral access requires insertion of a balloon device to create a working space [1].

General anesthesia and full muscle relaxation is essential. The insufflation of carbon dioxide in the initial phase should generally be at 0.5 l/min. The surgeon, the target organ, and the monitor should be in line to facilitate ergonomics (Figure 18.1). Failure to position the

Pediatric Urology: Surgical Complications and Management. Edited by Duncan T. Wilcox, Prasad P. Godbole and Martin A. Koyle. © 2008 Blackwell Publishing, ISBN: 978-1-4051-6268-5.

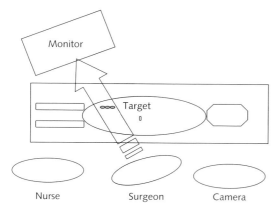

Figure 18.1 Alignment of surgeon, target organ, and monitor to maximize ergonomic performance.

patient correctly and orient the target organ monitor and surgeon in an ergonomic fashion results in major complications. There is no question that task performance is severely compromised by obtuse operating angles, and the failure to observe basic ergonomics is likely to result in poor task performance. These factors need to be considered prior to the commencement of any laparoscopic case.

The surgeon must be completely familiar with all associated equipment, including the insufflation machine, the camera processor, the light source, and carbon dioxide. It is the surgeon's responsibility to be able to troubleshoot and rapidly identify problems with the equipment. In depth training on each individual device is essential prior to commencement of any endoscopic surgery. Failure to achieve this level of competency can result in serious errors and can be a factor in a major complication. Familiarity with the equipment is essential [1,2].

The use of the Veress needle is contraindicated in children due to the risk of inadvertently injuring a hollow viscus such as bowel or blood vessels. It is accepted that this risk is small, however perforation may be unrecognized and catastrophic [3–5]. The initial port should be placed under direct vision, generally transumbilically. The exception to this is the blind balloon insufflation/port introduction of the retroperitoneal technique. Secondary instrument ports are always introduced under direct vision. Radially dilating ports (i.e. those with an expandable sheath inserted over a needle) improve port fixation and reduce CO_2 leakage. These ports are preferred for complex and difficult procedures.

Complications

Complications in laparoscopy can be summarized under the following headings:
- Port site
- Insufflation
- Inadvertent injury
- Tissue approximation
- Other patient-related complications
- Surgeon-related complications

Port sites
Port site herniation is a surprisingly common complication of laparoscopy in infants and children. Herniation can occur even through a 3 mm port site. To prevent this the following points are noted:

1 Most port site herniations occur from a mid line trocar site, particularly the umbilicus. There is usually omentum entrapped within the port site, possibly exacerbated by a rush of CO_2 at the time of trocar withdrawal. All port sites should be closed if possible. Meticulous attention, particularly to the umbilical port, is essential to avoid this complication.

2 A port site herniation is usually identified by omentum appearing in the wound in the first 24 h of surgery. The patient needs to be returned to the operating theater, have the omentum ligated and removed, and the port site reclosed.

Insufflation
Pneumoperitoneum
Carbon dioxide is a relatively inert gas and is well tolerated as a pneumoperitoneum agent. The potential complications are as follows:

- High-pressure pneumoperitoneum will lead to diaphragmatic splinting, reduced tidal volume, and retention of CO_2. Whilst end tidal carbon dioxide often remains elevated during laparoscopy, experienced anesthetic support is required to minimize this complication.

- Gas embolism: Gas embolism is possible, particularly if an open viscus has been perforated. Fortunately, this is extremely rare in pediatric surgery. Immediate conversion to laparotomy is required if this is suspected. If gas embolism occurs, immediate insertion of a central venous catheter and aspiration of affected gas is required by the anesthetist. Gas embolism is most likely to occur by a misplaced Veress needle, and as discussed previously, this should not be used.

- Hypothermia can occur as a result of excessive CO_2 utilization. This is best avoided by utilizing an insufflation device that warms the gas, particularly in lengthy procedures.

Leakage of carbon dioxide into adjacent body spaces

Carbon dioxide pneumoperitoneum may escape into the:
1 subcutaneous space (subcutaneous emphysema),
2 pleural space (pneumothorax), and
3 mediastinum (pneumomediastinum).
Small pneumothoraces and leakage of air into the chest cavity can be treated conservatively and the operation can be continued. A major pneumothorax requires insertion of an intercostal drain and adequate consideration as to the cause. Subcutaneous emphysema is often a result of the gas spreading between the abdominal wall and the skin and will resolve in the next 24 h. The pneumoperitoneum disappears within 24 h on an erect abdominal X-ray. It is not the cause of air under the diaphragm after 24 h and a viscus perforation should be suspected if this sign is present [4].

Inadvertent injury
Blood vessel perforation

Perforation of a major blood vessel requires immediate laparotomy and hemostasis. Urgent vascular surgical opinion should be requested.

Bowel perforation

If a perforation is recognized during laparoscopy it may be repaired endoscopically at that time. Open laparotomy is not essential, however if the surgeon has minimal tissue approximation skills, or if the leak cannot be identified laparoscopically, then converting to open surgery is recommended. Delayed peritonitis due to viscus rupture may be treated either laparoscopically or by open surgery based on the experience of the surgical team. In most instances the perforation should be sutured, extensive saline lavage performed, and triple antibiotic therapy instigated [6].

Unrecognized energy delivery

There are now a wide variety of instruments for dissection and energy delivery. It is important that each surgeon becomes familiar with the equipment available. Specific training on energy sources is required and all surgeons performing laparoscopy surgery should have full training as to the risks of electrosurgery and associated energy sources, prior to the commencement of any procedure. Full knowledge and training is the key to avoiding complications in this area.

Diathermy

Damage to adjacent organ structures by electrosurgical equipment is a common problem in advanced endoscopic surgery and a source of major complications.

Diathermy injury is best avoided, utilizing the following points:
1 The operating surgeon must control the foot pedal of the affected device and not the assistant and/or scrub nurse.
2 Short bursts of electrosurgery utilizing direct tissue contact are essential.
3 An electrosurgical monitoring device should be fitted to each diathermy machine to detect electrosurgical leakage along the shaft of the diathermy instrument.
4 All operating centers should have a program of testing and maintaining the electrosurgical hook equipment on a regular basis.
5 The surgeon must understand and avoid capacitive coupling prior to the commencement of any laparoscopic procedure.

Alternative energy sources

There are now a variety of energy sources involving high frequency oscillating devices. The instrument delivering this type of energy often remains at temperatures in excess of 100°C, particularly at the tip of the instrument. Inadvertent damage to adjacent structures from direct contact with a heated tip is common and must be avoided. The surgeon must fully understand the basic physics and ergonomics of any alternate energy source prior to its utilization. Prior training on inert tissue is recommended.

Unrecognized injury to adjacent structures is an acknowledged complication of laparoscopic surgery. The emergence of this complication may be delayed for several days and can even lead to unrecognized intra-abdominal infection and subsequent death. The child may recognize a delayed viscus rupture. This involves the sudden occurrence of a warm sensation in the abdominal cavity followed by significant pain and then a feeling of unwellness. Early recognition of these symptoms by the treating clinical team is essential.

This complication is best avoided by utilizing the following techniques:
1 The surgeon must be fully trained in the use of energy sources and instrumentation prior to the performance of any surgical procedure.
2 The surgeon must be able to relax within his level of competence and perform a tissue manipulation in a slow, smooth, and ergonomic fashion.

3 Clear visualization, an adequate working space, and a careful, meticulous dissection technique are essential.

Tissue approximation

The ability to join tissue structures is an essential skill of any advanced endoscopic surgeon. In most cases suturing of the affected tissues is required, generally using interrupted technique. There are associated techniques including fibrin glue and endoscopic staples.

The following recommendations are made in order to prevent leakage from tissue approximation:

1 The surgical team should be fully trained in endoscopic suturing, and this is best performed by training on both simulators and on laboratory bench top. Mastery of this skill must be achieved in the skills laboratory prior to any surgeon undertaking this on a human. It is inappropriate to train a surgeon in suturing on live human tissue without full competence being achieved in a skills laboratory setting.

2 Clear visualization, an adequate working space, and excellent ergonomics all contribute to accurate tissue approximation. The combination of these factors can influence the outcome of the procedure and the surgeon must be fully trained in these aspects of surgical care prior to commencing the task.

3 In advanced tissue approximation procedures such as laparoscopic pyeloplasty a mentoring approach is essential, with an experienced surgeon accompanying the surgeon through the first few cases.

Leakage from endoscopic stapled anastomosis can be prevented by:

1 Ensuring the operator is completely familiar with the stapling device, and understands the staple depth and the maximum tissue thickness.

2 Cautious usage in inflamed bowel (particularly inflammatory bowel disease).

3 Accurately closing the enterotomy sites with interrupted sutures.

Other complications
Severe pain

Shoulder pain is a common complaint after laparoscopy, particularly with longer procedures. Occasionally children undergoing laparoscopy demonstrate unexpectedly severe pain following the procedure unresponsive to narcotic administration. The likely cause of this pain is rapid pneumoperitoneum with associated high intra abdominal pressure, resulting in distension and triggering of pain fibers. This complication results in not only significant shoulder tip pain, but generalized abdominal

pain as well. Narcotic and other associated analgesic infusions including Ketamine may be required to control pain. The estimated incidence of this is one to two per thousand laparoscopies.

Tissue retrieval

The complications of tissue removal are as follows:

1 Tumor spillage into the peritoneal cavity and port site, resulting in implantation and metastasis. This is best avoided by ensuring all potential tumors are appropriately placed in a retrieval bag and removed through a generous port site incision.

2 Bag rupture during specimen removal: It is essential that the surgeon is fully familiar with the usage and operation of a retrieval bag. The surgeon must ensure that the specimen retrieval bag is opened fully and any rolled up portion of the bag is fully unfurled prior to placement of the specimen within the bag. A port site must be appropriately enlarged to enable easy withdrawal of the specimen to prevent rupture [7].

If rupture does occur then widespread lavage and collection of all visible specimen is required. This is particularly of significant risk during removal of the spleen where splenic implantation may result in ongoing hemolysis.

Hematuria

Isolated hematuria has been reported after a variety of laparoscopic procedures, including appendicectomy and Meckel's diverticulectomy. This complication appears to be self-limiting and usually occurs for 2 to 3 days after the procedure. A renal and bladder ultrasound is essential to ensure that no underlying secondary pathology such as a PUJ obstruction has been missed. The mechanism of the hematuria is uncertain, is probably related to pneumoperitoneum, and it usually self resolves.

Complications specific to retroperitoneal surgery

Retroperitoneal surgery is often required for advanced urological surgery. The following table outlines the complication and the proposed methodology for overcoming it (Table 18.1).

Injury and trauma to the operating surgeon

There is no question that laparoscopic surgery is a demanding skill. Significant injuries to surgeons have been documented over the last decade [8–10].

The following complications can occur:

1 Radial nerve injury particularly involving the thumb. This can occur by placing the thumb continually through

Table 18.1 Retroperitoneal complications.

	Cause	Action
Failure to achieve access	Balloon expands into muscle or subcutaneous space	Enlarge wound, separate muscle with deep retractors, and place balloon deeper.
Peritoneal perforation	Instrument or trocar damage	Advise anesthetist, increase flow rate to 3–4 l/min, widen tear to allow peritoneal space to equilibrate, continue task. Convert to intraperitoneal procedure if poor visibility.
Duodenal perforation	Excessive diathermy dissection, failure to recognize renal structures (often confused with a small multicystic kidney)	Nasogastric tube, triple antibiotics, direct endoscopic suture if recognized and possible. Laparotomy if anatomy uncertain or closure difficult.
Poor exposure/visibility	Small working space and inadequate dissection, possible CO_2 leak from trocar	Check trocars, increase pressure and flow rate, blunt dissect peritoneum to create larger space, insert additional port if possible.

the looped end of the needled holder and squeezing tightly. Digital pressure on the radial nerve may result and surgeons are advised to develop a relatively tension-free grip on instruments so that this does not occur.

2 Shoulder strain and rotator cuff injury. This injury is reasonably common and results from the surgeon holding his or her shoulders in an abducted position for prolonged periods of time. This has resulted in significant loss of function, neurapraxia, and muscle pain, particularly if there is associated lateral rotation of the spine during the procedure. This complication is best avoided by lowering the patient's position, ensuring the monitor is in a gaze down position, and avoiding prolonged periods of fixed stance.

3 Anterior osteophyte formation and spinal degeneration. It is becoming increasingly clear that surgeons adopt fixed neck positions during endoscopic surgery and this may result in associated vertebral damage. Once again, the ability to relax and achieve mastery with advanced endoscopic surgery is essential.

Endoscopic surgery does place significant stress on the operator. During prolonged cases it is recommended that two competent surgeons be present and that they rotate as the main operator during the case. In our practice, we have both found that to achieve complex difficult surgery particularly during the early stages of our careers, it made an enormous difference to have two surgeons there who could reflect difficulties on each other and exchange as the main operator. It certainly reduces the physical damage to the surgeon.

Optimizing laparoscopy

We believe that laparoscopic surgery is enhanced by creating a team atmosphere in the operating room, and being aware of when one's limitations as a surgeon have been reached.

Surgical team approach to improving overall laparoscopic performance

Surgical performance is best improved by taking notice of the ten golden rules as outlined below. Any unit undertaking laparoscopic surgery must have a meticulous attitude to training and preparation for this type of surgery. A team approach is recommended with two surgeons of similar standing and competence being involved, particularly in difficult cases. The surgical team must have the ability to clearly question the dissection moves of the main operator and challenge any operative decision at any point. To achieve excellent outcomes, it is important to avoid significant time pressure and never rush complex endoscopic surgery. Tired surgeons, particularly with fatigue from lack of sleep, result in worse outcomes. There is clear evidence that these team approaches and combined attitudes influence decisions.

Elective versus emergency conversions

Converting a procedure from a laparoscopic to an open one can be a difficult clinical decision. We firmly feel that a surgeon should be able to determine that on a particular day, with a particular patient, with that surgeon's particular ability, if they are unable to achieve completion of the task laparoscopically then an elective conversion to an open procedure should ensue. While we do not place firm time limits on this occurring, one must recognize that after 2 h of advanced endoscopic operating, fatigue is likely to have set in. The outcome from a patient who has been electively converted to an open procedure is excellent.

Emergency conversion in the face of significant bleeding, major perforation or adjunct organ damage, represents a more difficult situation. Emergency conversions usually occur after a long series of errors including poor vision, poor port placement, failing instrumentation, and unclear anatomy. This scenario needs to be recognized that conversion occurs at an elective stage rather than at emergency. The outcome for emergency conversion has been documented as worse in several large adult series [10,11].

In summary, multiple complications can occur from laparoscopic surgery. Paramount to preventing these is a well-prepared and trained surgical team. Competent surgeons who approach these tasks in a methodological fashion with adequate surgical skills training are unlikely to commit major errors.

Ten golden rules for safe laparoscopy

1 Achieve complete training in all endoscopic equipment and energy sources.

2 Understand the ergonomics of task performance.

3 Always use an open initial port insertion technique.

4 Correct any deterioration of visibility or working space early.

5 Work as a team, in a team environment. Encourage other surgeons and nurses to question/comment on the dissection.

6 Do not aim to complete the operation laparoscopically at all cost, remember that elective conversions are far safer than emergency conversions.

7 Proceed to advanced surgery with another colleague, share the operating time and work together.

8 Plan your surgery well, do not apply list pressure or operate fatigued.

9 Recognize that to achieve mastery, a calm cautious approach is required.

10 Remember the ego of the surgeon must always be subservient to the patient's welfare.

References

1 Lee ACH, Stewart RJ. Diagnostic laparoscopy in operative endoscopy and endoscopic surgery in infants and children. In Edited by Najmaldin et al. Paediatric Endoscopic Surgery London: Holder Arnold, 2005: pp. 197–201.

2 Hanna GB, Kimber C, Cuschieri A. Ergonomics of task performance in endoscopic surgery. In *Endoscopic surgery in Children*, Edited by Bax, Rothenberg and Valla et al., Berlin: Springer, 1999: pp. 35–52.

3 Soderstrom RM. Injuries to major blood vessels during endoscopy. *J Am Assoc Gynecol Laparosc* 1997;4:395–8.

4 Bax NMA, vander Zee DC. *Complications in Laparoscopic Surgery in Children in Endoscopic Surgery in Children*. Berlin: Springer, 1999: pp. 357–68.

5 Byron JW, Markenson G, Miyazawa K. A randomized comparison of Verres needle and direct trocar insertion for laparoscopy. *Surg Gynecol Obstet* 1993;177:259–62.

6 Schafer M, Lauper M, Krahenbuhl L. Trocar and Veress needle injuries during laparoscopy. *Surg Endosc* 2001;15:275–80.

7 Mathew G, Watson DI, Ellis T *et al.* The effect of laparoscopy on the movement of tumor cells and metastasis to surgical wounds. *Surg Endosc* 1997;11:1163–6.

8 Vereczkei A, Feussner H, Negele T *et al.* Ergonomic assessment of the static stress confronted by surgeons during laparoscopic cholecystectomy. *Surg Endosc* 2004;18:1118–22.

9 Matern U, Eichenlaub M, Waller P, Ruckauer K. MIS instruments. An experimental comparison of various ergonomic handles and their design. *Surg Endosc* 1999;13:756–62.

10 Giger UF, Michel JM, Opitz I *et al.* Risk factors for perioperative complications in patients undergoing laparoscopic cholecystectomy: Analysis of 22,953 consecutive cases from the Swiss Association of Laparoscopic and Thoracoscopic Surgery database. *J Am Coll Surg* 2006;203:723–8.

11 Deziel DJ, Millikan KW, Economou SG *et al.* Complications of laparoscopic cholecystectomy: A national survey of 4,292 hospitals and an analysis of 77,604 cases. *Am J Surg* 1993;165:9–14.

19

Laparoscopy for the Upper Urinary Tract

J.S. Valla

Key points

- Minimally invasive surgery can introduce complications.
- Prevention of complications is paramount.
- Conversion and complication rate is related to:
  - laparoscopic experience of the surgical team
  - access technique → avoid blind technique

- size of patient → great care in infants
- extent of the disease → try to improve before operation
- complexity of the procedure → ask for expert's assistance.
- If risk-to-benefit ratio is carefully assessed, laparoscopy should be tried to minimize morbidity.

The most common operations performed on the upper urinary tract in children are total nephrectomy, partial nephrectomy, and pyeloplasty; these procedures are indicated for nonmalignant disease and could be performed by using minimally invasive techniques [1].

The goal of these new techniques is to get the same result as with classical open surgery but with less morbidity, less complications. Paradoxically, laparoscopy introduces a new range of potential complications; moreover not one of these operations, except perhaps total nephrectomy, are now validated as the gold standard procedure [2–4].

Minimally access surgery of the upper urinary tract is exposed to two kinds of complications:
• Those related to the disease, already studied in the previous chapters of this book.
• Those related to the technique, which will be discussed here. Prevention is the most important element of this chapter; the pediatric urologist must keep in mind all the possible complications before surgery, during each step of the procedure, and also deal with possible postoperative complications.

Pediatric Urology: Surgical Complications and Management. Edited by Duncan T. Wilcox, Prasad P. Godbole and Martin A. Koyle. © 2008 Blackwell Publishing, ISBN: 978-1-4051-6268-5.

During the preoperative period

Informing the family

The parents and the patient may overlook that laparoscopic surgery for the upper urinary tract is a major surgical procedure with possible attendant complications and that the operation may have to be converted to an open procedure. The family must be aware of the benefits of minimally invasive surgery but also of complications related to the disease and related to the technique; informed consent is essential in the pediatric population, as the reported benefits of the laparoscopic approach have not been firmly established. Alternative management options should be discussed and the patient should be informed about the laparoscopic experience of the surgeon.

Training of the surgical team

The surgeon's training and experience is of paramount importance but in pediatric urology the surgeon is faced with several limiting factors: the number of indications is small, and tutoring is more difficult than with traditional open surgery, so the learning curve likely will be longer in mastering technical skills such as suturing and knot tying. This can be especially challenging when one attempts to use finer suture material in a reduced working space.

The experience of all members of the team is also important, as the assistants, nursing support, and the experience of the anesthesiologists all can impact the operating surgeon and the smooth transition from standard open techniques to the laparaoscopic approach.

Checking the material

The pediatric urologist must check that all the needed devices are working well and appropriate for the size of the child; that is, just like in open surgery, instruments and materials should be individualized for each given patient. It is imperative, especially as one is gaining experience, that all team members are prepared to convert to an open approach and hence, all appropriate instruments must be available.

Contraindications and specific indications

Indications and contraindications are summarized in Table 19.1. There are no absolute contraindications to perform a technique laparoscopically, but the technique should be chosen that is most appropriate to each case. For example, severe retroperitoneal inflammation is classically considered as a contraindication or at least a significant risk to laparoscopy. However, experienced teams have successfully performed laparocopic nephrectomy, even in the face of xanthogranulomatosis pyelonephritis [5].

Table 19.1 Indications and contraindications for minimal access surgery of the upper urinary tract in children.

Indications	
Kidney surgery	• Renal biopsy
	• Total nephrectomy
	• Partial nephrectomy
	• Renal cyst
Upper urinary tract reconstructive surgery	• Pyeloplasty
	• Ureteropyelostomy
	• Retrocaval ureter
Stone	• Nephrectomy, pyelotomy, ureterostomy
Contraindications	
General	• Uncontrolled coagulopathy
	• Significant cardiopulmonary risk
Local	• Multiple prior renal surgeries
	• Uncontrolled retroperitoneal inflammation of infection

In case of massive hydronephrosis or huge multicystic dysplastic kidneys, it might be beneficial to evacuate the urine percutaneously to maximize the working space and visibility. Arguments have been made that suggest a preference for a transperitoneal approach to the retroperineal approach: need for total nephroureterectomy, prior retroperitoneal surgery, horseshoe kidney, and size of the patient; under 6 months of age or 6 kg and the opposite in case of obese patients, the retroperitoneal access is more difficult [6].

Regarding access, the most significant limiting factor impacting laparoscopic reconstructive surgery is the size of the patient. The smaller the child, the smaller the working space and the more challenging the case will be; in the patient undergoing pyeloplasty, the minimum age varies between 2 months and 2 years, depending on the surgeon's experience [7–8].

Finally, due to the learning curve that is inherent in transitioning from open to laparoscopic surgery, procedures of increasing complexity should gradually be adapted to the surgeon's and his/her team's experience. For example, partial nephrectomy should be considered only after the team has developed a comfort level performing total nephrectomies. Once extirpative surgery has been mastered, then increasing complexities of reconstructive surgery can be attempted.

During the operation

In the operating room, the pediatric urologist must be aware of two things especially if the procedure is prolonged: (1) positioning is paramount as is protection of all pressure points, and (2) the comfort of the surgeon and the team must be ergonomically maximized: screens must be positioned that guarantee a comfortable view that allows almost a "straight plane" not only for the surgeon, but for the surgical assistant. It is important for the novice to realize that minimally invasive surgery at times can be much more tiring than classical open surgery and hence comfort is essential.

Access

Many complications deal with access techniques:
• In case of *transperitoneal access*, injury of the intestine or major blood vessels may be minimized by using the open access technique under visual control [9]. Dissection and handling of intraperitoneal structures to reach the kidney must be carried out in a meticulous fashion to avoid or at least minimize potential complications such as hollow viscus perforation and hemorrhage.

• In case of *retroperitoneal access*, whatever the position of the patient, lateral or prone, the most common complication is the accidental peritoneal perforation, which induces pneumoperitoneum and can further reduce the retroperitoneal working space and visibility [10]. The risk of peritoneal tear is particularly high in smaller children where the peritoneum is thinner and less protected by fat. The peritoneum is most vulnerable at the beginning of the procedure, when creating the working space. As for transperitoneal access, visual control represents the best guarantee against visceral and peritoneal injury even if this open technique is more time consuming, it allows a safe introduction of an atraumatic smooth trocar.

In children the cutaneous incision is invariably too small to enable finger dissection of the retroperitoneal space, so the options available to create an initial working space are: balloon insufflation (either commercially available or made in the operating room using a finger port from a surgical glove affixed to the end of a catheter) and formal blunt dissection from the initial port where the telescope essentially acts as an extension of the surgeon's finger to dissect the peritoneum out of harm's way. Once access has been achieved, the surgeon should get his/her bearings by identifying traditional anatomical landmarks: quadratus lumborum, psoas muscle, and posterior part of the kidney. The thick lateral and posterior abdominal wall cannot be distended by insufflation as well as the anterior abdominal wall; this explains why a good muscle relaxation is essential, so a sufficient operating space can only be achieved by pushing away peritoneum and intraabdominal organs and by dissecting the lateral peritoneal reflection at least to the anterior axillary line. The two additional operating trocars are introduced under laparoscopic vision; it is more judicious to first introduce the posterior port in the costospinal angle, far away from the peritoneum. A blunt laparoscopic instrument introduced through this posterior port allows the surgeon the ability to gently sweep the lateral peritoneal reflection anteriorly and medially. This is the safest method to allow the third inferior trocar to be introduced above the iliac crest. If in spite of all these precautions a peritoneal injury occurs at the beginning of the procedure, there are several potential solutions: the most elegant, but difficult, is to close the perforation with a purse-string 5/0 suture; the most simple is to desufflate the pneumoperitoneum continuously using Veress needle. If the working space is not improved by the previous maneuvers, then it is necessary [2] to open widely the peritoneum and to continue the procedure using a mixed approach retro- and intraperitoneal.

Another rare complication that could occur during access or insufflation is a pneumothorax due to diaphragmatic injury or excessive CO_2 insufflation pressure [6–12]. If a decrease in O_2 saturation is noticed by the anesthesiologist, a pneumothorax must be excluded and if present, evacuated.

Hemostasis

The crucial point during kidney surgery is vascular control; bleeding may occur at any time: dissection, clip or suture placement, or transection. It should not be forgotten that because of magnification, bleeding seems greater on the screen than in reality. Efficient suction – irrigating devices and a laparoscopic vascular clamp (DEBAKEY) – should be readily available. The surgeon must be accomplished in assuring temporary vascular control by compressing or clamping the concerned vessel to optimize visual inspection. As with open surgery, cauterizing blindly, in a field of blood, only exacerbates the situation. Placing an additional trocar is often necessary to assist the team in identifying and controlling the bleeding point. This accessory port allows a grasper to hold on the kidney or on the pedicle and to improve vision during aspiration. It is also useful to increase the gas in-flow which by itself may increase the compartment pressure and assist in controlling the bleeding diathesis. This must be done carefully and the anesthesiologist must monitor the patient closely. When controlling a difficult "bleeder," it is preferable to clamp the vessel using nondominant hand while clearing the operative field with the dominant hand using the suction device. When the bleeding structure is clearly identified, two scenarios are commonly distinguishable. If a small vessel is involved, it can be simply coagulated by monopolar, bipolar, or ultrasonic device. If a large vessel is involved, it must be dissected further to allow ligation of clip application. If however a major vessel is injured, only an accomplished surgeon should attempt to repair it using laparoscopic suturing techniques. In the scenario of uncontrolled bleeding or major vascular injury, the decision for conversion to open surgery is dictated by the hemodynamic conditions of the patient and the skills of the surgeon. While open conversion is being prepared for, the bleeding area should be compressed for as long as it takes to stabilize the patient, ready the operating theater, and assure that appropriate blood products, when thought necessary, are ready.

• For a total nephrectomy the renal vessels appear vertically in the operating field; they must be dissected in the inferior part of the field where there is only one artery and one vein and not too close to the kidney hilum where the vessels divide into segmental branches.

A sufficiently wide area of exposure (at least 1 cm) allows creation of a large window around vein and artery and to get a safe vascular control.

On the left side care is taken to avoid injury to the adrenal vein and tail of the pancreas; on the right side, one must be careful with the posterior wall of the duodenum which is contiguous to the anterior part of the vessels. On the right side, the renal vein could be misidentified and confused with the vena cava. This is especially so if the renal vein is short and if the camera has been rotated showing the vena cava vertical. Thus awareness of the degree of orientation is essential!

Partial nephrectomy

For partial nephrectomy, separation of the renal parenchyma, at least in hands, is made easier and safer by using ultrasonic or Harmonic scalpel. Usually there is minimal or no bleeding if the appropriate segmental vessels have been primarily ligated. The resection margin created by preliminary vessel ligation is assured and the line of excision is carefully incised. The remnant tissue can be grasped to provide counterattraction to simplify the remainder of tissue excision. The base of the stump is also cauterized or the Harmonic scalpel is used to scarify it and minimize bleeding.

If there is any doubt about a possible opening of a calyx, saline with or without methylene blue is injected via a whistle tip ureteric catheter that is often placed initially, specifically to deal with this situation. If the leak is confirmed and significant, caliceal suture repair is performed or biological adhesive is applied.

The most serious complication of partial nephrectomy, but not specific to minimally invasive surgery, is the loss of the functioning segment. This can be due to three causes. First, transection of the major blood supply because of misidentification. If recognized and repairable, immediate conversion to open procedure and reconstruction of the artery is mandated. Secondly, vasospasm due to excessive manipulation or traction on the vessels can occur. This complication is managed by local irrigation with warm saline and the application or injection of a vasodilatator such as papaverine. It is essential that the patient is also appropriately hydrated. Lastly, a compressive perirenal hematoma can occur. In the last situation the diagnosis is often delayed and there is little to be done to save the remaining parenchyma.

Extracting the kidney is rarely associated with problems. For larger specimens, where morcellation is required, it can be time consuming to master the placement of specimen within the bag.

Suture

For reconstructive surgery, such as dismembered pyeloplasty, the success depends upon delicate suturing. Such techniques are advanced, demanding, and time consuming, even for skilled laparoscopic surgeons. Appropriate orientation to prevent twisting the ureter, use of traction sutures, and an experienced camera assistant all are important in minimizing the potential for error.

Completion

All drains must be secured before exsufflation to avoid any untimely extraction.

At the end of the procedure, exufflation is progressively started. The following must be inspected to assure that hemostasis is secure. First, the operative area, particularly near the hilum or the pyeloureteral junction must be inspected during desufflation as even significant bleeding can be masked by the temporary tamponade associated with the insufflation pressure. Second, the cannula sites should be observed after each one is removed to minimize the risk of missing a small bleeder. It is a practice to close all port sites to avoid any visceral or omental evisceration.

During the postoperative period

None of the complications that arise postoperatively are specific to minimally invasive surgery other than those that might be associated with port placement. Careful adherence to technique and not attempting to take short cuts are paramount in reducing the potential for complication.
• Hemorrhage is suspected in the situation of pain, swelling of the abdominal wall, bleeding from a port site or through a drain. If significant, this will result in a decreased hematocrit. If visible hemorrhage does not stop rapidly or intra-abdominal bleeding is manifested by a drop in hematocrit that requires blood replacement or affects hemodynamic parameters, then exploration is indicated. It should be mentioned that an open exploration is mandatory in the case where a previous retroperitoneoscopic approach has been employed, as redo retroperitoneoscopy is often ineffective due to poor vision. In the instance where a transperitoneal laparoscopic approach has been used and if the hemodynamic

status of the patient is stable, a redo transperitoneal laparoscopic exploration can be considered.

• Urine leak may be evident in the early postoperative period and is confirmed radiologically. Assuring that the kidney itself is draining into the bladder is mandatory. Stent or percutaneous nephrostomy drainage should be considered. Large urinomas that have secondary affects or infected urinomas require drainage, either percutaneously or if necessary in complex scenarios, via an open approach. Asymptomatic urinomas are often noted incidentally at routine ultrasonographic follow-up after partial nephrectomy and usually are asymptomatic. Thus observation in most cases is all that is necessary.

• Intraperitoneal sepsis can be due to intraoperative unrecognized bowel perforation or some days later if due to thermal injury with a delayed necrosis. Clinical symptoms could be partly masked because of antibiotic and analgesic therapy. A second look by laparoscopy is justified to assess the damage and decide how to manage it according to its importance and the surgeon's laparoscopic experience.

• Finally, port site herniation is managed as usual.

Personal results

Our personal experience of complications after retroperitoneoscopic approach, which is our favorite, is summarized in Table 19.2.

The conversion rate rises from 0% for renal biopsy to 8.5% for partial nephrectomy. Operative incidents are still high, even if we always use an open technique (1 case of renal pelvis perforation [huge hydronephrosis], 10 cases of subcutaneous emphysema, 1 case of transient postoperative abdominal wall paralysis). The most frequent complication is peritoneal perforation during the access: 15%; however no vascular or bowel injury. All of these incidents have been managed laparoscopically.

Operative incidents related to dissection and hemostasis are as follows: 1 case of duodenal perforation during partial nephrectomy (conversion), 1 case of diaphragmatic tear (laparoscopic repair), 1 case of postoperative perirenal hematoma after partial lower pole nephrectomy with loss of function of the remaining upper pole (late diagnostic, no reoperation, surveillance), and 10 cases of postoperative urinomas (5 after pyeloplasty, 5 after partial nephrectomy) of which 2 needed reoperation for drainage.

Discussion

With experience the use of operative laparoscopy in pediatric urology has continued to expand. Improved technology, continued growth and experience by the surgeon and the demand by the public for minimally invasive techniques, have all contributed to the growth of this surgical option. Still, many pediatric urologists are still reluctant to employ laparoscopic techniques due to the steep learning curve and time commitment that are necessary to allow reconstructive surgery to be comfortably and reliably performed. Some cite the potential for complications, which were reported while these approaches were in their infancy [13]. Others argue that the advantages of this new surgery have not yet been demonstrated according to the criteria of evidence-based medicine. Indeed large pediatric comparative studies are still lacking. The published data mainly come from expert teams and are retrospective studies [14–19]. Is it logical to judge the

Table 19.2 Personal experience in retroperitoneoscopy including the learning curve.

Procedure	NB	Conversion	Complications		Reoperation
			Per OP	Post OP	
Renal biopsy	8	0	0	0	0
Total nephrectomy	110	2%	20%	2%	0
Partial nephrectomy	35	8.5%	26%	15%	1/35
Pyeloplasty	55	4%	13%	18%	7/55
Adrenalectomy	15	13%	20%	0	0
Stone	6	0	0	1	1
Retrocaval ureter	2	0	0	0	0
Total	231				

complication rate for all the procedures on the upper urinary tract or is it better to separate the simple procedures (biopsy, total nephrectomy) from the complex one (pyeloplasty, partial nephrectomy)? Is it logical to include in the complication rate the cases operated since the beginning of this new technique or it is more realistic to exclude the learning curve? What is the length of the learning curve for each procedure, which seems variable according to each team [20–21]? Should we separate the complications according to their seriousness: simple trouble like peritoneal perforation during retroperitoneoscopy, incident repaired by laparoscopy, accident like vascular or visceral injury which need conversion or reoperation, and disaster which could lead to death?

Concerning the adult literature [22–24], the conversion rate in open surgery is around 6%; the complications rate varies from 4.4% to 20.6%; in the comparative study of Fomara *et al.* [24], the complication rate was higher with open surgery (25.4%) than with laparoscopy (20.6%). The reintervention rate in the adult data is between 0.8% and 1.1%.

In the data of Ku *et al.* [25], which compared laparoscopy for congenital benign renal diseases in children and adults, the result looks better in children with less complications. However, in the pediatric group, as indicated before, the complication rate is best correlated to the age of the patient. In the study of Castellan *et al.* [26] 80% of complications were seen in patients younger than 1 year regardless of the access route, trans or retroperitoneal.

Concerning the pediatric literature [3–26], the complication rate varies between 2% and 10%, the reoperation rate between 0.39% and 12%.

In the multicentric data of Peters *et al.* [3], published 10 years ago, about 5428 cases of diagnostic and therapeutic procedures, significant complications occurred in 1.18% of cases. The significant predictors of complications include the experience of the operator and the access technique – open or Veress needle.

Conclusion

The goals of minimally invasive surgery are to maintain the principles of open procedures while minimizing morbidity for the young patient. But no method is risk free. As laparoscopic techniques increase in popularity and frequency so too will the intraoperative and postoperative complications associated with these treatments. As experience grows the rate of complication should decline. For each child, the risk-to-benefit ratio must be carefully assessed. However, in experienced hands, laparoscopy could today be considered as an essential part of the armamentarium of pediatric urologist in managing pathology of the upper urinary tract.

References

1 Esposito C, Valla JS, Yeung CK. Current indications for laparoscopy and retroperitoneoscopy in pediatric urology. *Surg Endosc* 2004;18:1559–64.

2 Peters CA. Complications of retroperitoneal laparoscopy in pediatric urology: Prevention, recognition and management. In *Retroperitoneoscopy and Extraperitoneal Laparoscopy in Pediatric and Adult Urology*. Edited by P Caione, LR Kavoussi, R Micali. Springer Italia, 2003: pp. 203–10.

3 Peters CA. Complications in pediatric urological laparoscopy: Results of a survey. *J Urol* 1996;155:1070–3.

4 Esposito C, Lima M, Mattioli G *et al.* Complications of pediatric urological laparoscopy: Mistakes and risks. *J Urol* 2003;169:1490–92.

5 Merrot T, Rodorica-Flores R, Steyaert H *et al.* Is diffuse xanthogranulomatous pyelonéphritis a contra-indication to retroperitoneoscopic nephroureterectomy? *Surg Lap Endosc* 1998;8:366–69.

6 Mulholland TL, Kropp BP, Wong C. Laparoscopic renal surgery in infants 10 Kg or less. *J Endourol* 2005;19:397–400.

7 Kutikov A, Reskick M, Casale P. Laparoscopic pyeloplasty in the infant younger than 6 months: Is it technically possible? *J. Urol* 2006;175:1477–9.

8 Cascio S, Tien A, Chee W *et al.* Laparoscopic dismembered pyeloplasty in children younger than 2 years. *J Urol* 2007;177:335–8.

9 Franc-Guimond J, Kryger J, Gonzalez R. Experience with the BAILEZ technique for laparoscopic access in children. *J Urol* 2003;170:936–8.

10 Valla JS. Videosurgery of the retroperitoneal space in children. In *Endoscopic Surgery in Children*. Edited by NMA. Bax, KE. Gerogeson, A. Najmaldin, JS. Valla. Springer Berlin Heidelberg, 1999: pp. 379–92.

11 Waterman BJ, Robinson BC, Snow BW *et al.* Pneumothorax in pediatric patient after urological laparoscopic surgery: Experience with 4 patients. *J Urol* 2004;171:1256–9.

12 Shanberg AM, Zagnoev M, Cloughert TP. Tension pneumothorax caused by the argon beam coagulator during laparoscopic partial nephrectomy. *J Urol* 2002;168:2162.

13 Duckett JW. Editorial pediatric laparoscopy: Prudence please. *J Urol* 1994;151:742–43.

14 Pulagari AV, Pattaras JG, Pugach JL *et al.* Pediatric/adolescent laparoscopic VS open dismembered pyeloplasty: Result on postoperative morbidity. *J Urol* 2000;163:81.

15 Bonnard A, Fouquet V, Carricaburu C *et al.* Retroperitoneal laparoscopy versus open pyeloplasty in children. *J Urol* 2005;173:1710–13.

16 Lee RS, Retik AB, Borer JG *et al.* Pediatric retroperitoneal laparoscopic partial nephrectomy: Comparison with an age matched cohort of open surgery. *J Urol* 2005;174:708–12.

17 Piaggio L, Franc-Guimond J, Figueroa TE *et al.* Comparison of laparoscopic and open partial nephrectomy for duplication anomalies in children. *J Urol* 2006;175:2269–73.

18 Valla JS, Breaud J, Carfagna L *et al.* Treatment of ureterocele on duplex ureter: Upper pole nephrectomy by retroperitoneoscopy in children based on a series of 24 cases. *Eur Urol* 2003;43:426–29.

19 Yeung CK, Tam YH, Sihoe JD *et al.* Retroperitoneoscopic dismembered pyeloplasty for pelvi-ureteric junction obstruction in infants and children. *BJU Int* 2001;87:509–13.

20 Cook A, Khoury A, Bagli D *et al.* The development of laparoscopic surgical skills in pediatric urologists: Longterm outcome of a mentorship – training model. *Can J Urol* 2005;12:2824–8.

21 Ku JH, Yeo WG, Kim HH *et al.* Laparoscopic nephrectomy for renal diseases in children: Is there a learning curve? *J Pediatr Surg* 2005;40:1173–6.

22 Fahlenkamp D, Rassweilerr J, Fornara P *et al.* Complications of laparoscopic procedures in urology: Experience with 2407 procedures in 4 German Centers. *J Urol* 1999;162:765–70.

23 Cadeddu JA, Wolfe JS, Nakada S *et al.* Complications of laparoscopic procedures after concentrated training in urological laparoscopy. *J Urol* 2001;166:2109–11.

24 Fornara P, Doehn C, Freidrich HJ *et al.* Nonrandomized comparison of open flank versus laparoscopic nephrectomy in 249 patients with benign renal disease. *Eur Urol* 2001;40:24–31.

25 Ku JH, Byun SS, Choi H *et al.* Laparoscopic nephrectomy for congenital benign renal diseases in children: Comparison with adults. *Acta Paediatr* 2005;94:1752–5.

26 Castellan M, Gosalbez R, Carmack AJ *et al.* Transperitoneal and retroperitoneal heminephrectomy. What approach for which patient? *J Urol* 176:1636–39.

20

Robotics in Pediatric Urology: Pyeloplasty

L. Henning Olsen and Yazan F. Rawashdeh

Key points

- Robotic surgery in pediatric urology is still in its infancy.
- Robotic assisted pyeloplasty is the commonest robotic procedure in pediatric urology.
- Robotic assisted pyeloplasty has outcomes comparable to those of open and laparoscopic procedures.

- Robot-related complications are not uncommon and include arm collisions, system failures, and complications related to lack of tactile feedback.
- Pyeloplasty-related complications are akin to those encountered in open and laparoscopic procedures.

Introduction

Although considered a novelty, the concept of robotics and computer-assisted surgical techniques in urology has been in existence for about 20 years. In 1989, at the Imperial College in London, Davies and his colleagues showed the feasibility of using a modified industrial robot for transurethral prostatic resection. Two years later the same group was able to carry out transurethral prostatectomies on five patients, marking the first time an active robot was used for resecting human tissue [1]. Other early milestones include the introduction of automatized, surgeon-controlled systems for placement of brachytherapy needles in prostatic tissue [2], for taking prostate biopsies [3], and for the percutaneous access of the kidney [4]. These systems were image guided, relying on coordinates designated by the surgeon and obtained from transrectal ultrasound, fluoroscopy, MRI, or CT images that were processed by the robot's integrated computer system, allowing highly precise trajectory calculation. Common for these robots were the facts that they all were active in the sense that they proceeded

Pediatric Urology: Surgical Complications and Management. Edited by Duncan T. Wilcox, Prasad P. Godbole and Martin A. Koyle.
© 2008 Blackwell Publishing, ISBN: 978-1-4051-6268-5.

autonomously once programmed and activated by the surgeon and that none of them achieved widespread clinical use especially not in the pediatric realm.

Commercialization of robotics came with the introduction of the Automated Endoscopic System for Optimal Positioning (AESOP, Intuitive Surgical, Sunnyvale, California) in 1993. It was however the advent of the master–slave telerobotic systems in the late 1990s that entailed a paradigm shift in the way minimally invasive surgery was to evolve at the turn of the century.

Master–slave telerobotic systems

Master–slave systems are designed to convey a surgeon's movements to robotic arms that replicate these movements via sophisticated end effectors connected to these robotic arms. The surgeon is therefore not in direct physical contact with the patient, thereby fulfilling the concept of telepresence surgery and enabling the potential of performing operative procedures remotely [5]. Of the different systems developed, the da Vinci and the ZEUS telemanipulators stand out as the most utilized robots. Originating from two different California-based manufacturers, the two companies merged in 2003 and since then da Vinci Surgical System has dominated the market.

Robots in pediatric urology

The da Vinci surgical system is undoubtedly the most utilized robot in pediatric urology. However due to its recent history of less than a decade and issues pertaining to high costs (initial investment premium in excess of one million euros and significant running costs of about 100,000 euros annually), applications are still somewhat limited and finding a niche for the da Vinci robot in pediatric urology has thus been a balancing act between need and reason. Robotic assisted pyeloplasty (RAP) is by far the commonest procedure described in a still modest body of literature, the bulk of which is class 4 evidence (case reports and case series) with no randomized controlled clinical trials. Other anecdotal uses have been reported and yet other applications have been contemplated and shown feasible in experimental studies (Table 20.1).

Robotic assisted pyeloplasty (RAP)

Laparoscopic pyeloplasty (LAP) has yielded results comparable to those of open pyeloplasty, which is considered the gold standard for treatment of ureteropelvic junction (UPJ) obstruction. In comparison with open pyeloplasty, LAP confers benefits of minimal morbidity, shorter convalescence, and better cosmesis [11]. LAP is however a cumbersome procedure with a long-learning curve, and requires a vast repertoire of laparoscopic skill, especially the ability to master the technically demanding intracorporeal suturing techniques. In direct juxtaposition with open pyeloplasty, RAP has also been shown to decrease hospital stay and lessen the need for analgesia in the perioperative period albeit with a few shortcomings pertaining to significantly longer operative times and higher costs [12]. With gaining experience, however, operative times tend to approach those of the open procedures [13]. Considering that functional outcomes and reported complications are similar by both procedures, and barring the issue of cost, the balance tips in favor of RAP. No direct comparisons between pediatric RAP and LAP have been published but if studies in adults can be taken as an indicator, no clear clinical advantages are evident for the experienced laparoscopic surgeon as operative outcomes, length of hospital stay, complications; and clocked operative times are virtually indistinguishable although there was a tendency toward shorter operative and anastomosis times in RAP [14–16]. The latter claim has since been discounted

Table 20.1 Other less-reported applications of robotics in pediatric urology.

Author	Procedure	Robotic system	Subjects and number	Median age	Complications	Comments
Olsen and Jorgensen et al. [6]	Retroperitoneoscopic heminephrectomy	da Vinci	14 girls	4.9	Two converted to open operation; one due to lack of progress and one due to bleeding	Median operative time 176 min
Pedraza et al. [7]	Appendicovesicostomy (Mitrofanoff)	da Vinci	1 boy	7	None	Operative time 6 h
Pedraza et al. [8]	Bilateral heminephroureterectomy	da Vinci	1 girl	4	None	Operative time 7 h 20 min. The robot was only used to dissect the renal hilum and the upper pole vessels bilaterally while the rest of the procedure was done laparoscopically
Olsen et al. [9]	Pneumovesical ureter reimplantation a.m. Cohen	da Vinci	8 pigs		Two port hernias	Procedure was successful in all
Yee et al. [10]	Reconstruction of traumatic UPJ disruption	da Vinci	1 boy	11	None	Operative time 8 h 50 min

in a recent study which prospectively compared LAP to RAP and found significantly longer operative and total operative theater times in the RAP patients in addition to a substantial cost increase of 2.7 times [17]. The authors of the mentioned study conclude, based on their findings, against the indiscriminate application of RAP especially for surgeons adept with intracorporeal suturing who stand to benefit little from the da Vinci.

RAP points of technique

Most surgeons will usually favor the transperitoneal approach to RAP because this access provides them with familiar landmarks that aid in orientation. In this procedure the patient is positioned supine with the affected side elevated on a 30° foam or gel wedge. The camera port is placed at the umbilicus using Hasson's technique. The abdomen is insufflated to 10–12 mmHg. Working ports are placed in the midline between the umbilicus and xyphoid and in the midclavicular line below the umbilicus. The table is angled to raise the affected side into a 60° flank position. The robot is positioned on the ipsilateral side of the patient, angled over their shoulder and the three robotic arms are engaged with the laparoscopic ports. A fourth port can be placed distal to the xyphoid to provide additional retraction, sutures, and suction. The UPJ can be exposed transmesenterically on the left in the larger pediatric patient or by mobilizing the colon along Toldt's line on either side. The surgical procedures follow the same rules as the open procedure [18–20].

For the retroperitoneal approach the patient is positioned in a semiprone position; infants and children are placed on a small gel sandbag placed under the contralateral iliac crest. The upper leg is extended, while the lower leg is flexed and the legs are padded with gel cushions to decrease undue stretch and to avert pressure sores in prolonged procedures. Excessive internal rotation of the upper leg should be avoided especially in older patients as this might be hazardous for the hip joint. Adolescent patients should be placed with their waist on the kidney rest and the operating table should be flexed in order to open the costovertebral angle. Since the robot fixes the ports and keeps them in position just a limited degree of flexion is needed in contrast to open and laparoscopic procedures. The first 15–20 mm skin incision is made one finger breadth above the iliac crest just posterior to the anterior iliac spine. The external fascia is incised and the muscles are split by blunt dissection under direct vision with small retractors. The lumbodorsal fascia is incised

sharply and with the index finger a *small* retroperitoneal recess is developed posterio-cranially. In adults and older children, a commercial dilating balloon trocar is inserted and the retroperitoneal space is dilated with 400–500 ml air. In infants and some smaller children, commercial trocars are too large and should be replaced by a homemade dilating balloon catheter. The balloon should remain inflated *in situ* for 5 min [21,22].

The first instrument port is placed under digital guidance just medial to the edge of the latissimus dorsi muscle and two finger breadth above the iliac crest. The medial instrument port is placed just below the costal margin in the anterior axillary line. An optional 5-mm port for assistance, suction, and suture delivery is inserted in the right or left iliac fossae. Blunt trocars through 70 mm radially dilating sleeves are preferred to the original cutting trocars of the da Vinci system. This diminishes the risk of bleeding and tissue/organ injury. Finally an airtight balloon tipped trocar is used in the primary incision for camera access; the balloon retains the tip of the trocar in the retroperitoneum, preventing it from retraction in between the abdominal muscle layers. The robot is then engaged, being wheeled in from the ipsilateral side at an angle of 45–60° from the patient's head depending on the expected localization of the UPJ. The retroperitoneum is then insufflated to 8–10 mmHg, which is slightly lower than pressures needed for transperitoneal access. As soon as the 0° telescope is inserted, Gerota's fascia is recognized, incised, and the remainder of the procedure is as with the open technique [21,22].

Robot-related complications and preventing them

Complications related to robotic movement envelope are not uncommon. Robotic arms colliding with each other, with the table, or even with the bedside surgical assistant are not only a nuisance that at best serves to prolong operations, but also pose a danger as collision with the vulnerable pediatric patient may cause injury or pressure sores, especially as the surgeon has limited tactile feedback preventing immediate collision recognition. The bedside assistant's role is therefore not limited to technical assistance but also extends to being the operator's second pair of eyes and ears.

Compared with pediatric patients the size of the da Vinci is overwhelming, and when fully engaged the robot may restrict the bedside surgical assistant's access to the patient while the arms are in use and may require the anesthesiology team to make special preparations to ensure prompt access to the patient's airway [23,24]. Moreover, some authors recommend special positioning of smaller patients <20 kg by elevating them upon foam padding to allow more lateral placement of instrument ports, thereby giving the arms and assistant surgeon more mobility, as the arms can pitch downwards to a greater extent without encountering the table [24]. Pelvic procedures on smaller patients also carry the risk of pressure injury to the upper body by excessive downward pivoting of the robotic arms. This can be prevented by protecting the upper body by strategically placing the metal railing of the anesthetists screen and by using a 30° camera which decreases the angle by which the robotic camera arm needs to be tilted.

The surgeon controls the amount of force applied by the da Vinci arms, which ranges from a fraction of an ounce of force for delicate suturing to the several pounds of force necessary to retract large tissue structures. Therefore lack of tactile feedback presents an important drawback to the inexperienced surgeon, as the instruments may be moved too forcefully resulting in tissue injury or suture breakage. Carelessly manipulating a needle between two needle holders can easily break the needle or to that effect instrument tips which may result in the untoward retaining of foreign bodies [25]. Lack of tactile feedback can be compensated for by the enhanced stereoscopic video imagery, which gives excellent visual cues of suture tension and tissue deformability. With experience and dedicated training, operators may further enhance their internal perceptual model of tissue consistency to correlate applied forces and tissue deflection [26].

The da Vinci employs a number of safety features aimed at preventing injury, for example, to start the procedure the surgeon's head must be placed in the console viewer. Otherwise, the system will lock and remain motionless until it detects the presence of the surgeon's head once again. During the procedure, a zero-point movement system prevents the robotic arms from pivoting above or at the entry incision, which could otherwise be unintentionally torn. System failures, whether mechanical or related to the system computer, are however known to occur and surgeons operating the robot have to be familiar with system troubleshooting. Depending on the type of failure, delays of up to hours can be incurred, as is the case when a malfunctioning robotic arm or a motherboard has to be replaced. Such delays are unacceptable and needless to say the procedure has to be completed laparoscopically or by open conversion. Surgeons are hence mandated to plan for such contingencies [27].

Procedure-related complications: Pyeloplasty

As with all other minimally invasive procedures, optimal port placement in RAP is paramount but can be challenging in the pediatric patient and requires detailed planning and more often than not nonconventional solution or lateral thinking. The manufacturer's recommended positioning between camera and instrument ports is triangular with at least 8 cm of distance between ports (Figure 20.1). It is however obvious that this distance cannot be kept in infants and smaller children especially when attempting the retroperitoneal approach. Additionally, the retroperitoneal space can be quite restricted especially in the initial steps of the procedure before opening Gerota's fascia, as is the case with the transperitoneal approach in infants [20]. The amount of intracorporeal working space required by instruments in order to be active further limits maneuverability especially when using 5-mm instruments with "snake wrist" technology which are limited by a >10 mm distance from the distal articulating joint and the instrument tip [24]. Ports should therefore not be inserted more than 0.5–1 cm below the inner fascial layer. This results in an instrument pivoting point laying at the skin level and consequently more pronounced arm movements with an increased risk of collisions between the arms (Figure 20.2). Considering these factors is thus crucial when planning port placement, so as to take full advantage of instrument dexterity and to avoid collisions between instruments (Figure 20.3), which may seriously limit a surgeon's ability and reach. Limitations in camera arm movement can make it impossible to visualize the UPJ in a large hydronephrosis and was in the author's experience the reason for open conversion in one such case. The camera port has since been moved closer to the iliac crest to avoid this shortcoming [21,22].

Orientation in the *retroperitoneal space* can be difficult for the beginner especially in obese and older children where it can be difficult to keep an overview and the right working direction. The few landmarks encountered

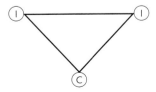

Figure 20.1 Optimal triangle between camera port (C) and instrument port (I) to avoid collisions between the robotic arms.

include the quadratus lumborum and psoas muscles. As the operator has no direct contact with the patient it is advisable to leave the console once in a while to check working direction judged by inspecting the instruments, as relying solely on imagery may be insufficient. Beginner pitfalls include mistaking the vena cava for a dilated renal pelvis and muscles under fatty tissue for the kidney. The *transperitoneal access* offers more familiar landmarks, however one should be careful to have the active part of both robotic instruments in sight especially when using monopolar cautery as even small serosal bowel lesions can have disastrous consequences. Both Yee [12] and Weise [16] describe postoperative ileus as a complication to the transperitoneal approach probably due to leakage of urine from the anastomosis.

JJ-catheter complications, whether related to placement or patency, have also been reported. The stent can be placed retrogradely prior to the procedure or preoperatively over a guidewire either through the accessory port [22] or percutaneuosly using an 18-gauge angiography needle [13,20]. The JJ-catheter should be placed after the first half of the anastomosis is completed. This stabilizes the ureter

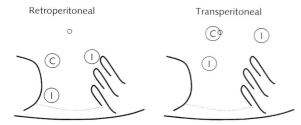

Retroperitoneal   Transperitoneal

Figure 20.2 Port placement for the transperitoneal and retroperitoneal route in pyeloplasties. (C) camera port (I) Instrument port.

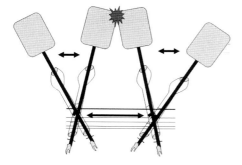

Figure 20.3 In children, the ports and instruments are inserted just a few centimeters apart with consequently more pronounced movements of the robotic arm outside the patient.

and facilitates insertion. Care should be exercised while maintaining countertraction on the ureter while inserting the stent as lack of haptic feedback may lead to inadvertent injury. In the authors series of 67 RAP procedures, 3 JJ-catheters were found in the distal ureter at cystoscopy after the operation [22]. Since children always are under general anesthesia when the JJ-catheters are removed, this complication rarely poses an additional risk as the displaced catheters can easily be removed with a dormia basket. Some authors advocate the use of blue dye instilled into the bladder to secure proper stent placement [13,20]. Assessment of the anticipated ureteral length and inserting a defined length of the guidewire into the ureter and the bladder may also reduce the risk of JJ-stent displacement. When placing the stent antegrade through the assistant port, the guidewire is fed through the assistant port and there from guided down the ureter by the operator using the DeBakey forceps and the needle holder. JJ-size choice depends on the estimated length of the ureter. For optimal placement, it is advisable with a controlled insertion. This is done by the assistant who as soon as the tip of the guide reaches the upper open end of the ureter, feeds a measured length of the guide, a little longer than the actual length of the JJ-stent. This ensures that the JJ-catheter reaches the bladder but does not go beyond. Countertraction is exerted on the JJ-stent by a semi-closed DeBakey forceps while the guidewire is removed in order to keep the stent in place. As soon as the JJ-stent has been placed, the posterior part of the anastomosis and – if necessary – the pelvic defect are closed.

Pelvis drainage in the early postoperative period is reliant on a patent anastomosis and/or stent when present. In the previously mentioned series from the authors' institute four patients needed postoperative nephrostomy. Two of them had an occluded JJ-catheter due to a blood clot while the remaining two who were unstented were believed to be obstructed due to postoperative edema. Three of them resolved spontaneously within a few days while one had to be reoperated due an overlooked crossing vessel [22]. Meticulously washing out the renal pelvis prior to completing the anastomosis reduces the risk of blood clot formation and is routinely done at the author's institute.

Surgical outcome

The few series reporting on RAP in children have a failure rate of 0–6% increasing with the number of patients reported (Table 20.2) [13,20–22,28]. Lee *et al.* reported in their series one patient out of 33 who required a

Table 20.2 Surgical outcomes and complications of the pediatric RAP series published to date.

Author	Number	Age (range)	Operative time minutes (range)	Follow-up months (range)	Complication rate (N)	Complications (N)	Failure rate (N)	Failure cause (N)
Atug et al. [28]	7	(6–15) years	184 (165–204)	10.9 (2–18)	14.3 % (1)	Prolonged drainage	0%	–
Yee et al. [12]	8	9.8 (6.0–15.6) years	248 (144–375)	14.7 (2–24)	0%	–	0%	–
Kutikov et al. [20]	9	5.6 (2–8) months	122.8 (NA)	6 (NA)	0%	–	0%	–
Lee et al. [13]	33	7.9 (0.2–19.6) years	219 (133–401)	10 (0.4–28)	3% (1)	Overlooked crossing vessel	3% (1)	Overlooked crossing vessel (1) redo
Olsen et al. [21,22]	67		146 (93–300)	12.1 (0.9–49.1)	17.9 %	Conversion (1) Postoperative nephrostomy catheter (4) Hematuria (2) UTI (2) Displaced JJ-catheter (3)	6%	Overlooked crossing vessel (1) redo Kinking ureter (2) redo Re-stenosis (1) balloon dilatation

redopyeloplasty due to an overlooked crossing vessel [13]. This was their only patient done by a retroperitoneal approach and similar to the abovementioned case from the author's series [22]. This complication, at least in children, seems to be peculiar to retroperitoneal access and is best avoided by completely exposing the lower pole of the kidney.

In the authors' series two further patients needed redo-pyeloplasties due to significantly decreasing differential function. An open redo-pyeloplasty in both cases revealed a kinking ureter, which in hindsight was probably related to extensive straightening caused by the stay sutures in the pelvis and the upper end of the ureter during the primary procedure. Positioning stay sutures should therefore be used with caution since they may leave the ureter and the pelvis in an unfavorable position once released and allowed to fall back. Other series in children do not report failures, which lead to reoperations [12,20,28]. However minor complications such as postoperative hematuria and urinary tract infections are reported. There is no difference with regard to hospital stay, outcome, failure, and complications between the reported series. However, outcome can be defined in various ways as described elsewhere in this volume.

Conclusions

Robotic surgery in pediatric urology is still in its infancy. But with the rapid pace of events leading to this juncture, it is unquestionable that major refinements and revelations are in store. At this point in time, however, indications for use of robots in pediatric urology are quite limited and pertain mainly to areas where conventional laparoscopy's shortcomings have been a major hindrance as in reconstructive procedures such as pyeloplasty. Initial experience here has revealed functional outcomes and complication rates similar to those of laparoscopy. Operators are nonetheless faced with new challenges that need to be tackled: complications that are yet to be reported and economic issues that need to be addressed before robotics become commonplace in pediatric urology.

References

1 Muntener M, Ursu D, Patriciu A, Petrisor D, Stoianovici D. Robotic prostate surgery. *Expert Rev Med Devices* 2006;3:575–84.

2 Fichtinger G, Burdette EC, Tanacs A, Patriciu A, Mazilu D, Whitcomb LL *et al.* Robotically assisted prostate brachytherapy with transrectal ultrasound guidance – Phantom experiments. *Brachytherapy* 2006;5:14–26.

3 Rovetta A. Tests on reliability of a prostate biopsy telerobotic system. *Stud Health Technol Inform* 1999;62:302–7.

4 Bauer J, Lee BR, Stoianovici D, Bishoff JT, Micali S, Micali F *et al.* Remote percutaneous renal access using a new automated telesurgical robotic system. *Telemed J E Health* 2001;7:341–6.

5 Satava RM. Emerging technologies for surgery in the 21st century. *Arch Surg* 1999;134:1197–202.

6 Olsen LH, Jorgensen TM. Robotically assisted retroperitoneoscopic heminephrectomy in children: initial clinical results. *J Ped Urol* 2005;1:101–4.

7 Pedraza R, Weiser A, Franco I. Laparoscopic appendicovesicostomy (Mitrofanoff procedure) in a child using the da Vinci robotic system. *J Urol* 2004;171:1652–3.

8 Pedraza R, Palmer L, Moss V, Franco I. Bilateral robotic assisted laparoscopic heminephroureterectomy. *J Urol* 2004;171:2394–5.

9 Olsen LH, Deding D, Yeung CK, Jorgensen TM. Computer assisted laparoscopic pneumovesical ureter reimplantation a.m. Cohen: Initial experience in a pig model. *APMIS Suppl* 2003;109:23–5.

10 Yee DS, Klein RB, Shanberg AM. Case report: Robot-assisted laparoscopic reconstruction of a ureteropelvic junction disruption. *J Endourol* 2006;20:326–9.

11 Klingler HC, Remzi M, Janetschek G, Kratzik C, Marberger MJ. Comparison of open versus laparoscopic pyeloplasty techniques in treatment of uretero-pelvic junction obstruction. *Eur Urol* 2003;44:340–5.

12 Yee DS, Shanberg AM, Duel BP, Rodriguez E, Eichel L, Rajpoot D. Initial comparison of robotic-assisted laparoscopic versus open pyeloplasty in children. *Urology* 2006;67:599–602.

13 Lee RS, Retik AB, Borer JG, Peters CA. Pediatric robot assisted laparoscopic dismembered pyeloplasty: Comparison with a cohort of open surgery. *J Urol* 2006;175:683–7.

14 Gettman MT, Peschel R, Neururer R, Bartsch G. A comparison of laparoscopic pyeloplasty performed with the da Vinci robotic system versus standard laparoscopic techniques: Initial clinical results. *Eur Urol* 2002;42:453–7.

15 Bhayani SB, Link RE, Varkarakis JM, Kavoussi LR. Complete da Vinci versus laparoscopic pyeloplasty: Cost analysis. *J Endourol* 2005;19:327–32.

16 Weise ES, Winfield HN. Robotic computer-assisted pyeloplasty versus conventional laparoscopic pyeloplasty. *J Endourol* 2006;20:813–19.

17 Link RE, Bhayani SB, Kavoussi LR. A prospective comparison of robotic and laparoscopic pyeloplasty. *Ann Surg* 2006;243:486–91.

18 Lee RS, Borer JG. Robotic surgery for ureteropelvic junction obstruction. *Curr Opin Urol* 2006;16:291–4.

19 Passerotti C, Peters CA. Robotic-assisted laparoscopy applied to reconstructive surgeries in children. *World J Urol* 2006;24:193–7.

20 Kutikov A, Nguyen M, Guzzo T, Canter D, Casale P. Robot assisted pyeloplasty in the infant-lessons learned. *J Urol* 2006;176:2237–9.

21 Olsen LH, Jorgensen TM. Computer assisted pyeloplasty in children: The retroperitoneal approach. *J Urol* 2004;171:2629–31.

22 Olsen LH, Rawashdeh YF, Jorgensen TM. Pediatric robot assisted retroperitoneoscopic pyeloplasty: A 5-year experience. *J Urol* 2007;178:2137–41.

23 Mariano ER, Furukawa L, Woo RK, Albanese CT, Brock-Utne JG. Anesthetic concerns for robot-assisted laparoscopy in an infant. *Anesth Analg* 2004;99:1665–7.

24 Woo R, Le D, Krummel TM, Albanese C. Robot-assisted pediatric surgery. *Am J Surg* 2004;188:27S–37S.

25 Camarillo DB, Krummel TM, Salisbury JK, Jr. Robotic technology in surgery: Past, present, and future. *Am J Surg* 2004;188:2S–15S.

26 Bethea BT, Okamura AM, Kitagawa M, Fitton TP, Cattaneo SM, Gott VL *et al.* Application of haptic feedback to robotic surgery. *J Laparoendosc Adv Surg Tech A* 2004;14:191–5.

27 Hanly EJ, Marohn MR, Bachman SL, Talamini MA, Hacker SO, Howard RS *et al.* Multiservice laparoscopic surgical training using the da Vinci surgical system. *Am J Surg* 2004;187:309–15.

28 Atug F, Woods M, Burgess SV, Castle EP, Thomas R. Robotic assisted laparoscopic pyeloplasty in children. *J Urol* 2005;174:1440–2.

21

Lower Urinary Tract Laparoscopy in Pediatric Patients

Rakesh P. Patel, Benjamin M. Brucker and Pasquale Casale

Key points

- Preoperative voiding cystourethrograms (VCUG) to ensure bladder capacity more than 130 cc.
- Improve voiding habits and constipation prior to surgery.
- Cystoscopy with ureteral catheter placement prior to surgical positioning for laparoscopic

component is extremely helpful but not mandatory.
- Keep dissection away from pelvic plexus.
- Distended abdomen postoperatively is a bladder leak until proven otherwise.

Laparoscopic transvesical and extravesical ureteral reimplantation

Introduction

Minimally invasive ureteral reimplantation is being developed and becoming an alternative option to traditional open surgery as a standard of care in children with disorders such as vesicoureteral reflux (VUR), primary obstructive megaureter (POM), and other pathologies of the ureterovesical junction [1,2]. VUR occurs in approximately 30% of children with at least one febrile urinary tract infection (UTI) [3]. It has been well documented over the years that UTI in the presence of VUR can cause pyelonephritis and this potentially can lead to renal scarring with its associated sequelae [4].

Treatment modalities for VUR vary and depend on the patient's clinical course. There is currently no consensus among health care professionals regarding when

medical or surgical therapy should be used [5]. When surgery is warranted, open ureteral reimplantation has been the gold standard over the years. In the recent years, subureteric injection of implant material has shown considerable promise [6].

In the 21st century, laparoscopy, with or without robotic assistance, is being used increasingly to treat this condition and has helped to minimize morbidity of this major surgery [1,2,7]. Both, intravesical and extravesical antireflux techniques performed laparoscopically [8,9] have been shown to have good success rate and benefits.

Laparoscopic- and robotic-assisted extravesical reimplantation

In girls, the ureter can be seen cephalad to the uterus. The ureter is exposed by incising the peritoneum anterior to the uterus and sweeping the uterine ligament and pedicle posteriorly. In boys, the ureter is visualized and mobilized at the level of the iliac vessels. The vas deferens needs to be mobilized from the ureter and kept cephalad to the portion of the ureter to be placed in the detrusor tunnel. The ureter then is seen just outside the bladder, mobilized and cleared for approximately 4 or 5 cm. After filling the bladder partially through a preplaced Foley

Pediatric Urology: Surgical Complications and Management. Edited by Duncan T. Wilcox, Prasad P. Godbole and Martin A. Koyle. © 2008 Blackwell Publishing, ISBN: 978-1-4051-6268-5.

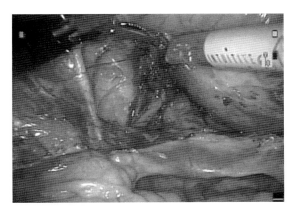

Figure 21.1 View of detrusor tunnel formation and left ureter for extravesicle robotic-assisted ureteral reimplantation.

catheter, a detrusor incision of approximately 2.5 cm is made up to the mucosa. A Y-shaped mobilization around the hiatus of the ureter is performed, but not circumferentially to avoid damage to the nerves. Detrusor muscle is then wrapped around the ureter with 3-0 or 4-0 absorbable suture. While doing the detrusorrhaphy, a "hitch stich" is passed through the periureteral sheath in order to stabilize the ureter and prevent recurrent reflux post surgery (Figure 21.1).

Outcomes

As this is a relatively new technique with only few specialized centers offering this procedure, large series and long-term outcomes are yet to be studied. However, preliminary results have been published.

Peters *et al.* published their initial experience with 17 patients, 15 girls, and 2 boys with a mean follow-up of 5–8 months and had two failures. Other complications in this series were two patients with bladder leakage; one with voiding dysfunction; one patient with a solitary kidney had obstruction, but did well with stent placement [10].

Riquelme *et al.* [11] had 15 patients in their series of pure laparoscopic transperitoneal Lich Gregoir extravesical ureteral reimplant. Fourteen of fifteen patients had success, which is comparable to open surgery. In three patients with mucosal perforation, Foley catheter was left for 3–4 days. Patients did not experience bladder spasms and gross hematuria. At follow-up of 15–49 months only one patient had UTI.

Complications

• *Voiding difficulties*: This technique when undertaken by an experienced surgeon should minimize the urinary

retention issues, in case of bilateral ureteral reimplant, as at time of dissection nerves are clearly seen and dissection is kept away from the nerves. None of the series published with this operation have recorded this problem.

• *Bladder leak*: Occurs in a small number of patients and is usually amenable to Foley catheter drainage.

• *Bleeding*: The authors have not seen any major bleeding problems in patients. With transperitoneal laparoscopy, there is the potential for bleeding to occur into a larger potential space than the contained space of the extraperitoneal pelvis.

• *Infection*: Prophylactic antibiotics are given in order to minimize this complication and it is our routine to also send a urine culture during initial cystoscopy.

• *Urinary obstruction*: Ureteral catheters may be placed to facilitate dissection and reimplantation. This is especially true in case of solitary kidney and prior stenting is recommended [10].

• *Persistent reflux*: Noted to be equivalent to open surgery.

Preventing complications

Preoperative

• Treat dysfunctional voiding to minimize recurrence.
• Treat any UTI.
• Cystoscopy and ureteral retrocatheter placement for visualizing bladder for any evidence of infection and to identify ureter at time of surgery with ease.

Intraoperative

• Adequate detrusorrhaphy to achieve good tunnel length.
• Minimize dissection around the nerves to prevent any postoperative bladder dysfunction.
• Good hemostasis, to improve visualization and meticulous dissection.
• Care should be taken not to violate the bladder mucosa.
• If there is a history of prior dextranomer/hyaluronic acid injection, this mound may need to be mobilized and dissected off in order to get a good tunnel length.

Postoperative

• Foley catheter/ureteral catheter drainage overnight, longer if bladder perforation is suspected.
• Adequate pain control; patients usually do not complaint of bladder spasms once the Foley catheter is removed, which is one of the advantages of this procedure.
• Patient should be voiding without problems prior to discharge.

Management of complications

• *Bladder dysfunction and leakage*: Usually amenable to drainage.

• *Persistent reflux*: Patient may outgrow or may be managed endoscopically; treat voiding dysfunction prior to surgery to minimize this complication. Failed conservative therapy may necessitate reoperative intervention.

Conclusions

Early results from these procedures are very encouraging. Robotic-assisted laparoscopy for treatment of reflux when undertaken by trained surgeons is a safe and effective procedure. Robotic-assisted laparoscopy has an added advantage of more magnification, elimination of hand tremors, and ease of tying knots. More training and clinical research is required prior to drawing definite conclusions.

Laparoscopic transvesical ureteral reimplantation

Introduction

Laparoscopic transvesical reimplantation with or without robotic assistance is currently being developed as another alternative to open surgery. This approach harbors the potential for decreased postoperative bladder spasms, reduced incisional pain, faster catheter removal, and improved cosmesis.

The operation is performed via pure laparoscopy using transvesical cross-trigonal ureteral reimplantation for VUR and Glenn-Anderson reimplantations for primary obstructing megaureters [1]. The patient is placed in the dorsal lithotomy position. Three 3 mm torcars are placed under cystoscopic guidance as described by Yeung *et al.* [2]. A pediatric feeding tube is placed through urethra and connected to a suction apparatus. Suction is clamped and unclamped as required during surgery. Excisional ureteral tapering may be performed in select cases (Figure 21.2).

Outcomes

In the authors' hands, of the 32 patients, four had complications and/or surgical failure [1]. Two patients had persistent reflux. In this series, bladder capacity was a factor (more or less than 130 ml) between success and failure/complications. The hypothesis is that larger the bladder capacity, more feasible the operation. There is also a technical problem with bladder contractions at time of important dissection secondary to a pneumovesicum above 6–8 mm of Hg. This may disrupt visualization at a

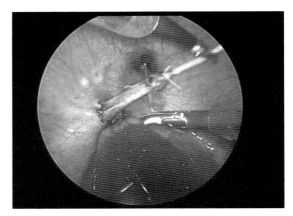

Figure 21.2 Vesicoscopic appearance of the left ureter being dissected after insertion of a ureteral catheter. Note the feeding tube at the bladder neck utilized as a suction device.

critical moment. This underscores the technical difficulty in performing this highly complex task in the limited space of the pediatric bladder. Peters *et al.* [10] had one patient with leakage that resolved after 1 week of maintaining an indwelling urethral catheter.

Complications

• Persistent reflux
• Leakage from the port site
• Infection
• Ureteral stricture
• Hematuria

Preventing complications
Preoperative

• *Patient selection*: The larger the bladder capacity, the more feasible the operation.
• Treat voiding dysfunction prior to surgery [12].

Intraoperative

• Preemptive placement of fascial sutures to facilitate a watertight closure.
• Fine balance between bladder distention with CO_2 and water to minimize bladder spasms that may disrupt vision.
• Extreme care when tapering POMs as they may have an ischemic segment and strictures may develop.
• Minimize bleeding or prompt control of bleeding to optimize visualization.

Postoperative

• Urethral catheter drainage until the next morning.
• Adequate hydration and pain/spasms control.
• Antibiotics.

Managing complications
- *Ureteral stricture*: endoscopic balloon dilation or redo reimplantation.
- *Leakage*: drainage with urethral catheter.
- *Persistent reflux*: endoscopic or redo reimplantation.

Conclusions
Laparoscopic intravesical ureteral reimplantation is in its infancy. At this time, caution should be used when considering this procedure for young patients with small bladder capacity (<130 cc), and for those who require ureteral tapering [1]. This technically challenging pediatric procedure with further experience may become part of each pediatric urologist's armamentarium.

Minimally invasive surgery for management of ureteral stumps

Introduction
VUR into a poorly functioning kidney, or a poorly functioning upper or lower pole of an ipsilateral duplex system, has been managed by nephrectomy and partial ureterectomy through a flank incision or a complete nephroureterectomy (NU) via an additional lower abdominal incision to remove distal ureter [10,13–15].

There have been two schools of thought regarding leaving ureteral stumps behind. Some authors agree to total ureterectomy and some leave behind ureteral stumps because of very low incidence of UTI [16–21]. Casale *et al.* [22] in their series found 19% (6/32) of all patients with refluxing stumps had symptomatic UTI and recommended NU or heminephroureterectomy (HNU) to the level of bladder hiatus. For those who required surgical intervention, the authors recommended laparoscopic distal ureteral stump removal.

Cystoscopy is performed and under fluoroscopic guidance the ureteral stump is imaged. A ureteral catheter is placed to aid in identification of the stump at time of laparoscopy. For a duplex system, the functional moiety is protected by placing an additional ureteral catheter. A urethral catheter is placed, and the open-ended catheter is secured to the urethral catheter. Three ports are placed including the camera port. The White line of Toldt is incised. The ureteral stump is filled with saline through open-ended catheter. The stump is then dissected to the distal intramural segment using sharp dissection. The detrusor defect is closed with an absorbable suture after removing the open-ended catheter [22] (Figure 21.3).

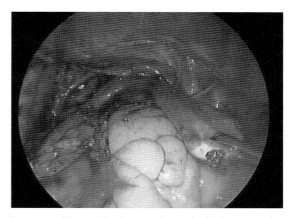

Figure 21.3 View of distal stump dissected off of the normal ipsilateral ureteral moiety.

Outcomes
Laparoscopic ureteral stump removal is a minimally invasive and effective way of dealing with symptomatic-retained ureteral stumps after simple partial or total nephrectomy and partial ureterectomy.

Complications
- Persistence of symptoms
- Injury to other ureter in case of duplex system requiring reimplantation
- Injury to nerves causing voiding symptoms (less likely secondary to unilateral insult)
- Infection
- Bleeding
- Bladder leak requiring prolonged catheter drainage.

Preventing complications
Preoperative
- Treat UTI.

Intraoperative
- Imaging of ureteral stump and placement of open-ended catheter for identification.
- Placement of double pigtail stent in the healthy ureter in case of duplex system.
- Use of an absorbable suture to tie the excised stump.
- Minimize dissection around nerves.

Postoperative
- Catheter drainage of the bladder until the first morning postoperative.
- Pain and bladder spasms control.
- Voiding cystourethrogram if signs of urinary leakage are present.

Conclusions

Laparoscopic ureteral stump removal is an effective way of treating symptomatic distal ureteral stumps. At time of primary surgery, some authors leave behind ureteral stumps because of low incidence of symptomatic UTI (5%). However, when indicated an NU or HNU should be performed minimally up to the bladder hiatus.

Complicated urachal remnants

Introduction

The urachus is the fibrous cord that represents the embryonic remnant of the communication between the bladder and the umbilicus [23]. Anomalies of the urachus include urachal sinus, urachal cyst, patent urachus, and urachal diverticulum. The most common is the urachal cyst that occurs in 1/5000 births [24]. Laparoscopic treatment of these symptomatic urachal remnants has been described since 1993 [25,26]. Presentation of these complicated remnants include: infection, drainage from the umbilicus, abdominal distention, and abdominal pain. The gold standard for the treatment of these remnants of the allantois has been complete open surgical excision from the umbilicus to the bladder. Complete excision is advocated because of the high incidence of recurrent symptoms and the potential for malignant transformation in the remaining tissue [27].

There have been various techniques that have been employed for successful excision of the remnant tissue. Though the port placement is surgeon dependent, the general consensus is that a three port approach should be used. The dissection should be carried out starting just caudal to the umbilicus, taking down the urachus and the obliterated umbilical arteries [28]. The dissection should be carried out to the bladder that has been distended with the help of a urethral catheter. In most cases it is appropriate to take a small cuff of urinary bladder. The bladder closure should be carried out in two layers with absorbable sutures (Figure 21.4).

Outcomes

Given the rare nature of these anomalies there have been no large series that are available to accurately assess outcomes. There are only three small series that give preliminary insight into the safety and effectiveness of laparoscopic intervention for urachal remnants [28–30]. Only one of these is a series of four patients that are exclusively a pediatric population [29]. Table 21.1

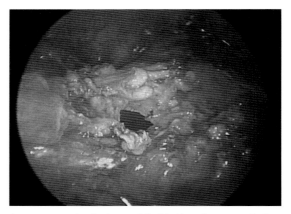

Figure 21.4 Defect in dome of the bladder after removal of urachal remnant.

summarizes the outcomes and complications of the laparoscopic approach to excision of the symptomatic urachal remnant.

Complications

Complete excision to the urachal tissue is paramount for insured success. Persistent drainage or repeat infection should be considered as a complication of the procedure. Port placement must be done to facilitate complete resection.

In an attempt to completely resect the cephalad aspect of the remnant, care must be taken not to damage the umbilicus. The distance to the visible umbilicus is often small and extensive use of cautery can cause thermal injury. Some have questioned the utility of such an approach for excision of urachal cysts because of the already small excision that the open approach utilizes verses potentially three small incisions [6]. With any laparoscopic manipulation and excision of the bladder the potential for a bladder leak exists.

Preventing complications
Preoperative
• Avoid acute infection when possible. Infection of the remnant may be the presenting symptom in many cases. If the child is acutely infected the dissection and success of the repair have the potential to be compromised. The acute inflammatory reaction often obscures tissue planes that could potentially lead to a wider excision than is necessary. Further, the inflammatory process that exists in the surrounding tissue has the potential to alter wound healing, resulting in persistent urine leak or possibly even a fistula.

Table 21.1 Summary of laparoscopic urachal remnant outcomes.

Study	Number of cases reported	Age range	Mean operative time	Reported complications	Mean time to discharge	Mean time to catheter removal
Khurana *et al.*	4	5 months to 10 years	n/r	None	n/r	1.6 days*
Cadeddu *et al.*	4	29–66 years	180 min	None	2.75 days	7 days
Cutting *et al.*	5	2–43 years	n/r	Intraoperative: no complication Postoperative: 1 Small periumbilical hematoma 2 Persistent umbilical drainage 3 Pyrexia	<3†	n/r

*Information not available on one of the patients.
†Not reported as a mean.
n/r, not reported.

Intraoperative

• *Port placement*: The port placement is important to insure the complete resection. Khurana and Borzi [29] note that the working ports should be placed at a more acute angle than usual to aid in the umbilical dissection. Cutting *et al.* [27] have further proposed a lateral view and lateral port placement to aid in complete visualization of the tract. They suggest placing three ports lateral to the rectus belly and then using a small incision under the umbilicus to remove the specimen.

• *Urethral catheter*: Urethral catheterization must be used in this laparoscopic approach to avoid bladder injury, aid in dissection, and ensure adequate bladder closure. In addition to minimizing the chance of bladder injury with port placement, the catheter facilitated filling the bladder to help define the appropriate plane on the peritoneal reflection to make a bladder cuff. The catheter can also be used to fill the bladder after repair in order to inspect the suture line for a watertight closure.

Postoperative

• *Foley catheter drainage*: The appropriate length of catheter drainage is not well studied and ultimately must be a decision that is made by the surgeon. Some advocate a cystogram while others maintain that a watertight closure intraoperatively is more than adequate to remove the catheter without further studies, although there has been no formal study evaluating these theories.

• *Anticholinergics*: Administered to reduce frequency and amplitude of involuntary bladder contractions that can occur from the dissection and catheter irritation.

Managing complications

The management of the persistence of drainage or infection unfortunately may necessitate a repeat resection. In cases with a urine leak secondary to a defect in the bladder closure can be handled with prolonged catheter drainage. One must remember that the laparoscopic approach is an intraperitoneal operation. Thus, in severe cases of bladder leaks, an open reoperation may be necessary.

Conclusion

The laparoscopic approach to the urachal remnant and its complications has been shown to be a safe effective approach. There are no randomized trials or large series that have been published on this topic. Further investigation into patient satisfaction, long-term outcomes, cost and operative time need to be performed before this technique gains popular acceptance.

Reconstructive bladder surgery

Introduction

Major reconstructive operations of the bladder in pediatric urology are still considered challenging endeavors

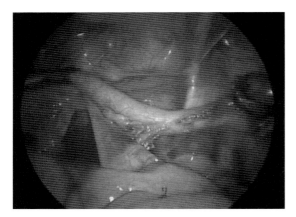

Figure 21.5 View of the appendix for appendicovesicostomy mobilized off the cecum. The drawback is that the patency test can only be done after appendiceal transaction.

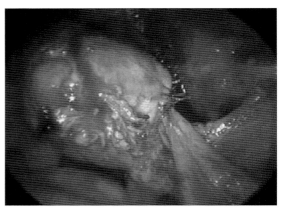

Figure 21.6 Appendix anastomosed to the bladder and aligned to the right lower quadrant for externalization.

even for the advanced laparoscopist. These operations may in fact be the last frontier for the lower urinary tract [6]. The first report of an enterocystoplasty that was preformed entirely intracorporally was in 1995 by Docimo *et al.* [31]. Though there have been no large series reported on the entirely intracorporeal technique, the laparoscopic-assisted reconstructive surgery has gained support in the literature [31,32].

The proposed advantage of incorporating laparoscopic techniques into large reconstructions is to allow the surgeon to perform the repair through a less morbid and more cosmetically pleasing Pfannenstiel incision [33]. Large abdominal scars may in fact have an emotional and social impact on younger patients, and a Pfannenstiel incision which can be covered by underwear or bathing suits is thought to be less traumatic [33,34].

The laparoscopic role in reconstructive surgery has included mobilization of the right colon, appendiceal harvesting for an appendiceal Mitrofanoffs, mobilization of the kidney and dilated ureter for ureterocystoplasty, harvest of stomach tissue for gastrocystoplasty, lysis of adhesions, and mobilization of the sigmoid [31–33,35] (Figures 21.5 and 21.6).

There have been reports of pure laparoscopic procedures that include an ileal cystoplasty, autoaugmentation of the bladder, and a robotically assisted appendicovesicostomy [36–38].

Outcomes

The largest published pediatric laparoscopic-assisted reconstructive surgery series includes 31 patients ranging in age from 1 to 36 years [32]. This series notes no intraoperative complications. One patient with a history of ventriculoperitoneal (VP) shunt was found to have dense adhesion and required a conversion to open antegrade continent enema (ACE), Monti sigmoid vesicostomy. In this series, 39 stomas were created and 94.9% were continent and easily catheterizable at a mean follow-up of 32 months. 25.6% of the new stomas created required minor procedures including: dilation and collagen injection.

The author reported five postoperative complications that were not related to the stomas created. These postoperative complications included a small bowel obstruction, traumatic bladder perforation, a delayed ileus, deep vein thrombosis, and a wound infection.

Hedican *et al.* [33] report laparoscopic-assisted reconstructive surgery with eight patients in their series. This series had no intraoperative complications reported and noted excellent cosmesis utilizing the Pfannenstiel or lower midline incision and using the trocar sites to mature the stomas and place drains. They had one patient who required re-exploration for a prolonged ileus and was found to have a knuckle of ileum passing between the crossed mesenteries of the appendiceal mitrofanoff and ileal antegrade continence enema stoma.

The experience of the complete laparoscopic- and robotic-assisted approach is still in its infancy. The outcome results are difficult to interpret given the scan numbers reported. Large series and controlled series are still needed. Further long-term outcomes are not yet established, however the data to date does support the safety and effectiveness of using laparoscopy.

Preventing complications
Preoperative
• *Patient selection*: Be aware of comorbidities such as prior abdominal surgery, severe kyphosis, and VP shunt placement. These comorbidities do not preclude a laparoscopic approach.
• *Ureteral catheters*: In order to avoid injury to the ureteral orifices, placement of externalized ureteral stents is advisable. This may also help during the postoperative period to divert the patient's urine output away from the healing anastomosis.

Intraoperative
• Recreate anatomic angles to ensure ease of catheterization. If stomas are created with pneumoperitoneum, the angle necessary for catheterization may change upon deflation.
• *Avoid visual estimation*: During the isolation on section of bowel for use in the reconstruction, care must be taken to accurately judge the appropriate length of bowel that the surgeon is going to use. The magnification of the laparoscope can make gross visual estimates difficult. Using premeasured vessel loops can help accurately measure segments of bowel and prevent taking segments of inappropriate length.
• *Irrigate port site*: Irrigation is a basic principle in open surgery and laparoscopic surgery. This deserves mention in light of the fact that port site infection has been noted as a complication of these procedures.
• *Choose a cosmetically conscious incision*: Though surgical success is paramount, the surgeon should strive to perform the procedure through small concealable incisions which is possible when undertaking laparoscopy-assisted reconstruction as long as they do not compromise the procedure. These are usually in areas that can be covered by undergarments.

Postoperative
• *Insure catheter drainage*: In order to insure adequate healing, catheters and drains must be used to divert urine flow. This includes the use of irrigation if reconstructions include mucous secreting surfaces. Preventing mucous plugs and thus preventing functional obstructions will insure that fresh anastomosis is not put under unsafe pressures.
• *Early recognition of stomal narrowing*: The inability to catheterize the stoma of a urinary bladder that otherwise has no other means of releasing a pressurized system can have serious consequences. The patient and family must be comfortable with stoma care and catheterization so that problems can be recognized and dilation or revision can take place prior to serious emergent situations.

Managing complications
The complications that arise from performing these reconstructive procedures are not managed differently than those that arise from purely open procedures. Management may however be easier in patients that had laparoscopic assistance or pure laparoscopic procedures. Not only does laparoscopy have potentially reduced incidence of postoperative problems such as ileus (from decrease bowel manipulation) and incisional hernias, the potential to decrease adhesion formation may allow for less technically difficult reexploration or revision if necessary. There have been reports of bladder perforation, bowel obstructions, and ileus in the series sited above. The details of the management can be found in basic surgical and urologic texts.

Conclusion
The laparoscopic procedures in reconstructive pediatric urology are technically possible and seem to be as safe as open procedures with the caution that the data is small and long-term outcomes are still to be studied. There is a role for pure laparoscopic reconstructions such as augments, bladder neck closure, catheterizable channels; however, the majority of literature favors using laparoscopic assistance and a cosmetically favorable incision. This approach may not only lessen morbidity, but may also be a more attractive option to some patients.

References

1 Alexander K, Thomas JG, Daniel JC, Pasquale C. Initial experience with laparoscopic transvesical ureteral reimplantation at the children's hospital of Philadelphia. *J Urol* 2006;176:2222–5,discussion 2225–6.
2 Yeung CK, Sihoe JD, Borzi PA. Endoscopic cross-trigonal ureteral reimplantation under carbon dioxide bladder insufflation: A novel technique. *J Endourol* 2005;19:295–9.
3 Stansfeld JM. Clinical observations relating to incidence and etiology of urinary tract infections in children. *Br Med J* 1966;1:631–5.
4 Rollenston GL. Relationship of infantile vesicoureteric reflux to renal damage. *Br Med J* 1970;1:460–3.
5 Elder JS. Guidelines for consideration for surgical repair of vesicoureteral reflux. *Curr Opin Urol* 2000;10:579.
6 Puri P, Chertin B, Velayudhan M, Dass L, Colhoun E. Treatment of vesicoureteral reflux by endoscopic injection of detranomer/hyaluronic acid copolymer: Preliminary results. *J Urol* 2003;170:1541–4,discussion 1544.

7 Guilherme CL, Soroush R-B, Richard EL, Louis RK. Laparo-scopic ureteral reimplantation: A simplified dome advance-ment technique. *J Endourol* 2005;19:295–9.

8 Olsen LH, Deding D, Yeung CK, Jorgensen TM. Computer assisted laparoscopic pneumovesical ureter reimplantation a.m. Cohen: Initial experience in a pig model. *APMIS Suppl* 2003; 109:23–5.

9 Gill IS, Ponsky LE, Desai M, Kay R, Ross JH. Laparoscopic cross-trigonal Cohen ureteroneocystotomy: Novel tech-nique. *J Urol* 2001;166:1811–14.

10 Peters CA. Robotic assisted surgery in pediatric urology. *Pediatr Endosurgery Innovat Technol* 2003;7:403–13.

11 Riquelme M, Aranda A, Rodriguez C. Laparoscopic extra-vesical transperitoneal approach for vesicoureteral reflux. *J Laparoendosc Adv Surg Tech A* 2006;16:312–16.

12 Higham-Kessler J, Reinert SE, Snodgrass WT, Hensle TW, Koyle MA, Hurwitz S, Cendron M, Diamond DA, Caldamone AA. A review of failures of endoscopic treatment of vesicoureteral reflux with dextranomer microspheres. *J Urol* 2007;177:710–14,discussion 714–15.

13 Persad R, Kamineni S, Mouriquand PD. Recurrent symp-toms of urinary tract infection in eight patients with reflux-ing ureteric stumps. *Br J Urol* 1994;74:720–2.

14 Krarup T, Wolf H. Refluxing ureteral stump. *Scand J Urol Nephrol* 1978;12:181.

15 Ahmed S, Boucat HA. Vesicoureteral reflux in complete ure-teral duplication: Surgical options. *J Urol* 1988;140:1092.

16 Ubirajara B, Jr., Adriano AC, Miguel ZF. The role of reflux-ing distal ureteral stumps after nephrectomy. *J Pediatr Surg* 2002;37:653–6.

17 De Caluwé D, Chertin B, Puri P. Fate of the retained ureteral stump after upper pole heminephrectomy in duplex kid-neys. *J Urol* 2002;168:679–80.

18 De Caluwé D, Chertin B, Puri P. Long-term outcome of the retained ureteral stump after lower pole heminephrectomy in duplex kidneys. *Eur Urol* 2002;42: 63–6.

19 Plaire JC, Pope JC, IV, Kropp BP, Adams MC, Keating MA, Rink RC, Casale AJ. Management of ectopic ureters: Experience with the upper tract approach. *J Urol* 1997;158:1245–7.

20 Androulakakis PA, Tephanidis A, Antoniou A: Christophoridis C. Outcome of the distal ureteric stump after (hemi)nephrectomy and subtotal ureterectomy for reflux or obstruction. *BJU Int* 2001;88:586–9.

21 Cain MP, Pope JC, Casale AJ, Adams MC, Keating MA, Rink RC. Natural history of refluxing distal ureteral stumps after nephrectomy and partial ureterectomy for vesicoureteral reflux. *J Urol* 1998;160:1026–7.

22 Casale P, Grady RW, Lee RS, Joyner BD, Mitchell ME. Symptomatic refluxing distal ureteral stumps after neph-roureterectomy and heminephroureterectomy. What should we do? *J Urol* 2005;173:204–6,discussion 206.

23 Pomeranz A. Anomalies, abnormalities, and care of the umbilicus. *Pediatr Clin North Am* 2004;51:819–27.

24 Berman SM, Tolia BM, Laor E, Reid RE, Schweizerhof SP, Freed SZ. Urachal remnants in adults. *Urology* 1988;31:17–21.

25 Madeb R, Knopf JK, Nicholson C, Donahue LA, Adcock B, Dever D, Tan BJ, Valvo JR, Eichel L. The use of robotically assisted surgery for treating urachal anomalies. *Br J Urol* 2006;98:838–42.

26 Trondsen E, Reiertsen O, Rosseland AR. Laprascopic exci-sion of urachal sinus. *Eur J Surg* 1993;159:127–8.

27 Cutting CW, Hindley RG, Poulsen J. Laparoscopic man-agement of complicated urachal remnants. *Br J Urol Int* 2005;96:1417–21.

28 Cadeddu JA, Boyle KE, Fabrizio MD, Schulam PG, Kavoussi LR. Laparoscopic management of urachal cysts in adult-hood. *J Urol* 2000;164:1526–8.

29 Khurana S, Borzi PA. Laparoscopic management of compli-cated urachal disease in children. *J Urol* 2002;168:1526–8.

30 Kim TW, Chung H, Yang SK, Lee TU, Woo SH, Kim HS. Laparoscopic management of complicated urachal rem-nants in a child. *J Korean Med Sci* 2006;21:361–4.

31 Docimo S, Moore R, Adams J, Kavoussi L. Laparoscopic blad-der augmentation using stomach. *Urology* 1995; 46:565–9.

32 Chung S, Meldrum K, Docimo S. Laparoscopic assisted reconstructive surgery: A 7-year experience. *J Urol* 2004;171,372–5.

33 Hedican SP, Schulam PG, Docimo SG. Laparoscopic assisted reconstructive surgery. *J Urol* 1999;161:267–70.

34 Abdullah A, Blankeney P, Hunt R, Broemeling L, Phillips L, Herndon DN, Robson MC. Visible scars and self esteem in pediatric patients with burns. *J Burn Care Rehabil* 1994;15:164.

35 Cilento BG, Diamond DA, Yeung CK, Manzoni G, Poppas DP, Hensle TW. Laparoscopically assisted ureterocystoplasty. *Br J Urol* 2003;91:525–7.

36 Pedraza R, Weiser A, Franco I. Laparscopic appendicovesi-costomy (mitrofanoff procedure) in a child using the DaVinci robotic system. *J Urol* 2004;171:1652–3.

37 Pedraza R, Weiser A, Franco I. Laparoscopic appendi-covesicostomy (mitrofanoff procedure) in a child using the DaVinci robotic system. *J Urol* 2004;171:1652–3.

38 Elliott SP, Meng MV, Anwar HP, Stoller ML. Complete laparoscopic ileal cystoplasty. *Urology* 2002;59:939–43.

VI Genitalia

22

Hernia and Hydrocele Repair

Henrik Steinbrecher

Key points

- Inguinal hernias come in different shapes and sizes.
- Hernia repair in children should not be automatically relegated to junior surgeons to operate.
- The overall complication rate is up to 10%.
- A thorough understanding of the inguinal anatomy, varying risks, and operative methods will enable the surgeon to minimize their complication rate.
- Modern advances in surgery, specifically laparoscopic surgery, are bringing with them new and perhaps better techniques, but also new risks and complications.
- The best treatment for complications is prevention.

Introduction

Inguinal hernia repair and correction for hydroceles in children are some of the commonest operations performed in the life of a pediatric surgeon. Much has been written about the age incidence and distribution, male to female ratio, laterality, and incarceration rate such that the reader is directed to comprehensive reviews for this data [1–3]. Controversies continue as to the role of identifying a patent processus vaginalis to pre-emptively treat a potential future hernia and whether laparoscopic surgery is the way forward [4].

Surgical techniques

A number of approaches are utilized for repair of inguinal hernias but the essential principles are the same. In the open procedure the hernial sac is identified, dissected off the surrounding structures (testicular cord in males, round ligament in females) to the deep inguinal ring or site of origin, assessed for contents that are reduced and dealt with appropriately (divided and transfix ligated if complete sac into scrotum/labia, transfix ligated if incomplete sac). The wound is finally closed after ensuring that the testis (in the male) is pulled down into the scrotum with the cord lying lax in the wound.

Over recent years newer techniques such as laparoscopic herniotomy have brought with them a new set of potential problems.

Inguinal herniotomy/ligation of PPV

The traditional operation of pediatric inguinal herniotomy is well described [5]. A number of alternative approaches can be adopted in selected clinical cases (Table 22.1) such

Table 22.1 Approaches commonly in use for inguinal herniotomy.

Approaches	References
Standard approach	[5]
Scrotal "Bianchi" approach	[6]
Laparoscopic	[7–10]
Preperitoneal	[11–13]
Transperitoneal ring closure (incarcerated hernia)	[14]

Pediatric Urology: Surgical Complications and Management. Edited by Duncan T. Wilcox, Prasad P. Godbole and Martin A. Koyle. © 2008 Blackwell Publishing, ISBN: 978-1-4051-6268-5.

as strangulation [13,15], the "difficult" hernia [16], and the bilateral hernia [17]. The scrotal approach has been adopted by some to avoid opening the inguinal canal and thereby reducing accompanying risks of damage to the cord structures [6].

Laparoscopic herniotomy

One of the first reported laparoscopic herniotomy in girls was published in 1998 [7]. Subsequently, it became clear that the laparoscopic approach could be taken in boys as well [8]. A randomized blinded comparative study has shown that laparoscopic herniotomy can give less pain and better wound cosmesis than an open approach, although the operation takes longer [10]. Many modifications of laparoscopic techniques have evolved [9,18,19] ultimately aiming at completely reproducing the open procedure with suture ligation and division of the peritoneum, or reproducing the same results as open surgery.

Large "dumbbell" hydrocele/ abdominoscrotal hydrocele

This type of hydrocele was first described by Dupytren in 1834 as "L'hydrocele en bissac." Until 1981 only eight pediatric cases had been described in children [20]. Its etiology and operative approach have been described in a number of papers [21] and includes complete excision of the abdominal element with an addition Jaboulay or Lord's procedure for the scrotal element. The operative treatment of this type of hydrocele has developed over the years such that now even the laparoscopic approach is being advocated [22].

The neonatal inguinal hernia

It is clear that the neonatal inguinal hernia operation is a highly specialized operation that can challenge the most experienced pediatric surgeon. The tissues are thin, often edematous and friable. Neonatal inguinal hernias often present incarcerated, making subsequent operation, usually carried out during the same admission or soon afterwards, more difficult. The surgical approach is usually the same as for a hernia in an older child although it has to be remembered that the internal and external ring may overlie each other and that the tissue planes may not be as easily defined due to edema. Many anesthetists prefer to give neonates a spinal or caudal anesthesia with some sedation (glucose dummy, etc.) [23,24], so abdominal movement is also an hindrance to the surgeon in these cases.

The "sliding hernia"

In this type of hernia the bowel such as the appendix, the fallopian tube, or even the bladder wall can be intimately associated with one wall of the hernial sac such that it is impossible to separate the two. In this case, simple transfixion ligation is unsafe. To avoid damaging the viscus a transfixion suture may be placed distal to the sliding element and then the whole stump may be invaginated, reducing the viscus and the hernial sac together. A purse-string narrowing (in boys) or closure (in girls) of the internal ring is then performed. An alternative method is to initially invaginate the sliding part of the sac and then purse-string it at the base of the invagination [25].

The incarcerated hernia

An incarcerated inguinal or femoral hernia can be a real test of surgical skill and a number of alternative techniques have been developed to facilitate easy reduction of the hernia and subsequent adequate surgical treatment. The preperitoneal approach was described well over 30 years ago [12] and has more recently been redescribed [13]. A transperitoneal approach with ligation of the internal ring avoids tackling of the cord, allows inspection of the gut, and can aid hernial reduction [14].

The pediatric hydrocele/patent processus vaginalis

Surgery for the common pediatric hydrocele, which is in effect a persistent patent processus vaginalis (PPV) is to all intents and purposes identical to that of the hernia and will not be considered separately here. Minor variations such as the hydrocele of the cord (male)/canal of Nuck (female), epididymal cysts need no separate explanation as regard to complications. A number of variations of the standard procedure have been expounded in the literature to reduce the risk of vasal damage. These include division and nonligation of the sac [26] and nondivision with ligation only.

The pediatric distal hydrocele

The distal hydrocele – be it part of a large dumbell hydrocele or a secondary hydrocele – either missed or as a result of other surgery, e.g. varicocoele surgery is usually surgically treated by the Lords method [27].

Femoral hernia repair

The standard operative procedure for femoral hernia repair – the "low approach" has been well documented and attributed to Langenbeck [5]. This relatively straightforward inferior approach is safe if a nonacute diagnosis and procedure is carried out. The better approach for strangulation is the "high approach," which involves more generous dissection of the inguinal canal proper, possibly weakening it. The hernia is approached from above, extraperitoneally, by drawing up the cord, conjoint tendon, and dividing the transversalis fascia to expose the hernial sac [28]. A more medial "high approach" is the McEvedy technique, which tackles the sac from above but more medially than through the canal. An incision is made medial to the semilunaris line in the anterior rectus sheath and an extraperitoneal approach is taken to the neck of the sac [29].

Outcomes

The overall success rate for inguinal herniotomy, with success being defined as one operation with no complications, is about 95%. A number of factors determine whether complications or not are likely to occur.

Outcomes by age

It is well recognized that hernia repair in the premature and young infant is a different entity to that in an older child. The recurrence rate of neonatal herniotomy has been shown to be higher than that accepted for non-neonatal hernias [30] with recurrence rate in this series of 92 herniotomies in children <44 weeks gestation being 8.6%. At the other end of the spectrum, a recent paper has noted a much higher recurrence rate in teenagers [3], which the author could not explain.

Outcomes by presentation method

Emergency herniotomy and incarceration has a higher complication rate than routine surgery [31,32]. It is not clear whether this is due to surgical expertise in operating on emergency cases, or the inherent difficulty of the procedure, although the latter is more likely since an emergency pediatric hernia is usually carried out by a senior surgeon. Although not strictly an operative complication but nonetheless a "surgical" one, is a missed diagnosis of androgen insensitivity when dealing with female inguinal hernias especially in bilateral cases. A missed diagnosis can lead to devastating sequelae in later life [33]. Only 53% of femoral hernias are said to be diagnosed correctly at initial presentation so that the recurrence rate of 13% is higher than that of inguinal herniae [34].

Outcomes by approach

The different approaches used to repair inguinal hernias attest to the surgeon's desire to facilitate success and reduce complications as much as possible. High approaches in incarcerated cases potentially reduce the risk of damage to the cord structures. Proper diagnosis of a dumbell hernia will allow the surgeon to choose the correct approach. Laparoscopic surgery is being hailed as an approach that allows easier reduction of contents under direct vision, nonhandling of edematous and friable tissue reducing the long-term risks; however, most series report higher recurrence rates than in the open method [35] although even in the field of laparoscopic surgery, newer techniques have reduced the recurrence rate to less than 1% [36]. One would expect the laparoscopic approach to have a lower risk of atrophy and vasal damage than the open approach but data are certainly not yet available to verify this in the long term in view of this relatively new technique.

Complications and prevention of complications associated with surgery

Pediatric inguinal herniotomy forms a substantial part of any pediatric surgeon's practice. It is often classed as a "training operation" although it is not without its problems and the overall historical complication rate is said to be between 1% and 8% [37,38]. Complications that are well recognized are listed in Table 22.2.

Meticulous attention to precise surgical technique is mandatory.

• Keloids are prevented by keeping the incision within Langer's lines/skin creases, utilizing the knife rather than the diathermy for making the incision, and avoiding wound infections. A monofilament absorbable suture is said to be less keloid forming.

• Bruising and hematoma formation occur due to immediate damage to vessel and inadequate diathermy/arrest of those that are bleeding. The commonest vessels to damage are the superficial inferior epigastric vein and the deep epigastric artery. The superficial vein should be diathermied or on occasions ligated.

Bipolar diathermy utilization is safer than monopolar as in the latter current may inadvertently travel along the testicular cord potentially damaging the testicular blood supply.

• Wound infection, though uncommon has been associated with the use of both nonabsorbable sutures such as silk [39] and absorbable sutures [3]. Avoiding a knot at either end of the skin subcuticular suture by burying it a number of times is said to reduce this [45].

• The ilioinguinal nerve encroaches on the inguinal canal in varying degrees.

Table 22.2 Complications associated with pediatric inguinal herniotomy.

Type	Specifics	Incidence	References
Wound complications	Incision scar keloid formation		
	Bruising/hematoma		
	Infection/abscess	0.6–1.5%	[3,39]
Neuropraxia	Ilio-inguinal nerve, genitofemoral nerve/division or entrapment		
Missed hernia			
Recurrent hernia		0–3.8%	[3,25]
Hydrocele	Postherniotomy	14%	[40,41]
Intra–abdominal obstruction	Adhesions		[42]
Bladder damage			[43]
Iliac vessel/femoral vessel damage	False aneurysms		
Testicular complications	Ascending testis, atrophy, damage to vas		[44]
Undiagnosed androgen insensitivity syndrome			[33]

The main nerve originally courses between the internal and external oblique muscles before entering the distal third of the inguinal canal. The genital branch of the genitofemoral nerve arrives in the inguinal canal via the internal ring or by piercing the fascia transversalis. It then runs along the back of the spermatic cord to the scrotum supplying the cremaster muscle in the male. In the female it accompanies the round ligament where it ends. Both nerves may easily be damaged on incising the canal. Localization of the nerves before dissection, diathermy, or ultimately closing the canal reduces possible damage risk.
• A hernia may be missed due to a number of factors. An incision that is too low can give a false impression of having exposed the inguinal canal fully and having reached the inferior epigastric artery (the site of the deep ring). The presence of a lipoma of the cord can mislead the surgeon into thinking that the sac has been identified. A lipoma is usually lateral and inferior to the testicular vessels whereas a hernial sac is lying anterior to the vessels. Incomplete exploration of the inguinal canal by identifying the cord at the external ring without opening up the inguinal canal can lead to a missed hernia higher up.
• Recurrent inguinal hernia is more frequent in neonatal hernia operations.

Recurrence is usually early in the first few days and weeks after the initial surgery. The recurrence rate after inguinal herniotomy is reported to be between 0.8% and 3.8% [25]. More than 50% occur in the first year postoperatively and more than 90% by 5 years postoperatively. It is greater if the operation is for incarceration. Grosfeld

and colleagues in their work expound a number of reasons for recurrent hernia some of which include: failure to ligate high, a large internal ring, injury to the floor of the inguinal canal, weakness due to comorbidity such as malnutrition, increased intra–abdominal pressure such as the presence of a VP shunt, and deferred orchidopexy.

The medial wall of the inguinal canal may be stretched sufficiently to weaken it as well as give a wide internal ring through which a further hernia may occur. This risk may be reduced by consciously narrowing the internal ring with an interrupted vicryl suture once the sac has been dealt with or by carrying out a formal approximation of the sleeves of the internal spermatic fascia that has been breached during herniotomy. This has led to a recurrence rate of 0% in 10 years for 945 male herniotomies [46].

An indirect recurrence occurs either because the ligation suture has come off the sac or the inguinal sac had been torn.
• A residual hydrocele following an inguinal herniotomy is occasionally a cause of concern as it is not clear as to whether a hernia has been missed, or whether the distal sac, usually large at initial operation, has reaccumulated fluid. An avoidance technique for this dilemma includes opening up the distal sac longitudinally during the initial operation although a randomized trial involving 798 males has suggested that there is no difference in hydrocele rate if the sac is split or left [41]. Evacuating any residual fluid at initial operation using a syringe or pressure on the scrotum is a good method of avoiding reaccumulation, although it may only serve to reassure

the parents postoperatively that an operation has actually been carried out!

• Intra-abdominal adhesion formation is rare. Failure to make sure that the sac has no contents could lead to incorporation of the contents into the ligature around the neck of the hernial sac with ultimate consequences of omental ischemia or bowel ischemia depending on what is caught. It is good practice to view the inside of the hernial sac once identified and reduce any contents rather than automatically twisting the sac and ligating it. In a complete sac this is easily done by placing two clips on either side of the sac once divided and opening it up, prior to dissecting it back to the internal ring.

• Damage to the bladder is rare and usually occurs if an incision is too low and medial [43], confusing the surgeon with the bulge of the bladder mimicking a hernial sac.

• Iliac and femoral vessel damage is also rare and commoner in older children.

It results from the sutures of the canal closure at the level of the lower border of the external oblique being placed too deep. It is good practice to see the metal of the needle at all times during placement of these sutures.

• Testicular ascent is usually caused by insufficient dissection of the sac to the deep ring or by failure to make sure that the testis is pulled down into the scrotum at the end of the operation, causing snagging of the cord under the external oblique layer of the canal and subsequent adhesion to it. It is said to occur in 0.8–2.8% [44]. Attention to these points reduces the risk of ascension.

• Testicular atrophy occurs as the blood supply to the testis is compromised, either acutely during the operation or subsequently due to scar formation. Its incidence may be underestimated as accurate measurements of pre- and postherniotomy testicular volume are rarely taken [40,47].

• Damage to the vas is similarly reduced if it is not grasped between forceps and only dissected off using one blade of a nontoothed forceps or not touched at all [48].

Specific complications of laparoscopic herniotomy

One of the largest personal series of laparoscopic inguinal hernia repair in children has shown a recurrence rate of 3.7% (20/542), a hydrocele rate of 0.7% (3/542), and a testicular atrophy rate of 0.2% (1/542, a child with a previous incarcerated hernia) [35]. In this series the hernial sac was not transected and was only closed from inside using a purse-string type of "N" stitch with nonabsorbable suture laparoscopically. In this series, the recurrence rate was lower in the last 100 cases

than at the beginning, suggesting a definitive learning curve for the technique. It also seems clear that using an absorbable suture does not increase the recurrence rate [49] although a different series of 972 repairs using the LPEC (laparoscopic percutaneous extraperitoneal closure) carried out in 3 centers had a recurrence rate with absorbable sutures of 5/40 (12.5%) and 0/932 with nonabsorbable sutures [36].

Management of complications

Obvious management is avoidance. Any immediate complications should be dealt with accordingly once recognized.

• *Bleeding should be stopped at the time of surgery*. The treatment of wound abscess may be conservative with antibiotics or surgical with incision and drainage.

• Recurrences are best dealt with sooner rather than later and methods include high ligation of the recurrent sac, snugging the internal ring (McVey repair), and preperitoneal repair in multiple recurrences [25].

• *Vasal injury*. Vasal injury identified at the time of surgery may be treated in two surgical ways but first and foremost, the onus is on the surgeon to be honest and tell the parents that this damage has occurred [50]. This can be during the time of surgery to allow discussion of the options of subsequent treatment or afterwards. Options for repair include primary repair using microscopic anastomosis [51,52] or delayed repair at an older age, in which case the vasal ends should be marked with a permanent suture to perform vaso-vasotomy after puberty although results with this method are poorer than straightforward vasectomy reversal operations [53].

• *Testicular atrophy*. Avoidance of initial damage is maximized by not grasping the vessels, not stripping all the tissue off the vessels, and only prudently using the diathermy, if at all. Some centers advocate no usage of the diathermy during this procedure and will omit it from the lay up set.

Summary

The operation of inguinal hernia repair in children is recognized by specialists to be one of the most taxing procedures encountered, depending on the age of the patient and the mode of presentation. The overall complication free operation rate is over 90% in most cases and modern techniques continue to be developed to try and improve the long-term outcome with reference to testicular damage, vasal damage, recurrence, and associated injuries.

References

1 Gross RE. *The Surgery of Infancy and Chidlhood.* Saunders: Philadelphia, 1972, pp. 417–22.

2 Skoog SJ, Conlin MJ. Pediatric hernias and hydroceles: The urologist's perspective. Common problems in pediatric urology. *Urol Clin North Am* 1995;22:119–30.

3 Ein S, Njere I, Ein A. Six thousand three hundred sixty-one pediatric inguinal hernias: A 35 year review. *J Pediatr Surg* 2006;41:980–86.

4 Parkinson E, Pierro A. Inguinal and umbilical hernias. In *Paediatric Surgery and Urology: Long term outcomes.* Edited by M Stringer, K Oldham, P Mouriquand. Cambridge University Press, UK, 2006, pp. 286–95.

5 Grosfeld JL. Hernias in children. In *Rob and Smith's Operative Surgery – Pediatric Surgery,* 5th edn. Edited by L Sitz, A Coran, 1995. Chapman and Hall, UK.

6 Koyle MA, Walsh R, Caruso A, Wilson E. Scrotal (Bianchi) approach to patent processus vaginalis in children. *Tech Urol* 1999;5:95–9.

7 Schier F. Laparoscopic herniorrhaphy in girls. *J Pediatr Surg* 1998;33:1495–7.

8 Montupet P, Esposito C. Laparoscopic treatment of congenital inguinal hernia in children. *J Pediatr Surg* 1999;34:420–3.

9 Becmeur F, Philippe P, Lemandat-Schultz A, Moog R, Grandadam S, Lieber A *et al.* A continuous series of 96 laparoscopic inguinal hernia repairs in children by a new technique. *Surg Endosc* 2004;18:1738–41.

10 Chan KL, Hui WC, Tam PKH. Prospective randomized single-center, single-blind comparison of laparoscopic vs open repair of pediatric inguinal hernia. *Surg Endosc* 2005;19:927–32.

11 Fowler R. Preperitoneal repair of inguinal hernias in infancy and childhood. *Aust Paediatr J* 1973;9:85–9.

12 Jones PF, Towns GM. An abdominal extraperitoneal approach for the incarcerated inguinal hernig of infancy. *Br J Surg* 1983;70:719–20.

13 Kamaledeen SA, Shanbhogue LK. Preperitoneal approach for incarcerated inguinal hernia in children. *J Pediatr Surg* 1997;32:1715–6.

14 Misra D, Hewitt G, Potts SR, Brown S, Boston VE. Transperitoneal closure of the internal ring in incarcerated infantile inguinal hernias. *J Pediatr Surg* 1995;30:95–6.

15 Koga H, Yamataka A, Ohshiro K, Okada Y, Lane GJ, Miyano T. Pfannenstiel incision for incarcerated inguinal hernia in neonates. *J Pediatr Surg* 2003;38:E16–18.

16 Applebaum H, Bautista N, Cymerman J. Alternative method for repair of the difficult infant hernia. *J Pediatr Surg* 2000;35:331–3.

17 Raine PA, Young DG. Single incision for bilateral inguinal herniorrhaphies in female children. *J Pediatr Surg* 1995;30:901.

18 Harrison MR, Lee H, Albanese CT, Farmer DL. Subcutaneous endoscopically assisted ligation (SEAL) of the internal ring for repair of inguinal hernias in children: A novel technique. *J Pediatr Surg* 2005;40:1177–80.

19 Oue T, Kubota A, Okuyama H, Kawahara H. Laparoscopic percutaneous extraperitoneal closure (LPEC) method for the exploration and treatment of inguinal hernia in girls. *Pediatr Surg Int* 2005;21:964–8.

20 Black RE, Cox JA, Han B, Babcock DS. Abdominoscrotal hydrocele – Casue of abdominal mass in children. *Pediatrics* 1981;67:420–22.

21 Squire R, Gough DCS. Abdominoscrotal hydrocele in infancy. *Br J Urol* 1988;61:347–9.

22 Kinoshita Y, Shono T, Nishimoto Y *et al.* A case of abdominoscrotal hydrocele surgically treated under laparoscopic assistance. *J Pediatr Surg* 2006;41:1610–12.

23 Gallagher TM, Crean PM. Spinal anaesthesia in infants born prematurely. *Anaestheia* 1989;44:434.

24 Frumiento C, Abajian JC, Vane DW. Spinal anesthesia for preterm infants undergoing inguinal hernia repair. *Arch Surg* 2000;135:445–51.

25 Grosfeld JL, Minnick K, Shedd F, West KW, Rescorla FJ, Vane DW. Inguinal hernia in children: Factors affecting recurrence in 62 cases. *J Pediatr Surg* 1991;26:283–7.

26 Mohta A, Jain N, Irniraya KP *et al.* Non-ligation of the hernial sac during herniotomy: A prospective study. *Pediatr Surg Int* 2003;19:451–2.

27 Lord PH. Bloodless surgical procedures for the cure of idiopathic hydrocoele and epididymal cyst (spermatocoele). *Prog Surg* 1972;10:94–108.

28 Johnstone JMS, Rintoul RF. Operations for hernia. In *Farquharson's Textbook of Operative Surgery.* Edited by RF Rintoul. Churchill Livingstone, UK, 1986, pp. 480–503.

29 McEvedy PG. Femoral hernia. *Ann R Coll Surg Engl* 1950;7:484.

30 Phelps S, Agrawal M. Morbidity after neonatal inguinal herniotomy. *J Pediatr Surg* 1997;32:445–7.

31 Morecroft JA, Stringer MD, Higgins M, Holmes SJ, Capps SN. Follow-up after inguinal herniotomy or surgery for hydrocele in boys. *Br J Surg* 1993;80:1613–14.

32 Steinau G, Treutner KH, Feeken G *et al.* Recurrent inguinal hernia in infants and children. *World J Surg* 1995;19:303–06.

33 Hughes IA, Lim HN, Ahmed SF. Clinical aspects of androgen insensitivity. *Clin Pediatr Endocrinol* 2002;11:9–15.

34 De Caluwe D, Chertin B, Puri P. Childhoosd femoral hernia: A commonly misdiagnosed condition. *Pediatr Surg Int* 2003;19:608–09.

35 Schier F. Laparoscopic inguinal hernia repair – A prospective personal series of 542 children. *J Pediatr Surg* 2006;41:1081–4.

36 Takehara H, Yakabe S, Kameoka K. Laparoscopic percutaneous extraperitoneal closure for inguinal hernia in children: Clinical outcome of 972 repairs done in 3 pediatric surgical institutions. *J Pediatr Surg* 2006;41:1999–2003.

37 Harvey M, Johnstone M, Fossard D. Inguinal herniotomy in children: A 5 year survey. *Br J Surg* 1985;72:485.

38 Rescorla F, Grosfeld J. Inguinal hernia repair in the perinatal period and early infancy: Clinical Considerations. *J Pediatr Surg* 1984;19:832.

39 Nagar H. Stitch granulomas following inguinal herniotomy: a 10 year review. *J Pediatr Surg* 1993;28:1505–7.

40 Davies BE, Frase N, Najmaldin AS *et al*. A prospective study of neonatal inguinal herniotomy: The problem of the postoperative hydrocoele. *Pediatr Surg Int* 2003;19:68–70.

41 Gahukamble DB, Khamage AS. Prospective randomized controlled study of excision versus distal splitting of hernial sac and processus vaginalis in the repair of inguinal hernias and communicating hydroceles. *J Pediatr Surg* 1995;30:624–5.

42 Stanley-Brown EG. Adhesion causing intestinal obstruction 13 years after herniorraphy. *J Pediatr Surg* 1972;7:438.

43 Koot VC, de Jong JR, van der Zee DC, Dik P. Subtotal cystectomy as a complication of infant hernia repair. *Eur J Surg* 1998;164:873–4.

44 Surana R, Puri P. Iatrogenic ascent of the testis: An under recognized complication of inguinal hernia operation in children. *Br J Urol* 1994;73:580–1.

45 Mahabir RC, Christense B, Blair GK *et al*. Avoiding stitch abscesses in subcuticular skin closures: The L-stitch. *Can J Surg* 2003;46:223–4.

46 Yokomori K, Ohkura M, Kitano Y *et al*. Modified marcy repair of large indirect inguinal hernia in infants and children. *J Pediatr Surg* 1995;30:97–100.

47 Leung WY, Poon M, Fan TW *et al*. Testicular volume of boys after inguinal herniotomy: Combined clinical and radiological follow-up. *Pediatr Surg Int* 1999;15:40–1.

48 Parkhouse H, Hendry WF. Vasal injuries during childhoos and their effect on subsequent fertility. *Br J Urol* 1991;47:91–5.

49 Schier F, Montupet PH, Esposito C. Laparoscopic inguinal herniorrhaphy in children: A three-centered experience with 933 repairs. *J Pediatr Surg* 2002;37:395–7.

50 UK-GMC 2006. *The Duties of a Doctor*. General Medical Council: UK, 2006.

51 Lamesch AJ, Dociu N. Microsurgical vasovasostomy. *Eur Surg Res* 1981;13:299–309.

52 Ozen IO, Bagbanci B, Demirtola A, Karabulut R, Ozen O, Demirogullari B *et al*. A novel technique for vas deferens transection repairs. *Pediatr Surg Int* 2006;22:815–19.

53 Matsuda T, Muguruma K, Hiura Y *et al*. Seminal tract obstruction caused by childhood inguinal herniorrhaphy: Results of microsurgical anastomosis. *J Urol* 1998;159:837–40.

23

Orchidopexy and Orchidectomy

Kim A.R. Hutton and Indranil Sau

Key points

- Congenital undescended testis is a common condition with palpable testes managed via open surgery with an inguinal or scrotal approach.
- Laparoscopic orchidopexy is becoming the gold standard for impalpable testes with a success rate >90%.
- Initial position of the testis affects surgical outcome; there are higher complication rates with intra-abdominal testes.
- Most common complications are testicular re-ascent and atrophy.

- Repeat orchidopexy is technically demanding and aided by adequate exposure, good lighting, optical magnification, and a clear understanding of inguinal anatomy.
- Acquired undescended testis is an increasingly recognized condition – the ascending testis – and may be managed nonoperatively.
- Altered body image following orchidectomy in childhood may lead to the request for a testis prosthesis later.
- Orchidectomy following acute torsion may result in subsequent infertility.

Introduction

The undescended testis is a common problem in pediatric urological practice with 3–5% of newborns affected, although the majority descend in the first few months of life resulting in an incidence of 0.8–1.1% at one year of age [1]. Treatment options are hormone manipulation and surgery. Surgical procedures for the palpable testis include the standard inguinal and more recently described scrotal orchidopexy. The impalpable testis can be managed by open surgery with testicular vessel preservation or an open one- or two-staged Fowler–Stephens procedure. Microvascular transfer of the intra-abdominal testis with anastomosis of the testicular artery and vein to the inferior epigastric vessels is a viable option for successful orchidopexy. Increasingly, however, the intra-abdominal testis is being managed laparoscopically via a one-stage orchidopexy, or if necessary a laparoscopic

Pediatric Urology: Surgical Complications and Management. Edited by Duncan T. Wilcox, Prasad P. Godbole and Martin A. Koyle. © 2008 Blackwell Publishing, ISBN: 978-1-4051-6268-5.

Fowler–Stephens procedure performed in one or two stages. This chapter will not cover these laparoscopic techniques as they are discussed in Chapter 24. Controversies in the management of cryptorchidism include age at operation, surgical approach, management of complications, and follow-up. Orchidectomy is performed for small, dysplastic undescended testes or for nonviable testes at exploration for acute torsion. The aim of this chapter is to look at the outcomes of these surgeries, to document the range of surgical complications that occur, and to provide advice on how to prevent and manage these complications.

Outcomes for orchidopexy

The success of orchidopexy can be measured from an anatomical or functional perspective. In the former, the surgeon aims to relocate the testis in a dependent position within the scrotum, with preservation of testicular volume indicating a lack of testicular atrophy. Most of the present literature describes outcomes in these terms and relates success to initial testis position and operative technique. In the latter, the objectives are to maximize and preserve future spermatogenic and endocrine functions of the testis. These data are often difficult to acquire, as patients must be followed through adulthood and long-term prospective, randomized and controlled studies to determine the optimal age and technique of orchidopexy from both an anatomical and functional standpoint have yet to be published.

Outcome by testis location

The excellent review by Docimo in 1995 summarizes the importance of preoperative testis position on successful orchidopexy [2]. Of over 300 articles and book chapters, a final assessment was limited to 64 reporting 8425 orchidopexies that contained sufficient data for analysis. Of 2491 testes, where a preoperative position and postoperative result were reported, a successful outcome was noted in over 90% located beyond the external ring and increasing failure rates observed with progressively higher testes (Figure 23.1). These results are expected when related to the increased complexity of surgical techniques required to bring peeping and intra-abdominal testes to the scrotum. In the past decade, success of orchidopexy has increased to >95% for inguinal testes and >85–90% for abdominal testes [3,4].

Fertility potential after orchidopexy in unilateral ectopic, canalicular, and emergent testes, as long as surgery is performed in early childhood, is good (>90%) and fertility for most cases of unilateral intra-abdominal testis and patients with unilateral anorchia or vanishing testis is expected, whereas the majority of patients with bilateral intra-abdominal testes are infertile [5].

Outcome by age

The age at orchidopexy has been decreasing steadily over the years with most surgeons now recommending surgery at 6–12 months of age. The drive for earlier orchidopexy has come from histological data documenting germ cell degeneration during the second year of life [6,7] and findings of delayed and defective prepubertal maturation of germ cells in cryptorchid testes [8]. To address possible concerns of earlier orchidopexy and specifically any increased risk to testicular vessel integrity, Wilson-Storey *et al.* retrospectively reviewed their results in 100 orchidopexies under and 100 over 2 years of age [9]. Results were similar in both groups with an atrophy rate of 5%. In a prospective randomized controlled study of 70 infants having surgery at 9 months of age, there were no re-operations and only one case of testicular atrophy (1.4%) [10].

Although it is too early to know if orchidopexy in the first year of life will improve long-term outcomes, a few studies suggest earlier surgery may be beneficial. In a randomized controlled study of 149 boys, 70 were randomized to surgery at 9 months and 79 to orchidopexy at 3 years of age. Over the first 24 months of life testes operated at 9 months showed statistically significant better growth, as assessed by ultrasound measured testicular volumes than nonoperated boys [10]. A previous study by Nagar and Haddad of 190 boys documented testis size before and after orchidopexy and noted testis growth in 11.6%, and this was statistically more likely when surgery was performed before 18 months of age [11]. Hadziselimovic *et al.* have published data on infertility in 218 cryptorchid men correlating testis biopsy findings and

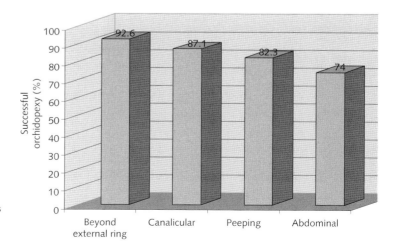

Figure 23.1 Historical success rates for orchidopexy in relation to preoperative testis location. (Data from literature review by Docimo, 1995 [2].)

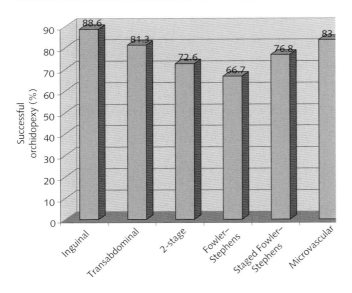

Figure 23.2 Historical success rates for orchidopexy in relation to type of orchidopexy. (Data from literature review by Docimo, 1995 [2].)

age at orchidopexy with total sperm counts. If transformation into Ad spermatogonia (the adult stem cell pool) had occurred, age-related differences in fertility outcome were observed, with earlier surgery resulting in higher sperm counts. Age at surgery had no effect in the group of cryptorchid men having no type A dark spermatogonia at the time of orchidopexy and this failure of germ cell maturation predicted infertility and azoospermia [12].

When orchidopexy is delayed to later childhood, subclinical decreases in Leydig cell function have been documented [13]. Surgery before the age of 2 results in higher inhibin B levels in adulthood, implying better-preserved Sertoli cell function [14].

Outcomes for palpable testes

Inguinal orchidopexy

The majority of undescended testes are amenable to a standard inguinal orchidopexy including division of cremasteric fibers, ligation and division of the processus vaginalis, and retroperitoneal dissection through the internal ring with division of lateral fascial bands as required. Saw *et al.* reported on 1057 palpable testes operated via an inguinal approach and 943 (89%) were in the bottom of the scrotum at the end of surgery, a further 67 (6%) in the middle, 41 (4%) in the top of the scrotum, 1 in the groin, and 5 boys underwent orchidectomy [15]. In Docimo's literature review inguinal orchidopexy was successful in 88.6% of cases (Figure 23.2) [2].

Scrotal orchidopexy

The advantage of this technique is said to be reduced postoperative pain due to the single incision used, improved cosmesis as the incision is placed in the inguinoscrotal crease or a high rugosal fold of the scrotum and reduced operative time as compared to a standard inguinal approach as there is only one incision to make and close.

The technique has been applied by some authors to all patients with palpable testes, while others have been more selective and restricted its use to testes that can be manipulated, albeit with difficulty, into the scrotum and therefore the results of individual studies are not directly comparable. However, conversion to an inguinal exploration is reported in 0–20% of cases, immediate complication rates are 0–6%, mainly wound infection and scrotal hematomas and successful orchidopexy is achieved in 94–100% of cases (see Table 23.1 and refs [16–21]). In the series reported by Parsons *et al.*, a low scrotal incision was used with an inguinal incision if a patent processus was identified, thereby explaining the high inguinal conversion rate [20]. With the higher scrotal approach, as used in the other series, dissection of the processus vaginalis from the cord is not usually a problem, although requiring more time and skill than surgery via a standard inguinal incision.

Despite technical demands, an average operative time of 15 min for patients with primary undescended testes and 35 min for patients with secondary ascent or iatrogenic ascent following previous inguinal surgery has been reported [22].

Table 23.1 Selected papers on scrotal orchidopexy documenting range of outcomes and complications. Early complications were related to scrotal hematoma, wound cellulitis, or wound infection.

Author	Year	Patient age in years	Number of operated testes	Inguinal conversion (%)	Early complications (%)	Need for redo orchidopexy (%)	Testis hypoplasia/ atrophy (%)
Bianchi and Squire [16]	1989	2–12	120	5 (4.2)	4 (3.3)	0	0
Iyer et al. [17]	1995	0.1–15.5	367	14 (3.8)	7 (1.9)	13 (3.5)	3 (0.8)
Lais and Ferro [18]	1996	0.4–14 (mean 5)	50	3 (6)	3 (6)	1 (2)	2 (4)
Russinko et al. [19]	2003	0.5–24 (median 4.5)	85	1 (1.2)	2 (2.4)	1 (1.2)	1 (1.2)
Parsons et al. [20]	2003	16 <2 years 19 2–6 years 17 >6 years	66	13 (20)	0	0	0
Bassel et al. [21]	2007	0.5–13 (mean 4.5)	121	0	4 (3.3)	0	0

Outcomes for impalpable testes

Inguinal approach and preperitoneal orchidopexy

In a number of series, management of the nonpalpable testis with open surgery has proved successful. Kirsch et al. reported on 1866 boys with undescended testes of which 447 (24%) were impalpable [23]. Surgery was successful in identifying testis location or blind-ending vas and vessels in 100% of cases. Of 91 intra-abdominal testes 33 were managed with inguinal orchidopexy and transperitoneal mobilization of the vas and vessels without vessel transection. Results were excellent (good scrotal position and size) or acceptable (palpably normal testis in the high scrotum) in 32/33 (97%). Youngson and Jones published on 90 boys with an impalpable testis utilizing a muscle-splitting preperitoneal orchidopexy for 28 intra-abdominal and 42 canalicular testes with success in 66 (94%) at 1 year [24]. However, on late follow-up after a mean of 11 years (range 6–16 years) this figure had reduced to 81%, with only 57% of the testes normal in size. Gheiler et al. have described initial laparoscopy and a subsequent open Jones orchidopexy for intra-abdominal testes with success in 18 of 19 (94%) cases [25].

Staged orchidopexy

In Docimo's analysis of the literature staged orchidopexy was successful in 180/248 (72.6%) testes [2] (see Figure 23.2). However, staged ochidopexy can result in high failure rates. Corbally et al. reported on 33 boys who had two orchidopexies on the developing testis and documented a high failure rate for intra-abdominal and canalicular testes with testis atrophy in 40% and a mean volume loss of 46% in the majority of remaining testes [26]. The role of staged orchidopexy has become largely historical, as successful one-stage techniques for transfer of the high intra-abdominal testis have emerged, e.g. laparoscopic orchidopexy, Fowler–Stephens orchidopexy, and microvascular transfer.

Fowler–Stephens orchidopexy

In some cases the high intra-abdominal testis may not be amenable to either extensive mobilization or staged orchidopexy because of an extremely short vascular pedicle. In these circumstances the testis can be mobilized on a vasal/peritoneal mesentery containing collateral circulation having divided the testicular vessels well above the body of the testis. The testis continues to be perfused by branches of the deferential and cremasteric arteries as described by Fowler and Stephens [27]. Some authors have suggested an advantage to staging this operation with testicular vessel ligation with minimal testicular handling as a first procedure and gonadal vessel transection, testicular mobilization, and orchidopexy several months later following robust collateral vessel development [28].

The results for these open one- and two-stage procedures are variable. Smolko et al. reported on seven patients with a poor result in five all four with an intra-abdominal testes and one of three with a preperitoneal testis (71% failure rate) [29]. They commented on the need to use vessel transection as a primary maneuver, without prior dissection

Table 23.2 Historical and contemporary results for open one- and two-stage Fowler–Stephens orchidopexy: results from articles published in the last decade combined.

	Number successful (%)	
	Literature review prior to 1995 (Docimo [2])	Current articles 1996–2006 [30–34]
One-stage Fowler–Stephens	214/321 (66.7)	64/73 (87.7)
Two-stage Fowler–Stephens	43/56 (76.8)	73/75 (97)

or skeletonization of the cord and linked its use to patients with prune belly syndrome and/or a long-looped vas. In Docimo's extensive review of the literature of 321 undescended testes treated with a single-stage Fowler–Stephens procedure, 214 (66.7%) had a successful result. Of 56 cases performed in two stages, 43 (76.8%) were successful [2] (see Figure 23.2). In more contemporary publications of open Fowler–Stephens orchidopexy, higher success rates have been reported (Table 23.2). Horasanli *et al.* [30] performed open single-stage Fowler–Stephens orchidopexy using optical magnification in 24 testes with success in 21(87.5%) and O'Brien *et al.* had a good result with one-stage mobilization and testicular vessel transection in 18 (82%) of 22 testes [31]. Using an open second stage mobilization following initial laparoscopic clipping of the testicular vessels, Law *et al.* reported viability, based on testicular size and consistency compared to the normal contralateral testis, in 19 (95%) of 20 testes [32]. Their only failure was in a case with an absent vas deferens. Dhanani *et al.* achieved excellent results with an open two-stage technique with 54 (98%) of 55 testes in a dependent scrotal position and testis size equivalent to the contralateral mate at a median of 1 year follow-up [33].

An interesting technical variation incorporating low spermatic vessel ligation, straightening of the looped vas and preservation of collateral circulation has been reported by Koff and Sethi [34]. In their series of 33 patients with intra-abdominal testes or testes visible at the internal inguinal ring, low vessel ligation resulted in successful orchidopexy in 38 of 39 testes (97%) examined at 1 month and 25 of 27 (93%) at 1 year follow-up.

Microvascular orchidopexy

From a logical point of view testicular autotransplantation should, by maintaining a full blood supply to a high inguinal/intra-abdominal testis, maximize the potential of future testis development and avoid the significant testicular loss and atrophy rates seen with staged and Fowler–Stephens orchidopexy. First described by Silber and Kelly in 1976

[35], the technique of microvascular transfer is technically demanding, requires specialized instrumentation, and is time-consuming (total operative time 2.5–3 h). These factors have undoubtedly played a role in limiting its widespread application. Preoperative assessment involves prior laparoscopy to document the presence and position of the testis. More recent studies have reported extending the role of endoscopy by performing laparoscopically assisted testicular autotransplantation [36].

Infants as young as 6 months of age have undergone microvascular transfer successfully which fits in with a desire for early orchidopexy to prevent subsequent degenerative testicular change. Occasionally, the vas deferens is also short and a scrotal position cannot be achieved despite microvascular transfer. A novel technique of vasal mobilization and testicular inversion has been described to overcome this pitfall [37]. In addition, in cases where the establishment of arterial inflow proves difficult, the testis will often survive on collateral circulation provided a successful venous anastomosis is performed – the "refluo" technique [38].

Most large series report good results with an adequately sized testis in the scrotum in 80–90% of patients postsurgery (see Table 23.3, Figure 23.2, and refs [2,36,39–42]). Less successful results could reflect a learning curve for this technically demanding surgery.

Complications of orchidopexy

Intraoperative
- Failure to achieve a dependent position in the scrotum
- Tearing of the hernial sac
- Injury to vas and/or testicular vessels
- Inadvertent torsion of spermatic vessels during testicular tunnelling
- Tension on vascular pedicle
- Avulsion of testicular vessels
- Ilio-inguinal nerve injury.

Table 23.3 Results of microvascular orchidopexy including laparoscopic testicular autotransplantation.*

Author	Year	Patient age (mean) in years	Number of testes	Number successful (%)
Wacksman et al. [39]	1982	1.9–20 (9.7)	7	6 (86)
Upton et al. [40]	1983	2–18	10	6 (60)
Bianchi [41]	1995	2–15	51	47 (92)
Boeckx et al. [42]	1998	3.25–15.75 (7.9)	25	24 (96)
Tackett et al.* [36]	2002	0.5–13 (3.6)	17	15 (88)

Early postoperative
• Pain
• Bleeding
• Hematoma
• Local edema
• Wound separation
• Wound infection.

Late postoperative
• Testicular malposition or re-ascent
• Testicular atrophy
• Torsion of testis
• Inguinal hernia
• Hernia alongside peritonealized vas after Fowler–Stephens orchidopexy – rare complication reported only as isolated case report
• Ureteral obstruction due to vasal compression after Fowler–Stephens orchidopexy – rare complication reported only as isolated case report
• Impaired spermatogenesis and infertility
• Testicular malignancy.

Preventing complications of orchidopexy

The complications of orchidopexy can be prevented by appropriate case selection, choosing the right surgical procedure for the individual patient, and by adhering to a philosophy of gentle tissue handling and meticulous surgical technique.

Preoperative considerations
Retractile testes
It is important to make an accurate diagnosis and correctly identify retractile testes as the majority end up in a satisfactory position long term without surgery [43] and

as reported by Puri and Nixon [44] these patients have normal fertility following conservative treatment.

Nonpalpable testes, contralateral hypertrophy, and initial scrotal exploration
In patients with nonpalpable testes, lubrication of the examining hands with liquid soap may assist in identifying a difficult to feel testis and avoid further investigation or inappropriate laparoscopy [45]. Most pediatric urologists and surgeons prefer laparoscopy for the assessment of the impalpable testis but in cases with a nonpalpable testis, and contralateral hypertrophy an initial scrotal incision may be more appropriate as 90–100% of patients have features consistent with the "vanishing testis syndrome" and perinatal torsion [45–48]. In the study by Hurwitz and Kaptein [45] in patients with a unilateral nonpalpable testis, hypertrophy with a testis length 1.8 cm or greater predicted monorchia with an accuracy of approximately 90% and in the series published by Belman and Rushton [48] of 22 boys with a left nonpalpable testis and hypertrophied right testis 19 (86.4%) were found to have scrotal nubbins on initial scrotal exploration. Laparoscopy was reserved for three cases where scrotal exploration was negative, with two vanishing testes and one intracanalicular testis found.

Snodgrass et al. [49] have taken this scrotum-first approach for the nonpalpable testis further with the suggestion that laparoscopy be reserved for cases where a scrotal nubbin is not identified and in patients where a patent processus vaginalis is found. In their series of 40 boys with a unilateral impalpable testis managed with an initial scrotal incision followed by laparoscopy, the scrotal exploration revealed 22 (55%) scrotal nubbins, 4 (10%) extra-abdominal testes, and 6 (15%) patients with a long looping vas associated with an intra-abdominal testis. Laparoscopy documented 13 (32.5%) intra-abdominal testes and one intra-abdominal vanished testis. Interestingly, laparoscopy falsely diagnosed an intra-abdominal vanished testis in 6 (15%) boys who had scrotal nubbins [49]. Not all palpable testes will be felt in the outpatients and a careful examination under anesthesia, and prior to a surgical procedure, should be performed as 18% of impalpable testes become palpable with the patient asleep [50].

The ascending testis

The entity of acquired undescended testis, where a previously normal scrotal testis retracts into an ectopic position, is a recently described phenomenon [51–53] with a prevalence of 1.2% age 6, 2.2% age 9, and 1.1% age 13 [54]. There is no consensus on etiology or correct management for these cases although recent data supports a conservative approach. Hack *et al.* [55] described a prospective study of 44 boys with 50 acquired undescended testes and noted spontaneous descent at puberty in 42 (84%) with a testicular volume appropriate for age. A more recent publication from the same group followed 139 boys with 164 acquired undescended testes [56]. Spontaneous descent occurred at puberty in 76% of testes (early puberty in 71.4% of these, 26.5% mid puberty, and 2.1% late puberty) and their expectant policy for the ascending testis has reduced orchidopexy rates in their hospital by 61.8% [57]. Whether this conservative management will affect future sperm counts, fertility, or malignancy risks in boys with acquired undescended testes is yet to be investigated.

Benefit of preoperative investigation

Ultrasound and standard magnetic resonance imaging (MRI) are unreliable for investigating the impalpable testis. Two different groups of investigators have, however, documented the accuracy of gadolinium (Gd)-enhanced MRI, with sedation, in localizing intra-abdominal testes, canalicular testes, hypoplastic/atrophic testes, and vanishing testes, with a sensitivity between 96% and 100% [58–60]. One article looking at a cost/risk analysis suggests that with MR angiography and observation of testicular nubbins, a substantial number of boys could forego operative intervention with minimal additional risk and no increased health care costs [61]. So far, although clearly Gd-MRI can be very reliable in experienced hands, it has yet to replace laparoscopy as the investigation of choice for the impalpable testis.

Operative considerations
Surgical technique

A good understanding of the operative principles for orchidopexy is required to prevent complications. The technique of inguinal orchidopexy was first reported by Bevan [62], with modifications described by Gross and Jewett [63], and subsequently by Koop and Minor [64]. For a contemporary description of orchidopexy, the reader is referred to a major operative pediatric surgery textbook [65].

Complications can be prevented by:

- Early identification of the testis, once Scarpa's fascia is opened. This will prevent inadvertent testis injury and can often be achieved by passing an index finger down into the scrotum in preparation for the future subdartos pouch. On removing the finger the palpable undescended testis usually pops directly into view within the operative field.
- Division of all attachments, including the gubernaculum, the cremasteric fibers, and the lateral spermatic fascia.
- Identification of the patent processus vaginalis in the anteromedial surface of the cord, and performing a high ligation. The sac/processus is usually divided and twisted prior to transfixion and division, and it is important not to trap the vas or vessels.
- Gentle handling of the vas and gonadal vessels. On no account they should be held or picked up with forceps.
- Prevention of tension on the cord structures which is likely to lead to ischemia or re-ascent.
- Creation of a subdartos pouch and if possible avoidance of suture fixation.
- Careful assessment of the orientation of the vascular pedicle prior to testicular tunnelling to prevent torsion and subsequent ischemia.
- Positive identification of the ilio-inguinal nerve just beneath the external oblique and its preservation.

Full mobilization of the testis with division of the hernia sac or processus and adequate retroperitoneal dissection are key to a satisfactory outcome. Davey [66] studied the relative importance of each step in 313 orchidopexies and found that sac/processus division accounted for 60% of increased cord length, while the remaining 40% was related to dissection within the internal ring and division of tethering lateral bands. A thorough knowledge of inguinal and retroperitoneal anatomy is required to prevent complications, and failure to achieve a satisfactory dependent scrotal position for the testis is often related to inadequate retroperitoneal mobilization. The reader is referred to the articles published by Hutcheson *et al.* [67] and Redman [68] on the applied anatomy of this region. If despite full mobilization there is still insuffi-cient length, the cord structures can be redirected medi-ally to the inferior epigastric vessels for a shorter route to the scrotum – the "Prentiss" maneuver [69,70].

In cases being assessed for a Fowler–Stephens orchidopexy, the procedure should be avoided when major ductal anomalies are present. Any case with absence or atresia of a segment of the vas or non-union of the vas and testis is likely to have inadequate collateral testis blood supply following testicular vessel transec-tion. In addition, the Fowler–Stephens procedure should be avoided in cases with an intrinsically short vas [71] and in reoperative cases [72].

With intra-abdominal testes it can be difficult to decide which procedure would be best suited to achieve a depend-ent scrotal position. Banieghbal and Davies [73] have used testicular mobility assessed at laparoscopy as a guide to management, and of 20 intra-abdominal testes that could be stretched to the contralateral internal inguinal ring a successful conventional orchidopexy was achieved. Other surgeons have predicted a successful orchidopexy with-out vessel division when the testis lies within 2 cm of the internal ring. When a small dysplastic intra-abdominal testis is present, orchidectomy is the best option. For microvascular orchidopexy a major problem can be the size discrepancy between the larger deep inferior epigas-tric artery and testicular artery. This can be overcome with accurately placed mattress sutures [42] or by creat-ing an arteriovenous fistula between the inferior epigas-tric artery and vena comitans, which increases run off and prevents microanastomotic thrombi within the trans-planted testis [74].

The creation of a subdartos pouch provides the best form of testis fixation [75,76]. In infants, when perform-ing the orchidopexy through a small 1.5–2.0 cm inguinal skin crease incision, there may be little space to pass an index finger down to the scrotum for pouch preparation without compressing and traumatizing the cord struc-tures in the corner of the wound. A novel and commer-cially available testicular tunneler (Surgical Innovations Limited, UK) can assist in creating a direct path to the scrotum (Figure 23.3). Once the tunneler has been passed from the inguinal incision and out through the scrotum, the testis is guided into position following the placement of a suture between the gubernaculum and end eye of the tunneler. The testis is then placed in the prepared subdar-tos pouch. Re-ascent may be further prevented by nar-rowing the subdartos fascia at the scrotal neck, but care is required not to constrict the testicular vessels [77]. On occasion the surgeon may deem it necessary to suture the

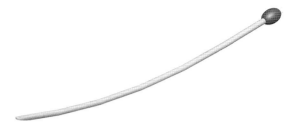

Figure 23.3 Lambert testicular tunneler. (Courtesy of Nick Robinson, Production Engineer and Claire Brook, Marketing Manager of Surgical Innovations Limited, Clayton Park, Clayton Wood Rise, Leeds, LS16 6RF, England, UK.)

testis to the midline scrotal septum to prevent re-ascent although there may be inherent risks.

Coughlin *et al.* [78] have reported a link between suture fixation at orchidopexy and infertility in previ-ously cryptorchid men (relative risk 7.56; 95% CI, 1.66, 34.39), and experimental studies performed by Bellinger *et al.* [79] in rats have documented inflammatory and necrotic changes after suture fixation. It is unclear, how-ever, if these findings can be extrapolated to humans as follow-up imaging studies have noted very minimal changes despite suture fixation at orchidopexy. Ward *et al.* [80] performed testicular ultrasound on 22 men operated in childhood with suture fixation and showed a single tunica albuginea calcification (1–2 mm) in 7 (32%) and a further 3 (14%) patients with a single hyp-oechogenic subtunical cyst (1–2 mm). The remaining 12 (54%) patients had normal scans and no difference was noted in testis size between the normally descended and operated testes in any patient. Theoretically breach-ing the tunica with a suture may lead to disruption of the blood/testis barrier and antibody formation, but in a study by Mirilas *et al.* [81] on 22 pubertal males (aged 12.1–17.7 years) operated for cryptorchidism before puberty sera were negative for anti-sperm surface anti-bodies in all patients. If a suture is required, PTFE may be ideal due to its softness and specific handling charac-teristics [82]. Fibrin glue as an alternative to sutures has been described in a rat model [83].

Postoperative considerations

There are no specific precautions in infants. In older boys, most surgeons advise restricted physical activities (riding a bike, kicking a football) for several weeks after orchidopexy until healing has fixed the testis in the sub-dartos pouch.

Managing complications of orchidopexy

Initial

A torn hernial sac requires careful identification and dissection free from the other cord structures prior to proximal transfixion. Micromosquito forceps are invaluable in holding the edges of delicate sac while control is achieved. Inadequate closure or failure to spot a torn sac may lead to a subsequent inguinal hernia. Although a transected vas is a rare event, the correct management is primary microsurgical vasovasostomy. If a testis cannot be placed in the scrotum, despite full mobilization and a Prentiss maneuver, it should be positioned as low as possible with a planned second procedure after 6–12 months. Small wound hematomas are likely to settle with conservative treatment and wound infection will respond to antibiotics and if necessary wound drainage.

Definitive

If there has been a vascular insult at the time of orchidopexy resulting in atrophy, the testis is lost. Some boys decide to have a testis prosthesis at puberty for cosmetic concerns. Postoperative hernias are uncommon and managed by herniotomy and herniorraphy if there is a direct component. Testis torsion after previous orchidopexy is rare but requires emergency exploration with de-torsion and repeat fixation or orchidectomy if the testis is nonviable [84].

Re-ascent of the testis requires a redo orchidopexy, which can be performed via the original inguinal incision [85,86] or with a scrotal approach [22,87]. Surgery is usually made difficult because of scar tissue, and careful dissection is required to prevent vas or testicular vessel injury. In both techniques early identification of the testis is important, with retrograde dissection of the cord structures to gain adequate length. When an inguinal approach is used, a strip of external oblique aponeurosis overlying the cord may be left attached, thus avoiding difficult dissection between the scarred external oblique, related to previous incision and closure, and the anterior aspect of the spermatic cord [86,88,89]. The previously divided hernia sac needs to be separated from the vas and vessels, the peritoneum swept away and retroperitoneal dissection completed. If scar tissue around the deep inguinal ring makes dissection problematic, opening the peritoneum above the ring and dissecting down from above may avoid potential vas or vessel injury [86,88]. A Prentiss maneuver may be required to achieve a dependent scrotal position and good operative exposure, excellent lighting, optical magnification, and tension-free placement within a scrotal subdartos pouch are important in achieving a satisfactory outcome.

Outcome of redo orchidopexy

Most papers on repeat orchidopexy include patients who had initial surgery for inguinal hernia, hydrocele, or cryptorchidism and results for these different groups are often amalgamated. A successful result has been documented in 92–100% of cases [22,85–92] (Table 23.4). In most series, the length of follow-up has been short or not stated. In the report by Pesce *et al.* [91] of 20 boys followed beyond puberty 65% had significantly reduced ultrasound-determined testicular volumes (when compared to controls, $p < 0.005$, although volumes were respectable, study group mean 12.7 ml SD 3.96; controls mean 15.4 ml SD 3.11). With regard to fertility 7 (35%) of the 20 had slightly impaired and 3 (18.7%) severely impaired sperm analysis [91].

Orchidectomy

The removal of a testis in childhood is usually for nonviability after acute torsion, for small dysplastic undescended testes, for testicular nubbins related to a nonpalpable testis, or for atrophy documented at exploration for a previously failed orchidopexy. Immediate complications following orchidectomy are related to wound hematoma and infection. In cases of torsion the contralateral testis is fixed using a subdartos pouch or suture fixation to prevent metachronous torsion. Opinion is divided whether the contralateral testis should be fixed in other cases requiring orchidectomy. Implantation of a testicular prosthesis is available at puberty for boys with a solitary testis and cosmetic concerns or psychological issues [93]. Complications include infection, hematoma, extrusion, unsatisfactory size or positioning, and implant rupture. A groin incision is usually preferred for insertion because of lower risks for infection and extrusion. Saline filled prostheses can deflate but appear safe and well tolerated [94]. Testicular torsion in adolescents and young adults is complicated by abnormalities of spermiogenesis and infertility with semen analysis normal in only 5–50% of patients on long-term follow-up [95]. In contrast, although data is limited, torsion in prepubertal boys does not seem to affect subsequent fertility [96].

Conclusion

Considerable operative expertise is required for successful infant orchidopexy. Inguinal or scrotal approaches to

Table 23.4 Results of redo orchidopexy.

Author	Year	Patient age in years	Number of operated testes	Follow-up in years	Complications (%)	Successful redo surgery (%)
Maizels et al.[*] [85]	1983	1–15 (median 6)	36 (2 orchidectomies)	Not stated	0	34 (100)
Cartwright et al.[*] [86]	1993	1.4–11	25	≥0.33	1 (4) re-ascent 1 (4) hypoplasia	23 (92)
Cohen et al.[*] [88]	1993	2–12 (mean 7.25)	27	0.5–1.5 (mean 0.74)	0	27 (100)
Palacio et al.[*] [89]	1999	4–16 (mean 7.2)	29	0.67–3.2 (mean 1.75)	0	11 (100)[†]
Redman [90]	2000	mean 4.8	13	1–5.1 (mean 2.6)	0	13 (100)
Caruso et al.[*,‡] [22]	2000	2–14 (average 9)	15	0.12–1	1 testicular infarction (6.7)	14 (93.3)
Pesce et al. [91]	2001	6–15 (mean 9.3)	41 (7 orchidectomies)	2–15	1 testis atrophy (2.9)	33 (97.1)
Rajimwale et al.[§] [87]	2004	–	25	0.12–1	1 re-ascent (4)	24 (96)
Ziylan et al. [92]	2004	Mean 6.8	32 (1 orchidectomy)	1–7 (mean 3.8)	2 high scrotal (6.5)	29 (93.5)

[*]Study included patients with an undescended testis following previous orchidopexy, inguinal herniotomy, or division of patent processus vaginalis for hydrocele.
[†]Results reported only for patients undergoing cordopexy (suturing of retained external oblique aponeurosis on anterior surface of cord to the pubic bone or tendinous part of the gracilis muscles).
[‡]Surgery performed via a scrotal approach. Three cases (20%) required inguinal conversion.
[§]Paper included 85 patients undergoing 100 "Bianchi" scrotal orchidopexies with mean age 3.2 years, age of patients with secondary trapped testes not provided separately, 3/25 (12%) of trapped testes required inguinal conversion for success.

the palpable undescended testis are successful in >95% of the cases. The impalpable testis can be managed by a variety of techniques with success in >85–90% of cases. Testis atrophy is avoided by careful dissection, gentle tissue handling, and meticulous surgical technique. Although uncommon, the failed orchidopexy is successfully salvaged by redo surgery in >90% of the cases. In cases where an orchidectomy is performed, the possibility of testicular prosthesis insertion should be discussed.

References

1 Berkowitz GS, Lapinski RH, Dolglin SE et al. Prevalence and natural history of cryptorchidism. Pediatrics 1993;92:44–9.
2 Docimo S. The results of surgical therapy for cryptorchidism: A literature review and analysis. J Urol 1995;154:1148–52.
3 Thorup J, Haugen S, Kollin C, Lindahl S, Lackgren G, Nordenskjold A, Taskinen S. Surgical treatment of undescended testes. Acta Paediatr 2007;96:631–7.
4 Taran I, Elder JS. Results of orchiopexy for the undescended testis. World J Urol 2006;24:231–9.
5 Murphy F, Paran TS, Puri P. Orchidopexy and its impact on fertility. Pediatr Surg Int 2007;23:625–32.
6 Huff DS, Hadziselimovic F, Duckett JW, Elder JS, Snyder HM. Germ cell counts in semithin sections of biopsies of 115 unilaterally cryptorchid testes: The experience from the Children's Hospital of Philadelphia. Eur J Pediatr 1987;146: S25–7.
7 Huff DS, Hadziselimovic F, Snyder 3rd, HM, Blythe B, Duckett JW. Histologic maldevelopment of unilaterally cryptorchid testes and their descended partners. Eur J Pediatr 1993;152:S101–14.
8 Huff DS, Fenig DM, Canning DA, Carr MCG, Zderic SA, Snyder 3rd, HM. Abnormal germ cell development in cryptorchidism. Horm Res 2001;55:11–17.
9 Wilson-Storey D, McGenity K, Dickson JA. Orchidopexy: The younger the better? J R Coll Surg Edinb 1990;35:362–4.
10 Kollin C, Hesser U, Ritzen EM, Karpe B. Testicular growth from birth to two years of age, and the effect of orchidopexy at age nine months: A randomized, controlled study. Acta Paediatr 2006;95:318–24.

11 Nagar H, Haddad R. Impact of early orchidopexy on testicular growth. *Br J Urol* 1997;80:334–5.

12 Hadziselimovic F, Hocht B, Herzog B, Buser MW. Infertility in cryptorchidism is linked to the stage of germ cell development at orchidopexy. *Horm Res* 2007;68:46–52.

13 Lee PA, Coughlin MT. Leydig cell function after cryptorchidism: Evidence of the beneficial result of early surgery. *J Urol* 2002;167:1824–7.

14 Coughlin MT, Bellinger MF, Lee PA. Age at unilateral orchiopexy: Effect on hormone levels and sperm count in adulthood. *J Urol* 1999;162:986–8.

15 Saw KC, Eardley I, Dennis MJS, Whitaker RH. Surgical outcome of orchiopexy. I. Previously unoperated testes. *Br J Urol* 1992;70:90–4.

16 Bianchi A, Squire BR. Transscrotal orchidopexy: Orchidopexy revised. *Pediatr Surg Int* 1989;4:189–92.

17 Iyer KR, Kumar V, Huddart SN, Bianchi A. The scrotal approach. *Pediatr Surg Int* 1995;10:58–60.

18 Lais A, Ferro F. Trans-scrotal approach for surgical correction of cryptorchidism and congenital anomalies of the processus vaginalis. *Eur Urol* 1996;29:235–8.

19 Russinko PJ, Siddiq FM, Tackett LD, Caldamone AA. Prescrotal orchiopexy: An alternative surgical approach for the palpable undescended testis. *J Urol* 2003;170:2436–8.

20 Parsons JK, Ferrer F, Docimo SG. The low scrotal approach to the ectopic or ascended testicle: Prevalence of a patent processus vaginalis. *J Urol* 2003;169:1832–3.

21 Bassel YS, Scherz HC, Kirsch AJ. Scrotal incision orchiopexy for undescended testes with or without a patent processus vaginalis. *J Urol* 2007;177:1516–18.

22 Caruso AP, Walsh RA, Wolach JW, Koyle MA. Single scrotal incision orchiopexy for the palpable undescended testicle. *J Urol* 2000;164:156–8.

23 Kirsch AJ, Escala J, Duckett JW, Smith GH, Zderic SA, Canning DA, Snyder 3rd, HM. Surgical management of the nonpalpable testis: The Children's Hospital of Philadelphia experience. *J Urol* 1998;159:1340–3.

24 Youngson GG, Jones PF. Management of the impalpable testis: Long-term results of the preperitoneal approach. *J Pediatr Surg* 1991;26:618–20.

25 Gheiler EL, Barthold JS, Gonzalez R. Benefits of laparoscopy and the Jones technique for the nonpalpable testis. *J Urol* 1997;158:1948–51.

26 Corbally MT, Quinn FJ, Guiney EJ. The effect of two-stage orchiopexy on testicular growth. *Br J Urol* 1993;72:376–8.

27 Fowler R, Stephens FD. The role of testicular vasculature anatomy in the salvage of high undescended testes. *Aust New Zeal J Surg* 1959;29:92–106.

28 Ransley PG, Vordermark JS, Caldamone AA, Bellinger MF. Preliminary ligation of the gonadal vessels prior to orchiopexy for the intra-abdominal testicle: A staged Fowler–Stephens procedure. *World J Urol* 1984;2:266–8.

29 Smolko MJ, Kaplan GW, Brock WA. Location and fate of the nonpalpable testis in children. *J Urol* 1983;129:1204–6.

30 Horasanli K, Miroglu C, Tanriverdi O, Kendirci M, Boylu U, Gumus E. Single stage Fowler–Stephens orchidopexy: A preferred alternative in the treatment of nonpalpable testes. *Pediatr Surg Int* 2006;22:759–61.

31 O'Brien MF, Hegarty PK, Healy C, DeFrietas D, Bredin HC. One-stage Fowler–Stephens orchidopexy for impalpable undescended testis. *Ir J Med Sci*. 2004;173:18–19.

32 Law GS, Perez LM, Joseph DB. Two-stage Fowler–Stephens orchiopexy with laparoscopic clipping of the spermatic vessels. *J Urol* 1997;158:1205–7.

33 Dhanani NN, Cornelius D, Gunes A, Ritchey ML. Successful outpatient management of the nonpalpable intra-abdominal testis with staged Fowler–Stephens orchiopexy. *J Urol* 2004; 172:2399–401.

34 Koff SA, Sethi PS. Treatment of high undescended testes by low spermatic vessel ligation: An alternative to the Fowler–Stephens technique. *J Urol* 1996;156:799–803.

35 Silber SJ, Kelly J. Successful autotransplantation of an intra-abdominal testis to the scrotum by microvascular technique. *J Urol* 1976;115:452–4.

36 Tackett LD, Wacksman J, Billmire D, Sheldon CA, Minevich E. The high intra-abdominal testis: Technique and long-term success of laparoscopic testicular autotransplantation. *J Endourol*. 2002;16:359–61.

37 Yunusov Yu, Kajumchodzaev AA. Microsurgery of cryptorchidism. I. Lengthening the short vas deferens. *Ann Plast Surg* 1993;31:149–50.

38 Domini R, Lima M, Domini M. Microvascular autotransplantation of the testis: The "refluo" technique. *Eur J Pediatr Surg* 1997;7:288–91.

39 Wacksman J, Dinner M, Handler M. Results of testicular autotransplantation using the microvascular technique: experience with 8 intra-abdominal testes. *J Urol* 1982;128:1319–21.

40 Upton J, Schuster SR, Colodny AH, Murray JE. Testicular autotransplantation in children. *Am J Surg* 1983;145:514–19.

41 Bianchi A. Microvascular transfer of the testis. In *Rob and Smith's Operative Surgery: Pediatric Surgery*, 5th edn. Edited by L Spitz, AG Coran. London: Chapman and Hall, 1995: pp. 726–33.

42 Boeckx W, Vereecken R, Depuydt K. Microsurgery for intra-abdominal testicular retention. *Eur J Obstet Gynecol Reprod Biol* 1998;81:191–6.

43 La Scala GC, Ein SH. Retractile testes: An outcome analysis on 150 patients. *J Pediatr Surg* 2004;39:1014–17.

44 Puri P, Nixon HH. Bilateral retractile testes – subsequent effects on fertility. *J Pediatr Surg* 1977;12:563–6.

45 Hurwitz RS, Kaptein JS. How well does contralateral testis hypertrophy predict the absence of the nonpalpable testis? *J Urol* 2001;165:588–92.

46 Koff SA. Does compensatory testicular enlargement predict monorchism? *J Urol* 1991;146:632–3.

47 Mesrobian HG, Chassaignac JM, Laud PW. The presence or absence of an impalpable testis can be predicted from clinical observations alone. *BJU Int* 2002;90:97–9.

48 Belman AB, Rushton HG. Is an empty left hemiscrotum and hypertrophied right descended testis predictive of perinatal torsion? *J Urol* 2003;170:1674–5.

49 Snodgrass W, Chen K, Harrison C. Initial scrotal incision for unilateral nonpalpable testis. *J Urol* 2004;172:1742–5.

50 Cisek LJ, Peters CA, Atala A, Bauer SB, Diamond DA, Retik AB. Current findings in diagnostic laparoscopic evaluation of the nonpalpable testis. *J Urol* 1998;160:1145–9.

51 Atwell JD. Ascent of the testis: Fact or fiction. *Br J Urol* 1985;57:474–7.

52 Eardley I, Saw KC, Whitaker RH. Surgical outcome of orchidopexy. II. Trapped and ascending testes. *Br J Urol* 1994;73:204–6.

53 Thayyil S, Shenoy M, Agrawal K. Delayed orchidopexy: Failure of screening or ascending testis. *Arch Dis Child.* 2004;89:890.

54 Hack WW, Sijstermans K, van Dijk J, van der Voort-Doedens LM, de Kok ME, Hobbelt-Stoker MJ. Prevalence of acquired undescended testis in 6-year, 9-year and 13-year-old Dutch schoolboys. *Arch Dis Child* 2007;92:17–20.

55 Hack WW, Meijer RW, van der Voort-Doedens LM, Bos SD, Haasnoot K. Natural course of acquired undescended testis in boys. *Br J Surg* 2003;90:728–31.

56 Sijstermans K, Hack WW, van der Voort-Doedens LM, Meijer RW, Haasnoot K. Puberty stage and spontaneous descent of acquired undescended testis: Implications for therapy? *Int J Androl* 2006;29:597–602.

57 Hack WW, van der Voort-Doedens LM, Sijstermans K, Meijer RW, Pierik FH. Reduction in the number of orchidopexies for cryptorchidism after recognition of acquired undescended testis and implementation of expectative policy. *Acta Paediatr* 2007;96:915–18.

58 Lam WW, Tam PK, Ai VH, Chan KL, Cheng W, Chan FL *et al*. Gadolinium-infusion magnetic resonance angiogram: A new, noninvasive, and accurate method of preoperative localization of impalpable undescended testes. *J Pediatr Surg* 1998;33:123–6.

59 Yeung CK, Tam YH, Chan YL, Lee KH, Metreweli C. A new management algorithm for impalpable undescended testis with gadolinium enhanced magnetic resonance angiography. *J Urol* 1999;162:998–1002.

60 Lam WW, Tam PK, Ai VH, Chan KL, Chan FL, Leong L. Using gadolinium-infusion MR venography to show the impalpable testis in pediatric patients. *AJR Am J Roentgenol* 2001;176:1221–6.

61 Eggener SE, Lotan Y, Cheng EY. Magnetic resonance angiography for the nonpalpable testis: A cost and cancer risk analysis. *J Urol* 2005;173:1745–9.

62 Bevan AD. Operation for undescended testis and congenital inguinal hernia. *J Am Med Assoc* 1899;33:773–7.

63 Gross RE, Jewett TC, Jr. Surgical experiences from 1,222 operations for undescended testis. *J Am Med Assoc* 1956;160:634–41.

64 Koop CE, Minor CL. Observations on undescended testes. II. The technique of surgical management. *AMA Arch Surg* 1957;75:898–905.

65 Hutson JM. Orchidopexy. In *Operative Pediatric Surgery*, 6th edn. Edited by L Spitz, AG Coran. London: Hodder Arnold, 2006: pp. 861–9.

66 Davey RB. Orchidopexy: The relative importance of each step of mobilisation. *Pediatr Surg Int* 1997;12:163–4.

67 Hutcheson JC, Cooper CS, Snyder 3rd, HM. The anatomical approach to inguinal orchiopexy. *J Urol* 2000;164:1702–4.

68 Redman JF. Applied anatomy of the cremasteric muscle and fascia. *J Urol* 1996;156:1337–40.

69 Prentiss RJ, Weickgenant CJ, Moses JJ, Frazier DB. Undescended testis: Surgical anatomy of spermatic vessels, spermatic surgical triangles and lateral spermatic ligament. *J Urol* 1960;83:686–92.

70 Ayub K, Williams MP. A simple alternative technique of orchidopexy for high undescended testis. *Ann R Coll Surg Engl* 1998;80:69–71.

71 Perovic S, Janic N. A short vas deferens limiting successful laparoscopic testicular descent. *Br J Urol* 1997;79:120–1.

72 Papparella A, Noviello C, Amici G, Parmeggiani P. Laparoscopic Fowler–Stephens procedure is contraindicated for intraabdominal testicular major duct anomalies. *Surg Endosc* 2004;August 24, Epub ahead of print.

73 Baniegbhal B, Davies M. Laparoscopic evaluation of testicular mobility as a guide to management of intra-abdominal testes. *World J Urol* 2003;20:343–5.

74 Yunusov MYu. Microsurgery of cryptorchidism. II. Managing arterial caliber discrepancy. *Ann Plast Surg* 1993;31:151–3.

75 Schoemaker J. Uber Kryptorchismus und seine Behandlung. *Der Chirurg* 1932;4:1–3.

76 Lattimer JK. Scrotal pouch technique for orchiopexy. *J Urol* 1957;78:628–32.

77 Arda IS, Ersoy E. The place of the technique of narrowing neck of the dartos pouch on the ascent of testis after surgery. *Scand J Urol Nephrol* 2001;35:505–8.

78 Coughlin MT, Bellinger MF, LaPorte RE, Lee PA. Testicular suture: A significant risk factor for infertility among formerly cryptorchid men. *J Pediatr Surg* 1998;33:1790–3.

79 Bellinger MF, Abromowitz H, Brantley S, Marshall G. Orchiopexy: An experimental study of the effect of surgical technique on testicular histology. *J Urol* 1989;142:553–5.

80 Ward JF, Cilento BG, Jr., Kaplan GW, Velling TE, Puckett M, Stock J. The ultrasonic description of postpubertal testicles in men who have undergone prepubertal orchiopexy for cryptorchidism. *J Urol* 2000;163:1448–50.

81 Mirilas P, Mamoulakis C, De Almeida M. Puberty does not induce serum antisperm surface antibodies in patients with previously operated cryptorchidism. *J Urol* 2003;170:2432–5.

82 Steinbecker KM, Teague JL, Wiltfong DB, Wakefield MR. Testicular histology after transparenchymal fixation using polytetrefluoroethylene suture: An animal model. *J Pediatr Surg* 1999;34:1822–5.

83 Sencan A, Genc A, Gunsar C, Daglar Z, Yilmaz O, Ulukus C *et al*. Testis fixation in prepubertal rats: Fibrin glue versus transparenchymal sutures reduces testicular damage. *Eur J Pediatr Surg* 2004;14:193–7.

84 Nesa S, Lorge F, Wese FX, Njinou B, Opsomer RJ, Van Cangh PJ. Testicular torsion after previous orchidopexy for undescended testis. *Acta Urol Belg* 1998;66:25–6.

85 Maizels M, Gomez F, Firlit CF. Surgical correction of the failed orchiopexy. *J Urol* 1983;130:955–7.

86 Cartwright PC, Velagapudi S, Snyder 3rd, HM, Keating MA. A surgical approach to reoperative orchiopexy. *J Urol* 1993;149:817–18.

87 Rajimwale A, Brant WO, Koyle MA. High scrotal (Bianchi) single-incision orchidopexy: A "tailored" approach to the palpable undescended testis. *Pediatr Surg Int* 2004; 20:618–22.

88 Cohen TD, Kay R, Knipper N. Reoperation for cryptorchid testis in prepubertal child. *Urology* 1993;42:437–9.

89 Palacio MM, Sferco A, Garcia Fernanndez AE, Vilarrodona HO. Inguinal cordopexy: A simple and effective new technique for securing the testes in reoperative orchiopexy. *J Pediatr Surg* 1999;34:424–5.

90 Redman JF. Inguinal reoperation for undescended testis and hernia: Approach to the spermatic cord through the cremaster fascia. *J Urol* 2000;164:1705–7.

91 Pesce C, d'Agostino S, Costa L, Musi L, Manzi M. Reoperative orchiopexy: Surgical aspects and functional outcome. *Pediatr Surg Int* 2001;17:62–4.

92 Ziylan O, Oktar T, Korgali E, Nane I, Ander H. Failed orchiopexy. *Urol Int* 2004;73:313–15.

93 Bodiwala D, Summerton DJ, Terry TR. Testicular prostheses: Development and modern usage. *Ann R Coll Surg Engl* 2007;89:349–53.

94 Turek PJ, Master VA, Testicular Prosthesis Study Group. Safety and effectiveness of a new saline filled testicular prosthesis. *J Urol* 2004;172:1427–30.

95 Visser AJ, Heyns CF. Testicular function after torsion of the spermatic cord. *BJU Int* 2003;92:200–3.

96 Puri P, Barton D, O'Donnell B. Prepubertal testicular torsion: Subsequent fertility. *J Pediatr Surg* 1985;20:598–601.

24

Laparoscopic Orchidopexy

Derek J. Matoka, Michael C. Ost, Marc C. Smaldone
and Steven G. Docimo

Key points

- Laparoscopy is the gold standard for localizing the nonpalpable testis.

- Laparoscopic orchidopexy is a logical extension of diagnostic laparoscopy with results and morbidity at least equal, and perhaps superior to its open counterpart.

- Primary laparoscopic orchidopexy is successful in 97% of cases.

- Meticulous technique and recognition of anatomical landmarks are essential in avoiding unintended injury.

- Testicular atrophy is the most common complication.

- Compliance of the pediatric abdomen increases risk to intra-abdominal structures.

Introduction

Laparoscopic orchidopexy is a well-established, safe, and effective approach for both the diagnosis and management of the nonpalpable testis. Cryptorchidism is present in 0.8–1.8% of 1-year-old boys. Although a testicle may be palpated in the groin in the majority of these boys, a nonpalpable testis occurs in 20% of this group [1]. The location of the testis may be intra-abdominal, either in the normal path of embryologic descent or ectopic, canalicular or absent. Historically, laparotomy was performed to localize an intra-abdominal testis or diagnose blind-ending vessels if cord vessels were not observed on initial inguinal exploration [2]. This was most often accomplished with a high inguinal approach (i.e. Jones incision) or Pfannenstiel incision. It is now standard practice to proceed with diagnostic laparoscopy when the testicle is nonpalpable. Subsequent laparoscopic

orchidopexy, whether staged or not, has consistently demonstrated equivalent and superior success rates to historical open series.

Cortesi first reported diagnostic laparoscopy for the evaluation of a nonpalpable testicle in 1976 [3]. Since that time the application of laparoscopy has evolved into a highly successful treatment option. In 1991, Bloom reported using laparoscopy to ligate the testicular vessels in the first stage of a Fowler–Stephens approach [4]. Jordan further advanced the role of laparoscopy as a therapeutic modality when he reported the first laparoscopic orchidopexy in 1992 [5]. Laparoscopy is now widely regarded as the gold standard in localizing nonpalpable testis and has gained prominence as the procedure of choice for relocating the abdominal testicle into the dependent scrotum.

Diagnostic laparoscopy is performed to evaluate for the presence of nonpalpable testicular tissue with the advantage of tailoring subsequent therapy based on the findings [6]. Findings of diagnostic laparoscopy include blind-ending testicular vessels and vas deferens located proximal to the internal ring indicating the diagnosis of a vanishing testis with no further intervention

Pediatric Urology: Surgical Complications and Management. Edited by Duncan T. Wilcox, Prasad P. Godbole and Martin A. Koyle. © 2008 Blackwell Publishing, ISBN: 978-1-4051-6268-5.

required. This may be found in 20% of evaluations for a nonpalpable testis. A normal appearing vas deferens and testicular vessels may exit a closed inguinal ring. In this presentation, exploration of the groin or scrotum may be warranted by either an open or laparoscopic approach, although this is somewhat controversial if the vessels appear atretic. Proponents of exploration note that 10% of testicular nubbins may contain viable germ cells [7]. If, on the other hand, the internal ring is open, an attempt to "milk" a canalicular (peeping) testicle in a retrograde fashion into the abdomen may be attempted. The groin should always be explored in light of a patent processus if this maneuver is unsuccessful in identifying a testicle. A blind-ending vas may be noted without the presence of testicular vessels indicating gonadal disjunction. Diagnostic laparoscopy should continue with emphasis on identifying the testicular vessels as they will lead to the gonad, if present [8]. Finally, in 50–60% of nonpalpable cases, an intra-abdominal or peeping testicle is identified.

Proceeding with therapeutic laparoscopy provides a logical and smooth transition in the management of a nonpalpable testis. The appearance of the testicle, an assessment of its mobility and vascular supply as well as careful inspection of the vas deferens are essential in planning a therapeutic surgical approach. The desired outcome is permanent fixation of the testicle in the scrotum, although removal of compromised testicular tissue is occasionally indicated. Ultimately, the goals of improving fertility, decreasing the potential for malignant transformation, easier examination of the scrotal testis, and prevention of testicular torsion are identical for both laparoscopic and open orchidopexy.

Surgical technique

The goal of laparoscopic orchidopexy is to adequately lengthen the testicular vessels and vas deferens to enable relocation of the testicle to the orthotopic scrotal position. Initial surgical "success" of laparoscopic orchidopexy will therefore be measured by maintenance of the testicle in a proper scrotal position without evidence of atrophy. Equally important is avoiding the associated complications inherent to this laparoscopic procedure. In light of this, it is critical to know the different steps that will maximize successful outcomes.

Some authors advocate universally performing primary laparoscopic orchidopexy without division of vessels in one stage [9,10] or in two stages with division

of vessels [11]. The majority of clinicians tend to manage each case on a more selective basis, determining their approach based on the ability to obtain sufficient length to place the testis in the scrotum [12–16]. Baker *et al.* completed a multi-institutional analysis to evaluate the outcomes of laparoscopic orchidopexy. They found that primary laparoscopic orchidopexy was successful in 97.2% of cases. One- and two-stage Fowler–Stephens orchidopexy was successful in 74.1% and 87.9% of cases, respectively. Such information is important in counseling patients prior to surgery [13].

Blind access for pneumoperitoneum with a Veress needle or trocar is less commonly used in the pediatric population as an overly compliant abdomen may increase the risk of injury to intra-abdominal structures. It is our preference to use the Bailez Technique for open access [17], modified to employ the use of a radially dilating trocar [18]. In our current technique, a 2-0 vicryl suture is first placed in the skin of the umbilicus to provide continual anterior tension. A 3 mm hidden infraumbilical incision is made in the skin and a scissor is then used at an approximate 15–20° angle in a superior direction to cut through the umbilical fascia into the underlying adherent peritoneum. Alternatively, the rectus fascia and underling peritoneum may be entered sharply at 90° under direct vision.

Exposure is facilitated by initially placing the patient in Trendelenburg position with the ipsilateral side of the table tilted up. Mobilization of the spermatic vessels begins with a peritoneal incision lateral to these vessels which is carried just over the internal ring and continued lateral and superior to the vas deferens. The triangle of peritoneum between the vas and vessels is maintained to preserve the rich anastomotic blood supply to the testicle. The peritoneal pedicle is elevated with the testicular vessels, vas, and testicle, creating a plane between these structures and the external iliac vessels. By retracting the testicle rostrally, the processus vaginalis and the gubernaculum are brought into the abdomen. The gubernaculum is thinned and sharply transected with cautery taking care to remain distal to a looping vas deferens. At this point, length may be assessed. It is helpful at this point in the procedure to deliver the testis through a neocanal as described below to get an accurate assessment of the available length. If additional mobilization is indicated, the peritoneum is dissected lateral to the vessels in a cephalad direction as proximal as possible. A perpendicular "relaxing" incision in the peritoneum that overlies the testicular vessels at the superior extent of the dissection is then delicately made to optimize length. In the unlikely event that length remains inadequate, a decision to divide the testicular vessels and proceed with a Fowler–Stephens orchidopexy can be made. Testes located proximal to the iliac vessels are more likely to require a Fowler–Stephens procedure to obtain adequate length [15] and are probably best managed with a planned, staged approach.

Various methods to deliver the testicle into the scrotum have been described. The technique described by our group employs 2 or 3 mm instruments and a radially dilating trocar system [18]. A 12 mm ipsilateral scrotal incision is first made and a subdartos pouch is created. A 2 mm laparoscopic grasper is placed through the ipsilateral 3 mm lateral trocar directed toward the scrotal incision. Care is taken to place the instrument over the pubis and between the medial umbilical ligament and epigastric vessels. The surgeon's free hand should palpate the pubic area and scrotal incision to ensure the instrument is being guided over the pubis and through the scrotal incision. After the instrument is passed through the scrotum the Foley catheter is checked for hematuria. Although rare, a bladder injury would most likely occur during this step of the procedure. Proper placement of the instrument in the position described above, as well as presence of a Foley catheter, should minimize the likelihood of this complication. The Step sheath is then passed onto the end of the 2 or 3 mm instrument *ex vivo* and brought through the scrotum. The 5 or 10 mm trocar obturator, depending on the size of the testicle, is then inserted creating the neoinguinal hiatus. A locking grasper is introduced into the abdomen through the scrotal trocar. The testicle is then grasped at the gubernaculum and delivered into the scrotum (Figure 24.1). It is imperative for the surgeon to visually monitor the tension on the cord during scrotal delivery so the vessels are not avulsed.

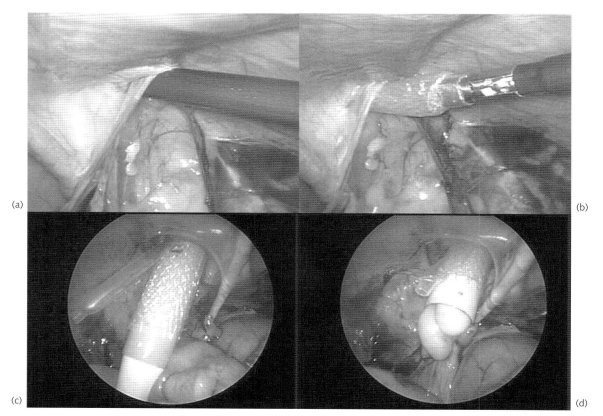

(a) (b) (c) (d)

Figure 24.1 Delivering the testicle into the scrotum requires developing a neohiatus (a–c) to facilitate passage of the testicle, epididymis, and cord structures into the scrotum without resistance. Using a 5–10 mm scrotal trocar opens a neohiatus with minimal resistance minimizes the risk of an avulsion injury (d).

Timing of surgery

At birth, the undescended testis has been shown to have normal histology. Although this may continue into the first year of life, delayed germ cell development has been described by 6–8 months of age. These changes are progressive with both light and electron microscopy demonstrating histologic changes consistent with deterioration of the germ cell population detectable by 18 months [19]. However, spontaneous testicular descent has been noted postnatally at 4–6 months. Therefore, in order to allow adequate time for a testis to descend spontaneously while minimizing the risk for irreversible developmental damage, the generally accepted recommendation is to perform orchidopexy at 6–18 months of age [8].

Outcomes

Laparoscopic orchidopexy has matured into a logical extension of diagnostic laparoscopy for the evaluation and management of the nonpalpable testis. The overall success rate, defined as a testis in an intrascrotal position with no atrophy, has consistently shown itself to be equal or better than its open equivalent with minimal associated morbidity in experienced hands. Docimo performed a meta-analysis in which success rates of various open orchidopexy techniques were compared (inguinal 89%; one-stage Fowler–Stephens 67%; two-stage Fowler–Stephens 73%; transabdominal 81%; microvascular 84%) [20]. These results substantiated a need for improved management alternatives opening the door for greater utilization of the laparoscopic approach. Several multi-institutional reviews and numerous single institutional papers have reported improved success rates over an open approach (Table 24.1). Baker *et al.* completed a multi-institutional analysis to evaluate the outcomes of laparoscopic orchidopexy. They found that primary laparoscopic orchidopexy was successful in 97.2% of cases. One- and two-stage Fowler–Stephens orchidopexy were successful in 74.1% and 87.9% of cases, respectively (Table 24.1). A 3% incidence of major complications and a 2% incidence of minor complications were reported [13]. When compared to the open approach, success rates were higher with decreased morbidity. Lindgren *et al.* compiled the experiences of several institutions. This group was more likely to perform a Fowler–Stephens type approach when the testis was located at or proximal to the iliac vessels. In addition, older boys were more likely to require ligation of the vessels. A 100% success rate was reported for primary orchidopexy as well as both one- and two-stage Fowler–Stephens procedures. However, in two cases where previous testicular surgery had been performed, the redo

Table 24.1 Laparoscopic orchidopexy.

Study	N	Mean operative time (min)	Testicular atrophy (%)	Unsatisfactory scrotal position (%)
Lindgren *et al.* (1998)	44	n/a	0* 4.5†‡	7
Baker *et al.* (2001)	310	124	2* 22† 10‡	1* 7† 2‡
Chang *et al.* (2001)	101		0* 15†‡	0 16† 14‡
Radmayr *et al.* (2003)	57	49* 38/53‡ (by stage)	0* 7‡	n/a
Samadi *et al.* (2003)	197	n/a	0* 7‡	9* 0‡

*Primary laparoscopic.
†One-stage Fowler–Stephens.
‡Two-stage Fowler–Stephens.

Fowler–Stephens procedure resulted in testicular atrophy. They described no complications [15].

Chang *et al.* reviewed their series and describe an overall success rate of 91% with more than 6 months of follow-up. For primary laparoscopic orchidopexy, first-stage, and second-stage Fowler–Stephens, the success rate was 94%, 84%, and 86%, respectively. Excluding those testicles involved in a previous exploration, the first-stage Fowler–Stephens success rate improved to 100%. The overall atrophy rate was 4% and only 1% in those with no prior exploration. Other minor complications were noted in 5% of their series [21]. This series was expanded by Samadi *et al.* to include 203 procedures. An overall success rate of 95% was reported. A viable testicle located within the scrotum was reported in 97% of cases undergoing primary laparoscopic orchidopexy at a minimum of 6 months of follow-up. In none of these cases was testicular atrophy observed. The Fowler–Stephens approach was successful in 90% of the cases. Atrophy was noted on follow-up in 4 of 58 procedures, 2 of which had undergone previous testicular surgery [22]. Radmayr *et al.* published their series of patients who had undergone laparoscopic orchidopexy. Technique was chosen based on location of the testis. They reported an overall success rate of 97%, 100% with primary orchidopexy, and 93% with a Fowler–Stephens approach. No complications were reported in this series [23]. Twenty-five patients were followed by Esposito *et al.* after undergoing laparoscopic orchidopexy. All testes were brought into the scrotum primarily except one which required a two-stage Fowler–Stephens procedure. A success rate of 96% with one intraoperative complication (4%) was reported [14]. The complication was an iatrogenic rupture of the testicular vessel. This testicle was noted to be atrophic 1 month after surgery.

Abolyosr conducted the only known prospective, randomized study between open and laparoscopic orchidopexy for the management of abdominal testes. In comparing success, the two procedures had similar results. The success of primary orchidopexy was 100% for both modalities, while the success rate was 85% and 90.5% for open- and laparoscopic-staged Fowler–Stephens orchidopexy, respectively. However, they demonstrated that there was significantly less associated morbidity with laparoscopy than the matched open procedure with respect to resuming a diet, hospital stay, and resumption of normal activities [24].

Docimo [25] and Riquelme [26] have described laparoscopic orchidopexy for the palpable undescended testis. The ability to achieve extensive vascular dissection, enhanced visibility when mobilizing the proximal testicular vessels, and the ability to create a neointernal ring are the same advantages identified for management of the intra-abdominal testis. Both authors report a success rate of 100%. Docimo reported no complications, while Riquelme reported a complication rate of 13.3%, comparable to that reported for an open procedure (12.2%) [27].

Complications

The number of complications associated with laparoscopic orchidopexy compares quite favorably to that of an open approach. In a large multi-institutional review, Baker reported a major complication rate of 3.0% and a minor complication rate of 2.0%. Major complications that have been reported include acute testicular atrophy, bowel perforation [28], cecal volvulus, bladder perforation [29], ileus, laceration of the vas, testicular vessel avulsion leading to a one-stage Fowler–Stephens orchidopexy, and wound separation/infection. It is important to note that complications during laparoscopic procedures are reflective of surgical experience [30]. Experience with approximately ten laparoscopic cases is necessary to reduce such risk [31]. Early recognition of such complications will help to limit their occurrence in the future. This discussion highlights the more common complications associated with laparoscopic orchidopexy.

The prevention of complications associated with laparoscopy starts with proper positioning and padding to reduce the risk of neuromuscular injuries. Although injuries are less likely to occur with pelvic laparoscopy, extremes in table positioning are often necessary. Close attention to placement of straps and/or tape and adequate padding should limit positioning-related injuries.

Complications related to access are a common concern. Indeed, the most frequent identifiable cause of complications associated with pediatric laparoscopy has been the method used for abdominal access. The pediatric abdomen is very compliant and limited in space. For this reason, open peritoneal access has been associated with fewer complications than when a Veress needle is used [30]. As previously mentioned, we prefer to gain access using an open technique. Regardless of the access technique used, preperitoneal insufflation may still occur. This complication can readily be identified when there is characteristically high opening pressure at low volumes. Additional sharp dissection and entry into the peritoneal cavity followed

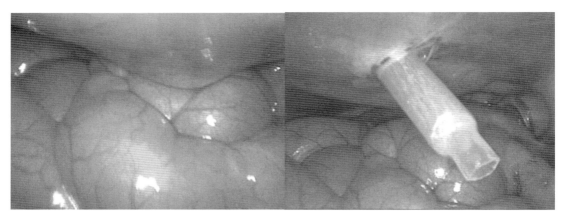

Figure 24.2 Despite maximal insufflation pressure, the great compliance of the pediatric abdomen makes trocar placement difficult. Small forces applied to the abdominal wall will distort the anatomy and place organs vulnerable to injury in close proximity to trocar trajectories.

by repositioning of the trocar is necessary if this occurs. Prior to placing additional working ports, areas vulnerable to trocar injuries must be mapped and noted with the laparoscope. Due to great abdominal wall compliance, the epigastric vessels, iliac vessels, and bowel all come into close proximity to access trajectories (Figure 24.2). Immediate inspection of these loci before and after port placement is mandatory (Figure 24.3).

A major vascular injury during access or additional trocar placement should be recognized immediately to prevent catastrophic sequelae. Injury to the aorta and vena cava may occur during umbilical access, while injury to the major pelvic vessels may occur with introduction of the lateral trocars. Upon removal of the trocar, brisk blood flow will be evident. The obturator should be replaced to tamponade the hemorrhage and guide the eventual repair. Immediate laparotomy is often indicated and a consult to a vascular specialist should be considered. Immediate resuscitation and communication with anesthesia is critical to avoid significant morbidity and mortality [32].

Bowel injury is also an important consideration during both access, instrument passage, and the use of cautery. Inner mucosa of the bowel may be noted on insertion of the laparoscope or trauma may occur to the bowel along the path of previously obtained access. Serosal tears or isolated bowel injuries may be repaired primarily by an experienced laparoscopist [21]. More extensive injuries may warrant formal laparotomy. Regardless, the entire bowel should be run and examined circumferentially if bowel injury occurs or is suspected.

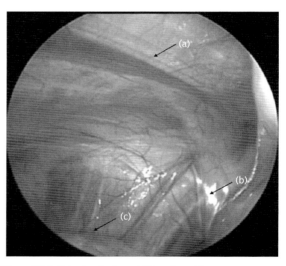

Figure 24.3 Prior to placing additional working ports, areas vulnerable to trocar injuries must be mapped and noted. Due to great abdominal wall compliance, the epigastric vessels (a), iliac vessels (b), and bowel (c) all come into close proximity to an access trajectory. Immediate inspection of the loci after port placement is mandatory.

Abdominal wall hemorrhage may be encountered. The epigastric vessels usually lie behind the rectus sheath and can be avoided by careful placement of the trocars. If hemorrhage is suspected, examination both externally and with the laparoscope may help to isolate the bleeding vessel. If visualized, it may simply be cauterized.

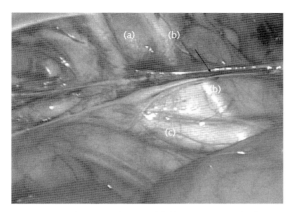

Figure 24.4 Pelvic view during a left laparoscopic orchidopexy. During medial mobilization of the vas deferens the cord structures (arrow) are held cranially and laterally. Care must be taken not to injure the iliac vein (a), iliac artery (b), and/or ureter (c) that lie immediately posterior to the mobilized peritoneal flap.

If the vessel cannot be visualized, various suture techniques may be utilized. Bhayani and Kavoussi describe obtaining circumferential control of the vessel using either the Carter–Thompson fascial closure device (Inlet Medical Inc., Eden Prairie, Minnesota) or a Keith needle that is initially passed percutaneously and grasped laparoscopically. It is then guided back through the skin on the other side of the vessel [33].

Surgical planning and an appreciation of the anatomical landmarks within the pelvis will aid in avoiding unintended difficulty. During testicular mobilization, care must be taken to avoid injury to the vas, testicular, femoral and iliac vessels, and the ureter. When mobilizing the vas on the medial aspect of the peritoneal flap these structures lay directly posterior and medial (Figure 24.4). In general, complications can be limited by careful intra-abdominal mobilization, using cautery in short bursts, and execution of meticulous technique. The laparoscopic approach helps to facilitate this by allowing extensive and high retroperitoneal mobilization of the testicular vessels in an atraumatic manner. Magnification plays a significant role, allowing for visualization of the vessels and vas deferens and precise dissection. Less traction on the cord is required and it is easier to preserve the perivascular tissue and avoid over skeletonization of both the vessels and the vas. If the colon needs to be mobilized, this can also be easily accomplished [10].

Omental herniation through a 3 mm umbilical trocar site has been reported [34]. However, this is a rare complication of laparoscopy with an incidence of 0.15% in over 5400 laparoscopic cases [30] and it is not mandatory to close the fascia of 3 mm incisions. At the time of incisional port closure, care must be taken not to incorporate intra-abdominal contents into the 5 mm wounds. This complication can be avoided by closing the fascia under direct visualization and elevation with the suture when tying knots to avoid entrapping bowel or omentum. Additionally, the laparoscope should be reintroduced after abdominal desufflation and the cannula removed over the laparoscope. These measures help to prevent entrapment of omentum or bowel at port sites [34].

Testicular atrophy is the most common long-term complication associated with laparoscopic orchidopexy. The frequency of this occurrence is dependent on the initial position of the testicle and the chosen technique for performing the orchidopexy. Generally, primary orchidopexy has the lowest atrophy rate, ranging from 0 to approximately 5% in larger series. Atrophy rates are highest for a one-stage Fowler–Stephens procedure, approaching 25% [5,14,23]. Finally, atrophy is observed in 0–15% of testicles after the two-stage Fowler–Stephens procedure [14,23,35].

Atrophy of the delivered testicle is closely monitored at the time of follow-up. There is a constant drive to improve the laparoscopic technique to limit the potential of an atrophied testis as a long-term outcome. It is universally acknowledged that minimizing the handling of the testis and vas and limiting the dissection in proximity to their blood supply with judicious use of cautery is crucial in reducing the risk of injury to these structures and subsequent atrophy of the testis [21]. To accomplish this goal, preserving the distal peritoneal triangle between the vas deferens and vessels has been described [8]. This allows for the greatest collateral vasculature and optimizes blood supply to the testis not only in a standard orchidopexy but also if the need for subsequent vascular division of the testicular vessels is required.

Utilizing the gubernacular tissue as a handle for maneuvering the testicle also aids in the dissection. By medially retracting the testis, dissection of the peritoneum lateral to the testicular vessels is facilitated, allowing for a wide and intact vascularized peritoneal window with optimized collateral blood supply [22,23]. This also enhances the ability to achieve a high ligation of the testicular vessel in those situations where this is necessary. As previously described, a perpendicular incision in the peritoneum at the superior aspect of the testicular vessel dissection may provide additional length. Lindgren has suggested that the "relaxing" incision in the peritoneum should be made prior to bringing the testis into the scrotum to decrease the risk of gonadal vessel injury [31]. In our hands, delivery of the testis through the neocanal is always done before incising the peritoneum in order to identify the extent of the required incision and to provide a "third hand" for distal retraction. The risk of spermatic pedicle injury should be very low with a careful peritoneal incision.

Avulsion of the spermatic vessels due to excessive traction placed on the testicle has been reported [9,14,21]. Conversion to a Fowler–Stephens approach is necessary in this situation but testicular atrophy is often reported following unintended disruption of the vessels.

Transection of a looped vas deferens is a potential complication. To avoid injury to the vas, one must be constantly aware of the possibility for a long looping vas to exist. The vas deferens should generally be left on the peritoneum and rarely dissected free. Overly aggressive dissection of the vas off of the peritoneum can result

in vasal injury, testicular atrophy, and rarely ureteral obstruction [8,36].

Injury to the bladder is most likely to occur when creating the neoinguinal hiatus (Figure 24.5). The risk is increased if the neohiatus is not formed superior to the pubis in a plane lateral to the medial umbilical ligament and medial to the epigastric vessels. Remaining cognizant of these pelvic landmarks is essential in preventing injury to the bladder, epigastric or femoral vessels [22]. If it appears that excessive force is required during antegrade establishment of the hiatus, the instrument is likely headed in the wrong direction and the path should be reexamined. Placement of a urinary catheter to maintain a decompressed bladder will also help to prevent bladder injury. It may also serve to alert the physician of a possible injury to the bladder if grossly bloody urine is detected in the drainage bag.

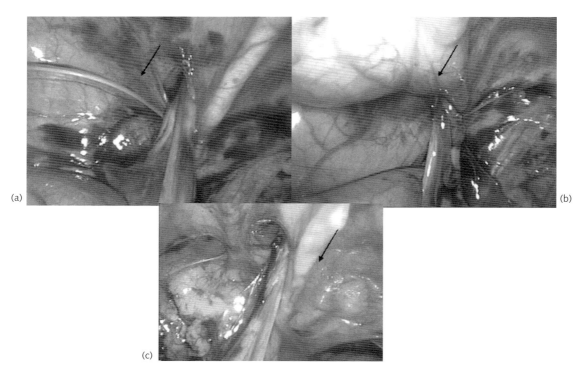

Figure 24.5 During delivery of the testicle into the scrotum, the bladder edge (arrows) is at increased risk for perforation. The risk is increased if the neoinguinal hiatus is not formed superior to the pubis in a plane lateral to the medial umbilical ligament and medial to the epigastric vessels. Following delivery of the testicle in a right laparoscopic orchidopexy there was concern that the bladder was perforated (a). Filling the bladder demonstrated no evidence of a leak (b). After delivery of the testicle through a 12 mm scrotal trocar in the final stage of a left laparoscopic orchidopexy, there is little concern of a bladder injury. The neohiatus was created in a plane lateral to the medial umbilical ligament and medial to the epigastric vessels (c).

Torsion of the testicular vessels following delivery to the scrotum has been reported [36]. This complication may be avoided by thoroughly examining the vessels after placement of the testicle into the scrotum to confirm the absence of torsion. If torsion is identified, the testicle is carefully repositioned in the scrotum until the vessels and vas have a normal interrelationship.

Ileus has rarely been reported after laparoscopic orchidopexy. Conservative management, consisting of limiting oral intake, intravenous fluids, and nasogastric suction when indicated has resulted in resolution of symptoms [8].

When performing laparoscopic orchidopexy, the associated hernia sac is not ligated and the internal ring is generally not formally closed [13]. However, Metwalli and Cheng describe an indirect inguinal hernia following laparoscopic orchidopexy. In their series, this complication has occurred in 1 of 25 procedures or 4%. While they do not advocate for closure of the internal ring in all cases, they suggest that this may be appropriate in select cases where a large internal ring defect is evident [37]. Considering that this is the only reported inguinal hernia after laparoscopic orchidopexy, the risk appears to be well under 1% overall.

Finally, Kim *et al.* describe a clinical scenario in which a testis was missed on diagnostic laparoscopy. Despite evidence of a closed processus vaginalis, an absent vas and blind-ending vessels above the internal ring, a testicle was later found while the patient was undergoing an unrelated procedure [38]. Given the concern for carcinoma *in situ* in the postpubertal cryptorchid patient, obtaining a definitive diagnosis by laparoscopy is imperative [39]. If a testis is not initially found and neither the vas nor the vessels are identified, the patient should be placed in an exaggerated Trendelenburg position to enable inspection all the way to the kidney. Placement of an additional trocar allows for a more complete examination under direct vision with minimal added morbidity. It is the responsibility of the surgeon to identify the vas and vessels with their associated anatomical end point before concluding the diagnostic portion of the procedure. Kim reported that the vessels were not accompanied by a vas. In addition, an ipsilateral multicystic dysplastic kidney was noted. They have suggested that this should raise suspicion for an ectopic testis and an exhaustive search with necessary mobilization should be performed before declaring the testis absent [38]. Cisek describes several unique cases in which thorough examination utilizing an additional port demonstrated a high intra-abdominal testis at or above the level of the renal

fossa in three ipsilateral renal anomalies that included multicystic dysplastic kidney and agenesis [6].

Conclusion

Advances in laparoscopic instrumentation and refinement in technique have contributed to the development of laparoscopic orchidopexy as the preferred treatment of the intra-abdominal testis in the pediatric population. The reported success of laparoscopic orchidopexy for delivering a viable testicle to the scrotum with minimal postoperative morbidity is consistently reported as superior to that of the open approach. In addition, the benefits of improved cosmesis, shorter convalescence, and increased magnification allowing for better visualization have driven laparoscopic-directed management as the standard approach for the undescended testis.

References

1 Berkowitz GS, Lapinski RH, Dolgin SE, Gazella JG, Bodian CA, Holzman IR. Prevalence and natural history of cryptorchidism. *Pediatrics* 1993;92:44–9.

2 Sweeney DD, Smaldone MC, Docimo SG. Minimally invasive surgery for urologic disease in children. *Nat Clin Pract Urol* 2007;4:26–38.

3 Cortesi N, Ferrari P, Zambarda E, Manenti A, Baldini A, Morano FP. Diagnosis of bilateral abdominal cryptorchidism by laparoscopy. *Endoscopy* 1976;8:33–4.

4 Bloom DA. Two-step orchiopexy with pelviscopic clip ligation of the spermatic vessels. *J Urol* 1991;145:1030–3.

5 Jordan GH, Winslow BH. Laparoscopic single stage and staged orchiopexy. *J Urol* 1994;152:1249–52.

6 Cisek LJ, Peters CA, Atala A, Bauer SB, Diamond DA, Retik AB. Current findings in diagnostic laparoscopic evaluation of the nonpalpable testis. *J Urol* 1998;160:1145–9; discussion 50.

7 Grady RW, Mitchell ME, Carr MC. Laparoscopic and histologic evaluation of the inguinal vanishing testis. *Urology* 1998;52:866–9.

8 Mathews R, Docimo SG. Laparoscopy for the management of the undescended testis. *Atlas Urol Clin* 2000;8:91–102.

9 Esposito C, Vallone G, Settimi A, Gonzalez Sabin MA, Amici G, Cusano T. Laparoscopic orchiopexy without division of the spermatic vessels: Can it be considered the procedure of choice in cases of intraabdominal testis? *Surg Endosc* 2000;14:658–60.

10 Rodriguez A, Freire U, Orpez R, Lorenzo G. Diagnostic and therapeutic laparoscopy for nonpalpable testis. *Surg Endosc* 2003;17:1756–8.

11 Godbole PP, Najmaldin AS. Laparoscopic orchidopexy in children. *J Endourol* 2001;15:251–6.

12 Peters CA. Laparoscopy in pediatric urology. *Curr Opin Urol* 2004;14:67–73.

13 Baker LA, Docimo SG, Surer I *et al*. A multi-institutional analysis of laparoscopic orchidopexy. *BJU Int* 2001; 87:484–9.

14 Esposito C, Damiano R, Gonzalez Sabin MA *et al*. Laparoscopy-assisted orchidopexy: An ideal treatment for children with intra-abdominal testes. *J Endourol* 2002;16:659–62.

15 Lindgren BW, Franco I, Blick S *et al*. Laparoscopic Fowler–Stephens orchiopexy for the high abdominal testis. *J Urol* 1999;162:990–3;discussion 4.

16 Papparella A, Parmeggiani P, Cobellis G *et al*. Laparoscopic management of nonpalpable testes: A multicenter study of the Italian Society of Video Surgery in Infancy. *J Pediatr Surg* 2005;40:696–700.

17 Docimo SG. Re: Experience with the Bailez technique for laparoscopic access in children. *J Urol* 2004;171:806.

18 Ferrer FA, Cadeddu JA, Schulam P, Mathews R, Docimo SG. Orchiopexy using 2 mm laparoscopic instruments: 2 Techniques for delivering the testis into the scrotum. *J Urol* 2000;164:160–1.

19 Taran I, Elder JS. Results of orchiopexy for the undescended testis. *World J Urol* 2006;24:231–9.

20 Docimo SG. The results of surgical therapy for cryptorchidism: A literature review and analysis. *J Urol* 1995;154:1148–52.

21 Chang B, Palmer LS, Franco I. Laparoscopic orchidopexy: A review of a large clinical series. *BJU Int* 2001;87:490–3.

22 Samadi AA, Palmer LS, Franco I. Laparoscopic orchiopexy: Report of 203 cases with review of diagnosis, operative technique, and lessons learned. *J Endourol* 2003;17:365–8.

23 Radmayr C, Oswald J, Schwentner C, Neururer R, Peschel R, Bartsch G. Long-term outcome of laparoscopically managed nonpalpable testes. *J Urol* 2003;170:2409–11.

24 Abolyosr A. Laparoscopic versus open orchiopexy in the management of abdominal testis: A descriptive study. *Int J Urol* 2006;13:1421–4.

25 Docimo SG, Moore RG, Adams J, Kavoussi LR. Laparoscopic orchiopexy for the high palpable undescended testis: Preliminary experience. *J Urol* 1995;154:1513–15.

26 Riquelme M, Aranda A, Rodriguez C, Villalvazo H, Alvarez G. Laparoscopic orchiopexy for palpable undescended testes: A five-year experience. *J Laparoendosc Adv Surg Tech A* 2006;16:321–4.

27 Moul JW, Belman AB. A review of surgical treatment of undescended testes with emphasis on anatomical position. *J Urol* 1988;140:125–8.

28 Caldamone AA, Amaral JF. Laparoscopic stage 2 Fowler–Stephens orchiopexy. *J Urol* 1994;152:1253–6.

29 Wiener JS, Jordan GH, Gonzales ET, Jr. Laparoscopic management of persistent Mullerian duct remnants associated with an abdominal testis. *J Endourol* 1997;11:357–9.

30 Peters CA. Complications in pediatric urological laparoscopy: Results of a survey. *J Urol* 1996;155:1070–3.

31 Lindgren BW, Darby EC, Faiella L *et al*. Laparoscopic orchiopexy: Procedure of choice for the nonpalpable testis? *J Urol* 1998;159:2132–5.

32 Pemberton RJ, Tolley DA, van Velthoven RF. Prevention and management of complications in urological laparoscopic port site placement. *Eur Urol* 2006;50:958–68.

33 Permpongkosol S, Link RE, Su LM *et al*. Complications of 2,775 urological laparoscopic procedures: 1993 to 2005. *J Urol* 2007;177:580–5.

34 Yee DS, Duel BP. Omental herniation through a 3-mm umbilical trocar site. *J Endourol* 2006;20:133–4.

35 Law GS, Perez LM, Joseph DB. Two-stage Fowler–Stephens orchiopexy with laparoscopic clipping of the spermatic vessels. *J Urol* 1997;158:1205–7.

36 Gill IS, Ross JH, Sung GT, Kay R. Needlescopic surgery for cryptorchidism: The initial series. *J Pediatr Surg* 2000;35:1426–30.

37 Metwalli AR, Cheng EY. Inguinal hernia after laparoscopic orchiopexy. *J Urol* 2002;168:2163.

38 Kim C, Bennett N, Docimo SG. Missed testis on laparoscopy despite blind-ending vessels and closed processus vaginalis. *Urology* 2005;65:1226.

39 Rogers E, Teahan S, Gallagher H *et al*. The role of orchiectomy in the management of postpubertal cryptorchidism. *J Urol* 1998;159:851–4.

25

Varicocele

Ramnath Subramaniam and Eva Macharia

Key points

- Diagnosis of varicocele is essentially clinical.
- Treatment of varicocele for subfertility is controversial.
- Intervention options include venous occlusion or surgical ligation.
- Surgical ligation remains the preferred approach.

- Nonartery sparing technique has better success than artery sparing approach.
- Hydrocele formation is the most frequent complication regardless of approach.
- Lymphatic sparing techniques are promising in reducing morbidity; long-term outcomes are needed to validate results.

Introduction

Varicocele is the abnormal dilatation of the pampiniform plexus of veins within the scrotum. The plexus receives tributaries from the epididymal veins and lies posterior to the testes. The plexus then ascends around the vas deferens to the superficial inguinal ring, where venules coalesce to form 3–4 veins that lie within the spermatic cord in the inguinal canal.

In a unique study of over 4000 boys in Turkey, the prevalence of varicocele increased significantly with age from <1% in under 10 year olds compared to 7.7% in 11–14 year olds and 14.1% in the 15–19 year olds [1]. This suggests a probable causal relationship between increased blood flow to the pubertal testis and varicocele.

The relationship between varicocele, male subfertility, and testicular atrophy is what underlies the current practice of correction of varicocele in prepubertal males [2]. Yet the empirical varicocelectomy as a remote treatment for subfertility remains controversial. Although the effect of increased temperature caused by a varicocele seems well established, this effect appears to be in both the testes and not in the ipsilateral gonad. Increased thickness of the lamina propria, increased nitric oxide levels in the venous plexus, and impaired transformation of

the myofibroblasts to fibroblasts are some of the abnormal findings reported from research studies [3–5].

Current opinion maintains that although varicocele is commonly diagnosed in men with infertility, their infertility may be multifactorial. The varicocele may be considered a sentinel sign or as a cofactor in men with other genetic or molecular problems as the underlying cause of infertility.

Diagnosis

Diagnosis of varicocele has historically been clinical. Characteristic symptoms are of scrotal discomfort and heaviness, which is worse when standing or walking. Physical examination demonstrates a classic "bag of worms" feel and appearance of the affected scrotum. The ipsilateral testis can often be palpated separate to the varicocele and may be reduced in size when compared with the contralateral testicle. Varicocele is left-sided in 90% and bilateral in 10%. A unilateral right-sided varicocele is exceedingly rare [1].

Traditionally, varicoceles have been classified clinically based on the classification suggested by Dubin and Amelaar adopted by the WHO [6]:
- Grade I – Palpable by valsalva maneuver
- Grade II – Palpable without valsalva maneuver
- Grade III – Visible before palpation

Color Doppler ultrasonography (CDU) allows diagnosis of varicocele which may not be clinically apparent,

Pediatric Urology: Surgical Complications and Management. Edited by Duncan T. Wilcox, Prasad P. Godbole and Martin A. Koyle. © 2008 Blackwell Publishing, ISBN: 978-1-4051-6268-5.

although the significance of this finding is unclear. The venous reflux into the venous plexus is diagnosed using the Doppler color flow mapping in the supine and upright position, at quiet respiration, and with valsalva maneuver. Continuous reflux pattern during quiet inspiration (without valsalva maneuver or deep inspiration) is the main criterion for diagnosis of varicocele [7].

Testicular hypotrophy

Testicular hypotrophy may be determined by the atrophy index (AI: $[Vr − Vl/Vr] \times 100$; Vr and Vl volumes of right and left testicle, respectively) [8]. In adolescents and adults, testis size should approximately be equal on both sides with a standard deviation of not less than 2 cc on ultrasound examination, which uses the ellipsoid method of volume calculation ($0.523 \times HWL$). Ultrasound estimation of testicular size has been shown to be more accurate than the physical estimation using orchidometers [9].

The criterion for defining testicular hypotrophy is inconsistent in various reports with atrophy index ranging from 10% to 25% [10–11]. Also absolute volume differentials vary from 2 cc in some reports to 3 cc in others [12–13]. Therefore, the reported incidence of hypotrophy in varicocele varies from 30% to 70% [14–15]. However, studies have not been able to correlate testicular volume with fertility status in adult men with varicocele [2].

Testicular injury

Bach *et al.* reported that the sertoli cell function was impaired even in young men with medium to high-grade unilateral varicocele. By contrast, Leydig cell function seems to be undisturbed. They demonstrated that these men had an exaggerated GnRH test response with high-elevated FSH levels. The baseline FSH levels were elevated above 5.6 U/l. This could provide an easier way to predict the outcome of the GnRH test, which is labor intensive and expensive [16]. Other investigators have shown a mixed response to the GnRH test [13]. However, there is no evidence yet that GnRh test response correlates with fertility in the long term.

Indications for intervention

Kogan [17] divided the indications for repair into the following groups:

Absolute	A small hypotrophic testis (2–3 cc smaller than the other)
	Additional testicular condition affecting fertility
Relative	Abnormal semen analysis
	Bilateral palpable varicocele
	Large size (grade)
	Softer ipsilateral testis
	Pain
	Supranormal LH and FSH response to GnRH stimulation test
	Patient or parental anxiety
Minor	Abnormal scrotal appearance

The most common and absolute criterion is a small testicle indicating growth arrest [15]. The testis remains small if conservatively managed, while catch-up growth has been reported by several authors [8,15]. Parrott *et al.* reported reversal of hypotrophy in 53–90% postintervention [10]. Kocvara *et al.* argue that the so-called reversal of growth may be due to edema associated with division of lymphatic vessels [18]. Pinto *et al.* report no correlation between testicular hypotrophy and fertility [2], but others have demonstrated the complete opposite [8,15]. The criterion of softer testis is very subjective and there is little written about it in literature.

In our experience, pain and discomfort should be an absolute indication for intervention and surgery successfully alleviates the symptoms. Anxiety is another common feature in the adolescent boys and intervention often helps to reassure them. GnRH stimulation test is intensive and expensive and is a weak criterion as an indication for intervention in the absence of correlation with fertility.

Age at intervention

The argument for early intervention lies in the observation that as the testicle is still growing, testicular atrophy associated with varicocele can be overcome during the pubertal growth spurt [19]. Studies have also demonstrated that varicocele-related testicular hypotrophy is a developing condition [1]. Hypotrophy was not present in boys younger than 11 years. In 11–14 year olds, the incidence was 7.3% and in 15–19 year olds it increased to 9.3%. These results suggest that varicocele-related testicular hypotrophy increased with puberty, supporting the idea that prepubertal intervention is ideal.

Intervention methods and outcomes

Broadly, the options of intervention in varicocele are either venous occlusion or surgical ligation. Venous occlusion is by either embolization or sclerotherapy. Sclerotherapy can be performed antegrade or retrograde. Surgical ligation can take place at various levels at, above, or below the inguinal region. Furthermore, it can be either by an open or by a laparoscopic approach and also can take the form of microsurgery (Figure 25.1). We will discuss the pros and cons of artery sparing and lymphatic sparing techniques.

Classification of methods of intervention in varicocele

- Venous occlusion
  - percutaneous embolization/sclerotherapy
  - antegrade scrotal sclerotherapy
- Surgical ligation – standard or microsurgical; artery sparing; and lymphatic sparing techniques
- High (suprainguinal) – laparoscopic or open
- Inguinal
- Subinguinal

Percutaneous embolization/sclerotherapy

This is an alternative to surgical ligation whereby the internal spermatic vein is embolized. The materials used include metal coil, spiders, plastics, brushes, detachable balloons, and sclerosing agents. A catheter is percutaneously inserted into the femoral vein under radiological guidance and left renal vein is catheterized. The left spermatic vein

is identified and the catheter is advanced into it far enough to not allow the distal end of the coil near the renal vein. Embolization is then performed using the chosen material; preferably the metal coil is used in children [20].

Advantages

This procedure is both artery and lymphatic sparing. Rivilla *et al.* perform this procedure under local anesthesia in children (mean age in their study; 11 years) with no complications of hydrocele or hematoma reported. There is no mention of bilateral or right-sided cases in the study. Clarke *et al.* have reported 90% success with this procedure.

Disadvantages

This procedure will require the services of an interventional radiologist and this can be a limitation [21]. There is a risk of coil dislodgement, left renal thrombosis or pulmonary embolus [20]. Collateral veins from the left renal vein could lead to failure to cannulate the internal spermatic vein along with severe vasospasm [21] and the diameter of the coil could be larger than the target vein.

Antegrade scrotal sclerotherapy

Tauber *et al.* described this new technique of an antegrade approach to the internal spermatic vein combining surgery and sclerotherapy [22]. The procedure involves an incision at the root of the scrotum and isolation and cannulation of the spermatic vein to the level beyond the internal ring. The sclerosing agent is injected mixed with air (2–3 ml agent with air in 3:1 ratio; air block technique). Patient co-operation is required to achieve increased intra-abdominal pressure by valsalva during injection under fluoroscopic control.

Advantages

Can be performed under local anesthetic and is artery and lymphatic sparing. Therefore, hydrocele formation is rare after this procedure. Tauber *et al.* [21] have reported a large series of 285 patients with 9% failure rate. Mazzoni *et al.* recommend this method as first line for recurrent varicocele, where they have had a success rate of 96% [23].

Disadvantages

An interventional radiologist with sufficient expertise is required and patient co-operation is paramount [22]. Therefore, this procedure can be of limited use in children. Complications noted include scrotal hematoma,

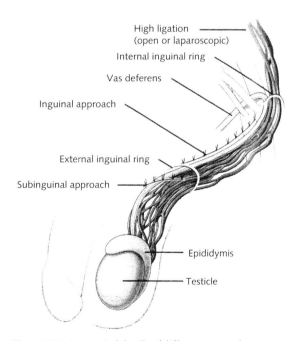

High ligation (open or laparoscopic)
Internal inguinal ring
Vas deferens
Inguinal approach
External inguinal ring
Subinguinal approach
Epididymis
Testicle

Figure 25.1 Anatomical details of different approaches.

epididymitis (3.8%), testicular atrophy, and left flank erythema [21,24]. Zaupa *et al.* report their experience with this technique highlighting the fact that the procedure can take longer to perform in children due to difficulty in cannulation [25]. They warn that focal testicular necrosis can occur rarely despite an uncomplicated primary procedure.

Subinguinal (microsurgical) ligation

In a study involving infertile men undergoing microscopic varicocelectomy (mean age 32 years), Hopps *et al.* describe the number and relationship of internal and external spermatic arteries, veins, and lymphatics within the subinguinal portion of the spermatic cord and compare it to the inguinal approach. They found that this approach was associated with more internal spermatic veins, more external spermatic veins greater than 2 mm in diameter, and more total spermatic arteries per dissection compared to the inguinal approach [26]. Goldstein *et al.* were the pioneers of this approach through a subinguinal incision and identify the veins, arteries, and lymphatics with the help of an operating microscope [27]. Schiff *et al.* have described the feasibility of this microsurgical approach in boys (<18 years old) with a low complication rate [28]. Chan *et al.* report accidental ligation of the artery despite the use of operating microscope in approximately 1% of cases [29]. They describe several reasons including men who have small sized arteries, aggressive manipulation leading to spasm, and the close proximity of the arteries to the venae comitantes. To increase detection of the lymphatics, the use of isosulfan blue has been proposed [30].

Advantages
Artery and lymphatic sparing approach using the microscope reduces the incidence of recurrent varicocele and hydrocele formation. In theory, preservation of the artery should lead to improved spermatogenesis as demonstrated by Cayan *et al.* probably by a positive effect on Leydig cell function [31].

Disadvantages
Dissection can be tedious [26]; accidental ligation is a possibility particularly in pediatric age group and necessitated the availability of an operating microscope.

Inguinal ligation

The inguinal approach was described by Ivanissevich in 1918. It involves opening the inguinal canal and ligating the dilated veins while allowing preservation of the spermatic artery with minimal morbidity. The reported success rate is approximately 85% with hydrocele formation in about 15% [9].

Hopps *et al.* observed that the inguinal approach was easier compared to the subinguinal technique [26]. This approach is best avoided if the integrity of the inguinal canal has been breached with some prior procedure.

Advantages
This approach provides a familiar anatomy, easy access to cord structures, identification, and preservation of the artery without compromising success rates.

Disadvantages
May not be suitable with previous inguinal surgery, hydrocele formation secondary to ligation of the lymphatics although this can be overcome by the use of isosulfan blue.

High (suprainguinal, retroperitoneal) ligation

This approach described by Palomo is performed via a high inguinal incision and is very popular. It has also been successfully adapted to use by the laparoscope. The spermatic vessels are mass ligated well above the pampiniform plexus, where only a few branches require ligation. Attempts at modification to this technique by an artery sparing method led to a higher incidence of recurrence. Kass and Marcol [32] reported 89% success with artery sparing compared to 98% with artery nonsparing original Palomo procedure. There is no evidence yet to prove that artery ligation affects testicular hemodynamics and function. Atassi *et al.* noted compensatory growth in both artery sparing and nonsparing groups with no detrimental growth effects such as testicular atrophy [33]. This technique spares the artery to the vas and therefore preserves the collateral blood supply to the testis. Secondary hydrocele formation varies from 3% to 36% in different series [34,35]. Oswald *et al.* [36] proposed the use of isosulfan blue to identify the lymphatics and Riccabona *et al.* [37] demonstrated a low recurrence rate of 2% with the lymphatic sparing approach and no hydrocele formation in their series.

Advantages
Extremely low recurrence rates, easy to perform, allows adaptation by minimally invasive methods, and very popular.

Disadvantages
Hydrocele formation is a problem due to lymphatic ligation but can be overcome using isosulfan blue to

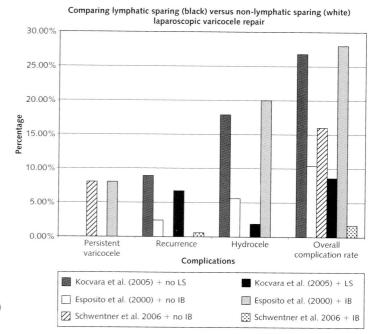

Figure 25.2 Comparing lymphatic sparing (black) versus nonlymphatic sparing (white) laparoscopic varicocele repair.

identify and preserve the lymphatics. Figure 25.2 shows the reported series in literature comparing lymphatic sparing and nonsparing approaches.

Laparoscopic varicocele ligation

As explained earlier, the Palomo procedure has been adapted to use by the laparoscopic approach with similar recurrence rates to the open procedure, as well as low morbidity and complication rates [24,38]. Incidence of hydrocele formation due to ligation of lymphatics with this approach [24,39] remains high (11–23%). Various modifications including the artery sparing and lymphatic sparing techniques have been described similar to the ones explained earlier [40]. Kocvara *et al.* describe the laparoscopic microsurgical approach using 10×–20× magnification to preserve the lymphatics [41]. This magnification is achieved by working quite close to the target. They showed that hydrocele formation and testicular hypotrophy occurred less with this technique, 1.9% and 2.9% respectively compared with 17.9% and 20.1% respectively in the conventional group, *p* = 0.0003. Poddoubny *et al.* have excellent results (99% success) with the laparoscopic artery and lymphatic sparing approach with no complications [42].

Advantages
Minimally invasive Palomo procedure with similar results.

Disadvantages
Similar to the Palomo procedure (see p. 196).

Management and prevention of complications

Hydrocele
Regardless of the surgical approach, the most frequent complication following an operation for varicocele is the formation of a hydrocele. In a large multicenter study involving 278 children between 7 and 17 years of age, Esposito *et al.* [43] showed that the median incidence of hydrocele following varicocele surgery is about 12%. This incidence was higher (17.6%) with artery nonsparing procedures compared to artery sparing procedures (4.3%) and is well demonstrated in Figure 25.2. Esposito *et al.* [43] have recommended noninvasive procedure like scrotal puncture for persistent hydrocele, which does not disappear after clinical observation. This successfully eliminated the hydroceles in 82% of the cases. The rest of the children (18%) required surgery to correct

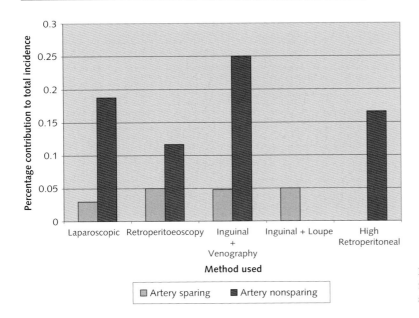

Figure 25.3 Incidence of hydrocele following artery sparing versus nonartery sparing technique.

the hydrocele. Hassan *et al.* [39] reported an incidence of 22.8% after laparoscopic varicocele ligation with a statistically significant decrease in hydroceles when the internal spermatic vein is simply ligated rather than ligated and divided. This possibly suggests that more lymphatics get divided by the latter approach. The general consensus is that the ligation or obstruction of the lymphatics is the cause for hydrocele formation and lymphatic sparing procedures have successfully reduced the incidence of this complication (Figure 25.3) [30,36,37,40].

Recurrent varicocele

It is difficult to ascertain the true incidence of persistence or recurrent varicocele in comparison to different techniques with most authors claming good success rates. However, some have suggested that efforts in trying to spare the artery result in an increased incidence of recurrent varicocele. Kass and Marcol [32] had better success with artery nonsparing Palomo procedure (98%) compared to artery sparing techniques (89%). Riccabona *et al.* [37] compared four different techniques and concluded that artery sparing procedures resulted in more recurrence rates as shown in Figure 25.4. However, others have shown excellent results with artery sparing methods [42]. There is little information available as to the best way to treat recurrence. Mazzoni *et al.* report that antegrade sclerotherapy was more successful in recurrent cases than as a primary procedure. They recommend this method as

the treatment of choice for recurrent varicocele particularly if the internal spermatic vein has been completely occluded in the primary treatment (percutaneous retrograde sclerotherapy or open and laparoscopic ligation).

Other complications

Chrouser *et al.* reported transient numbness following possible nerve injury in 4.8% of cases, which appeared within 10 days of surgery and resolved at an average of 8 months [44]. This study in boys with a mean age of 14 years had these symptoms around the anterior part of the ipsilateral thigh consistent with injury to the genitofemoral nerve. They recommend that cautery or harmonic dissection of the peritoneum overlying the spermatic cord and excessive traction on the tissues surrounding the cord should be avoided intraoperatively. Isolated cases of partial testicular necrosis have been reported [29] while others like sigmoid serosal tear are due to laparoscopic misadventure or effects of a laparoscopic learning curve [38].

Conclusions

Various surgical procedures have been used to ligate or obliterate the internal spermatic vein including the laparoscopic or open surgical ligation in the retroperitoneum or the venous plexus inguinally or subinguinally. The standard open surgical or laparoscopic

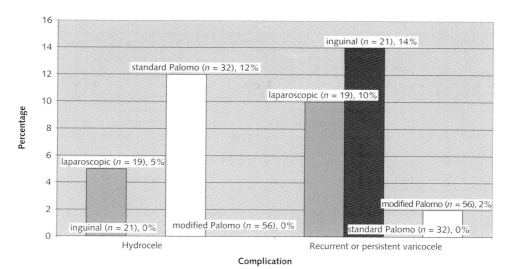

Figure 25.4 Optimizing the operative treatment of boys with varicocele: sequential comparison of techniques.

Palomo technique of nonartery sparing mass ligation remains popular with better success than the artery sparing approach. Hydrocele formation is the most frequent complication but lymphatic sparing measures seem to reduce its incidence. However, long-term studies with these techniques are needed to validate the results. Children who undergo varicocele surgery should be followed up for potential complications.

References

1 Akbay E, Cayan S, Boruk E, Deuce MN, Bozlu M. The prevalence of varicocele and the varicocele-related testicular atrophy in Turkish children and adolescents. *BJU Int* 2000;86:490–3.

2 Pinto K, Krrovand RL, Jarow JP. Varicocele related testicular atrophy and its predicted effect upon fertility. *J Urol* 1994;152:788–90.

3 Santoro G, Romeo C, Impellizzeri P, Arco A, Rizzo G, Gentile C. A morphometric and ultrastructural study of the changes in the lamina propria in adolescents with varicocele. *BJU Int* 1999;83:828–32.

4 Barbieri ER, Hidelgo ME, Venegas A, Smith R, Lissi EA. Varicocele-associated decrease in antioxidant defences. *J Androl* 1999;20:713–7.

5 Romeo C, Santoro G, Impellizzeri P *et al*. Myofibroblasts in adoloescent varicocele. An ultrastructural and immunohistochemical study. *Urol Res* 2000;28:24–8.

6 Dubin L, Amelaar RD. Varicocele size and results of varicocelectomy in selected subfertile men with a varicocele. *Fertil Steril* 1970;21:606–9.

7 Tasci AI, Resim S, Caskurlu T, Dincel C, Bayrakter Z, Gurbuz G. Color doppler ultrasonography and spectral

8 Paduch DA, Niedzielski J. Repair versus observation in adolescent varicocele: A prospective study. *J Urol* 1997;158:1128–32.

9 Diamond DA, Paltiel HJ, DiCanzio J *et al*. Comparative assessment of pediatric testicular volume: Orchidometer versus ultrasound. *J Urol* 2000;164:1111–14.

10 Parrott TS, Hewatt L. Ligation of the testicular artery and vein in adolescent varicocele. *J Urol* 1994;152:791–3.

11 Sayfan J, Siplovich L, Koltun L, Benyamin N. Varicocele treatment in pubertal boys prevents testicular growth arrest. *J Urol* 1997;157:1456–7.

12 Podesta ML, Gottlieb S, Medel R, Ropelato G, Bergada C, Quesada E. Hormonal parameters and testicular volume in children and adolescnts with unilateral varicocele: preoperative and postoperative findings. *J Urol* 1994;152:794–7.

13 Kass EJ, Freitas JE, Bour JB. Adolescent varicocele: Objective indications for treatment. *J Urol* 1989;142:579.

14 Thomas JC, Elder JS. Testicular growth arrest and adolescent varicocele: Does varicocele size make a difference? *J Urol* 2002;168:1689–91.

15 Kass EJ, Belman AB. Reversal of testicular growth failure by varicocele ligation. *J Urol* 1987;137:475–6.

16 Bach T, Pfeiffer D, Tauber R. Baseline follicle-stimulating hormone is a strong predictor for the outcome of the gonadotrophin-releasing hormone test in young men with unilateral medium or high grade varicocele. *BJU Int* 2006;98:619–22.

17 Kogan SJ. The pediatric varicocele. In *Pediatric Urology*, Edited by Gearhart J, Rink R, Mouriquand P. Philadelphia: WB Saunders Co, 2001, Chapter 48, pp. 763–74.

18 Kocvara R, Dolezal J, Hampl R, Povysil C, Dvoracek J, Hill M *et al*. Division of lymphatic vessels at varicocelectomy leads

to testicular oedema and decline in testicular function according to the LH-RH analogue stimulation test. *Eur Urol* 2003;43:430–5.

19 Cayan S, Akbay E, Bozlu M, Doruk M, Acar D, Ulusoy E. The effect of varicocele repair on testicular volume in children and adolescents with varicocele. *J Urol* 2002;168:731–4.

20 Rivilla F, Casillas JG, Gallego J, Lezana AH. Percutaneous venography and embolisation of the internal spermatic vein by spring coil for treatment of the left varicocele in children. *J Ped Surg* 1995;30:523–7.

21 Clarke SA, Agarwal N, Reidy J. Percutaneous transfemoral testicular vein embolisation in the treatment of childhood varicocele. *Ped Radiol* 2001;31:515–7.

22 Tauber R, Johnsen N. Antegrade scrotal sclerotherapy for the treatment of varicocele: technique and late results. *J Urol* 1994;151:386–90.

23 Mazzoni G, Minucci S, Gentile V. Recurrent varicocele: Role of antegrade sclerotherapy as first choice treatment. *Eur Urol* 2002;41:614–18.

24 May M, Johannsen M, Beutner S, Helke C, Braun KP, Lein M *et al.* Laparoscopic surgery versus antegrade scrotal sclerotherapy: Retrospective comparison of two different approaches for varicocele treatment. *Eur Urol* 2006;49:384–7.

25 Zaupa P, Mayr J, Hollwarth ME. Antegrade scrotal sclerotherapy for treating primary varicocele in children. *BJU Int* 2006;97:809–12.

26 Hopps CV, Lemer ML, Schlegel PN, Goldstein M. Intraoperative varicocele anatomy: A microscopic study of the inguinal versus subinguinal approach. *J Urol* 2003;170:2366–70.

27 Goldstein M, Gilbert BR, Dicker AP, Dwosh J, Gnecco C. Microsurgical inguinal varicocelectomy with the delivery of testis: An artery and lymphatics sparing technique. *J Urol* 1992;148:1808.

28 Schiff J, Kelly C, Goldstein M, Schelgel P, Poppas D. Managing varicoceles in children: Results with microsurgical varicocelectomy. *BJU Int* 2005;95:399–402.

29 Chan PTK, Wright JE, Goldstein M. Incidence and post-operative outcomes of accidental ligation of the testicular artery during microsurgical varicocelectomy. *J Urol* 2005;173:482–4.

30 Scwentner C, Oswald J, Lunacek A, Deibl M, Bartsch G, Radmayr C. Optimizing the outcome of microsurgical subinguinal varicocelectomy using isosulphan blue: A prospective randomized trial. *J Urol* 2006;175:1049–52.

31 Cayan S, Acar D, Ulger S, Akbay E. Adolescent varicocele repair: Long term results and comparison of surgical techniques according to optical magnification use in 100 cases at a single university hospital. *J Urol* 2005;174:2003–7.

32 Kass EJ, Marcol B. Results of varicocele surgery in adolescence: A comparison of techniques. *J Uol* 1992;148:694–6.

33 Atassi O, Kass EJ, Stinert BW. Testicular growth after successful varicocele correction in adolescents: Comparison of artery sparing techniques with the Palomo procedure. *J Urol* 1995;153:482–3.

34 Misseri R, Gershbein AB, Horowitz M, Glassberg KI. The adolescent varicocele II: The incidence of hydrocele and delayed recurrent varicocele after varicocelectomy in a long term followup. *BJU Int* 2001;87:494.

35 Szabo R, Kessler R. Hydrocele following internal spermatic vein ligation: A retrospective study and review of literature. *J Urol* 1984;132:924.

36 Oswald J, Korner I, Riccabona M. The use of isosulphan blue to identify lymphatic vessels in high retroperitoneal ligation of adolescent varicocele avoiding post operative hydrocele. *BJU Int* 2001;87:502.

37 Riccabona M, Oswald J, Koen M, Lusuardi L, Radmayr C, Bartsch G. Optimizing the operative treatment of boys with varicocele: Sequential comparison of 4 techniques. *J Urol* 2003;169:666–8.

38 Koyle MA, Ootamasathien S, Barqawi A, Rajimwale A, Furness III, PD. Laparoscopic Palomo varicocele ligation in children and adolescents: Results of 103 cases. *J Urol* 2004;172:1749–52.

39 Hassan JM, Adams MC, Pope JC, Demarco RT, Brock JW. Hydrocele formation following laparoscopic varicocelectomy. *J Urol* 2006;175:1076–9.

40 Schwentner C, Rdamayr C, Lunacek A, Gozzi C, Pinggera GM, Neururer R *et al.* Laparoscopic varicocele ligation in children and adolescents using isosulphan blue: A prospective randomized trial. *BJU Int* 2006;98:861–5.

41 Kocvara R, Dvoracek J, Sedlacek J, Dite Z, Novak K. Lymphatic sparing laparoscopic varicocelectomy: A microsurgical repair. *J Urol* 2005;173:1751–4.

42 Poddoubny IV, Dronov AF, Kovarski SL, Korznikova IN, Darenkov IA, Zalikhin DV. Laparoscopic ligation of testicular veins for varicocele in children. A report of 180 cases. *Surg Endosc* 2000;14:1107–9.

43 Esposito C, Valla JS, Najmaldin A, Shier F, Mattioli G, Savanelli A *et al.* Incidence and management of hydrocele following varicocele surgery in children. *J Urol* 2004;171:1271–3.

44 Chrouser K, Vandersteen D, Crocker J, Reinberg Y. Nerve injury after laparoscopic varicocelectomy. *J Urol* 2004;172:691–3.

26 Hypospadias Urethroplasty

Warren T. Snodgrass

Key points

- The commonest modern techniques for hypospadias repair include the TIP (tubularized incised plate) urethroplasty, onlay prepucial flaps, tabularized prepucial flaps, and two-stage repairs.
- Complications following hypospadias urethroplasty include urethrocutaneous fistula, meatal stenosis or neourethral stricture, diverticulum, and dehiscence.

- There is a greater incidence of these problems as the severity of the hypospadias defect increases regardless of surgical technique used.
- Ongoing performance is necessary to maintain competence.
- Use of optical magnification, delicate instruments, fine suture materials and needles, and careful, precise tissue handling are commonly advised to reduce complications.

Introduction

Hypospadias repair includes straightening associated ventral curvature (when present), urethroplasty, glansplasty, and skin closure with either circumcision or foreskin reconstruction. Although each step is an important determinant of outcome, most complications result from urethroplasty, which will be the focus of this review.

Modern options for primary hypospadias urethroplasty can be divided into several categories, including tubularizations of the urethral plate, supplementation of the urethral plate with prepucial flaps, or replacement of the urethral plate with prepucial flaps or grafts. Within each group are various specific techniques, but the most commonly performed today include TIP (tubularized incised plate), onlay prepucial flaps, tubularized prepucial flaps, and two-stage Byar's flaps [1].

The most common complications following hypospadias urethroplasty include urethrocutaneous fistula, meatal stenosis or neourethral stricture, diverticulum, and dehiscence. Generally there is a greater incidence of

these problems as the severity of the hypospadias defect increases regardless of surgical technique used. There is also variation in specific complications and their incidence between various repairs.

Most reviews of hypospadias outcomes emphasize short-term results and complications. While most problems are apparent within several months following surgery, ultimate function of the reconstructed penis cannot be determined until after puberty. Since most hypospadias repairs are done within the first year of life in the United States, and in early childhood throughout most the world, it is difficult to obtain data regarding micturition, sexual function, and patient's perception of outcome in adulthood. Furthermore, ongoing modifications of surgical techniques and introduction of new procedures means those reports on adults operated as children provide long-term results for repairs no longer in use. This chapter accordingly will emphasize short-term complications, but will also review limited long-term data available on modern techniques.

Etiologies of urethroplasty complications

Few randomized studies investigate factors associated with complications from hypospadias urethroplasty.

Pediatric Urology: Surgical Complications and Management. Edited by Duncan T. Wilcox, Prasad P. Godbole and Martin A. Koyle.
© 2008 Blackwell Publishing, ISBN: 978-1-4051-6268-5.

Those actively involved in these operations believe ongoing performance is necessary to maintain competence, although no standards have been established. Use of optical magnification, delicate instruments, fine suture materials and needles, and careful, precise tissue handling are commonly advised to reduce complications.

Fistula

Urethrocutaneous fistulas are the most common complication following urethroplasty. Several factors have been implicated in their occurrence, including apposing suture lines from neourethral and skin closure, distal obstruction from meatal stenosis or urethral stricture, turbulent urine flow, and locally impaired vascularity. Steps advised to reduce likelihood of fistula include in-turning epithelium into the neourethral lumen; two-layer closure of the neourethra using fine, absorbable sutures; and interposition of vascularized tissues as "barrier layers" between the neourethral and overlying skin suture lines.

Fistulas usually are apparent within the first few months after surgery, but occasionally develop years later. Some close spontaneously, but most require surgical correction.

Meatal stenosis

Meatal stenosis may result from poor distal vascularity and wound contracture, technical errors in meatoplasty, or less commonly, from balanitis xerotica obliterans (BXO). Regardless of urethroplasty technique, the neomeatus should be generously sized and oval, not rounded, allowing for minor postoperative contraction. This precaution especially applies to tubularization procedures where temptation to suture the neourethra too far distally can directly lead to stenosis. BXO is not commonly encountered after hypospadias repair in the United States, possibly due to preference for circumcision, but should be suspected when typical white scar involves the meatus.

Neourethral stricture

Strictures indicate focal regions of impaired neourethra vascularity, or contracture of the anastomosis between reconstructed urethra and proximal native urethra. A circumferential anastomosis is thought to have greater risk for constriction, although a comparison study of tubularized versus onlay prepucial flaps found no significant difference in strictures between the two techniques [2]. Despite initial concerns that the relaxing incision for TIP would create stricture, this complication has been only rarely encountered.

Diverticulum

Diverticulum formation may indicate distal obstruction, turbulent flow, and/or creation of too large neourethra. Genital skin is elastic to allow erection, and so may balloon proximally from fixed resistance of the nondistensible glanular urethra without anatomic obstruction when prepucial flaps are used for urethroplasty.

Dehiscense

Wound dehiscence results in partial or complete failure of urethroplasty, returning the neomeatus to a more proximal location. The main factor implicated in this complication is tension on approximated tissues, although impaired local vascularity and traumatic dislodgement of the urethral stent are other possible etiologies. While it is difficult to prove differences in outcomes based upon choice of suture materials and techniques, the incidence of wound separation was less after changing from chromic catgut horizontal mattress sutures to subepithelial polyglactin glansplasty (unpublished data).

Complications according to surgical technique

TIP

TIP urethroplasty was first described to correct distal hypospadias, but subsequently indications expanded to include midshaft and more proximal cases when associated ventral penile curvature can be straightened preserving the urethral plate. Incidence of complications varies significantly according to the severity of the hypospadias. Outcomes from reported series between 1994 and 2004, comprising the first decade of experience with the technique, are summarized in Table 26.1. My personal complication rate for the last 120 patients was 2.5%, including two fistulas and one glans dehiscence. This contrasts with a recently published 13% for midshaft repairs and 25% for proximal shaft to perineal defects [3]. Others have not subdivided patients with midshaft versus more proximal TIP repairs, but results from reported series are summarized in Table 26.2.

As seen from these tables, fistula, meatal stenosis, and glans dehiscence are the most common complications after TIP. It is not surprising that fistulas sometimes develop after TIP since the neourethra and shaft skin are both closed in the ventral midline. The fact that dartos flap barrier layers do not always prevent fistulas may indicate that inflammation to reabsorb suture can establish a tract from the neourethra through dartos to the skin. Meatal stenosis most often arises from technical

Table 26.1 TIP outcomes for distal hypospadias.

Authors	Year	Number of patients	Mean follow-up months	Patients total complications	Fistula	Meatal stenosis	Dehiscence	Stricture
Snodgrass [4]	1994	16	22	0	–	–	–	–
Snodgrass [5]	1996	129 (8 reoperations)	NS	10	5	3	2	–
Steckler and Zaontz [6]	1997	31	3	0	–	–	–	–
Ross and Kay [7]	1997	15	<12	0	–	–	–	–
Elbakry [8]	1999	21	20	4	4	4	–	–
Sugarman et al. [9]	1999	25	10	1	1	–	–	–
Oswald et al. [10]	2000	30	15	1	–	–	1	–
Holland et al. [11]	2000	60	27	9	6	3	–	–
Dayanc et al. [12]	2000	20	20	2	1	1	–	–
Guralnick et al. [13]	2000	28	9	8	6	2	–	–
Borer et al. [14]	2001	156	6–38	7	6	1	–	–
Smith [15]	2001	53	1	0	–	–	–	–
Cheng et al. [16]	2002	414	4–66	1	0	1	–	–
El-Sherbiny [17]	2003	64	6	9	7	2	–	–
Jayanthi [18]	2003	110	9	1	1	–	–	–
Samuel and Wilcox [19]	2003	65	4	4	3	–	1	–
Leclair et al. [20]	2004	1–62 (6 midshaft)	12	13	9	4	–	–
Elicevik et al. [21]	2004	324	6–60	75	39	32	12	3
Lorenz et al. [22]	2004	22	3–6	1	1	1	–	–
Total		1745		146 (8%)	89 (5%)	54 (3%)	16 (1%)	

NS, Not stated.

error, specifically tubularizing the neourethra too far distally. Urethral stricture is a rarely reported complication despite the midline urethral plate relaxing incision. Since flaps are not used to supplement the urethral plate, diverticulum should not occur, and have been only anecdotally noted in published series, possibly from incorporating adjacent shaft skin into the neourethra.

Onlay and tubularized prepucial flaps

Onlay prepucial flap today is used to correct midshaft and proximal shaft hypospadias when there is no ventral curvature >30° leading to transection of the urethral plate. However, when introduced in 1987 the operation was more commonly used for distal and midshaft repairs, and most reported outcomes reflect its use to correct these less severe defects. The original publication by Elder et al. included 44% distal and 54% midshaft

hypospadias [23]. A subsequent article from the same institution by Baskin et al. [24] stated 83% of their 374 patients undergoing onlay had mid to distal hypospadias. Results from series using onlay prepucial flap for proximal hypospadias are summarized in Table 26.3.

Similarly, the tubularized prepucial flap (transverse Island, TI) was introduced in the early 1980s before the urethral plate was identified as a distinct structure, and when "chordee excision" more often led to excision of the urethral plate. Today the urethral plate is much less commonly excised, typically only when ventral curvature >30° persists after the penis is degloved and ventral dartos contributing to bending is dissected. Early reports on tubularized prepucial flaps included patients with distal, sometimes glanular, hypospadias and so do not reflect current use of the technique primarily for proximal defects with persistent ventral curvature. Those specifically

Table 26.2 Prior reports of midshaft to proximal TIP.

Authors	Date	Number of patients	Ventral curvature (%)	Mean follow-up months	Total patient complications (%)	Fistula	Meatal stenosis	Stricture	Dehiscence	Recurrent curvature
Snodgrass et al. (multicenter) [25]	1998	16 midshaft 11 proximal	11 (69) 10 (91)	NS	3 (11)	1	1	0	1 complete	NS
Chen et al. [26]	2000	10 midshaft 27 proximal	9 (23)	12.5	2 (20) 5 (19)	2* 4*	1* 3*	0 0	NS NS	NS NS
Borer et al. [14]	2001	16 midshaft 9 proximal	NS	6–38	1 (6) 2 (22)	1 2	NS NS	NS NS	NS NS	NS NS
Snodgrass and Lorenzo [27]	2002	13 midshaft 20 proximal	5 (38) 13 (65)	9	2 (15) 9 (45)	1 6*	0 1*	1 0	0 1	0 2
Cheng et al. (multicenter) [16]	2002	100 "midshaft to penoscrotal"	NS	4–66	4 (4)	3	1	0	NS	NS
Samuels and Wilcox [19]	2003	18 proximal	4 (22)	4	4 (22)	1	0	0	3 glans	NS
Mustafa [28]	2005	1 midshaft 12 proximal	1 (100) 1 (8)	NS	4 (31)	3	1	0	NS	NS
Total		253			36 (14)					

NS, Not stated.

Table 26.3 Onlay, TI for midshaft to proximal hypospadias.

Authors	Date	Number of patients	Ventral curvature (%)	Mean follow-up months	Total patient complications (%)	Fistulas	Meatal stenosis	Dehiscence	Stricture	Diverticulum	Other
Onlay											
Mollard et al. [29]	1991	22	22	NS	0	–	–	–	–	–	–
Barroso et al. [30]	2000	12 midshaft 35 proximal	29	15	12	8	2	2	–	4	2
Samuel et al. [31]	2001	17	10	38	10	10	2	–	–	–	2
Total		86			22 (26%)	18 (21%)	4 (4%)	2 (2%)	–	4 (4%)	4 (4%)
TIP											
Chuang and Shieh [32]	1995	56	56	6	22	16	2	–	3	1	–
Ghali [33]	1999	148	148	23	48	22	17	–	13	–	17
MacGillivray et al. [34]	2002	24	24	62	10	9	–	–	1	–	–
Patel et al. [35]	2005	12	12	25	3	1	1	1	–	1	–
Total		240			83 (35%)	48 (20%)	20 (8%)	1 (0.4%)	17 (7%)	2 (1%)	17 (7%)

NS, Not stated.

reviewing outcomes of tubularized prepucial flaps for proximal hypospadias are listed in Table 26.3.

Steps to reduce likelihood of complications with these procedures have been described. Neourethra suture lines in-turn epithelium and are done in layers to ensure sound closure. The vascular pedicle to the flap can be advanced laterally over the neourethra to provide a barrier layer. The suture line for tubularized flaps is rotated dorsally against the corpora. Care is exercised to avoid making the neourethra too large, which promotes diverticula. Proximal and distal anastomoses are made obliquely to reduce concern for meatal stenosis or proximal stricture.

Byar's flaps

Two-stage urethroplasty today is reserved for proximal hypospadias when associated ventral curvature leads to urethral plate transection or excision to facilitate straightening. There are very few modern reports of Byar's flap outcomes. Retik *et al.* [36] published a series of 58 patients noting a 5% incidence of fistulas and no meatal stenosis. However, neither length of follow-up nor overall complications were reported. In contrast, Greenfield *et al.* [37] used a similar two-stage prepucial flap repair described by Belt-Fuqua in 39 patients and found that while only 2.5% of patients developed fistulas, 21% had diverticulum, and 18% strictures.

Byar's flaps may be more prone to diverticulum formation than are other skin flap urethroplasties. Onlay flaps are anchored to the urethral plate and tubularized prepucial flaps can be gently stretched to the desired length with any excess excised. However, the vascular pedicle of Byar's flaps does not fix to the underlying corpora cavernosa surface and are difficult to size precisely to the defect. Consequently, the resultant neourethra tends to be irregular, promoting turbulent flow, and poorly attached to the corpora, allowing expansion. Furthermore, glans closure creates a region of relatively fixed distal resistance to urinary flow, potentially stimulating distention of the prepucial skin tube along the penile shaft.

Diagnosis of complications

Presentation

Given that most primary hypospadias operations today are performed during infancy or early childhood, most complications are asymptomatic and sometimes are initially unrecognized. Unless a fistula is apparent on physical inspection or the child is observed voiding from more than one location, the defect may not become apparent until toilet training. Meatal stenosis or neourethral stricture is suspected when the patient appears to have stranguria. A visibly small meatus, however, does not necessarily indicate stenosis following hypospadias surgery. Diverticula usually are noted because of ballooning of the neourethra during voiding with subsequent dribbling. Glans dehiscence may be found by parents, but is asymptomatic until after toilet training when the abnormal meatus affects urinary direction.

Physical examination

Fistulas may occur at any point along the neourethra, and may be suspected during routine postoperative evaluations. They range in size from pinhole openings that emit tiny droplets of urine to defects of several millimeters through which most voided urine passes. The opening sometimes is not apparent despite a clear history of abnormal leakage.

Meatal stenosis results in a visible small opening. A white discoloration may indicate BXO, which complicates management as all affected tissues must be excised to prevent recurrence. As mentioned, a small appearing neomeatus is not necessarily indicative of obstructive stenosis, and a sound of age-appropriate size should be passed to rule out meatal stenosis. There are no external signs of urethral stricture, but a slow stream might be observed in the clinic. Similarly, failure of a sound to pass through the reconstructed urethra prompts additional investigation to detect obstruction.

Diverticula are readily observed when the neourethra balloons in size during voiding, and compression on the distended urethra expresses additional urine. These may be focal expansions of one segment along the penile shaft or can expand along the entire neourethra and into the scrotum.

Wound dehiscence sometimes is first noted when the dressings are removed postoperatively and the catheter is visible proximally. More often, presentation is less dramatic and may be overlooked unless the surgeon specifically confirms during examination that the glans wings are well-fused together. In some cases, the glans wings retract partially apart over time with only a thin bridge of skin giving the impression the glansplasty is intact.

Uroflowometry

Assessment of the neourethra by uroflowometry has been recommended as a noninvasive test for obstruction after urethroplasty. Testing is obviously limited to toilet-trained boys, who must void sufficient volume into the center of the funnel to validate the findings. Peak flow values most often are within expected range for age-matched controls, but a plateau-shaped curve, in contrast to the usual bell-shaped pattern, may be noted [38]. This finding possibly indicates decreased elasticity of the neourethra versus native urethras. Peak flows less than 5 cc/sec should be verified accurate and then prompt further investigation to exclude meatal stenosis or urethral stricture.

Imaging

Retrograde urethrography or voiding cystourethrography potentially is useful to detect neourethral obstruction or document a fistula or diverticulum. However, such testing is unnecessary for a history suspicious for fistula, and diverticula are apparent on physical examination. Meatal stenosis may complicate attempts to catheterize the urethra, and it can be difficult to pass a catheter even in the absence of obstruction because of a tortuous neourethra, narrowed but nonobstructing proximal anastomosis, or a prostatic utricle. Instrumentation of the neourethra could itself result in injury and is distressing to children. Accordingly, there is little role for diagnostic imaging to assess outcomes from hypospadias repair.

Intraoperative evaluation

Following induction of general anesthesia the hypospadias repair is evaluated for the suspected defect and potential coexisting complications. After visual inspection, a sound can be passed through the neomeatus followed by urethroscopy. When suspected fistulas are not detected, a catheter placed through the meatus allows injection of dilute methylene blue dye with simultaneous compression proximally to the native urethra until leakage is seen or absence of fistula is established. Regardless of preoperative assessments, thorough intraoperative evaluation should be done to detect comorbidities. For example, fistulas may occur due to distal obstruction or a diverticulum that also must be corrected for successful fistula repair. Similarly, a diverticulum may arise from distal obstruction.

Hypospadias reoperation

Timing of intervention

It is recommended that sufficient time elapse for tissue reaction to subside after urethroplasty before correction of complications. A period of 6 months is commonly

considered a minimum delay, and since most postoperative complications are asymptomatic or minimally bothersome this is feasible. Earlier intervention is required when high-grade obstruction causes severe stranguria or urinary retention. If relief of obstruction is required early postoperatively, temporizing solutions such as proximal urethrostomy or suprapubic tube placement may be necessary before definitive therapy.

Preoperative testosterone stimulation has also been considered to improve vascularity of tissues before reoperation. However, no study has randomized patients to determine potential impact of hormonal therapy.

Principles of correction
Fistulas

Fistula tracts are dissected to the urethra and excised at entrance into the lumen. The defect is closed with fine sutures turning epithelium into the urethra. Then a barrier flap of healthy tissue is developed to cover the repair before skin closure. Uncomplicated small fistulas can be corrected without postoperative urinary diversion, while larger defects and those associated with such other problems as meatal stenosis or diverticulum requiring more extensive surgery are stented.

Depictions of fistula repair emphasize rotational flaps to avoid overlapping suture lines. Another option is to excise fistulas through a longer midline incision through the median raphe, which facilitates access to the tract as well as regional dartos tissues for a barrier flap while concealing the scar.

Special considerations are needed when a fistula occurs very near to the corona. When these are small and there is neither meatal stenosis nor partial separation of the glans wings, it may not be necessary to redo the glansplasty, but rather to follow the steps mentioned above for repair [39]. When only a thin band of skin separates the neomeatus from a fistula, the fistula is more than approximately 1 mm, or there is meatal stenosis, then reoperative glansplasty should be performed as part of fistula closure.

A large fistula more than a few millimeters probably indicates ischemia and these defects may require additional urethroplasty to successfully close. When there is a paucity of regional dartos tissues to create a barrier flap, consideration should be given to harvesting tunica vaginalis as a pedicle flap from a testicle to cover the repair.

Meatal stenosis

Obstruction at the neomeatus requires reoperative glansplasty. The glans is opened through the meatus in the ventral midline proximally until healthy urethra is encountered. If there is any clinical suspicion of BXO, all tissues from the healthy region of the urethra distally must be aggressively excised and staged urethroplasty done using buccal mucosa graft. Unfortunately, intraoperative biopsy for frozen section may not be feasible to obtain a sufficient sample for diagnosis while preserving tissues for one-stage repair if BXO is not present. Dense scarring in the glans is another indication for two-stage buccal graft repair. If there appears to be less reaction, TIP or inlay grafting might be considered, with strong consideration to inlay grafting rather than relying upon scarred tissues to reepithelialize spontaneously. Graft taken dorsally is reliable even in the presence of dense fibrosis. Alternatively, in the absence of BXO, which is a contraindication to repair with skin flaps, meatal stenosis can be repaired using regional flaps, such as the Mathieu flip-flap [40]. Objections to flaps for reoperations include relative lack of well-vascularized skin and less cosmetic neomeatus.

Urethral stricture

Options for repair of neourethral stricture depend on length and density of fibrosis, with most of these strictures less than 1 cm. Urethral dilation sometimes is effective especially in the initial postoperative period, but the majority require surgery [41]. Optical urethrostomy has been used with overall success in approximately 25%, and in one series was most likely following onlay flap or urethral plate tubularizations [42]. Excision and reanastomosis could be considered as in adult urethral stricture repair, but may be a less attractive option after hypospadias surgery since blood supply to adjacent neourethra is less certain. Strictures less than 5 mm can be exposed through a midline ventral incision, with either TIP or dorsal inlay grafting as discussed for meatal stenosis. Longer strictures could require proximal urethrostomy with excision of the stricture and staged grafting to bridge the defect or replace the distal neourethra. Onlay or tubularized skin flaps have also been used, but following prior surgery there may be less skin available for these flaps, and their blood supply is less reliable [43].

Glans dehiscence

Separation of the glans wings with resultant proximal displacement of the meatus is approached using a "Y" shaped ventral incision extending along the junction of the glans and urethral plate on either side, joining 2 mm below the meatus, and extending proximally down the midline as far as the penoscrotal junction. Distal urethroplasty and repeat glansplasty are performed, a ventral dartos flap is dissected to cover the repair, and any excess shaft skin is removed to improve cosmesis.

Diverticulum

After excluding distal obstruction, a ventral midline skin incision is made over the ballooned neourethra. The diverticulum can also be opened in the midline, although an eccentric line of incision lateral to midline is preferred by some to avoid overlapping suture lines in the neourethra and overlying skin. Once the defect is opened, excess tissue is excised and the neourethra is closed in two layers over a catheter. A dartos or tunica vaginalis barrier flap covers the repair before skin closure.

Techniques for hypospadias reoperation

Operations used for primary hypospadias repair are adapted for reoperations as discussed below. Common to each is increased incidence of additional complications, and for both TIP and skin flap reoperation, these problems are encountered significantly more often than with initial surgery. Presumably this indicates vascularity to previously operated tissues is less certain, or other currently unknown factors in wound healing are adversely affected after prior intervention. Even experienced surgeons may be unable to predict health of residual tissues.

TIP

TIP is modified for reoperation when the urethral plate remains and appears minimally scarred. The technique is as described above for reoperative glansplasty, since dehiscence is the most common indication for the procedure. Published outcomes for TIP reoperation as summarized in Table 26.4. In these series most patients have failed two or fewer repairs. Previous urethral plate incision is not a contraindication unless there is gross scarring. Fistulas are the most common complication, with reduced incidence when a barrier flap covers the repair [44].

Skin flaps

Both onlay and tubularized flaps have been fashioned for reoperative urethroplasty. As with TIP, basic steps in the procedure resemble primary operations, except there may be less skin for a flap and vascularity appears diminished. Care must be taken to avoid incising across blood supply to preserve neourethra. Results of reoperations using skin flaps are listed in Table 26.5.

Table 26.4 TIP reoperations.

Authors	Number of patients	Mean number of prior operations (range)	Complication rate (%)	Fistula (%)	Meatal stenosis (%)	Stricture (%)	Diverticulum	Dehiscence (%)
Shanberg et al. [45]	13	2.5 (1–6)	15	8*	8	0	0	8
Borer et al. [14]	25	NS	24	20	4	0	0	0
Yang et al. [46]	25	2.5	NS	28	52	8	NS	NS
Snodgrass and Lorenzo [27]	15	1 (1–2)	20	13	0	0	0	6

NS, Not stated.
*One patient had both glans dehiscence and a fistula.

Table 26.5 Skin flaps.

Authors	Number of patients	Technique	Complication rate (%)	Fistula (%)	Meatal stenosis (%)	Stricture (%)	Diverticulum	Dehiscence (%)
Secrest et al.	69	35 ventral flap	29	3	6	8	–	11
		34 flip-flap	47	NS	NS	NS	NS	NS
Jayanthi et al.	44	8 tube flap	56	25	–	12	–	25
		8 onlay flap	–	–	–	–	–	–
		28 flip-flap	29	7	3	3	–	14
Simmons et al.	53	36 onlay	14	3	–	11	–	–
		17 flip-flap	24	18	–	–	–	6

NS, Not stated.

Inlay grafting

If the urethral plate previously was excised, a healthy skin strip sometimes can be conserved as a substitute urethral plate. It is incised in the midline, but rather than rely upon spontaneously reepithelialization, the resultant defect is grafted with buccal mucos, or other skin source if there is no BXO. This inlay graft is quilted into place, and then tubularization proceeds for a single-stage repair. Dorsal inlay grafting mimics current trends in adult urethral stricture repair, taking advantage of the reliable take that occurs when graft is secured dorsally to the corpora.

To date, only one series has reported more than anecdotal experience with inlay grafting, performing repairs in 31 patients with a mean of four failed operations. Complications developed in 16%, including one fistula and four proximal strictures [47].

Staged buccal grafting

When there is gross scarring of the urethral plate or residual skin flap, these tissues are excised and replaced with buccal graft for staged urethroplasty. In the first operation, unhealthy tissues from prior surgery are removed from the surface of the corpora and between glans wings, reestablishing a deep glans groove. A proximal urethrostomy is created and buccal graft harvested. Inner lip is used to resurface the glans, while cheek covers the penile shaft. The graft is quilted into place, using subepithelial stitches in the glans to avoid suture marks.

Following the first stage, focal contraction or scar develops in up to 20% of patients [48]. Partial graft contracture can be corrected by midline incision and buccal inlay grafting during the planned second stage urethroplasty. More extensive contracture or scarring requires a second operation to excise the unhealthy region and regraft. Urethroplasty is then performed 6 months later.

At the second stage, the now-vascularized buccal plate is tubularized turning epithelium into the lumen with a two-layer closure. The entire neourethra is covered with dartos and/or tunica vaginalis flaps, and then glansplasty and shaft skin closures proceed as described above for primary repairs.

In a series of 32 patients with a mean of four failed repairs (1–17) undergoing staged buccal graft reoperation, 19% had complications after the second stage, including one fistula, one meatal stenosis, and four glans dehiscences [48]. All glans disruptions occurred in prepubertal boys where grafted buccal tissue from the cheek appeared bulky. Subsequently thinner lip grafts have been used in the glans.

Long-term outcomes

The final outcome determination for hypospadias surgery is status of the penis in adulthood, including micturition, sexual function, and its appearance.

Micturition

The quality of the urinary stream after urethroplasty depends upon several factors, including its force and direction, as well as lack of post-void dribbling. While uroflowometry can be used to evaluate velocity, no objective test measures ability to aim or complete urination without dripping. Therefore patient questionnaires are needed to fully assess perceptions regarding micturition.

Since TIP was introduced in 1994, no studies have been reported to date characterizing patients' perceptions of voiding. Instead, surrogate evidence has been used to assure lack of obstruction, assuming patients with a well-healed neourethra should be able to void satisfactorily. One report [49] involved 21 boys re-evaluated from 17 months to 7 years (mean 36 months) after surgery by urethral calibration, finding no strictures. Uroflowometry in 17 of these patients, a mean of 45 months postoperatively, demonstrated peak flow rates above the fifth percentile in all cases. Similarly, Gurdal

et al. [50] obtained uroflowometry data of a mean of 3.5 years postoperatively in 19 boys, of whom 18 had normal flow while one with a peak flow between the 5th and 25th percentiles had meatal stenosis.

Greenfield *et al.* (51) recently published results from questionnaires answered by 27 patients 13 years after prepucial flap urethroplasty. Nearly all indicated some dissatisfaction with micturition, with 10 noting "minor" spraying, 10 needing to milk the urethra post-voiding to prevent dribbling, and 5 having a weak stream or straining to void.

Sexual function

Ventral penile curvature of varying degrees occurs in approximately 15% of distal hypospadias and over 50% of proximal cases. There is no data confirming straightening techniques currently used in children, primarily dorsal plication and/or ventral corporal grafting, remain effective during pubertal growth.

Patient-reported ejaculatory function has been infrequently surveyed, with no assessments after most repairs in use today. In Greenfield's series of prepucial flaps [51], half the patients who experienced ejaculation had to milk secretions from the urethra.

Cosmesis

Patients consider the appearance of the reconstructed penis as important as its function, and their opinion of the cosmetic result may vary from the assessment by the operating surgeon. In addition, when Mureau *et al.* [52] asked what factors influenced patient opinion, they found only some were potentially under the control of surgeons (meatal position, scars) whereas others (penile size, appearance of testes and scrotum) might not reflect technical issues.

Greenfield *et al.* also used questionnaire concerning appearance of the penis in adults after prepucial flap repairs in childhood. The authors reported 92% of patients responded, and they were pleased with the outcome, with 88% considering their penis normal. No such patient-derived data yet exists for TIP. However, a recent study in which photographs of the penis after TIP, Mathieu and onlay prepucial flap repairs were scored by a panel of health care workers reported TIP to create the most normal appearance of the glans and meatus. A recent questionnaire survey of parents was completed to determine their impression after TIP repair, using parents whose boys only underwent circumcision for controls [53]. There were no differences in responses between parents of hypospadias patients and circumcision controls, nor between parents and the operating surgeon.

References

1 Cook A, Khoury AE, Neville C *et al.* A multicenter evaluation of technical preferences for primary hypospadias repair. *J Urol* 2005;174:2354–7,discussion 2357.

2 Wiener JS, Sutherland RW, Roth DR *et al.* Comparison of onlay and tubularized island flaps of inner preputial skin for the repair of proximal hypospadias. *J Urol* 1997;158:1172–4.

3 Snodgrass W, Yucel S. Tubularized incised plate for mid shaft and proximal hypospadias repair. *J Urol* 2007;177:698–702.

4 Snodgrass W. Tubularized, incised plate urethroplasty for distal hypospadias. *J Urol* 1994;151:464.

5 Snodgrass W, Koyle M, Manzoni G *et al.* Tubularized incised plate hypospadias repair: results of a multicenter experience. *J Urol* 1996;156:839.

6 Steckler RE, Zaontz MR. Stent-free Thiersch-Duplay hypospadias repair with the Snodgrass modification. *J Urol* 1997; 158:1178.

7 Ross JH, Kay R. Use of a de-epithelialized local skin flap in hypospadias repairs accomplished by tubularization of the incised urethral plate. *Urology* 1997; 50:110.

8 Elbakry A. Tubularized-incised urethral plate urethroplasty: is regular dilatation necessary for success? *BJU Int* 1999; 84:683.

9 Sugarman ID, Trevett J, Malone PS. Tubularization of the incised urethral plate (Snodgrass procedure) for primary hypospadias surgery. *BJU Int* 1999; 83:88.

10 Oswald J, Korner I, Riccabona M. Comparison of the perimeatal-based flap (Mathieu) and the tubularized incised-plate urethroplasty (Snodgrass) in primary distal hypospadias. *BJU Int* 2000;85:725.

11 Holland AJ, Smith GH. Effect of the depth and width of the urethral plate on tubularized incised plate urethroplasty. *J Urol* 2000;164:489.

12 Dayanc M, Tan MO, Gokalp A *et al.* Tubularized incised plate urethroplasty for distal and mid-penile hypospadias. *Eur Urol* 2000;37:102.

13 Guralnick ML, al-Shammari A, Williot PE *et al.* Outcome of hypospadias repair using the tubularized, incised plate urethroplasty. *Can J Urol* 2000;7:986.

14 Borer JG, Bauer SB, Peters CA *et al.* Tubularized incised plate urethroplasty: expanded use in primary and repeat surgery for hypospadias. *J Urol* 2001;165:581.

15 Smith DP. A comprehensive analysis of a tubularized incised plate hypospadias repair. *Urology* 2001;57:778.

16 Cheng EY, Vemulapalli SN, Kropp BP *et al.* Snodgrass hypospadias repair with vascularized dartos flap: the perfect repair for virgin cases of hypospadias? *J Urol* 2002; 168:1723.

17 El-Sherbiny, MT. Tubularized incised plate repair of distal hypospadias in toilet-trained children: should a stent be left? *BJU Int* 2003;92:1003.

18 Jayanthi, VR. The modified Snodgrass hypospadias repair: reducing the risk of fistula and meatal stenosis. *J Urol* 2003; 170:1603.

19 Samuel M, Wilcox DT. Tubularized incised-plate urethroplasty for distal and proximal hypospadias. *BJU Int* 2003;92:783.

20 Leclair MD, Camby C, Battisti S *et al.* Unstented tubularized incised plate urethroplasty combined with foreskin reconstruction for distal hypospadias. *Eur Urol* 2004;46:526.

21 Elicevik M, Tireli G, Sander S. Tubularized incised plate urethroplasty: 5 years' experience. *Eur Urol* 2004;46:655.

22 Lorenz C, Schmedding A, Leutner A *et al.* Prolonged stenting does not prevent obstruction after TIP repair when the glans was deeply incised. *Eur J Pediatr Surg* 2004;14:322.

23 Elder JS, Duckett JW, Snyder HM. Onlay island flap in the repair of mid and distal penile hypospadias without chordee. *J Urol* 1987;138:376–9.

24 Baskin LS, Duckett JW, Ueoka K *et al.* Changing concepts of hypospadias curvature lead to more onlay island flap procedures. *J Urol* 1994;151:191–6.

25 Snodgrass W, Koyle M, Manzoni G *et al.* Tubularized incised plate hypospadias repair for proximal hypospadias. *J Urol* 1998;159:2129.

26 Chen SC, Yang SS, Hsieh CH *et al.* Tubularized incised plate urethroplasty for proximal hypospadias. *BJU Int* 2000; 86:1050.

27 Snodgrass WT, Lorenzo A. Tubularized incised-plate urethroplasty for hypospadias reoperation. *BJU Int* 2002; 89:98.

28 Mustafa M. The concept of tubularized incised plate hypospadias repair for different types of hypospadias. *Int Urol Nephrol* 2005;37:89.

29 Mollard P, Mouriquand P, Felfela T. Application of the onlay island flap urethroplasty to penile hypospadias with severe chordee. *Br J Urol* 1991;68:317.

30. Barroso U, Jr, Jednak R, Spencer Barthold J *et al.* Further experience with the double onlay preputial flap for hypospadias repair. *J Urol* 2000;164:998.

31 Samuel M, Capps S, Worth A. Proximal hypospadias. Comparative evaluation of staged urethroplasty (modified Thiersch Duplay followed by Mathieu) and single stage on-lay island flap repair. *Eur Urol* 2001;40:463.

32 Chuang JH, Shieh CS. Two-layer versus one-layer closure in transverse island flap repair of posterior hypospadias. *J Pediatr Surg* 1995;30:739.

33 Ghali AM. Hypospadias repair by skin flaps: a comparison of onlay preputial island flaps with either Mathieu's meatal-based or Duckett's tubularized preputial flaps. *BJU Int* 1999; 83:1032.

34 MacGillivray D, Shankar KR, Rickwood AM. Management of severe hypospadias using Glassberg's modification of the Duckett repair. *BJU Int* 2002;89:101.

35 Patel RP, Shukla AR, Austin JC *et al.* Modified tubularized transverse preputial island flap repair for severe proximal hypospadias. *BJU Int* 2005;95:901.

36 Retik AB, Bauer SB, Mandell J *et al.* Management of severe hypospadias with a 2-stage repair. *J Urol* 1994;152:749–51.

37 Greenfield SP, Sadler BT, Wan J. Two-stage repair for severe hypospadias. *J Urol* 1994;152:498–501.

38 Hammouda HM, El-Ghoneimi A, Bagli DJ *et al.* Tubularized incised plate repair: Functional outcome after intermediate followup. *J Urol* 2003;169:331–3,discussion 333.

39 Geltzeiler J, Belman AB. Results of closure of urethrocutaneous fistulas in children. *J Urol* 1984;132:734–6.

40 Teague JL, Roth DR, Gonzales ET. Repair of hypospadias complications using the meatal based flap urethroplasty. *J Urol* 1994;151:470–2.

41 Duel BP, Barthold JS, Gonzalez R. Management of urethral strictures after hypospadias repair. *J Urol* 1998;160:170–1.

42 Husmann DA, Rathbun SR. Long-term followup of visual internal urethrotomy for management of short (less than 1 cm) penile urethral strictures following hypospadias repair. *J Urol* 2006;176:1738–41.

43 Jayanthi VR, McLorie GA, Khoury AE *et al*. Can previously relocated penile skin be successfully used for salvage hypospadias repair? *J Urol* 1994;152:740–3,discussion 743.

44 Nguyen MT, Snodgrass WT. Tubularized incised plate hypospadias reoperation. *J Urol* 2004;171:2404–6,discussion 2406.

45. Shanberg AM, Sanderson K, Duel B. Re-operative hypospadias repair using the Snodgrass incised plate urethroplasty. *BJU Int* 2001;87:544.

46 Yang SS, Chen SC, Hsieh CH *et al*. Reoperative Snodgrass procedure. *J Urol* 2001;166:2342.

47 Shelton TB, Noe HN. The role of excretory urography in patients with hypospadias. *J Urol* 1985;134:97–9.

48 Snodgrass W, Elmore J. Initial experience with staged buccal graft (Bracka) hypospadias reoperations. *J Urol* 2004;172:1720–4,discussion 1724.

49 Snodgrass W. Does tubularized incised plate hypospadias repair create neourethral strictures? *J Urol* 1999;162:1159–61.

50 Gurdal M, Tekin A, Kirecci S *et al*. Intermediate-term functional and cosmetic results of the Snodgrass procedure in distal and midpenile hypospadias. *Pediatr Surg Int* 2004;20:197–9.

51 Lam PN, Greenfield SP, Williot P. 2-stage repair in infancy for severe hypospadias with chordee: Long-term results after puberty. *J Urol* 2005;174:1567–72,discussion 1572.

52 Mureau MA, Slijper FM, van der Meulen JC *et al*. Psychosexual adjustment of men who underwent hypospadias repair: A norm-related study. *J Urol* 1995;154:1351–5.

53 Ziada A, Snodgrass W. Patient and surgeon evaluation of outcome in hypospadias repair. *J Pedi Urol*, in press.

Phalloplasty for the Biological Male

Piet Hoebeke, Nicolaas Lumen and Stan Monstrey

Key points

- Congenital absence or loss of the penis is a devastating condition.
- Gender reassignment is no longer an option for this condition.
- Phalloplasty is the gold standard treatment for this condition.
- Maximal conservation of any penile tissue and incorporation in the phallus must be considered.
- Phalloplasty must be performed by experienced surgeons.
- Complication rate of phalloplasty is high.
- Erectile implants after phalloplasty are feasible.

The biological male without a penis or with an insufficient penis remains a major challenge. Failure of penile development, trauma, medically indicated penile amputations, and failed reconstructions of congenital anomalies are the main reasons for penile insufficiency (Table 27.1). Severe penile insufficiency and absence of a penis are devastating conditions for men with significant psychological and physical impact. Although uncommon, it is a challenging condition to treat.

Possible treatment options are gender reassignment, tailoring of the penile stump, penile reattachment, phallic reconstruction (phalloplasty), and most recently penile transplantation (Table 27.2). In the past, sex reassignment to the female gender had been offered based on the principles applied to newborns with disorders of sexual differentiation and ambiguous genitalia. There is no evidence to demonstrate that the outcome of this policy is satisfactory. Indeed, long-term evaluation of a few patients shows contradictory results, which have triggered great controversy of this therapy [1]. The issue of gender reassignment is beyond the scope of this chapter. However, some recent reports have alerted physicians to the high incidence of gender identity disorder in

Table 27.1 Conditions leading to severe penile insufficiency.

Congenital conditions (disorders of sexual development)
• Aphallia or penile agenesis
• Ideopathic micropenis
• 46 XY DSD
• Exstrophy
• Cloacal exstrophy
Genital trauma
• Injuries
• Surgery
Penile amputation

Table 27.2 Treatment options for severe penile inadequacy.

• Endocrinological treatment
• Penile reconstruction
• Penile replacement (phalloplasty)
• Gender reassignment
• "Penile transplantation"
• "Tissue engineering"

Pediatric Urology: Surgical Complications and Management. Edited by Duncan T. Wilcox, Prasad P. Godbole and Martin A. Koyle. © 2008 Blackwell Publishing, ISBN: 978-1-4051-6268-5.

gender reassigned children. Especially in cloacal exstrophy, the results have been disappointing [2,3]. Today sex reassignment is no longer considered treatment of choice.

Tailoring of the penile stump by means of penile degloving, division of the suspensory ligament, and rotational skin flaps has been reported [4,5]. However, this can only by applied to moderate penile injuries where there is still a reasonable penile stump. Penile reattachment can be attempted in the acute phase following traumatic amputation of the penis. The survival of the reattached penis depends on the viability of the amputated segment and the condition of the graft bed or penile stump. Reattachment must take place within 24-h. Current reattachment techniques rely on microsurgical approximation of the dorsal structures and cavernosal arteries with uniformly good results. In traumatic amputation, salvage of the amputated segment with reattachment is the primary treatment option [6]. The outcome of erectile function after reattachment is, however, not clear. Recently, a single unsuccessful case report has been published on penile transplantation [7]. This technique is still experimental and is not a current treatment option. Future options like tissue engineering are until today not in science but rather in science fiction.

Phallic reconstruction is another treatment option. The first phallic reconstruction was described by Bogoras in 1936 with a tubed abdominal flap [8]. Phalloplasty procedures have followed the evolution and advances made in plastic surgery. Originally, it was a complex, time-consuming, multistage procedure using tubed skin flaps or pedicled myocutaneous flaps with variable and suboptimal results [9–11].

In 1984, Chang completed the first successful microsurgical phalloplasty with a radial forearm free flap [12]. Since then the radial forearm flap has been widely accepted as the best donor site for penile reconstruction and is nowadays the gold standard in penile replacement for female-to-male transsexuals [13–15]. This technique can also be applied to boys without an adequate penis. Defining penile insufficiency is difficult. To base the definition of inadequacy on length and appearance alone is impossible especially in infants and young children. Penile inadequacy is an individual diagnosis that can only be made after puberty when sexual development is completed and the patient is sexually active. Puberty can change the final outcome of penile length and girth substantially. The number of children diagnosed with micropenis persisting into adulthood is limited [16].

As for penile reconstruction, many techniques have been described for penile augmentation. However,

the results of most of these surgeries are very limited, Indeed, the reported outcome is often poor [17].

In this chapter, we will focus on the phalloplasty. It is considered the gold standard for penile absence or severe penile inadequacy, when endocrinological therapy is not beneficial.

Phalloplasty

Surgical reconstruction of the penis (phalloplasty) is difficult because of the different cosmetic and functional requirements of the patients:

1 The reconstructed penis should be aesthetically acceptable, it must be as normal as possible in appearance (minimal scar, glandular reconstruction, etc.).

2 The penile shaft must contain a urethra that extends to the distal tip and must permit the patient to void in a standing position unless there is a concomitant condition that makes normal voiding impossible.

3 The penile shaft should allow the implantation of a penile stiffener in order to regain the possibility of sexual intercourse. Therefore, protective and erogenous sensation is needed.

4 The donor area should cause minimal morbidity with an acceptable scar that is easy to conceal.

Many of these objectives could not be obtained with the older methods in which phallic reconstruction required a complex multistaged procedures. Nowadays, microvascular free flap techniques come closer to achieving these objectives. Despite the multitude of free flaps that have been published (frequently as a case report), the radial forearm free flap is universally considered the gold standard in penile reconstruction [13–15,18].

Surgical technique

At the Ghent University Hospital, more than 300 consecutive patients have undergone phallic reconstruction using a radial forearm flap. This experience is mainly in female to male transsexuals. We describe our current technique as well as the different changes and refinements made like we use it in the reconstruction for the biological male in this radial forearm phalloplasty procedure.

Depending on the underlying condition we try to preserve any useful penile and cavernosal tissue. The urethral stump if available is prepared for connection with the phallic urethra and if available a dorsal penile nerve is identified. A free vascularized flap of the forearm and the creation of a phallus with a tube-in-a-tube technique is performed with the flap still attached to the

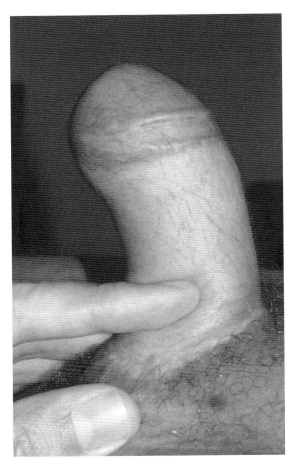

Figure 27.1 End result with glandular reconstruction and tattooing of the glans.

forearm by its vascular pedicle. A small skin flap and skin graft are used to create a corona and imitate the glans of the penis (Figure 27.1).

The free flap is then transferred to the pubic area where first the urethral anastomosis is performed. The radial artery is then microsurgically connected to the common femoral artery in an end-to-side fashion usually with an interpositional vein graft taken at the ankle. The venous anastomosis is performed between the cephalic vein and the greater saphenous vein. One forearm nerve is connected to the ilioinguinal nerve for protective sensation, and the other nerve is anastomosed to one of the dorsal penile nerves for erogenous sensation. All patients receive a suprapubic urinary diversion postoperatively.

The defect on the forearm was covered in the first 50 patients with full-thickness skin grafts taken from the groin area and in the later patients with split-thickness skin grafts harvested from the medial and anterior thigh.

The patients remain in bed for 1 week after which the transurethral catheter is removed. Three to five days later the suprapubic catheter is clamped and voiding is started. It sometimes takes more days before good voiding is observed. The average admission period for the phalloplasty procedure is approximately 2.5 weeks.

Tattooing of the glans can be performed after a 2–3 month period, before sensation returns to the penis (Figure 27.1).

Sexual function

Sexual function and pleasure is one of the goals in phallic reconstruction. For this purpose in biological males, any sensitive penile tissue left must be incorporated. Any glans tissue present can be incorporated in the base of the neophallus. This is important for sexual stimulation and pleasure. Further erogenous and tactile sensation of the neophallus is obtained by microscopic anastomosis of respectively one dorsal phallic nerve and one ilioinguinal nerve to the cutaneous nerves of the flap [19].

Obtaining sufficient rigidity of the penis to allow penetration is extremely difficult because there is no good substitute for the unique erectile tissue of the penis. The radial forearm flap is too soft and can even demonstrate some atrophy of the subcutaneous fat with a loss of more than 20% of circumference. The use of bone or cartilage grafts has often resulted in complications and failure because of resorption, curving, or fracture [20,21]. For sexual penetration, a penile stiffener is needed, and fortunately, the radial forearm flap has a sufficient subcutaneous bulk to permit incorporation of a penile prosthesis. Incorporation of a penile stiffener can only be done after the phallus is endowed with sufficient protective sensation, which usually takes at least 12 months. Good protective sensation is critical in preventing breakdown and erosion of an internal stiffener [22,23]. Next to sensitivity urethral function also has to be considered. Implantation of a penile prosthesis must be withheld until the urethra is stable, and the patient is free of voiding symptoms and urinary tract infection [22].

Unfortunately, high erosion rates (20–50%) are reported [13,22]. One of the reasons could be the less vascularized skin and subcutaneous tissue of the neophallus (in comparison with a native impotent penis), which can lead to chronic ischemia after implantation of a stiffener and subsequently diminished resistance against infection and perforation.

Despite the complications and difficulties, the satisfaction rate after phalloplasty is high and the results cosmetically pleasing (Figure 27.2). None of our patients regret the surgery. An important boost concerning the

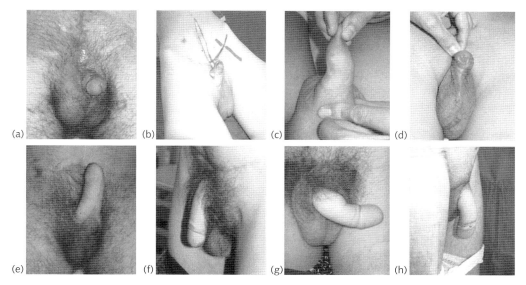

Figure 27.2 Results of phalloplasties in biological males. Cripple exstrophy (a, b), epitheloied sarcoma of penis (c), cripple hypospadias with absence of corpora (d). (a)–(d) Before surgery; (e)–(h) after surgery.

self-esteem level is observed in each patient, which is a very important outcome factor postoperatively.

Complications

Despite the good outcomes described with phalloplasty, this is associated with a high complication rate. Most complications are related to the urethral reconstruction. [13,24,25]. The main complications are fistulae and stenoses whenever the urinary tract is attached to the native urethra. Despite the high prevalence of these complications, the literature on treatment of these complications is sparse. Consequently always consider whether the urethral reconstruction is necessary, as some boys will not need urethral reconstruction as the bladder is augmented and diverted. In addition it is important to consider the ejaculation of the patient.

Is he actually ejaculating? Where? If so, do we want to reconstruct the urethra for ejaculation alone, or do we want to keep the ejaculation where it is? Preference should be given to keep the ejaculation where it is as reconstructing a urethra just for ejaculation can result in higher complications and possible anejaculation due to the length of the urethra and the weakness of the ejaculation due to the underlying condition.

Urethral fistulas

Remove all scar tissue and try to bring well vascularized tissue to the area that needs reconstruction. In radial forearm flap phalloplasty, we have to consider that the tissue of the urethra is skin and not mucosa. Larger stitches with cutting needles should be used. The duration of bladder drainage is unknown but in our practice we prefer to drain for 12 days. When using local skin flaps consider possible future hair growth in the urethra. A good alternative is the use of buccal mucosa [26].

Urethral stenosis

In our experience we first attempt an endoscopic incision of the stenosis, if the stricture is relatively short. We leave a catheter for 12 days, which is much longer than after urethrotomy for urethral stenosis in normal urethras. We have to remember that part of the urethra is composed of skin and healing of skin lesions is much slower than mucosal healing.

If endoscopic incision fails, we perform a formal urethroplasty. End-to-end anastomosis or Heineke-Mikulicz type reconstructions with longitudinal incision over the stenotic area closed transversally. For longer strictures or complex and repetitive stricture, two-stage urethroplasty (Johansson) must be considered. The stenotic area is longitudinally incised and the borders of the stricture are sutured to the surrounding healthy skin. The urethra remains opened until the skin and urethra are well healed, which usually takes a minimum of 3 months. During the second stage of the urethroplasty, the urethra is closed again and covered with skin.

Experience with phalloplasty in biological males

There are only a few series published on this topic. Perovic reported phalloplasty in 24 patients without a functional penis using the extended pedicle island groin flap. He suggests this technique as an available alternative to the microsurgical free tissue phalloplasty [27].

Sengezer *et al.* suggested total penile reconstruction with sensate osteocutaneous free fibula flap. With this technique, promising results were obtained in 18 patients without a functional penis for different reasons [28]. Gilbert *et al.* were the first to describe the application of a radial free forearm flap for phallic reconstruction in 11 boys without a functional penis. Satisfactory results were obtained [29].

We performed phalloplasty in eight males with the use of the radial forearm flap. Two boys with inadequate penis after exstrophy repair, one boy with penile loss after multiple hypospadias repair, one boy with Partial Androgen Insensitivity Syndrome (PAIS) and micropenis, one boy with a penile epithelioid sarcoma, and two men who traumatically lost their penis. There were no complications concerning the flap. Two complications were reported in the early postoperative period: one pulmonary embolism and one severe hematuria. Two patients developed urinary complications (stricture and/or fistula) for which a secondary procedure was necessary.

Patient satisfaction after surgery was high in seven cases and moderate in one case. Psychological evaluation confirms this, especially on the self-esteem level. Four patients underwent erectile implant surgery. In two patients, the erectile implant had to be removed because of infection (unpublished data).

In our series one adolescent patient presenting with epithelioid sarcoma of the penis, the phalloplasty was performed in a one-stage procedure with the penectomy. [30]. This could be an option for some patients undergoing penile amputation if oncologically acceptable.

The reported success of phalloplasty in boys without a functional penis has convinced us that penile reconstruction is the optimal treatment for this condition. It has extremely good results and improves self-esteem and their physical and psychological well-being. But the complication rate of the erectile implants is high.

Phalloplasty opens new horizons for the treatment of penile agenesis, micropenis, crippled penis, shrivelled penis, some disorders of sexual development (DSD) conditions, traumatic amputations in which the amputated segment is lost for replantation, iatrogenic amputations, and cloacal exstrophy.

References

1 Woodhouse CR. Sexual function in boys born with exstrophy, myelomeningocele, and micropenis. *Urology* 1998;52:3–11.
2 Reiner WG, Gearhart JP. Discordant sexual identity in some genetic males with cloacal exstrophy assigned to female sex at birth. *N Engl J Med* 2004;350:333–41.
3 Mayer-Bahlburg HF. Gender identity outcome in female-raised 46, XY persons with penile agenesis, cloacal exstrophy of the bladder, or penile ablation. *Arch Sex Behav* 2005;34:423–38.
4 Ochoa B. Trauma of the external genitalia in children: Amputation of the penis and emasculation. *J Urol* 1998;160:1116–19.
5 Amukele SA, Gene WL, Stock JA, Hanna MK. 20-Year experience with iatrogenic penile injury. *J Urol* 2003;170:1691–4.
6 Jezior JR, Brady JD, Schlossberg SM. Management of penile amputation injuries. *World J Surg* 2001;25:1602–9.
7 Hu W, Lu J, Zhang L, Wu W, Nie H, Zhu Y *et al.* A preliminary report of penile transplantation. *Eur Urol* 2006;50:851–3.
8 Bogoras NA. Uber die volle plastische wiederherstellung eines zum koitus fahigen penis (Penisplastica totalis). *Zentralbl Chir* 1936;22:1271.
9 Hoopes JE. Surgical reconstruction of the male external genitalia. *Clin Plast Surg* 1974;1:325.
10 Orticochea M. A new method of total reconstruction of the penis. *Br J Plast Surg* 1972;25:347.
11 Puckett CL, Montie JE. Construction of male genitalia in the transsexual, using a tube groin flap for the penis and a hydraulic inflation device. *Plast Reconstr Surg* 1978;61:523–30.
12 Chang TS, Hwang WY. Forearm flap in one stage reconstruction of the penis. *Plast Reconstr Surg* 1984;75:251.
13 Monstrey S, Hoebeke P, Dhont M, Selvaggi G, Hamdi M, Van Landuyt K *et al.* Radial forearm phalloplasty: A review of 81 cases. *Eur J Plast Surg* 2005;28:206–12.
14 Gilbert DA, Horton CE, Terzis JK, Devine CJ, Winslow BH, Devine PC. New concept in phallic reconstruction. *Ann Plast Surg* 1987;18:128.
15 Hage JJ, Bloem JJ, Suliman HM. Review of the literature on techniques for phalloplasty with emphasis on the applicability in female-to-male transsexuals. *J Urol* 1993;150:1093–8.
16 Lee PA, Houk CP. Outcome studies among men with micropenis. *J Pediatr Endocrinol Metab* 2004;17:1043–53.
17 Li CY, Kayes O, Kell PD, Christopher N, Minhas S, Ralph DJ. Penile suspensory ligament division for penile augmentation: Indications and results. *Eur Urol* 2006; 49:729–33.
18 Gottlieb LJ, Levine LA. A new design for the radial forearm free-flap phallic reconstruction. *Plast Reconstr Surg* 1993;92:276–84.
19 De Cuypere G, T'Sjoen G, Beerten R, Selvaggi G, De Sutter P, Hoebeke P *et al.* Sexual and physical health after sex reassignment surgery. *Arch Sex Behav* 2005;34:679–90.
20 Ali M. Surgical treatment of the male genitalia with special reference to the use of periosteal bone graft in constructing the penis. *J Int Coll Surg* 1957;27:352.

21 Khouri RK, Young VL, Casoli VM. Long-term results of total penile reconstruction with a prefabricated lateral arm free flap. *J Urol* 1998;160:383–8.

22 Jordan GH, Alter GJ, Gilbert DA, Horton CE, Devine CJ. Penile prosthesis implantation in total phalloplasty. *J Urol* 1994;152:410–14.

23 Hoebeke P, Decuypere G, Ceulemans P, Monstrey S. Obtaining rigidity in total phalloplasty: Experience with 35 patients. *J Urol* 2003;169:221–3.

24 Hage JJ, Bloem JJ. Review of the literature on construction of a neourethra in female-to-male transsexuals. *Ann Plast Surg* 1993;30:278–86.

25 Hoebeke P, Selvaggi G, Ceulemans P, De Cuypere G, T'Sjoen G, Weyers S *et al.* Impact of sex reassignment surgery on lower urinary tract function. *Eur Urol* 2005;47:398–402.

26 Rohrmann D, Jakse G. Urethroplasty in female-to-male transsexuals. *Eur Urol* 2003;44:611–4.

27 Perovic S. Phalloplasty in children and adolescents using the extended pedicle island groin flap. *J Urol* 1995;154:848–53.

28 Sengezer M, Öztürk S, Deveci M, Odabaçi Z. Long-term follow-up of total penile reconstruction with sensate osteocutaneous free fibula flap in 18 biological male patients. *Plast Reconstr Surg* 2004;114:439–50.

29 Gilbert DA, Jordan GH, Devine CJ, Winslow BH, Schlossberg SM. Phallic construction in prepubertal and adolescent boys. *J Urol* 1993;149:1521–6.

30 Hoebeke PB, Rottey S, Van Heddeghem N, Villeirs G, Pauwels P, Schrauwen W *et al.* One-stage penectomy and phalloplasty for epithelioid sarcoma of the penis in an adolescent. *Eur Urol* 2006; 51 (5): 1429–32.

28 Female Genital Reconstruction I

Sarah M. Creighton

Key points

- The success of genital reconstructive surgery in sexual function and reproduction may not be tested until many years after the initial surgical procedure.

- Long-term complications of genital reconstructive surgery are common and the most frequent complication is vaginal stenosis.

- Assessment of the long-term complications of genital surgery must include sexual function evaluation.

- The vagina has no role in the prepubertal girl and vaginal surgery can safely be deferred until puberty if a uterus is present and later still if a uterus is not present.

- Revision surgery for vaginal stenosis is necessary in the majority of those undergoing vaginoplasty in early childhood.

- Clitoral surgery damages sexual sensation and has a negative impact on sexual function.

Introduction

Female genital reconstruction is a highly controversial and emotive topic. While short-term surgical complications of such procedures occur and are important to manage correctly, it is the long-term complications that have caused such concern and debate. Correlation of any particular surgical procedure to its later success or failure can be almost impossible. Complications of genital surgery such as vaginal stenosis may make intercourse painful or impossible, but the pediatric surgeon responsible for the initial vaginal reconstruction will never have the opportunity to follow patients into adult life when such complications become apparent. The success of genital reconstruction in sexual function and reproduction is often not tested until many years after the procedure. Surgeons and procedures change and adult patients may have had operations that have long been modified or abandoned in favor of something else. In addition, the contribution of genital reconstructive surgery to gender identity or psychological well-being is poorly understood and even more difficult to quantify.

Despite these difficulties, researchers around the world are striving to provide long-term outcome data. If surgery continues to be an option for families and patients, it is essential that clinicians working with families are aware of what information is currently available and also the limitations and uncertainties of these data.

Types of surgery

Reconstructive genital surgery is most commonly performed in the following two situations:
- To create a neovagina in conditions where the genitalia are female and the uterus and vagina are absent, i.e. Rokitansky Syndrome, Complete Androgen Insensitivity Syndrome (CAIS).
- To feminize the genitalia when a child with ambiguous genitalia is assigned to a female sex of rearing. A uterus may be present such as in congenital adrenal hyperplasia (CAH) or may be absent such as in 46XY disorders of sex development (DSD).

Pediatric Urology: Surgical Complications and Management. Edited by Duncan T. Wilcox, Prasad P. Godbole and Martin A. Koyle. © 2008 Blackwell Publishing, ISBN: 978-1-4051-6268-5.

Creation of a neovagina

Congenital vaginal agenesis can be seen in women with Rokitansky Syndrome and Androgen Insensitivity Syndrome (AIS). Presentation with these two conditions can be at any time throughout childhood but if the external genitalia are normal, then presentation at puberty is commonest. Congenital vaginal absence can also be part of complex genital anomalies affecting the lower urinary and intestinal tract such as anorectal and cloacal anomalies [1].

Timing of vaginoplasty

The vagina has no function in the prepubertal girl. If a uterus is present, then a passageway for menstruation is required at puberty. If the uterus is absent, then the vagina is not required until sexual activity is planned. If presentation is at adolescence with primary amenorrhea, then the timing of any vaginal reconstruction is uncontroversial. The procedure can be discussed with the patient and planned to fit in with need for intercourse and academic and/or work commitments. Nonsurgical alternative treatments such as vaginal dilation can be offered and may make surgery unnecessary.

However, if the diagnosis of vaginal agenesis is made at birth or during childhood, the situation is more controversial. In the past, creation of a neovagina was often recommended during early childhood. Progressive passive vaginal dilation is not appropriate for children, which left surgery as the only option. Intestinal vaginoplasty has been used most commonly in this group. However, short- and long-term complications of this procedure are not uncommon and include persistent vaginal discharge, bleeding, and colitis. While these complications may perhaps be acceptable and manageable in an adult woman for whom surgery has facilitated a normal sex life, these complications are wholly unacceptable in a prepubertal child for whom the vagina has no current function. In addition, the need for repeat reconstructive surgery at adolescence has also been demonstrated whatever method of vaginal construction is used [2].

In the neonate with associated complex urinary and gastrointestinal anomalies, vaginal reconstruction is usually performed at the primary reconstructive procedure. The rationale for this is that there may be only one opportunity to access the pelvis, as surgery will be highly complex and re-entry to the abdomen at a later stage hazardous. Although this sounds logical, the few studies on this group of patients have shown that despite early vaginoplasty, obstructed menstruation is common and repeat vaginoplasty often required [3]. Consideration should be given to following the same principles in this group of girls and deferring surgery until puberty in the presence of a uterus or until sexual activity if the uterus is absent.

Assessment of outcome

The long assessment of vaginoplasty outcomes can be difficult. Complications of the procedure such as vaginal stenosis or persistent vaginal discharge may be troublesome many years after the primary procedure. Patients' satisfaction will be influenced not only by the procedure but also by the clinical and psychological implications of their underlying condition as well as other treatments such as hormonal or steroid therapy. Other factors such as infertility will in most cases cause additional distress.

When assessing outcomes of pediatric vaginal reconstruction it is important to remember that the major aim of surgery is to allow the adult patient to have comfortable and pleasurable sexual intercourse. Anatomical success as quantified by a surgeon does not guarantee success in sexual function. Motivation for reconstruction is often based on aspirations for normality not just in sexual anatomy but behavior and experiences [4]. Female sexual function and dysfunction is based not only on biological but on psychosocial components as well. Long-term assessment of vaginal reconstruction must include such information; otherwise the whole point of surgery is missed and the data meaningless. Other outcome measures include a passageway for menstruation and tampon use. Although these outcomes should be easier to assess, there is still little data. Some authors have graded the outcome as "excellent" if the vagina was thought to be suitable for intercourse, and "satisfactory" if the vagina permitted menstrual flow but did not allow intercourse [5]. This may appear logical but women may not perceive being unable to have penetrative intercourse as a satisfactory outcome of vaginoplasty.

Techniques for creation of a neovagina

Vaginal dilation

Nonsurgical vaginal dilation for vaginal agenesis was first reported by Frank in 1938, who described the use of vaginal molds of increasing width and length to successfully create a neovagina suitable for intercourse [6]. Since that time vaginal dilation has become accepted as first line treatment in women with an absent vagina and no previous genital surgery. The avoidance of surgical and anesthetic complications makes this ostensibly a low-risk choice. However, even this treatment modality cannot be considered complication free. Dilators are time consuming and may be distasteful to women [7]. Dilation therapy can be painful and acts as a constant reminder of abnormality. The commitment from the patient is considerable and nursing and psychological support essential. It is important that dilators receive the same evaluation as any other surgical technique to reconstruct the vagina. Anatomical enlargement of the vagina must be correlated with sexual function assessment. Success rates of 80–90% efficacy have been reported but the majority of these studies are retrospective studies and do not assess sexual function [8,9].

Vaginal dilation can only be performed in adolescent and adult women and is not appropriate for children. The option of deferring vaginal reconstruction until the patient is old enough to comply with dilation should be discussed with parents, especially in conditions such as Rokitansky Syndrome and CAIS where dilators work very well.

Surgical options for vaginal creation

Intestinal vaginoplasty

Intestinal vaginoplasty lines the neovagina with a segment of bowel keeping the vascular pedicle intact. The procedure is usually performed via a laparotomy although the laparoscopic approach has been reported [10]. The main advantage of this procedure is the low risk of vaginal stenosis and the avoidance of postoperative vaginal dilatation. Dilation is occasionally required at the perineal anastomosis but the vaginal canal itself should retain its original size. Other advantages include adequate vaginal length and natural lubrication.

Long-term complications are, however, common. Persistent mucous discharge is almost inevitable. This can be foul smelling and lead to problems with self-esteem and confidence. In some cases this will respond to treatment by vaginal irrigation using short-chain fatty acids and steroid enemas. A significant number of women will need to douche regularly and always wear a pad [11]. Symptomatic diversion colitis has been reported postoperatively and can lead to heavy vaginal discharge with bleeding [12]. In some cases removal of the

intestinal vagina is the only solution. Unsightly prolapse of the mucosa and a stoma-like perineal appearance can be upsetting to the patient and in rare cases complete prolapse of the sigmoid neovagina can occur.

There are several case reports in the literature of adenocarcinoma affecting the intestinal vagina, with a reported time to development of carcinoma anywhere from 7 to 50 years after the initial procedure [13,14]. Although these complications are uncommon, treatment is difficult and can lead to removal of the entire neovagina.

Satisfactory sexual function outcomes have been reported in women with intestinal vaginoplasty [11]. However, these results should be balanced against the risks of major surgery with high associated morbidity and persistent symptoms. In many cases – especially in the absence of prior genital surgery – women will achieve satisfactory sexual function with less invasive techniques such as dilation. Intestinal vaginoplasty should be reserved for those women who have failed previous vaginal reconstruction or have other associated complex bowel and urinary anomalies, where dilation and less invasive procedures are not possible. It should not be used as a first line treatment for vaginal agenesis.

When an intestinal vaginoplasty is the only option, surgery should where possible be deferred until adulthood. This means that potential problems of vaginal discharge and bleeding do not trouble the patient during childhood. In addition the risks of malignancy are deferred and adult women are more able to comply with the extra vaginal examinations required for surveillance of an intestinal vagina.

McIndoe–Reed procedure

The McIndoe (Abbe–McIndoe–Reed) technique is still commonly performed throughout the world, as it does not require abdominal surgery and is of a relatively low initial morbidity. A potential neovaginal space is created between the rectum and the bladder. A split-thickness skin graft is then taken from the thigh, buttock, or abdomen and is mounted on a mold and left in the neovaginal space for 7 days. The graft will then epithelize lining the neovaginal space.

Immediate morbidity is low although complications such as urethral and rectal fistulae have been reported, especially with older, firmer vaginal molds. One troublesome complication of the McIndoe technique is the formation of visible scars at the origin of the skin graft site and this may be unacceptable to some young women.

Overall the main long-term complication of this procedure is vaginal stenosis, which has been reported in up to 50% of women [15]. Stenosis can lead to painful intercourse or no intercourse at all, and it is imperative that the patient maintains her neovagina postoperatively by regular sexual intercourse or dilator use. Repeat surgery after a failed McIndoe–Reed procedure is difficult as the use of an intestinal segment can be hampered by excess scarring. Satisfactory long-term results have been reported for the McIndoe operation with up to 100% sexually active after the procedure [16]. There is, however, scanty information in the literature on sexual function or sexual pleasure in this group. As with intestinal vaginoplasty, there have been several case reports of carcinoma developing in the neovagina – in this situation a squamous cell carcinoma [17]. Prolonged postoperative follow-up is necessary with regular vaginal examination and prompt attention to any unusual onset of bleeding or discharge.

The risks of stenosis, need for dilation, and potential malignancy risk make this procedure also unsuitable for children, and surgery should be deferred until late adolescent or adulthood. With the increasing use of dilators and the advent of laparoscopic procedures such as the Vecchietti and Davydov procedures, it is probably that the McIndoe–Reed procedure will become less popular.

Laparoscopic Vechietti and Davydov procedures

The Vecchietti procedure allows creation of a neovagina by passive traction rather than dilation [18]. An acrylic "olive" with attached tension threads is placed at the vaginal dimple. The threads are passed under laparoscopic control from the vaginal dimple through the abdominal cavity and then to a traction device on the abdominal wall. The tension threads are tightened daily to stretch the vagina. This procedure requires elasticity of the vaginal skin and is not suitable for women with vaginal scarring from previous genital reconstruction. The Davydov procedure is also performed laparoscopically [19]. A perineal incision is made first to create a neovaginal space. Then peritoneum from the pelvic sidewalls and the Pouch of Douglas is freed and directed down toward the vaginal incision to line the sidewalls of the vagina. The top of the vagina is created by suturing a vaginal "roof" of large bowel and peritoneum. This procedure is more suitable for those women with previous vaginal scarring, as the vaginal skin is not required to stretch.

The short-term morbidity of these procedures is low although ureteric damage can occur [19]. Good short-term anatomical and functional results have been reported [18,19]. Long-term results for complications and ongoing sexual success are not available. It is probably that these laparoscopic procedures will become more widely used in future as an alternative to both intestinal and skin graft neovaginal creation.

Feminizing genital surgery for ambiguous genitalia

Background

In most children with ambiguous genitalia assigned female, feminizing clitoral and vaginal surgery is carried out as a "one-stage" procedure at 6–8 months of age. The aims of surgery are to achieve a pleasing feminine appearance, to allow menstruation if a uterus is present, to preserve sensation and permit normal sexual function, to promote normal psychosocial and psychosexual development, and to prevent urological sequelae. Whether or not these aims have been achieved is usually not apparent until the individual has reached adulthood.

As for vaginal reconstruction discussed above, immediate complications of feminizing genitoplasty need prompt and appropriate attention. However, it is the long-term complications that will impact upon the success of the procedure. Long-term complications may be easy to identify such as a poor cosmetic appearance or vaginal stenosis. They may also be more difficult to assess such as sexual dysfunction and poor psychosexual and psychosocial well-being.

Complications
Cosmetic appearance

The cosmetic appearance after genital surgery is variable, but up to 40% of women are reported to have an unsatisfactory genital appearance [20]. While immediate cosmetic outcomes may be good, the postpubertal appearance may be very different. Significant scarring and pubertal change may lead to irregular and lop-sided external genitalia. Poor steroid control in CAH may contribute to clitoral regrowth and hypertrophy.

Urinary complications

The anatomical changes present in those born with ambiguous genitalia may lead to incomplete bladder emptying and pooling of urine in the common urogenital sinus. This may lead to reflux and subsequent urinary tract infections as well as postmicturition dribbling. Pediatric studies have reported persistent urinary symptoms including incontinence and reduced bladder capacity [21]. Studies looking at the long-term outcomes of adult CAH patients have shown incontinence as well as high levels of lower urinary tract symptoms with 70% of women complaining of troublesome lower urinary tract symptoms [22]. These studies, were all observational questionnaire studies and more definitive urodynamic evaluation would be helpful to establish what the role of surgery is in causing or preventing urinary dysfunction.

Vaginal stenosis

Vaginal stenosis is the commonest long-term complication occurring in over 90% of cases [23]. In many cases multiple repeat operations are performed during childhood and adolescence in an attempt to treat recurrent stenosis. Despite specialist care in centers of excellence, total reconstruction is rarely adequately achieved by a single procedure in childhood. Furthermore, repeated attempts at surgical correction limit subsequent successful reconstruction by resulting in excessive scar tissue. Repeat surgery is of course associated with higher levels of complications. Frequent vaginal stenosis leading to repeat surgical correction is associated with an increased level of anxiety regarding intercourse and up to one-third of women experiencing specific difficulties with orgasm [24]. Other complications of multiple repeat procedures include recurrent urinary tract infections and persistent malodorous vaginal discharge. Menstruation may be obstructed and lead to hematocolpos requiring formal drainage and yet more vaginal surgery [25]. Deferral of reconstructive vaginal surgery until adolescence would avoid these complications during childhood.

Sexual function

Sexual function is likely to be affected by both vaginal size and clitoral sensation. Vaginal stenosis leading to pain or the inability to have penetrative intercourse will of course lead to poor sexual satisfaction. The clitoris has only one role – to contribute to sexual pleasure – and yet there is increasing evidence of the detrimental effect of clitoral surgery on sexual sensation and satisfaction.

Until recently, sexual function outcome data following childhood feminizing genitoplasty procedures has been sparse, with details on the assessment process often limited. Increasing concern from adult women who have undergone feminizing surgery has led to a recent focus of research on sexual function. Questionnaire studies assessing women after feminizing surgery demonstrate high levels of sexual dysfunction in all women after surgery when compared to normal controls [26]. When compared to women with ambiguous genitalia who had not undergone clitoral surgery, 39% of participants demonstrated specific difficulties with sensation and orgasm [27]. Subsequent objective sensation testing for women with CAH who had undergone genitoplasty procedures in childhood has demonstrated significantly impaired sensation to the clitoris in all women following genital surgery, when compared with normal controls, and this correlates to poorer sexual satisfaction [28].

Psychological outcomes

Genital surgery is likely to have an impact on psychosexual development and functioning although there is scanty information on either positive or negative outcomes. An accepted aim of surgery is to improve psychological well-being and failure to do so could be considered a complication. There is some evidence that in those who have undergone genital surgery, social and sexual milestones are reached later than age-matched controls and that these women are less sexually experienced and have expressed a lower level of sexual interest than control groups [29]. However, the specific contribution of genital surgery to these problems is difficult to separate from other factors associated with the various conditions assessed.

Conclusion

The short- and long-term complications of childhood reconstructive surgery on the clitoral and vagina are well recognized and documented in the medical literature. Surgeons operating on the genitals of children have constantly refined their techniques over the years in an attempt to find procedures with lower complication rates and better outcomes. However, the nature of pediatric surgery means that any improvements will not be put to the test until many years later. There is at present no evidence that more modern techniques are less morbid or have a more positive contribution to make long-term outcomes. In addition, the constant focus on surgical techniques and interventions can mean that the psychosexual and psychosocial aspects become neglected.

The majority of women with vaginal agenesis and/or genital ambiguity will wish to have genital reconstruction prior to sexual activity. There is, however, little evidence to support any benefits of such surgery during childhood. Deferring reconstructive surgery until later in life means that unavoidable surgical complications – which can be significant – do not happen in childhood. Informed consent can be taken and complications may be better managed in an adolescent or adult woman who can weigh these up risks and balance them against her requirements for a functional vagina.

References

1 Davies MC, Creighton SM, Wilcox DT. Long term outcomes of anorectal malformations. *Pediatr Surg Int* 2004;29:567–72.

2 Davies MC, Creighton SM, Woodhouse CRJ. The pitfalls of vaginal construction. *BJUI* 2005;95:1293–8.

3 Warne SA, Wilcox DT, Creighton S, Ransley PG. Long-term gynecological outcome of patients with persistent cloaca. *J Urol* 2003;170:1493–6.

4 Boyle ME, Smith S, Liao LM. Adult genital surgery for intersex: A solution to what problem? *J Health Psychol* 2005;10:573–84.

5 Powell DM, Newman KD, Randolph J. A proposed classification of vaginal anomalies and their surgical correction. *J Pediatr Surg* 1995;30:271–5.

6 Frank RT. The formation of artificial vagina without operation. *Am J Obstet Gynecol* 1938;35:1053–5.

7 Liao L, Doyle J, Crouch NS, Creighton SM. Dilation as treatment for vaginal agenesis and hypoplasia: A pilot exploration of benefits and barriers as perceived by patients. *J Obstet Gynaecol* 2006;26:144–8.

8 Roberts CP, Haber MJ, Rock JA. Vaginal creation for mullerian agenesis. *Am J Obstet Gynecol* 2001;185:1349–52.

9 Rock JA, Reeves LA, Retto H, Baranki TA, Zacur HA, Jones HW, Jr. Success following vaginal creation for Mullerian agenesis. *Fertil Steril* 1983;39:809–13.

10 Darai E, Toullalan O, Besse O, Potiron L, Delga P. Anatomic and functional results of laparoscopic – perineal neovagina construction by sigmoid colpoplasty in women with Rokitansky's syndrome. *Hum Reprod* 2003;18:2454–9.

11 Hensle TW, Shabsigh A, Shabsigh R, Reilly EA, Meyer-Bahlburg HF. Sexual function following bowel vaginoplasty. *J Urol* 2006;175:2283–6.

12 Syed HA, Malone PS, Hitchcock RJ. Diversion colitis in children with colovaginoplasty. *BJU Int* 2001;87:857–60.

13 Hiroi H, Yasugi T, Matsumoto K, Fujii T, Watanabe T, Yoshikawa H, Taketani Y. Mucinous adenocarcinoma arising in a neovagina using the sigmoid colon thirty years after operation. *J Surg Onc* 2001;77:61–4.

14 Lawrence A. Vaginal neoplasia in a male-to-female transsexual: Case report, review of the literature and recommendations for cytologic screening. *Int J Transgenderism* 2001;5:1.

15 Cali RW, Pratt JH. Congenital absence of the vagina; long-term results of vaginal construction in 175 cases. *Am J Obstet Gynecol* 1968;100:752–63.

16 Roberts CP, Haber MJ, Rock JA. Vaginal creation for mullerian agenesis. *Am J Obstet Gynecol* 2001;185:1349–52.

17 Schult M, Hecker A, Lelle R, Senninger N, Winde G. Recurrent rectovaginal fistula caused by an incidental squamous cell carcinoma of the neovagina in Mayer-Rokitansky-Kuster-Hauser Syndrome. *Gynaecol Oncol* 2000;77:210–12.

18 Fedele L, Bianchi S, Zanconato G, Raffaelli R. Laparoscopic creation of a neovagina in patients with Rokitansky syndrome: Analysis of 52 cases. *Fertil Steril* 2001;74:384–9.

19 Giannesi A, Marchiole P, Benchaib M, Chevret-Measson M, Mathevet P, Dargent D. Sexuality after laparoscopic Davydov in patients affected by congenital complete vaginal agenesis associated with uterine agenesis or hypoplasia. *Hum Reprod* 2005;20:2954–7.

20 Creighton S, Minto C, Steele SJ. Feminising childhood surgery in ambiguous genitalia: Objective cosmetic and anatomical outcomes in adolescence. *Lancet* 2001;358:124–5.

21 Celayir S, Ilce Z, Danismend N. Effects of male sex hormones on urodynamics in childhood: Intersex patients are a natural model. *Pediatr Surg Int* 2000;16:502–4.

22 Davies MC, Crouch NS, Woodhouse CRJ, Creighton SM. Congenital adrenal hyperplasia and lower urinary tract symptoms. *BJU Int* 2005;95:1263–6.

23 Alizai NK, Thomas DFM, Lilford RJ, Batchelor AGG, Johnson N. Feminizing genitoplasty for congenital adrenal hyperplasia: What happens at puberty? *J Urol* 1999;161:1588–91.

24 Krege S, Walz KH, Hauffa BP, Korner I, Rubben H. Long-term follow-up of female patients with congenital adrenal hyperplasia from 21-hydroxylase deficiency, with special emphasis on the results of vaginoplasty. *BJU Int* 2000;86:253–8.

25 Sotiropoulos A, Morishima A, Homsy Y, Lattimer JK. Long-term assessment of genital reconstruction in female pseudo-hermaphrodites. *J Urol* 1976;115:599–601.

26 May B, Boyle M, Grant D. A comparative study of sexual experiences. Women with diabetes and women with congenital adrenal hyperplasia. *J Health Psychol* 1996;1:479–92.

27 Minto CL, Liao KLM, Woodhouse CRJ, Ransley PG, Creighton SM. The effect of clitoral surgery on sexual outcome in individuals who have intersex conditions with ambiguous genitalia: A cross sectional study. *Lancet* 2003;361:1252–7.

28 Crouch NS, Minto CL, Liao LM, Woodhouse CRJ, Creighton SM. Genital sensation following feminising genitoplasty for congenital adrenal hyperplasia; a pilot study. *BJU Int* 2004;93:135–8.

29 Kuhnle U, Bullinger M. Outcome of congenital adrenal hyperplasia. *Pediatr Surg Int* 1997;12:511–15.

Female Genital Reconstruction II

Jeffrey A. Leslie and Richard C. Rink

Key points

- The decision of surgery versus observation should be "led" by the physicians, not "made" by the physicians.
- A multidisciplinary approach is essential to manage these patients effectively.
- Altered clitoral sensation from older surgical techniques is common; outcome from more modern methods appears better.

- Reoperation after vaginal surgery is common.
- Partial urogenital mobilization results in good early success.
- It is important to remember that surgery does not cure intersex patients.

Introduction

Management of disorders of sexual differentiation (DSD) (previously known as "intersex" conditions), pure urogenital sinus (UGS) anomalies, and cloacal anomalies represent some of the most challenging tasks the pediatric urologist will face. In addition to the complicated surgical aspects of treatment of these patients, complex emotional issues often exist. Unfortunately, despite significant advances over the past few decades in surgical techniques and improved knowledge of the anatomy and innervation of the female genitalia, few well-designed studies exist to provide definitive guidance for the reconstructive surgery. For these reasons, we strongly advocate a multidisciplinary approach to the management of these children, including an endocrinologist, psychologist, psychiatrist, geneticist, pediatric urologist, and most importantly the patient and/or the patient's family. It is beyond the scope of this chapter to fully address the myriad pros and cons of these controversies, and the need for further well-designed studies is acknowledged. There is a common belief that all surgeons believe

children with DSD should undergo reconstruction and that all non-surgeons generally recommend observation. It is our hope that neither of these occur. What in fact should happen is that the parents and patients should be informed of all the risks and options available, as well as the psychosocial and surgical debates that exist based on the current state of knowledge. They should have the opportunity to discuss their child's situation with the multidisciplinary committee as well as with lay and support groups, such as the CARES Foundation (Congenital Adrenal Hyperplasia Research Education and Support) and ISNA (Intersex Society of North America). The decision of surgery versus observation should be "led" by the physicians, not "made" by the physicians.

While there are very few areas as controversial as surgery for any DSD, this chapter assumes that after discussing all aspects of observation versus surgery, as well as timing of surgery and the controversies involving the various aspects of surgery, the family desires surgical reconstruction. This chapter therefore focusses on the surgical management of the most common disorder of sexual differentiation, that is congenital adrenal hyperplasia (CAH). Pure UGS anomalies will also be briefly addressed, as the surgical management is similar to that of CAH in many respects. For the majority of patients, feminizing genitoplasty requires three distinct operative components: clitoroplasty, labioplasty, and vaginoplasty (for detailed

Pediatric Urology: Surgical Complications and Management. Edited by Duncan T. Wilcox, Prasad P. Godbole and Martin A. Koyle. © 2008 Blackwell Publishing, ISBN: 978-1-4051-6268-5.

discussion see refs [1–21]). We will not discuss reconstruction along male lines. This chapter will concentrate on preoperative management and on postoperative care, outcomes, complications, and their subsequent management. It is of note that in our experience with patients with CAH, that we see from throughout the United States, virtually all parents have decided on early surgery prior to visiting our institution. After discussion of all aspects, pros and cons, and meeting with us and our endocrinologists, they continue to desire early reconstruction.

Preoperative considerations

Prior to surgery, in addition to multidisciplinary counseling and family input mentioned previously, all children should undergo renal/bladder and pelvic ultrasonography, as well as genitography by a pediatric radiologist. Particular attention must be made to delineate the size of the vagina, and most importantly, the level of the confluence of the vagina with the UGS. This information is invaluable in preoperative planning as well as for counseling parents regarding the extent of surgery required for vaginoplasty.

The pediatric endocrinologist must be involved in the CAH child's care to ensure they are metabolically stable and are under good endocrinologic control. Additionally, these children require "stress dose" steroids at the time of surgery. At a minimum, all children should undergo an enema, and if a more significant vaginoplasty is anticipated, a full mechanical bowel preparation may be warranted, as well as preoperative antibiotics. Endoscopic evaluation is essential. Measurements of the distance from the perineum to the vaginal confluence (length of the UGS) and the confluence and the bladder neck (functional urethral length) should be made, with the latter more important in determining the type and extent of vaginoplasty necessary. The size and number of vaginas and the presence of a cervix should be noted. This information should then be correlated with the radiographic studies to confirm the anatomy. These measures aid in achieving a satisfactory cosmetic and functional outcome.

Outcomes and complications

Clitoroplasty

Results from genitoplasty should focus not only on cosmetic appearance but more importantly on maintenance of normal sexual function. Unfortunately, the follow-up data in most earlier studies focussed on the former, and long-term data with accurate information regarding the exact procedure performed, severity of virilization preoperatively and quality of endocrinologic control is lacking. Additionally, surgical techniques to reduce the prominence of the clitoris have dramatically improved in recent years, as a result of the improvement in current knowledge of clitoral neuroanatomy.

Alizai et al. [22] reported follow-up on 13 girls who underwent clitoral surgery at the time of feminizing genitoplasty, of which 12 of these surgeries were performed at a mean age of 2.5 years at four different centers. Nine of these girls reportedly underwent a nerve sparing reduction clitoroplasty, but it is not clear from the follow-up data presented which patients received this procedure. All were reconstructed prior to Baskin's description of the neural anatomy. The anatomical outcome was deemed unsatisfactory in 46% (6 of 13); however, one of these 13 girls underwent intentional clitoridectomy at the time of genitoplasty. One (8%) of the 12 girls who underwent clitoral reduction had residual prominence, while four (33%) had atrophy. The remaining seven (58%) were felt to have an acceptable clitoral appearance. No one has yet defined what "acceptable appearance" is, however. Gearhart and colleagues evaluated that pudendal nerve evoked potentials in six patients after clitoroplasty and noted that modern clitoroplasty techniques preserve nerve conduction in the dorsal neurovascular bundle [23]. Recent studies by Poppas have also demonstrated normal sensitivity. In a response to the Gearhart study, Chase reported a patient who underwent infant clitoridectomy with preserved pudendal latency testing in adulthood, who is nevertheless anorgasmic. She also reported several patients who underwent clitoral surgery prior to the advent of modern techniques who have preserved subjective clitoral sensation but have difficulty in attaining orgasm or have developed pain following orgasm [24]. Minto et al. [6], in a cross-sectional study, reported the results of genital examination in 13 patients who underwent clitoral surgery. Of these 13, nine had undergone clitorectomy, one a recession, two a reduction, and in one the procedure was unknown. In the two patients undergoing reduction, one was felt to have a "very large" clitoris and the other a "large" clitoris. Interestingly, of the nine patients who had undergone prior clitorectomy, only four had an "absent" clitoris on exam, with the remainder having a varied appearance, including "small," "normal," and "large." Also of note, the median age of first clitoral surgery in these patients was 3.5 years

(0.1–42). Results from a sexual satisfaction questionnaire revealed that difficulties with sensuality, communication, and avoidance were higher in those patients having undergone clitoral surgery compared with the nonoperated group. However, both groups had difficulties with orgasm. Nevertheless, 5 of the 18 women who had had clitoral surgery reported severe difficulties with orgasm, compared with none of the 10 women who had not undergone clitoral surgery. Unfortunately, as mentioned previously, many of these women had undergone clitorectomy or recession, rather than the modern technique of neurovascular sparing clitoral reduction, calling into question the interpretation of these disappointing results with respect to modern techniques. In a pilot study, this same group of investigators subsequently reported vibratory and temperature sensitivity data on six women who had all undergone prior clitoral reduction. Five of these women had undergone one clitoroplasty, and the other required two procedures. Two patients had no identifiable glans tissue at the time of testing, and the scarred area was subsequently assumed to be the clitoral position and thus stimulated. Five patients had abnormal warmth sensation and all had abnormal cold sensation. Five of the six had abnormal vibratory sensation. None of the patients had a sufficient introitus to accept the 2.8 cm diameter thermal probe, while three of the six could accept the 2.4 cm vibratory probe. Vibratory sensation was intact for these three women. On questionnaire analysis of the five sexually active women, four reported problems achieving orgasm and avoidance behaviors. Three had vaginal penetration difficulties and issues with sensuality. Interestingly, only two of the five expressed dissatisfaction with their sexual relationships, highlighting the difficulties in interpreting such data [5]. Additionally, five of these six patients had initial surgery 15 years or more prior to this study, when more modern techniques and, more importantly, knowledge of the precise neuroanatomy of the clitoris were not yet available. Many of those who advocate no clitoral surgery in CAH, when clitoral hypertrophy is the norm, then report results of clitoroplasty as the patient having a large clitoris and report this as unsatisfactory.

Frost-Arner et al. [25] reported on eight women with CAH (mean age of 20) who had undergone neurovascular bundle-sparing clitoroplasty prior to 3 years of age, without a vaginoplasty (done at or prior to puberty). Vibratory and light-touch/deep-pressure sensitivity of the clitoris was analyzed and compared to a control group of six healthy women. One of these patients had undergone a second clitoral reduction at 7 years of age. Six of the women were having intercourse successfully and did not report dryness or other coital problems. All the women considered the anatomy of the external genitalia to be normal. The authors reported no abnormalities in the appearance of size of the clitoris in any patient. Most notably, there was no difference in vibration or light-touch/deep-pressure between those seven women who had undergone early clitoroplasty when compared to the controls. The one patient who had undergone a second clitoroplasty did have reduced vibratory sensation, however. Stikkelbroeck et al. [26] reported long-term data on eight patients with CAH who underwent early (0.1–3.7 years) clitoral surgery, with dorsal resection of the corpora in all patients, with preservation of the ventral portion only. Interestingly, orgasms by clitoral stimulation were confirmed in four patients (50%). The authors hypothesized that clitoral sensation had been preserved at least partially by the remaining ventral nerve structures or that re-innervation had occurred.

Vaginoplasty

As in the case for clitoroplasty, outcomes from vaginoplasty should also focus not only on cosmetic appearance, an adequate outlet for menstrual flow, and ease of tampon insertion, but more importantly on sexual function, ease of intercourse, and maintenance of adequate lubrication. While surgery for correction of UG sinus anomalies is not as controversial as clitoroplasty, the appropriate timing of vaginoplasty is widely debated. This debate has evolved due to the high rates of secondary vaginal surgery reported in follow-up studies after infant or early childhood vaginoplasty. Jones et al. [27] noted in 1976 that 25 of 84 patients undergoing vaginoplasty required a secondary procedure to allow intercourse; 5 of these 25 subsequently required a third procedure. The authors reported that the poor results were caused by failure to exteriorize the vagina initially or by scar formation. Similarly, Sotiropoulos et al. [28] found that all patients undergoing prepubertal vaginoplasty required a revision at puberty. Azziz et al. [29], in 1986, reported that satisfactory coitus was noted in 62% of 42 women with CAH, 23 years after vaginoplasty. They noted a less favorable outcome when the initial procedure was performed before 1 year of age. Thirty secondary procedures were needed to achieve these results, however. These data have been widely quoted, but almost all of these patients underwent a cutback procedure initially, which is a procedure that has since been abandoned as it does not open the narrowed distal vagina adequately, and thus will almost always lead to stenosis. The revision performed in these patients was a flap vaginoplasty, which is the procedure that would be performed initially today. In a series from Johns Hopkins,

22 of 28 patients (78.6%) needed further vaginal surgery. The authors noted that if secondary surgery was needed for stenosis, success rates were high if the procedure was performed near puberty [30]. Nihoul-Fekete et al. [31] noted that 30% of 43 CAH patients required secondary surgery. Hendren and Atala reported on 16 patients with a high confluence, in whom six of nine adults had satisfactory coitus and two had stenosis [9].

More recent studies have not demonstrated much improvement in the rates of secondary vaginoplasty for stenosis. Alizai et al. [22] reported results of examination under anesthesia on a group of 14 CAH patients who underwent initial vaginoplasty at a mean age of 2.5 years. They found that 13 of the 14 girls required further vaginal surgery. Stenosis was present in 43% and a persistent UGS with or without fibrosis in 50%. Minto et al. [6] found that 39% of 28 patients required secondary surgery and 11% required a third procedure. Bocciardi et al. [32] recently reported long-term follow-up on 66 patients with ambiguous genitalia who underwent a one-stage Passerini-Glazel feminizing genitoplasty. Examination under anesthesia was performed in 46 patients (70%) at mean age of 10 years for those who underwent early vaginoplasty (6 months to 8 years) and at 2 years postoperatively in those who underwent later vaginoplasty (9 years or older). The authors reported a good result of vaginoplasty in 20 girls (43%), with no stenosis at the suture line. Mild stenosis at the suture line which could be easily dilated with Hegar dilators was noted in 10 girls (22%). Significant stenosis, requiring secondary Y-V vaginoplasty, was found in 16 girls (35%). Of these 16, 10 (45.5%) had undergone early vaginoplasty and 6 (25%) later vaginoplasty. All mothers and patients reported satisfaction with external genital appearance and the vaginal introitus was located in a physiologic location in all patients. Additionally, mean operative time for revisional vaginoplasty was 20 min and most patients were discharged home 3 days postoperatively. Repeat examination one year later confirmed no recurrent stenosis in all patients. Despite the higher rate of secondary vaginoplasty in the girls who had early vaginoplasty (45.5% versus 25%), the authors concluded that genitoplasty including vaginoplasty should be performed in early infancy, as secondary vaginoplasty can be successfully performed easily in those patients in whom it is required with a minor revision. Interestingly, Eroglu et al. [33] actually noted less vaginal stenosis in those who underwent early one-stage vaginoplasty (3.4%) than in those who underwent late surgery (42.8%). Krege et al. [34] reported results on 27 CAH patients, 25 of whom underwent vaginoplasty. In 20 patients a one-stage procedure

was performed at a mean age of 3.6 years, while five patients underwent a two-stage procedure. Nine (45%) of the 20 patients who underwent early flap vaginoplasty developed vaginal stenosis requiring secondary vaginoplasty, while none of the five (four flap vaginoplasties and one pull-through) who underwent a two-stage procedure developed significant stenosis. From these data, the authors recommended that in children with more severe virilization (Prader III–V) the vaginoplasty should be deferred to a second operation at the beginning of puberty. Stikkelbroeck et al. [26] reported long-term outcome of early (0.1–3.7 years) genitoplasty in eight patients, seven of which included early one-stage clitorovaginoplasty. Six (86%) of these seven patients required additional vaginal surgery in puberty due to stenosis. Six patients participated in a structured psychosexual interview at last follow-up. All six patients reported reaching sexual milestones such as falling in love, kissing, and petting. Five of the six had had coitus and four of these reported an adequate introitus, although two had mild vaginal strictures on gynecological examination. Vaginal depth was considered adequate in all five patients who had had coitus, both by the patient and gynecologist. The patient who had not yet had coitus reported pain with tampon use and was found to have a vaginal stricture and partial fusion of the labia.

Taken together, the aforementioned studies highlight several issues: (1) outcomes from vaginoplasty, whether done early or peri-pubertally, vary significantly, likely due to differences in both surgical techniques and experience, as well as by the examiner; (2) objective data such as mild vaginal stenosis or stricture on examination do not always correlate to problems with intercourse or sexual function for the patient; and (3) "single-stage" early vaginoplasty is a misnomer, as the majority of these children will require a secondary procedure at puberty and this should be expected and parents should be counseled accordingly. Our preference currently is for early (infant) clitorovaginolabioplasty, with the understanding that a simple introitoplasty will likely be required in the postpubertal period. Delaying the vaginoplasty but proceeding with early clitoral and labial surgery as advocated by some is by definition always at least a two-stage procedure. Our rationale for this approach is based on several factors, including availability of the excess prepucial skin for construction of the introitus and labia minora; relative ease of vaginal mobilization in the infant compared with the mature, deeper female vagina and pelvis; the benefits of residual maternal estrogen effect on genital tissue; as well as the psychosocial aspects of major genital surgery done postpubertally compared to in infancy. It should be noted, however, that we occasionally defer the vaginoplasty to a postpubertal age when the vagina is small or rudimentary, with the hope that some dilation of the vaginal vault will occur with time and menarche with subsequent menstrual flow.

It seems clear to us that the overwhelming majority of CAH patients are identified as females, and both the families and the children desire reconstruction. This is in agreement with the recent consensus report of world leaders in this field [35]. Unfortunately, the appropriate timing remains to be defined. While some have advocated no surgery until the patient can decide, no one knows the psychological effects of this approach. Rather than argue timing, we should be defining the best techniques to achieve normal sensation and sexual function, documenting the initial anatomy and the endocrinologic control so that results truly can be compared. It is logical to believe that the more severely affected patients will have more complex surgery and complications. Regardless, each family should always be presented with all known data, risks, pros and cons, as well as access to advocacy groups such as CARES and ISNA. They should be active in the decision-making process. Most importantly, it is imperative to understand that neither observation nor surgery cure DSD.

Labioplasty

Little data exists on the outcome from labioplasty, other than cosmetic appearance. In the series of 66 patients who underwent Passerini-Glazel genitoplasty, Bocciardi et al. [32] reported good cosmetic results at the 1-year postoperative examination, except for four patients who developed postoperative wound infections resulting in large brown scars. Nevertheless, all mothers reported satisfaction with the genital appearance of their child. At the time of examination under anesthesia peri-pubertally, all mothers and patients continued to report satisfaction with the cosmetic result, even in those with scarring, which the authors attributed was likely due to pubic hair growth. Creighton et al. [4] reported that 26 (59%) of 44 patients had good or satisfactory (minor abnormalities, unlikely to be recognized by a non-medically trained person) cosmetic result. Regarding the labia specifically, 61% were deemed normal, 30% were poor or scrotalized, 5% were partially fused, and one patient (2%) had total fusion. In the series reported by Eroglu et al. [33], 2 of 36 patients had labial abnormalities noted: presence of extraresidual scrotal skin and a large labium minoris.

As mentioned previously, one of the main reasons we advocate early clitorovaginoplasty is to allow construction of the introitus and labia minora with the redundant dorsal prepuce present in females with significant clitoromegaly. This skin has been shown to be second only to the clitoris in sensitivity [15], and therefore is the ideal tissue for creation of labia minora based on its sensitivity as well as good vascular supply, as evidenced by its widespread and successful use as hypospadias surgery (e.g. Byer's flaps, onlay repairs).

Urogenital mobilization

At Riley Hospital for Children, we have recently reviewed our data on Total Urogenital Mobilization (TUM) and Partial Urogenital Mobilization (PUM), focusing on urinary continence, cosmetic results, and vaginal stenosis. A total of 18 children have undergone TUM, of whom only seven are neurologically normal. A total of 26 patients have had a PUM procedure, of whom 25 are neurologically normal. All neurologically normal children >3 years of age are continent. Of those neurologically impaired, two are dry voiding, seven are dry with CIC, and two are wet. Only 1 of 44 has vaginal stenosis on short-term follow-up. We have been pleased with the cosmetic outcomes. Farkas et al. [36] reported follow-up data on 46 patients who underwent TUM, with mean follow-up of 4.7 years. Intraoperative rectal injury occurred in one patient, which was managed by immediate closure without further sequelae. Three developed a mild infection of the buttock area. All patients had successful cosmetic and early functional results. Girls who had reached puberty had normal menstruation, a wet and wide introitus and no evidence of scarring or fibrosis of the perineum. The younger girls' vaginal orifice could be easily calibrated with a 20 or 22 Fr bougie. No patients have had problems with urinary tract infections and all are continent. None of the girls had had intercourse yet, and so further functional data regarding sexual satisfaction or coitus were not known. Jenak et al. [37] reported early results of TUM in six girls. With mean follow-up of 3.7 months, all patients had a satisfactory cosmetic appearance and all who were continent preoperatively remained continent after TUM. Vaginal calibration was performed in four patients and ranged from 6 to 14 Hegar (mean 10.5). Kryger et al. also reported encouraging data on 13 girls who underwent TUM, seven of whom had not reached the age of achieving continence and six who were continent preoperatively. Five of the seven girls who had not yet been toilet trained achieved continence normally. One was only 27 months old at the time of the report and remained incontinent day and night, with no interest in toilet training yet. The other girl was 3 years old and only experiencing nocturnal enuresis twice weekly. The mean age of the six girls who had achieved continence prior to TUM was 53 months. One of these patients was lost to follow-up, but the other five regained continence immediately postoperatively and had remained free of infections, urgency, or frequency, and all had no postvoid residual urine by bladder scanning. Cosmetic outcomes were good.

Prevention of complications

Clitoroplasty

Complications from clitoroplasty range from partial or total loss of sensation to atrophy or clitoral loss/necrosis. As mentioned previously, techniques of clitoral surgery have evolved dramatically over the past several decades, with subsequent decreases in these complications. The precise neuroanatomical information provided by Baskin *et al.* [14] in 1999 has been invaluable in improving outcomes in clitoral surgery, and long-term results from modifications in techniques should be forthcoming.

Avoidance of the neurovascular bundle found dorsally along Buck's fascia cannot be overemphasized. The incisions in the corpora cavernosa to remove the spongy erectile tissues of the corpora must be made ventrally only, with careful attention paid to avoid perforating the dorsal tunica during dissection. Once the erectile tissue has been resected, the flaccid corpora should be folded, securing the glans to the ligated proximal corporal stumps. The folded corporal tunics should be secured to the suprapubic fascia very carefully, to avoid injury or entrapment of nerve tissue. If the glans clitoris is very large and requires reduction, tissue should only be excised ventrally (similar to incisions made in hypospadias surgery). As mentioned, there is no evidence that a larger glans clitoris is detrimental to sexual function, and therefore aggressive attempts to make it smaller surgically should be tempered by this knowledge. We have not found it necessary to reduce the size of the glans in most cases. Additionally, excision of glanular epithelium to conceal the glans should be avoided, as the sensory neuropeptides are located just beneath this layer.

Vaginoplasty

The most common complication from vaginoplasty in virtually all series is stenosis (see section "Outcomes and complications"). When performed in infancy, this "complication" should not be unexpected, as most children will require a secondary vaginoplasty at or after puberty. In our experience, these secondary procedures are usually minor and easily performed. Nevertheless, a few key points should be mentioned in order to minimize stenosis when early vaginoplasty is performed and eliminate it when performed later.

Selection of the appropriate technique of vaginoplasty cannot be overstated. The cut-back procedure should not be used, except for simple labial fusion. Flap procedures should not be used for a "high" confluence. Regardless of the technique chosen, ensuring that the distal stenotic segment of the native vagina has been opened to the point of normal vaginal caliber is paramount to ensure a good result. The flap should then be advanced into the apex of this incision without tension. If the vagina is not adequately opened, it will appear stenotic. Herein lies the advantages of TUM or PUM for the higher confluence. These techniques allow the surgeon to move the vagina closer to the perineum, improving visualization, shortening the length of the perineal skin flap required to reach the apex of the posterior vaginal incision, and thus decreasing the chances for stenosis while improving cosmetics. Unfortunately, it will be years before long-term results are known.

When a high confluence is present, requiring separation of the vagina from the UGS, stenosis is much more likely as a circumferential anastomosis to the perineum is required. Furthermore, urethrovaginal fistulae can occur,although this complication is infrequent. Rink *et al.* [12] reported 6-month to 5-year follow-up on eight patients with a high confluence who underwent an early perineal approach for separation of the urethra from the vagina, noting only one (12.5%) urethrovaginal fistula which did not affect continence or voiding and for which the patient subsequently did not desire repair. Krege *et al.* [34] noted that 1 of 25 patients who underwent vaginoplasty developed a urethrovaginal fistula after meatoplasty. Eroglu *et al.* [33] reported that 3 (8.3%) of 36 patients developed fistulae, all of which required repair.

The dissection to separate the urethra from the vagina and subsequent closure of the urethra can be very challenging due primarily to poor exposure or visualization. We have found this dissection and closure of the urethra to be much more easily performed after TUM or PUM has been performed. Additionally, positioning the child supine with a circumferential body sterile prep allows the surgeon to rotate the child prone, further enhancing visualization of this area, without the need to divide the rectum [12].

Summary

In closing, there are a number of issues we believe are important for the reader to understand. The management of DSD, UGS, and cloacal anomalies is complex from both a surgical and psychosocial standpoint. It is clear that surgery does not cure intersex conditions. Furthermore, the exact psychological impact of surgery versus no surgery is poorly understood at this time. We believe that vaginal dilation is never indicated in children nor is vaginal surgery repeated during childhood. We fully recognize that many patients who undergo vaginoplasty as an infant may require secondary vaginoplasty at puberty but we believe this is more easily done and is a less significant procedure than primary vaginoplasty in the adult. In those situations where a neovagina is required such as in Mayer–Rokitansky patients, the vaginoplasty should always be postponed until after puberty. A multidisciplinary approach is mandatory for children with any degree of DSD. Family support, education, and counseling are critical to a good functional outcome. If surgical reconstruction is elected, it requires precise knowledge of each child's unique anatomy, delicate and precise tissue handling, and lifelong commitment by the surgeon. In the CAH patients, excellent endocrinologic management is mandatory for optimal results. DSD and cloacal anomalies occur in a spectrum of complexity, and the more difficult cases should be handled only in centers with expertise and experience in these areas. This is particularly true of those with a high vaginal confluence where a pull-through vaginoplasty may be necessary. With this procedure, dissection occurs between the vagina and the bladder which we believe creates the greatest risk to continence and vaginal and clitoral sensation. Lastly, in spite of significant advances there is still much to be learned. Long-term outcomes are difficult to obtain but are necessary and should look at not just adequate vaginal caliber and cosmetics but also at any change in clitoral or vaginal sensation, orgasm potential and ability to have enjoyable, painless intercourse.

References

1 America ISoN. Recommendations for Treatment, 2007. Available at www.isna.org.

2 Creighton SM. Adult female outcomes of feminising surgery for ambiguous genitalia. *Pediatr Endocrinol Rev* 2004;2:199–202.

3 Creighton SM. Long-term outcome of feminization surgery: The London experience. *BJU Int* 2004;93:44–6.

4 Creighton SM, Minto CL, Steele SJ. Objective cosmetic and anatomical outcomes at adolescence of feminising surgery for ambiguous genitalia done in childhood. *Lancet* 2001;358:124–5.

5 Crouch NS, Minto CL, Laio LM, Woodhouse CR, Creighton SM. Genital sensation after feminizing genitoplasty for congenital adrenal hyperplasia: A pilot study. *BJU Int* 2004;93:135–8.

6 Minto CL, Liao LM, Woodhouse CR, Ransley PG, Creighton SM. The effect of clitoral surgery on sexual outcome in individuals who have intersex conditions with ambiguous genitalia: A cross-sectional study. *Lancet* 2003;361:1252–7.

7 de Jong TP, Boemers TM. Neonatal management of female intersex by clitorovaginoplasty. *J Urol* 1995;154:830–2.

8 Gonzalez R, Fernandes ET. Single-stage feminization genitoplasty. *J Urol* 1990;143:776–8.

9 Hendren WH, Atala A. Repair of the high vagina in girls with severely masculinized anatomy from the adrenogenital syndrome. *J Pediatr Surg* 1995;30:91–4.

10 Mandell J, Haskins JM, Hammond MG. Surgical correction of external genitalia and lower genitourinary tract of markedly virilized child. *Urology* 1988;31:234–6.

11 Passerini-Glazel G. Vaginoplasty in severely virilized CAH females. *Dialogues Pediatr Urol* 1998;21:2–3.

12 Rink RC, Pope JC, Kropp BP, Smith ER, Jr., Keating MA, Adams MC. Reconstruction of the high urogenital sinus: Early perineal prone approach without division of the rectum. *J Urol* 1997;158:1293–7.

13 Kogan SJ, Smey P, Levitt SB. Subtunical total reduction clitoroplasty: A safe modification of existing techniques. *J Urol* 1983;130:746–8.

14 Baskin LS, Erol A, Li YW, Liu WH, Kurzrock E, Cunha GR. Anatomical studies of the human clitoris. *J Urol* 1999;162:1015–20.

15 Schober JM, Ransley P. Anatomical description and sensitivity mapping of adult women based on the SAGASF survey. *BJU Int* 2002;83:39–50.

16 Rink RC, Adams MC. Feminizing genitoplasty: State of the Art. *World J Urol* 1998;16:212–18.

17 Pena A. Total urogenital mobilization–an easier way to repair cloacas. *J Pediatr Surg* 1997;32:263–7,discussion 7–8.

18 Rink RC, Adams MC. Evaluation and suegical management of the child with intersex. *Prog Paediatr Urol* 1999;2:67–88.

19 Rink RC, Cain MP. *Further Uses of the Mobilized Sinus in Total Urogenital Mobilization Procedures.* Paper presented at the American Academy of Pediatrics, Boston, 2002.

20 Gosalbez R, Castellan M, Ibrahim E, DiSandro M, Labbie A. New concepts in feminizing genitoplasty–is the fortunoff flap obsolete? *J Urol* 2005;174:2350–3, discussion 3.

21 Rink RC, Metcalfe PD, Cain MP, Kaefer M, Casale AJ, Meldrum KK. *Partial Urogenital Mobilization: The Advantages without the Risks.* Paper presented at the annual meeting of European Society for Pediatric Urology and American Academy of Pediatrics, Uppsala, Sweden, 2005.

22 Alizai NK, Thomas DF, Lilford RJ, Batchelor AG, Johnson N. Feminizing genitoplasty for congenital adrenal hyperplasia: What happens at puberty? *J Urol* 1999;161:1588–91.

23 Gearhart JP, Burnett A, Owen JH. Measurement of pudendal evoked potentials during feminizing genitoplasty: Technique and applications. *J Urol* 1995;153:486–7.

24 Chase C. Re: Measurement of pudendal evoked potentials during feminizing genitoplasty: Technique and applications. *J Urol* 1996;156:1139–40.

25 Frost-Arner L, Aberg M, Jacobsson S. Clitoral sensitivity after surgical correction in women with adrenogenital syndrome: A long term follow-up. *Scand J Plastic Reconst Surg*

Hand Surg [Nordisk plastikkirurgisk forening [and] Nordisk klubb for handkirurgi] 2003;37:356–9.

26 Stikkelbroeck NM, Beerendonk CC, Willemsen WN, Schreuders-Bais CA, Feitz WF, Rieu PN *et al.* The long term outcome of feminizing genital surgery for congenital adrenal hyperplasia: Anatomical, functional and cosmetic outcomes, psychosexual development, and satisfaction in adult female patients. *J Pediatr Adolesc Gynecol* 2003;16:289–96.

27 Jones HW, Jr., Garcia SC, Klingensmith GJ. Secondary surgical treatment of the masculinized external genitalia of patients with virilizing adrenal hyperplasia. *Obstet Gynecol* 1976;48:73–5.

28 Sotiropoulos A, Morishima A, Homsy Y, Lattimer JK. Long-term assessment of genital reconstruction in female pseudohermaphrodites. *J Urology* 1976;115:599–601.

29 Azziz R, Mulaikal RM, Migeon CJ, Jones HW, Jr., Rock JA. Congenital adrenal hyperplasia: Long-term results following vaginal reconstruction. *Fertil Steril* 1986; 46:1011–14.

30 Bailez MM, Gearhart JP, Migeon C, Rock J. Vaginal reconstruction after initial construction of the external genitalia in girls with salt-wasting adrenal hyperplasia. *J Urol* 1992;148:680–2,discussion 3–4.

31 Nihoul-Fekete C, Philippe F, Thibaud E, Rappaport R, Pellerin D. Continued evaluation of results of surgical management of female congenital adrenal hyperplasia. Report on 48 cases [author's trans.]. *Archives francaises de pediatrie* 1982;39:13–16.

32 Bocciardi A, Lesma A, Montorsi F, Rigatti P. Passerini-glazel feminizing genitoplasty: A long-term followup study. *J Urol* 2005;174:284–8,discussion 8.

33 Eroglu E, Tekant G, Gundogdu G, Emir H, Ercan O, Soylet Y *et al.* Feminizing surgical management of intersex patients. *Pediatr Surg Int* 2004;20:543–7.

34 Krege S, Walz KH, Hauffa BP, Korner I, Rubben H. Long-term follow-up of female patients with congenital adrenal hyperplasia from 21-hydroxylase deficiency, with special emphasis on the results of vaginoplasty. *BJU Int* 2000;86:253–8,discussion 8–9.

35 Hughes IA, Houk C, Ahmed SF, Lee PA. Consensus statement on management of intersex disorders. *Arch Dis child* 2006;91:554–63.

36 Farkas A, Chertin B, Hadas-Halpren I. 1-Stage feminizing genitoplasty: 8 years of experience with 49 cases. *J Urol* 2001;165:2341–6.

37 Jenak R, Ludwikowski B, Gonzalez R. Total urogenital sinus mobilization: A modified perineal approach for feminizing genitoplasty and urogenital sinus repair. *J Urol* 2001;165:2347–9.

30

Persistent Cloaca

Stephanie Warne and Duncan T. Wilcox

Key points

- Renal impairment occurs in up to 50% of patients.
- Normal voiding continence is uncommon.
- Social urinary continence can be created in up to 95% of patients.

- Gynecological problems frequently occur at puberty and should be anticipated.
- Patients with a long common channel have a poorer prognosis.

Introduction

Cloacal malformation is a rare, complex malformation with an incidence of 1 in 50,000 [1–4] (Figure 30.1). The defect is usually classified by the length of the common channel: short common channel <3 cm measured endoscopically and long common cloacal channel >3 cm which represents a more severe defect. Persistent cloaca remains a difficult reconstructive challenge but with advances in surgical technique and perioperative medical care it is now possible to anatomically correct the defect in the majority of patients [3].

The ideal goals of the primary surgical reconstruction for patients with persistent cloaca are the achievement of bowel and urinary control for the child and normal sexual function in adult life [1]. However, data on the long-term functional outcome for these patients is sparse as the published literature tends to concentrate on various complex surgical techniques.

Reconstructive surgery

In 1989, the preliminary report of the posterior sagittal anorecto vaginourethroplasty (PSARVUP) for repair of cloaca was described [5]. Using this technique the cloaca

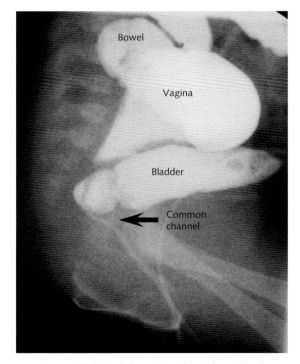

Figure 30.1 Radiological illustration of an infant with a long common channel cloaca.

can be repaired by complete separation of the three structures [5,6]. During the posterior sagittal approach the rectum is separated from the urogenital sinus and the vagina is then dissected from the urinary tract and

Pediatric Urology: Surgical Complications and Management. Edited by Duncan T. Wilcox, Prasad P. Godbole and Martin A. Koyle. © 2008 Blackwell Publishing, ISBN: 978-1-4051-6268-5.

both rectum and vagina are mobilized from below (and above where necessary) in an attempt to place both in their normal positions. The previous common channel is used to create a neourethra [5,6]. This procedure is difficult and time-consuming with significant risk of complication from urethral and vaginal ischemic complications during separation of the vagina from the urethra. Pena reports stenosis or fistula in 42 of 217 (19%) patients repaired by this procedure [7].

In 1997, the total urogenital sinus mobilization (TUM) technique was described, treating the urethra and the vagina as a single unit thus avoiding the dissection of the vagina from the urinary tract [8]. This technique reduced operative time considerably and simplified the procedure. In this modification, the rectum is separated from the vagina via the posterior sagittal approach and then the entire urogenital sinus is dissected and mobilized en bloc down to the perineum [8]. This circumferential mobilization usually extends anteriorly above the pubourethral ligament, laterally above the levator ani muscles, and posteriorly to the peritoneal reflection until enough length has been gained to connect the vaginal edges and urethra to the perineum [8,9]. In case of low confluence, the common channel can either be discarded or used to create a mucosal-lined vestibule. In patients with high-confluence, the sinus can be split and used to form the anterior vaginal wall or retubularized in patients with a short urethra [9].

Around two-thirds of cloacas can be repaired by perineal approach alone [7,9], but in cases of a long common cloacal channel a combined abdominal approach may be necessary [5–8]. In cases where the vagina is too short to anastomose to the perineum additional skin flaps, vaginal switch or intestinal replacement can be used to create a vagina [6–8].

Outcomes

Renal abnormalities and function

Structural abnormalities of the kidney are common in cloaca patients and are diagnosed in approximately 60% of patients at presentation [7,10]. Renal dysplasia, duplex systems, pelviureteric junction obstruction, and renal ectopia are the most frequently encountered anomalies [7,10–12].

There is a high incidence of renal failure observed in cloaca patients. In one large retrospective review, by 5.7 years half had chronic renal failure which was end stage, requiring renal transplantation in 19% [10]. Renal

impairment causes serious morbidity and there was an overall mortality rate of 6% from renal failure in this series [10]. Patients with structural abnormalities particularly renal dysplasia, solitary kidney, and vesicoureteric reflux were statistically more likely to develop chronic renal failure [10].

Postnatally it is important to relieve urinary tract obstruction early, correct upper tract abnormalities, prevent urinary tract infection, and treat bladder dysfunction thus dealing with the main preventable causes of renal deterioration [6,10]. Of greatest therapeutic importance are the infants with bilateral vesicoureteric reflux or those with vesicoureteric reflux and a contralateral abnormal kidney as these girls are at significant risk of renal deterioration [13]. A further decrease in renal function may be a result of hydronephrotic damage, or hypertensive changes [10].

Fecal continence

Approximately 60% of patients become continent of feces [1,7,14]. However, only 28% are continent by spontaneous bowel movements and have satisfactory control [1,7]. Almost one-third need rigorous bowel management programs in the form of rectal washouts [15] or antegrade enemas [16] to achieve social continence.

Urinary continence

The reported rate of social urinary continence varies from between 60% and 95% [1,6,14]. Hendren reported that 64% of his patients void spontaneously and are dry by voiding alone. In a more recent series only 22% void spontaneously and are dry [3]. A further 12% of that group have achieved continence by clean intermittent catheterization (CIC), but 46% of patients required reconstructive surgery [1]. Patients with short common channel and good bladder neck at presentation were much more likely to be continent by normal voiding [1]. This is supported by a recent review of 192 patients, where 48% of patients required an intervention to achieve social continence of urine [14]. Multiple procedures were often necessary to achieve satisfactory urinary continence and independence for the child.

The etiology of urinary incontinence in cloaca patients is multifactorial and may be secondary to: structural abnormalities of the bladder (including bladder atresia), bladder neck or urethra, and sacral dysplasia with neurovesical dysfunction. A high incidence of neurovesical dysfunction has been reported in cloaca patients and is often associated with lumbosacral bony abnormalities or intraspinal lesions [17,18]. Patients with a cloaca may potentially be at risk of iatrogenic nerve damage not only during the posterior sagittal approach to the rectum but also during the total urogenital mobilization procedure.

In a recent prospective study of anorectal patients, 90% of cloaca patients had bladder dysfunction on urodynamics at presentation [19]. The most common abnormal urodynamic finding overall was detrusor overactivity with bladder instability during the filling phase and high detrusor pressures during the voiding phase [19]. All patients then had a combination of PSARVUP and TUM performed. After reconstructive surgery there was a deterioration in bladder function in 5 of 10 (50%) of the cloaca group and in 1 in 20 (5%) of Anorectal malformation (ARM) patients that served as controls (Table 30.1). All six of these patients required intervention by CIC or urinary diversion and the observed change was statistically significant in the cloaca group [19].

In this study, four of the cloaca patients who had deterioration in bladder function postsurgery showed a change from detrusor overactivity preoperative to an inadequate bladder postoperative on urodynamics [19]. All four had a long common channel (>3 cm). This confirms earlier data in which 60% of patients with a cloaca were incontinent of urine [14], many were described as having large floppy and inadequate bladders. Several studies have shown that posterior sagittal anorectoplasty alone does not alter bladder function in anorectal patients [20]. It thus appears that deterioration in bladder function in cloaca patients may be associated with mobilization of the common channel to create a separate urethra and vagina. Pena reports urinary incontinence in 72% of those with a long common channel compared with 28% of those with a short common channel [2,7,14].

The finding of an atonic bladder after surgery suggests that there was damage to the nerve supply to the bladder at a lower motor neurone level. The urinary tract and vagina share a large common wall therefore some dissection between these structures cannot be avoided in repair of cloacal malformation [2]. In patients with a long common channel, significant dissection between the vagina, the urethra, and the bladder neck may be necessary. The peripheral nerve supplies are deficient in patients with sacral agenesis; therefore even minimal trauma to these nerves in patients with sacral agenesis can result in additional functional loss which may not have been the case in children with normal nerve fibers [21]. As the majority of cloaca patients have preexisting neurogenic bladder dysfunction it may be that minimal disruption during surgical repair results in denervation and an inadequate bladder.

Gynecological outcome

Cloaca patients have a high incidence of innate gynecological problems [22,23], but these may remain asymptomatic until the onset of menses or early adult life. The mullerian and vaginal abnormalities found in patients with cloacal malformation show great variation depending on whether the confluence is high or low. Sixty percent [14,22,24] of cloaca patients have some degree of septation of the uterus and vagina ranging from a partial septum in a large vagina with single cervix and uterus to a completely separated double vagina with double cervix and uteri.

In one long-term outcome study of 41 adult patients, two-thirds developed uterine function at puberty, whilst 20% had primary amenorrhea due to a vestigial uterus [22]. Thirty-two percent were menstruating normally and 15 (36%) presented with hematometra/hematocolpos typically had cyclical abdominal pain at puberty (Figure 30.2, Table 30.2). The most common cause of the obstructed uterus was stenosis of persistent urogenital sinus (no previous genital tract reconstruction), but a few developed vaginal stenosis of previous reconstruction. All patients who developed an obstructed uterus required surgical intervention [22]. This was supported by others in whom an obstructed uterus was seen in 41% of 22 cloaca patients [23].

The long-term outcome for the uteri left *in situ* is unknown and it has been suggested that endometriosis and infertility may be the result of an obstructed uterus [23,25]. There are also case reports in similar patients who were able to conceive and carry a pregnancy to term [26,27]. This should encourage surgeons to create a passage for effective uterine drainage and to preserve the uterus and fallopian tubes where possible.

Adult gynecological follow-up has been reported in 21 adult patients [22]. This reported that 86% had an adequate vagina with no menstrual problems and 12 (57%) are or have been sexually active. Half of these women

Table 30.1 Status of urodynamics after surgical reconstruction.

Bladder function	Stable	Improved	Worse
Cloaca $n = 10$	5	0	5
ARM $n = 20$	16	3	1

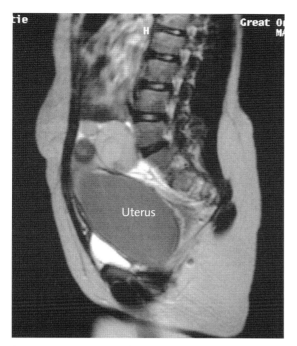

Figure 30.2 MRI scan of adolescent cloaca patient who presented with a 6-month history of cyclical abdominal pain.

Table 30.2 Outcome at menarche for 41 cloaca patients.

Outcome	n	%
Normal menstruation at puberty	13	32
Hematometra	15	36
Amenorrhea (vestigial uterus)	8	20
Early puberty (normal uterus and vagina)	3	7
Amenorrhea under investigation	2	5

progressed normally from their initial reconstructive procedure through menarche to adulthood without the need for further vaginal surgery [22]. An additional five (28%) had delayed primary vaginal reconstruction: three at puberty and two as adults which was adequate to allow sexual intercourse later in life [22]. However, 19% of adult cloaca patients required additional vaginal surgery to facilitate intercourse. Even if the girl has no problems at menarche her vagina may not be adequate to allow sexual intercourse later in life [22].

In only one series, so far, has there been reported a normal pregnancy and delivery of a healthy baby [6]. If pregnancy does occur, these women will require considerable support particularly those with impaired renal function, bladder augmentation, and catheterizable conduits [28]. Delivery by caesarean section is usually recommended in patients where vaginoplasty has been performed [27].

Complications

The TUM technique was initially reported as eliminating the complications of urethral and vaginal stenosis by preserving the blood supply to the urogenital sinus and improving the cosmetic result [7,8]. However, a recent report showed that 3 of 22 patients (14%) presented postoperatively with a surgical complication that required major redo perineal surgery [9]. Urethral stenosis was observed in two children, both with a long common channel, occurring after separation of the urethra from the vagina ($n = 1$) or after tubularization of the common channel ($n = 1$). These girls were treated by a vesicostomy to allow CIC in one case, and a Mitrofanoff channel after failure of a redo urethroplasty in the other case. Urethrovaginal fistula was diagnosed in one patient. Persistent minimal common channel (<0.5 cm) was present in three girls, of whom one required minor urethral revision to allow easier CIC. Distal vaginal closure or stenosis was observed in three cases: one girl with congenital diffuse perineal hemangioma presented with complete anal and vaginal closure, and underwent a successful redo-PSARP, and two children (including one with distal vaginal agenesis) have a tight introitus that may require further surgery. Anal stenosis was observed in five children, either managed with multiple dilatations ($n = 3$), or requiring VY anoplasty ($n = 2$).

Preventing complications

As the condition is rare little has been written on avoiding surgical complications. Surgical complications can be characterized:
1 *Ischemic complications to the common channel.* Ischemia to the common channel causes problems with fistulae and late urethral and vaginal stenosis. If the common channel is short little mobilization is required but with a long common channel extensive mobilization can lead to ischemia. This more frequently occurs if too much dissection is attempted from below. In a long common channel it is advisable to start the dissection from below

and then turn early to avoid skeletonizing the channel. If the common channel is not going to reach it is appropriate to use the common channel for the urethra alone. The vagina is then dissected free of the urethra, occasionally a vaginal flap can be made to create extra length, especially if the patient had previous hydrocolpos. If there is a bifid system by sacrificing one uterus the whole system can be tubularized and brought down. While skin flaps can avoid tension care must be given as they can lead to an unsatisfactory cosmetic appearance later.

2 *Nerve damage.* The bladder dynamics frequently change following surgical reconstruction [19]. This suggests neural damage, which can be minimized by staying in the midline, avoiding close dissection around the common channel, and using monopolar diathermy sparingly.

Conclusion

Although the majority of cloaca patients can achieve social fecal and urinary continence with the surgical reconstructive procedures performed today, a large number will require additional and sometimes multiple urological procedures not only to achieve continence but also to treat bladder dysfunction and to protect the upper tracts. Half develop renal failure so most patients particularly those with severe malformations will need regular review and lifelong surveillance. Due to the high incidence of associated gynecological problems all these girls should be reassessed at early puberty. Additional surgery may then be necessary to create a vagina for menstruation and for sexual intercourse, which is possible in the majority. As more of these patients reach adult life better data will become available on long-term outcomes. Persistent cloaca still remains one of the most challenging conditions to treat in pediatric surgery and urology and these patients should be cared for by a dedicated team with specialist experience in this area.

References

1 Warne SA, Wilcox DT, Ransley PG. Long-term urological outcome in patients presenting with persistent cloaca. *J Urol* 2002;168:1859–62.

2 Brock WA, Pena A. Cloacal abnormalities and imperforate anus. In *Clinical Pediatric Urology*, 3rd edn. Edited by Kelais PP, King LR, Belman AB. WB Saunders, 1992: Vol. 2, Chapter 19, Philadelphia, pp. 920–42.

3 Hendren WH. Urological aspects of cloacal malformations. *J Urol* 1988;140:1207–13.

4 Odibo AO, Turner GW, Borgida AF *et al.* Late prenatal ultrasound features of hydrometrocolpos secondary to cloacal anomaly: Case reports and review of the literature. *Ultrasound Obstet Gynecol* 1997;9:419–21.

5 Pena A. The surgical management of persistent cloaca: Results in 54 patients treated with a posterior saggital approach. *J Pediatr Surg* 1989;24:590–8.

6 Hendren WH. Cloaca, the most severe degree of imperforate. *Anus Ann Surg* 1998;228:331–46.

7 Pena A, Levitt MA, Hong A, Midulla P. Surgical management of cloacal malformations: A review of 339 patients. *J Pediatr Surg* 2004;39:470–9.

8 Peña A. Total urogenital mobilization – An easier way to repair cloacas. *J Pediatr Surg* 1997;32:263–8.

9 Leclair MD, Gundetti M, Kiely EM, Wilcox DT. The surgical outcome of total urogenital mobilization in cloaca. *J Urol* 2007;177:1492–5.

10 Warne SA, Wilcox DT, Ledermann SE, Ransley PG. Renal outcome in patients with cloaca. *J Urol* 2002;167:2548–51.

11 Pena A, Hong A. Advances in the management of anorectal malformations. *Am J Surg* 2000;180:370–6.

12 Rink RC, Herndon CD, Cain MP *et al.* Upper and lower urinary tract outcome after surgical repair of cloacal malformations: A three-decade experience. *BJU Int* 2005;96:131–4.

13 McLorie G, Sheldon M, Fleisher M *et al.* The genitourinary system in patients with imperforate anus. *J Pediatr Surg* 1987;22:1100–4.

14 Pena A. Anorectal malformations. *Semin Pediatr Surg* 1995;4:35–47.

15 Shandling B, Gilmour R. The enema continence catheter in spina bifida: Successful bowel management. *J Pediatr Surg* 1987;22:271–3.

16 Malone PS, Ransley PG, Kiely EM. Preliminary report: The antegrade continence enema. *Lancet* 1990;336:1217–18.

17 Boemers TM, Beek FJ, van Gool JD *et al.* Urologic problems in anorectal malformations. Part 2: Functional urologic sequlae. *J Pediatr Surg* 1996;31:634–7.

18 Rivosecchi M, Lucchetti M, De Gennaro *et al.* Spinal dysraphism detected by magnetic resonance imaging in patients with anorectal anomalies: Incidence and clinical significance. *J Pediatr Surg* 1995;30:488–90.

19 Warne SA, Godley ML, Wilcox DT. Surgical reconstruction of cloacal malformation can alter bladder function; A comparative study with anorectal anomalies. *J Urol.* 2004;172:2377–81.

20 Boemers TML, Bax KMA, Rövekamp MH, van Gool JD. The effect of posterior sagittal anorectoplasty and its variants on lower urinary tract function in children with anorectal malformations. *J Urol* 1995;153:191.

21 Scott JES. The anatomy of the pelvic autonomic system in cases of high imperforate anus. *Surgery* 1959;45:1028.

22 Warne S, Creighton S, Wilcox DT, Ransley PG. The long term gynaecological outcome of girls presenting with persistent cloaca. *J Urol* 2003;17:1493–6.

23 Levitt MA, Stein DM, Pena A. Gynecologic concerns in the treatment of teenagers with cloaca. *J Pediatr Surg* 1998;33:188–93.

24 Meyers RL. Congenital anomalies of the vagina and their reconstruction. *Clin Obstet Gynecol* 1997;40:168–80.

25 Golan A, Langer R, Bukovsky I. Congenital anomalies of the mullerian system. *Fertil Steril* 1989;51:747–53.

26 Moura MD, Navarro PA, Nogueira AA. Pregnancy and term delivery after neovaginoplasty in a patent with vaginal agenesis. *Int J Gynecol Obstet* 2000;71:215–16.

27 Edmonds ED. Vaginal and uterine anomalies in the pediatric and adolescent patient. *Curr Opin Obstet Gynecol* 2001;13:463–7.

28 Greenwell TJ, Venn SN, Mundy AR. Augmentation cystoplasty. *BJU Int* 2001;88:511–25.

Renal Impairment Surgery

31

Hemodialysis and Peritoneal Dialysis

Alun Williams

Key points

- Transplantation is the gold standard for the management of end-stage kidney disease. Dialysis is sometimes necessary.

- Choice of dialysis (hemodialysis or peritoneal dialysis, PD) depends on family preference, clinical and environmental circumstances. PD is more "child-centered."

- For hemodialysis, "no needle" dialysis via a central venous catheter is favored. Central

vessels should be reused as far as possible in cases of repeated access.

- For placement of peritoneal tubes, laparoscopy has the advantage of placement under direct vision, with an extraperitoneal tunnel to fix the catheter in the pelvis.

Introduction

Renal replacement therapy in childhood has evolved in tandem with the adult experience. While the ultimate aim is a kidney transplant, preferably without recourse to dialysis, hemodialysis and PD remain crucially important in the armamentarium of therapies for acute and end-stage chronic renal disease.

The ethos of providing dialysis in childhood has been to promote and support development as normally as possible in an environment familiar to the child: in practice, home PD is preferable in this sense. Pediatric dialysis units are regionalized, and twice- or three-times weekly trips to hospital for hemodialysis can be disruptive and expensive. In addition, the cardiovascular response to hemodialysis (with episodes of hypotension during treatment) may make this a less attractive option. There is also evidence that hemodialysis increases the risk of

subsequent allograft failure [1]. Techniques of peritoneal and vascular access will be considered separately.

Hemodialysis access

Technique

Generally, vascular access for dialysis can be by means of indwelling central venous catheter ("no needle") or by establishing a high-flow conduit which can be punctured for access (e.g. an arteriovenous fistula (AVF), a prosthetic graft or shunt).

In small children, needled conduits can be technically difficult to establish, maintain, and access requires repeated needling which can be traumatic for the child. In the author's institution, we have taken the stance of "no needle" hemodialysis by means of an indwelling catheter, and the following section considers this.

If dialysis can be anticipated for more than a few weeks, a tunnelled cuffed line is preferable, as they are considered to be more durable, more comfortable and less obtrusive, and have fewer complications such as displacement. In the acute setting, a percutaneously placed (by Seldinger technique) line is reliable in the short term

Pediatric Urology: Surgical Complications and Management. Edited by Duncan T. Wilcox, Prasad P. Godbole and Martin A. Koyle. © 2008 Blackwell Publishing, ISBN: 978-1-4051-6268-5.

[2,3], which can then be removed, or if longer-term access is required, revised with a tunnelled line.

The upper body central circulation is preferable, in particular the right internal jugular vein. Access to the catheter is easy, the route and distance to the heart is shorter, and the lower body vessels are preserved, for either future access or for transplantation. The vein is accessed either by needle and guidewire or by open approach through a small transverse neck crease incision. Current standards would recommend the use of ultrasound localization of the vein for puncture [4]. The line is tunnelled from a convenient exit site on the anterolateral chest wall. It is important to ensure a gentle curve from venotomy to exit site as an acute angle may cause a kink. The line must be sized approximately prior to this maneuver to ensure that the cuff is placed within the subcutaneous tissue. Reasonable surface landmarks for the right atrium include the mid-point between sternal notch and xiphoid, and the right nipple to indicate line length. When the line has been placed via the peel-away introducer, or directly through a venotomy, the tip position must be confirmed by on-table fluoroscopy.

Many hemodialysis lines have proximal and distal lumens (see Figure 31.1) (although dialysis may be performed through a single lumen), and so adequate flow must be ensured through both lumens. The largest line passable with ease is preferable, in accordance with Poisseille's law determining flow. The tip of the line frequently needs to be placed within the right atrium. A reasonable practical approach to estimating adequate flow is to manually withdraw blood using a 20 cc syringe: flow should be smooth and constant over a few seconds through both lumens. Some manipulation of the line is frequently required to maximize the flow; constant reconfirmation of tip position by fluoroscopy is therefore imperative. In very small infants, customized strategies

for achieving adequate flow may be required for hemodialysis access [5].

Outcome

Complications

Bleeding at the time of operation can usually be controlled by local measures, although it is reasonable to have blood grouped and saved. With ultrasound localization, the risk of hemo- or pneumothorax should be low, but a plain chest radiograph is recommended after Seldinger technique. Occasionally passage of the line toward the heart can be difficult. This is particularly so for left-sided access, or with redo lines. For redos it is reasonable to confirm patency of the central veins by Doppler ultrasound; a formal venogram is rarely required, although may be indicated by clinical features of central vein occlusion (such as prominent chest wall veins, or plethora, or chronic limb swelling) with equivocal Doppler studies. Flow may be poor in the line. This may be due to tip position (in the SVC), occasionally because of an acute angulation in the subcutaneous tunnel, or may be due to thrombus. Infection associated with the line may supervene at any time. The latter two are the commonest complications of central venous catheters [6].

Preventing and managing complications

As mentioned above, fluoroscopy is mandatory for line insertion, and it can be useful to manipulate the line under screening if difficult. The line may bend or kink at the confluence of internal jugular and subclavian, or may take a route into the contralateral neck or arm drainage. Usually, perseverance with manipulation under screening is adequate to place the line. Placing small amounts of torque on the catheter during manipulation may be helpful, as may be the suspension of ventilation. Elevation or depression of a shoulder may alter the configuration of a jugular/subclavian confluence sufficiently to allow a line to pass. We have found a hydrophilic guidewire (Terumo UK Ltd, Egham, Surrey) to be useful in manipulation into the right heart. The introducer sheath and/or catheter can then be passed over the guidewire.

We prefer the jugular veins for access. Subclavian puncture is possible, but may lead to a higher risk of arm venous thrombosis, which in turn might affect establishment of an AVF [7]. We prefer to try and preserve the arm veins if possible for the sake of creation of an AVF later in life. If the inferior vena cava needs to be used, the same principles of access apply, although the

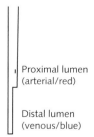

Proximal lumen
(arterial/red)

Distal lumen
(venous/blue)

Figure 31.1 Schematic showing separation of lumens of dual lumen hemodialysis catheter.

subcutaneous tunnel is often very awkward, as it either crosses the hip joint, putting the line at risk of kinking, or requires the line exit site to be on the thigh, which can be obtrusive and uncomfortable. Our preference is the left saphenofemoral junction or femoral vein, as the preferred site for the transplant kidney is on the right.

Where central veins become very narrowed (internal jugular vein stenosis is seen after 10% insertions, subclavian vein stenosis in over 40% [8]) or obliterated, with the so-called end-stage access, there may be a role for specialist interventional vascular radiology for access [7]. Line sepsis should be managed in the first instance with appropriate antibiotics, although clinical deterioration or failure to dialyze will necessitate removal of the line.

If dialysis is difficult because of poor flow (usually with high venous pressures), it is useful to confirm the tip position by means of plain radiography. A relatively "fresh" line (within a few days of its insertion) can be withdrawn safely with appropriate analgesia or sedation, if improved flow can be obtained in this way. A contrast study may also be helpful in demonstrating line thrombosis and venous run-off. Thrombolytic line locks (e.g. urokinase) may be useful, although more extensive thrombosis sometimes requires thrombolytic infusion (e.g. tissue plasminogen activator) with repeat contrast imaging to document progression.

If a line requires revision, within a few days of insertion the neck may be reopened and the line manipulated aseptically. We have found this generally unrewarding, however. Revising a line within 4 weeks or so of its insertion requires dissection of the vein for control above and below the venotomy. In an older line, when there is an established tract, it is reasonable to control the tract, and replace the line directly, or over a guidewire according to the surgeon's preference.

Symptoms or signs indicating a limb venous thrombosis require removal of the catheter; venous hypertension may warrant consideration of removal.

Other modes of hemodialysis access

As mentioned above, these require needle puncture access, although may be suitable for older children, or in transition to adult units where these modalities are more commonly encountered. The preferred technique is the arm AVF. If reasonable vessels exist at the wrist, it is advisable to fashion the anastomosis there, as this preserves the elbow brachiocephalic site for a later date. The fistula may fail to mature or thrombose later. Pseudoaneurysms may also form which require the access site to be abandoned. Generally, AVFs are fashioned in the nondominant arm, proceeding distal to proximal. If no native vessels are suitable for arteriovenous anastomosis, then a prosthetic loop graft may be used. These are most commonly used in the thigh. Graft thrombosis, aneurysm formation, and bleeding may occur.

Peritoneal dialysis access

Technique

As for hemodialysis access, catheters for PD may be intended for short- or longer-term use. The latter are usually cuffed and tunnelled to an abdominal wall exit site. There are three broad techniques for insertion:
- Closed (percutaneous)
- Open (minilaparotomy)
- Laparoscopic/laparoscopic assisted

The principles of the open and laparoscopic techniques are broadly similar but differ in terms of catheter fixation. This will be discussed later. In the setting of acute renal failure in a sick child, a catheter can be placed on the ward under sedation using local anesthesia. A needle puncture is made into the peritoneum (aspirating to ensure no visceral injury has occurred) in a similar way to the passage of a Verres needle for laparoscopic surgery, and a guidewire passed. After dilatation of the tract, the catheter is passed into the abdomen and flushed to ensure adequate influx and efflux of dialysate. PD may be commenced immediately. It is possible to tunnel the line if desired, but the usual indication for the percutaneous technique is for acute, short-term PD.

The open and laparoscopic techniques require general anesthesia. In the open approach, a small incision is made above the umbilicus, and the catheter placed into the pelvis. Many surgeons choose to perform an omentectomy to lower the potential risk of catheter entrapment and failure of dialysis. The abdomen is closed and the catheter tunnelled in a gentle curve to a suitable site on the abdominal wall. Again, as the preferred site for placing a transplant is in the right iliac fossa, it is usual to tunnel the PD catheter to the left iliac fossa.

The laparoscopic approach uses one or more ports to place the PD catheter, again with or without an omentectomy. At the author's unit, we prefer the laparoscopic-assisted approach described by Najmaldin [9]. The essence of the operation is a single supraumbilical incision, through which an omentectomy can be performed (in children the greater omentum tends to be flimsy and easy to manipulate through a very small hole), and a laparoscope is inserted. A needle and guidewire is then introduced to create a long extraperitoneal tunnel, through which a peel-away sheath is passed. The PD catheter is then seen to pass under direct vision into the true pelvis, fixed by a long extraperitoneal tunnel to avoid flipping (Figure 31.2). The catheter can then be tunnelled in the usual way, and the laparoscope port closed. PD catheters are available in a variety of configuration. We have used coiled double-cuffed tubes of which a variety of sizes are available, including very small tubes suitable for neonatal use (Figure 31.3).

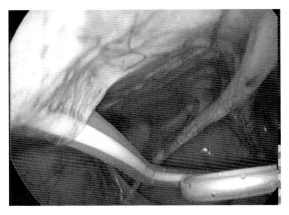

Figure 31.2 Intraoperative view of peritoneal dialysis catheter, showing position of coil, and fixation by extraperitoneal tunnel.

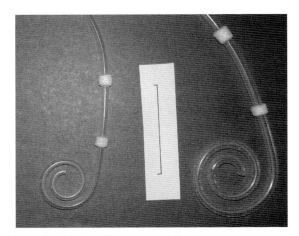

Figure 31.3 Coiled PD catheters suitable for neonatal use. Marker shows 5 cm.

Outcome

Dialysis can generally be commenced on the same day as operation if desired. This is useful for PD in acute renal failure, or the rapid establishment of PD in a child who becomes dialysis-dependant quicker than anticipated. Catheters used early (within days) tend to have more mechanical problems of which leak is the most important [10–12]. While the literature describes problems in the PD population in a variety of ways (percentage of patient population, catheter time, etc.), on average the frequency of problems with PD seems to be of the order of one episode per 6 "PD-months" [13]. Peritonitis, exit site and tunnel infections, and catheter occlusion make up the majority of the problems. Catheter survival is of the order of 80% at 12 months, 60% at 24 months, and 35% at 48 months [13,14]. Younger children (less than 2 years old) have increased risk of catheter removal for problems [14].

Complications

The presence of adhesions complicating previous surgery may make PD ineffective or impossible. Nonetheless, previous surgery is not necessarily a contraindication to PD. Bleeding or infection may occur early. Leak of dialysate may be seen early, and may necessitate suspension of PD. One innovative solution to dialysate leak has been the use of fibrin glue [15], although this is not widespread. Exit site infection or wound infection likewise may be seen early. PD peritonitis, characterized by cloudy (or fibrinous) PD effluent, pain, and fever may occur at any stage, and according to culture may or may not be rescuable with antimicrobials. Presentation with an acute abdomen can complicate PD, and sometimes the differentials (including acute appendicitis) can be difficult to exclude.

Dialysis (clearance) may become ineffective, reflecting peritoneal failure, or the child may have symptoms or fail to drain in or out. Fibrin sheath formation can occur causing a flap-valve effect. The tip of the PD catheter can migrate, or become entangled with intestine and omentum (if not excised) [13]. Occasionally, the subcutaneous cuff can erode through the skin.

Preventing and managing complications

Bleeding should be manageable by local control. One exception to this is the rare occurrence of visceral or blood vessel injury arising from closed technique puncture of the peritoneal cavity. Surgical exploration is mandatory if there is a suspected intra-abdominal injury. It is important to ensure that the field is relatively bloodless: clots may occlude the PD catheter and interfere with dialysis. Care needs to be taken when tunnelling the catheter, to ensure that the tube remains in the fat plane and does not transgress muscle. Laparoscopy has the advantage of allowing a thorough peritoneal inspection after the catheter has been inserted. Bleeding of sufficient magnitude to need re-exploration should be rare.

At our institution, we have always undertaken omentectomy. There is evidence regarding its efficacy [16], but in children, the greater omentum's mobility and flimsiness makes its removal a sensible step to obviate the risk of tube entanglement.

Dialysate leak is eminently manageable by lowering exchange volume, or suspending PD temporarily. A small volume leak may be inconsequential, especially if PD is crucial because of uremia or hyperkalemia. Our early experience mirrors that of others [17]: PD can be commenced satisfactorily within hours of insertion, rather than the traditional approach of allowing the catheter to "rest" for days.

Exit site, wound infection, or PD peritonitis should be managed conservatively in the first instance, according to culture. Intraperitoneal heparin is sometimes useful if the effluent is fibrinous. Rarely, fibrinolytics (e.g. urokinase) may be used. One important culture is fungal. Almost without exception, a PD catheter must be removed in the presence of fungal infection: even prolonged antifungal treatment is very unlikely to clear the organism. Likewise, recurrent bacterial infection may indicate revision of the catheter. Ideally, if a PD catheter is removed as a consequence of infection, it is prudent to wait a number of weeks prior to reinsertion.

Clarifying tube position, and fixation is one real advantage of the laparoscopic-assisted approach. It allows a thorough inspection of the peritoneum, and adhesiolysis if needs be, and the long extraperitoneal tunnel makes tip migration unlikely. It allows very accurate position, under direct vision, of the tip of the catheter in the true pelvis.

If PD becomes ineffective, or inflow and outflow are poor or symptomatic, a plain radiograph reveals the orientation and tip position. A contrast study may be helpful in demonstrating free flow (if a fibrin sheath or loculation is suspected). If the catheter has migrated or flipped out of the pelvis, under fluoroscopy the PD catheter can be manipulated by means of a guidewire. An unwell child, or one with abdominal symptoms and signs particularly those of intestinal obstruction, might indicate the presence of encapsulating sclerosing peritonitis. This can occur even after the removal of the PD catheter, and can be associated with significant morbidity of mortality [18].

Laparoscopic exploration of a malfunctioning catheter can be helpful [19], certainly if there is no associated infection. The tube can be released if it has become entangled or encased with fibrin. If excessively mobile, it can be looped within a suture placed at the dome of the bladder to further fix the tube (we have not seen this in laparoscopically placed tubes on account of the fixation afforded by the extraperitoneal tunnel). If the catheter requires revision with a new catheter, it is straightforward to use the peel-away Seldinger technique to create a new extraperitoneal tunnel.

Extrusion of the cuff is uncommon, but may be expected if the cuff is at the exit site, or if the tract is just under the skin rather than in the fat plane (or if the fat plane is attenuated, as in a neonate). Occasionally, chronic infection is seen in association with the cuff, rarely overgranulation or a pyogenic granuloma. A conservative approach to preserve the tube is to shave the cuff down to the level of tube (done simply with a regular blade) although there is a risk of tube puncture. If the symptoms associated with the cuff are refractory, or the tube is breached, a revision is required.

Conclusion

While the gold standard of renal replacement therapy is a successful kidney transplant, dialysis is an important mode of therapy, particularly in very small infants in whom a decision has been made to treat but renal replacement is required in the workup to transplantation. Many families opt for PD, and preservation of vascular access is one advantage *en passant* since these patients will almost inevitably require more intervention later in life. Nonetheless, dialysis is limited by peritoneal failure and by loss of central veins. The concept of "end-stage access" is very real and a cause of significant morbidity, or death. This is a major driving force toward early transplantation.

References

1 Goldfarb-Rumyantzev AS, Hurdle JF, Scandling JD *et al.* The role of pretransplantation renal replacement therapy modality in kidney allograft and recipient survival. *Am J Kidney Dis* 2005;46:537–49.
2 Oguzkurt L, Tercan F, Kara G *et al.* US-guided placement of temporary internal jugular vein catheters: Immediate

technical success and complications in normal and high-risk patients. *Eur J Radiol* 2005;55:125–9.

3 Kairaitis LK, Gottlieb T. Outcome and complications of temporary haemodialysis catheters. *Nephrol Dial Transplant* 1999;14:1710–4.

4 National Institute for Clinical Excellence. Final Appraisal Determination. Ultrasound locating devices for placing central venous catheters. *NICE guidelines*, August 2002. Available at www.nice.org.uk.

5 Everdell NL, Coulthard MG, Crosier J, Keir MJ. A machine for haemodialysing very small infants. *Pediatr Nephrol* 2005;20:636–43.

6 Bambauer R, Inniger R, Pirrung KJ *et al.* Complications and side effects associated with large-bore catheters in the subclavian and internal jugular veins. *Artif Organs* 1994;18:318–21.

7 Kovalik EC, Newman GE, Suhooki P *et al.* Correction of central venous stenosis: Use of angioplasty and vascular wall stents. *Kidney Int* 1994;45:1177–81.

8 Schillinger F, Schillinger G, Montagnac R *et al.* Stenosis veinuses centrales en hemodialyse: Etude angiographique comparative des acces soud-claviers et jugulaires internes. *Nephrologie* 1994;15:129–31.

9 Najmaldin A. Insertion of peritoneal dialysis catheter. In *Operative Endoscopy and Endoscopic Surgery in Infants and Children,* Edited by A Najmaldin, S Rothenburg, DC Crabbe, S Beasley. Hodder Arnold, London, 2005: Vol. 57, pp. 395–400.

10 Povlsen JV, Ivarsen P. How to start the late referred ESRD patient urgently on chronic APD. *Nephrol Dial Transplant* 2006;21:1156–9.

11 Donmez O, Durmaz O, Ediz B *et al.* Catheter-related complications in children on chronic peritoneal dialysis. *Adv Perit Dial* 2005;21:200–03.

12 Rahim KA, Seidel K, McDonald RA. Risk factors for catheter-related complications in pediatric peritoneal dialysis. *Pediatr Nephrol* 2004;19:1021–8.

13 Macchini F, Valade A, Ardissino G *et al.* Chronic peritoneal dialysis in children: Catheter related complications. A single centre experience. *Pediatr Surg Int* 2006;22:524–8.

14 Rinaldi S, Sera F, Verrina E *et al.* Chronic peritoneal dialysis catheters in children: A fifteen-year experience of the Italian Registry of Pediatric Chronic Peritoneal Dialysis. *Perit Dial Int* 2004;24:481–6.

15 Rusthoven E, van de Kar NA, Monnens LA, Schroder CH. Fibrin glue used successfully in peritoneal dialysis catheter leakage in children. *Perit Dial Int* 2004;24:287–9.

16 Nicholson ML, Veitch PS, Donnelly PK *et al.* Factors influencing peritoneal catheter survival in continuous ambulatory peritoneal dialysis. *Ann R Coll Surg Engl* 1990;72:368–72.

17 Williams AR, Hughes JMF, Lee ACH *et al.* Laparoscopic-assisted placement of peritoneal dialysis catheters: experience of a novel technique. *Arch Dis Child* 2003;88:A72.

18 Kawanishi H, Watanabe H, Moriishi M, Tsuchiya S. Successful surgical management of encapsulating peritoneal sclerosis. *Perit Dial Int* 2005;25:S39–S47.

19 Jwo SC, Chen KS, Lin YY. Video-assisted laparoscopic procedures in peritoneal dialysis. *Surg Endosc* 2003;17:1666–70.

Kidney Transplantation

Alun Williams

Key points

- Transplantation is the gold standard management of end-stage kidney disease.

- Pre-emptive transplantation is preferable: avoiding dialysis preserves access sites and may prolong graft life.

- Uropathies are disproportionally represented in the etiology of pediatric end-stage kidney disease. Pretransplant urological workup is therefore mandatory.

- Living donor kidneys are preferable.

- An abnormal urinary tract demands vigilance, but can be a safe means of drainage.

- Nonadherance with medication is commonplace and contributes to graft failure: transition to adult care needs attention.

Introduction

A successful kidney transplant is the gold standard renal replacement therapy independent of age. Although over time there has been a trend toward longer graft survival [1], a child who receives a transplant will almost inevitably require further renal replacement in due course. This is an important factor in timing a transplant in childhood. Pre-emptive transplantation is the counsel of perfection: avoiding dialysis may confer a survival benefit to the graft [2,3], preserves access sites for dialysis, and if native function can be preserved to some extent can avoid metabolic, biochemical, and fluid balance problems, and psychosocial issues associated with chronic hospitalization. At present between 20% and 30% on average children receive a pre-emptive kidney transplant in the United Kingdom and North America [4].

There is inevitably a period of medical and surgical workup before transplantation, and these issues (including HLA matching, virological and immunization protocols) are reviewed extensively elsewhere [5–10].

Uropathies constitute up to 20% of the pediatric kidney transplant population [1] in sharp contrast to adult programs, and peritransplant urological issues are considered later in the chapter. Kidneys are sourced from deceased and living donors. The latter is an increasing pool, particularly for the pediatric recipient where a donor is commonly a parent. Live donor programs introduce an additional element to work up in that stringent donor workup is necessary to ensure fitness for donation and assess in detail vascular anatomy. Organ allocation systems tend to prioritize children [1,11]. The median wait on the deceased donor list for a kidney in the United Kingdom in 2003 (all ages up to 18) was 164 days [11], and in the USA for the same period [1] was 360, 430, and 569 days (ages 1–5 years, 6–10 years, and 11–17 years, respectively).

After a thorough medical, surgical, and psychological workup, children enter either or both living donor or deceased donor transplant programs.

Urological workup of the recipient

The effect of an abnormal lower urinary tract on the kidneys is well recognized, and to assess the potential effect of the lower tract on a transplanted kidney, some

Pediatric Urology: Surgical Complications and Management. Edited by Duncan T. Wilcox, Prasad P. Godbole and Martin A. Koyle.
© 2008 Blackwell Publishing, ISBN: 978-1-4051-6268-5.

baseline information is mandatory. A "safe" bladder can be regarded as one that fills and stores at low pressure, and can be emptied at will. A "safe" bladder pressure has been variously defined, but on its original description represents a leak point pressure of <40 cm water [12]. There is evidence to suggest that 30 cm might represent a more "normal" value in childhood [13]. Drainage is preferably to completion, to lower the risk of infection in a residual volume of urine. Urodynamic studies are vital to demonstrate the bladder characteristics in children with uropathies. With the addition of radiographic screening (video-urodynamics), the presence of vesico-ureteric reflux (VUR) can be assessed. Appropriate measures to lower pressure, correct reflux if necessary and provide capacity and drainage can be instituted according to the urodynamic findings.

Several studies have demonstrated that transplantation into an abnormal urinary tract is safe if appropriate follow-up is in place, and is likewise safe into a reconstructed urinary tract [14–20]. It is generally accepted that pretransplant surgery is preferable to obviate the potential influence of immunosuppression in infection and healing. Some authors have commented that a dry augmented bladder can be problematic, and that major surgery in severely compromised renal function can precipitate end stage [21]. Although post-transplant urinary reconstruction is feasible and safe, logic dictates however that it is probably safer to transplant into a urinary tract that has been made "safe" beforehand.

VUR and transplantation have undergone a resurgence of interest in recent years. Certainly, VUR is a risk factor for urinary tract infection (UTI) which is the single commonest infectious complication following a kidney transplant, commoner still in those transplanted because of an underlying uropathy [22]. Many children will have had antireflux surgery of their native urinary tract before transplantation. Consideration should be given to pretransplant treatment for VUR if recurrent UTI is a problem. Also the effect of high-grade VUR should be borne in mind when interpreting urodynamics: much of the capacity may well be taken up into the upper tracts. Circumcision should also be borne in mind in boys with recurrent UTI [23].

Technique

There is some evidence to suggest that pediatric recipients fare better with pediatric donor kidneys [24]. Live donor kidneys undoubtedly fare better. Whether there

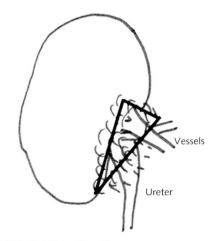

Figure 32.1 Forbidden dissection.

is any difference in outcome between laparoscopically retrieved kidneys or otherwise remains to be seen in the long term, although early to medium term results are equivalent [1]. The remainder of this section assumes that a donor kidney has been retrieved and is potentially usable.

The kidney is prepared on the backbench before induction of anesthesia to the recipient, to ensure that the organ is usable. The vessels are dissected toward (but not into) the renal hilum, taking care to preserve perinephric tissue associated with ureter (the so-called golden triangle shown schematically in Figure 32.1). Multiple vessels need to be given particular attention, as there may be an increased risk of thrombosis, although one multivariate analysis implicates donor atheroma as a risk factor, rather than multiple vessels *per se*, and that reconstruction does not necessarily disadvantage the graft [25,26]. Lower pole arteries are important to preserve because of the inevitable supply they give the transplant ureter. Small upper polar vessels can be tied safely. Where multiple vessels have been retrieved on a common vessel patch (Carrell patch), this can be used for the donor–recipient anastomosis, or the donor vessels anastomosed back-to-back or end-to-side (Figure 32.2) in a common anastomosis with the recipient vessel. It may be more convenient to do separate anastomoses of multiple vessels (e.g. using an inferior epigastric or internal iliac vessel), although this reintroduces the risk of thrombosis. For the venous drainage, a single large donor renal vein is sufficient, and accessory veins may be tied safely. However, vascular reconstruction of the renal veins is reasonable if circumstances dictate.

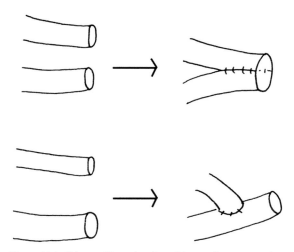

Figure 32.2 Side-to-side and end-to-side vessel reconstruction.

It is common practice to take a biopsy from the kidney pre-implantation. This can be helpful in establishing a baseline histological appearance, particularly if there is any concern over donor vascular disease.

The recipient undergoes general anesthesia and has a central venous line and urinary catheter placed. Induction antibiotics, immunosuppressive agents and steroids may be given at this point. Antibody induction agents, if used, are usually given before transfer to the operating theater. There has been a tendency to increased use of antibody induction agents over the last few years, as evidenced by the recent NAPRTCS review [1].

The choice of incision and approach for kidney transplantation is largely a matter of choice and experience. It has been commonplace to use a curved iliac fossa incision (modified Rutherford Morrison), approaching the iliac vessels in an extraperitoneal way. This is especially useful if the recipient is on peritoneal dialysis, since in the event of delayed graft function (DGF), dialysis can be continued. According to the habitus of the child, the incision can be elevated into a "hockey stick." Some surgeons prefer a transperitoneal approach, via a midline incision, in infants. This affords space, but has the potential disadvantage of transgressing peritoneum and can make subsequent access to the graft (e.g. for biopsy) difficult. In an extraperitoneal approach, the abdominal wall muscles may be cut, or mobilized in the pararectal plane, which we have found gives very good access to the retroperitoneum. The inferior epigastric pedicle is identified, and if it is not required for vascular anastomosis, is tied and divided. The spermatic cord in boys must be identified, preserved, and

retracted. The round ligament in girls can be divided. In the transperitoneal approach, the right colon and terminal ileum are mobilized to give access to the inferior vena cava inferior vena cava (IVC) and aorta. A retraction device such as an Omnitract can be useful. In small children, a competent assistant is just as effective, however.

In infants and small children (up to approximately 20 kg), the aorta and inferior vena cava are the preferred recipient vessels for anastomosis, and provide high-flow conduits. The common iliac veins are often of adequate caliber, the vein being the larger vessel. For ease of operation, the arterial and venous anastomoses are usually separated by a centimeter or two.

In recipients with vascular anomalies, or thrombosed venous drainage, the surgeon may need to be creative. A good "road map" of potential anastomotic sites is useful, and in the author's unit we have mandated that all recipients with previous "instrumentation" of the lower-body circulation (lines, nephrectomy, etc.) have detailed vascular imaging. Doppler ultrasound is straightforward and relatively noninvasive. Reconstructed computed tomography (CT) is useful but has a radiation dose, and can require contrast which might affect native renal function. Experience with magnetic resonance is evolving. However, we have found, anecdotally, that where venous drainage is adequate (whether through native "anatomical" vena cava or via collaterals) the transplant renal vein drains adequately. Small published series have articulated these issues [27,28]. Prothrombotic states, or concerns of caval thrombosis, might make postoperative anticoagulation advisable.

Vascular anastomosis is achieved using a continuous 5/0 or 6/0 nonabsorbable monofilament, taking care not to take the "back wall" of the recipient vessel inadvertently. It is useful to place curved bulldog-type clamps to the donor renal vessels to test the vascular anastomoses for leaks and then repair before reperfusing the kidney. At the time of arterial anastomosis we give a bolus of mannitol and frusemide. The warm ischemic time for the kidney is noted when the clamps are released. It is important to note the characteristics of reperfusion (uniform/patchy/absent), and whether or not urine is seen from the open distal end of the graft's ureter. Bleeding, not detected at the time of "anastomotic test," can be investigated and dealt with at this point.

The commonest mode of urinary drainage is to transplant ureter to native bladder (ureteroneocystostomy, UNC). Running in an irrigant through the bladder catheter is useful to distend the bladder to make it more easily identified, and additional reassurance can be sought

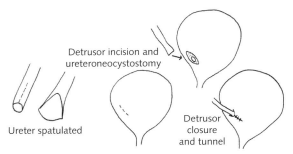

Figure 32.3 External ureteroneocystostomy.

Table 32.1 Graft survival (%) at 1, 3, and 5 years post-transplant according to year of transplant and organ source.

Cohort	Years post-transplant		
	1 (%)	3 (%)	5 (%)
LD 1987–1995	91	85	79
LD 1996–2005	95	90	85
DD 1987–1995	81	70	62
DD 1996–2005	93	84	77

LD, live donor; DD, deceased donor.
Source: NAPRTCS Annual Report 2006 [1].

by the use of dilute methylene blue. Particular care is needed in patients on peritoneal dialysis. The peritoneum is often very thick, there is often clear fluid within, and distinguishing this from a urinary bladder needs care. There are many ways to perform UNC: extra- or intravesical, stented, or unstented [29–31]. Our unit's preference is an extravesical anastomosis with a spatulated distal ureter, with reconstitution of a short detrusor tunnel over the UNC (Figure 32.3). The use of a stent is debatable, but wound drainage advisable.

If the native ipsilateral ureter is easy to identify, or the bladder is hard to distend or mobilize, a ureteroureterostomy may be used. Transplant ureters can be implanted safely into augmented or substituted systems, or into urinary diversions, although the risk of leak is higher [14–20,32].

After hemostasis has been assured, the wound is closed according to the surgeon's preference. Occasionally, especially in very small infants, the abdominal wall can be difficult to close primarily without raising concerns for the transplant's blood supply. In these children, it is reasonable to return after a few days for secondary closure of the abdominal wall (having closed the skin at the first operation). Some experience is evolving with prosthetic patches at primary closure [33].

Adequate maintenance of the recipient's central venous pressure and blood pressure makes high dependency or intensive care mandatory. Hypovolemia and hypotension are risk factors for thrombosis and DGF. Hypovolemia and prolonged operative time have also been shown to be independent risk factors for "slow" graft function, represented by slower than expected fall in creatinine post-transplant [34].

Subsequent recipient management, including immunosuppression, antibiotics, fluids and feeds are very individualized to units, and probably best managed on a protocol basis according to local preferences.

Outcome

Up to 95% of grafts function at one-year post-transplant: living donor kidneys have marginally better survival than deceased donor organs at one year, a difference that increases as time progresses [1]. Graft survival has been poorer in the under-fives, with a plateau into the early teens, thereafter falling until the early twenties [35]. Overall, there has been a trend to increasing graft survival over successive five-year cohorts. These are precised in Table 32.1.

In the 2006 NAPRTCS review [1], 2.6% of grafts had primary nonfunction DGF (or ATN – acute tubular necrosis as defined by NAPRTCS), which specifies the need for dialysis within the first week post-transplant. There was a sharp difference noted in DGF when comparing living donor (5.2%) and deceased donor (17%) kidneys. DGF impacts adversely on graft longevity.

Up to 50% of graft failure is accounted for by rejection. Acute rejection was reported to account for 12.9% graft failure in the 2006 NAPRTCS review. Again, there has been an improvement in probability of first acute rejection by year since the late 1980s, data shown in Table 32.2. Chronic allograft nephropathy (CAN) is a diverse collection of conditions, some of which are immunological, some drug-related, which requires monitoring when a "creeping creatinine" is noticed. Modulating the immunosuppressive regimen is useful, such as withdrawing calcineurin inhibitors, can be useful.

Kidney recipients with underlying uropathies seem to fare as well, in general, as those without. A recent survey of units in the United Kingdom [36] returned a cohort of 74 children (a total of 78 transplanted kidneys) with a spectrum of underlying urological abnormalities (the

Table 32.2 Twelve-month probability of first rejection by transplant year.

	Live donor (%)	Deceased donor (%)
1987–1990	54	69
1995–1998	33	41
2003–2005	13	16

Source: NAPRTCS Annual Report 2006 [1].

largest group being 39 boys with posterior urethral valves – PUVs) with a median follow-up of 36 months. Eleven were transplanted into a cystoplasty, 4 into a urinary diversion. Intermittent catheterization in 26 was via a Mitrofanoff stoma in 14. Three grafts were lost early to thrombosis, four lost later predominantly because of nonadherance to medicines. There were three ureteric complications (4%). Of 57 grafts that could be followed, 25/57 had recurrent UTI (44%). Thirty-nine of 57 had stable function (68%); of the 18 deteriorating grafts, 15/18 were in boys with PUV. The cause of graft deterioration in PUV children was multifactorial, although the survey highlighted the importance of pretransplant urodynamics in this group, as 9/39 boys with PUV had not had urodynamics. It is unlikely that any single factor can be amended to avoid graft failure in boys with PUV, although one study suggests that more conservative initial management of the boys with PUV as opposed to aggressive surgical intervention might be beneficial in terms of graft function [37].

A peculiarity of pediatric transplantation (in common with pediatric practice in most patients with chronic disease) is transition into adult medical care. Graft longevity has been observed to drop during adolescence [35], and there is common consensus that transition is, at best, a difficult time [38].

Complications

Bleeding is usually an immediate or early event. Vascular thrombosis occurs in up to 12% of recipients [39]. Although thrombosis can be immediate, it may manifest after several days, with nonfunction, no urine output, or graft tenderness, pain, and fever. Occasionally, a venous thrombosis can present very dramatically with a graft rupture and torrential hemorrhage. Urgent assessment of graft perfusion (with Doppler ultrasound and/or

isotope renography, e.g. MAG3) is mandatory if a vascular event is suspected. Later on in the postoperative course, stenosis of the renal artery can occur giving deterioration in graft function, and usually hypertension. Immediate immunological complications (such as hyperacute or early acute rejection) are thankfully fairly rare with detailed immunological pretransplant workup, modern donor–recipient matching, and evolving immunosuppression regimens.

Ureteric complications occur in up to 10% of transplants [40–42]. Urinary leak may present early, with increasing or prolonged wound drainage, or swelling around the graft. It can be sufficient to cause obstruction (urinary and vascular: to the graft and ipsilateral leg). Lymphocele can also present thus, and ultrasound is a useful way of imaging. Ureteric stenosis may manifest as deteriorating graft function secondary to obstruction, and a hydronephrosis may be apparent. In one series of modified Lich-Gregoir ureteric implantation [41], 1% had obstruction at the level of the UNC, responding well to stenting for several weeks. In one series of ureteroureteric anastomoses [42], 8.4% had a ureteric complication (14/166). Ultrasound, excretion renography, or even antegrade pyelogram may be useful in the diagnosis of ureteric stricture. Reflux into the graft may manifest as dilatation, or progressive scarring and deteriorating function if associated with UTI. Stones may occur in the graft. Particular note need to be taken if a ureter has been stented, to ensure its timely removal: retained stents may become encrusted.

Infection is common in a transplant recipient, and UTI is particularly common. In uropaths, urinary prophylaxis is a reasonable step because of this. Other infections as a consequence of immunosuppression demand vigilance.

Although immediate immunological events are uncommon, acute rejection is common, with a fine balance to be made between the risk of this and the risk of overimmunosuppression. The diagnostic gold standard is transplant biopsy, but frequently in pediatric practice, an empirical course of high-dose steroids is often given for a deterioration in graft function.

Gradual deterioration in the graft is again common, but multifactorial, encompassing the diagnostic potpourri that is CAN. Calcineurin inhibitors are well-recognized culprits, and careful thought needs to be given to ongoing immunosuppression in CAN. Recurrent UTI and lower urinary tract dysfunction are important to consider: this is the reason all children with urological antecedents must undergo urodynamics as a pretransplant baseline to document the "safety" of a recipient's bladder [36]. One of the biggest challenges in pediatric transplantation is the issue of nonadherance with medication.

Preventing and managing complications

As with all vascular anastomoses, technical problems with the anastomosis are the commonest cause of failure. Positioning the recipient arteriotomy and venotomy to allow comfortable anastomoses and allow the kidney the "sit" comfortably are important. "Fresh" vessel ends are important to avoid inclusion of adventitia within an anastomosis, and to avoid an intimal flap. Postoperative anticoagulation may be considered on the basis of a pre-existing prothrombotic state, if multiple vessels are present or if there has been perioperative hypotension. One recent report suggests that graft thrombosis might be prevented to a degree by the administration of interleukin-2 antagonists [43].

Ongoing bleeding after implantation requires re-exploration. Missed hilar vessels during bench preparation are common culprits and can be tied once identified. Loss of perfusion of a transplant kidney may be undetected for hours, although a sudden loss of urine output, or an acutely tender, swollen graft should alert to the possibility. Imaging may be helpful, but a vascular catastrophe requires re-exploration. Thrombectomy can be attempted but seldom seems to salvage the situation. Later deterioration in graft function (usually associated with hypertension) can be due to renal artery stenosis, which is usually just distal to the anastomosis. Interventional radiology with balloon dilatation is probably the method of choice in its management.

Lymphocele can manifest by prolonged wound drainage, perigraft or leg swelling, or deterioration in graft function. Small (or asymptomatic) lymphoceles can be managed expectantly. Symptomatic lymphoceles require drainage, either percutaneously, or fenestration into the peritoneum. Meticulous vascular dissection during preparation of the recipient vessels is to be commended to lower the risk of lymphocele.

Ureteric complications are usually a consequence of ischemia of the transplant ureter. Attention to the "golden triangle" of the ureter's blood supply, during bench preparation of the kidney, has been described earlier, and at the time of UNC it is useful to demonstrate an active blood supply to the cut end of the transplant ureter. Diathermy should be used sparingly and with caution.

An early ureteric leak may manifest as wound drainage: the drain effluent should be analyzed to determine whether it is urine or serum (lymph). Adequate bladder drainage must be ensured, especially in small infants, and some early leaks can reasonably be watched for a day or two, as they may settle. The use of stents is debatable, and studies demonstrate advantages to both stenting and not stenting [29,30]. One factor in pediatric transplantation that may be important as a decision-maker is that a child almost certainly requires a general anesthetic for removal of a stent. The author's preference is an unstented UNC.

A ureteric leak may be managed by early re-exploration or by temporizing transplant nephrostomy and later planned exploration. The latter demands dissection through scarred tissue which in itself can be hazardous to the blood supply of the kidney. If there is sufficient viable donor ureter, a redo UNC can be fashioned. If there is not sufficient viable ureter, the recipient native ureter can be used in the form of a ureteropyelostomy or ureteroureterostomy. With a capacious recipient bladder, a lateral bladder flap can be tubularized (Boari), or elevated to anastomose onto the transplant pelvis or ureter (similar in principle to the "bladder elongation psoas hitch" procedure [44]). Rarely an enteric interposition is required, or drainage into a cutaneous stoma.

Ureteric stenosis is again usually an ischemic phenomenon, although may present later in the post-transplant course. Stenting is a good option, although balloon dilatation has been reported with success [45]. Obstruction or stenosis refractory to stenting or dilatation requires revision as described earlier, or recourse to long-term stenting with intermittent stent changes.

Late operation for a ureteric complication is often difficult and hazardous, as the allograft becomes encased in scar tissue.

Urinary infection is an important early problem with pediatric transplant recipients, particularly those with underlying uropathies, and strategies for the management of VUR in the native urinary tract have been outlined earlier in the chapter. There has been interest in graft VUR and its effect. One report, using baseline DMSA imaging establishes a strong link between VUR, infection, and the acquisition of graft scars, and recommends initial UTI prophylaxis as well as vigilance for UTI [46]. Another suggestion of this study is antireflux urinary drainage. Many surgeons perform a modified Lich-Gregoir UNC as stated earlier. A traditional antireflux approach is the Leadbetter-Politano ureteric implantation, although this has been reported to have a higher incidence of ureteric complications [40], as well as the potential effects of an open bladder procedure. Uretero-ureterostomy is a potential consideration if the native ureters do not reflux. A potential "minimally invasive" approach mirroring that of native VUR is subureteric injection (commonly now with dextranomer/hyaluronic acid copolymer). Anecdotally this has been a valuable approach although obstruction and graft dysfunction have been reported, mandating caution [47].

Post-transplant care is as much multidisciplinary as that of pretransplant. Longer term sequelae of immunosuppression such as infection and malignancy, CAN, disease recurrence in an allograft, blood pressure control, lipid and glucose control, etc. require close collaboration between nephrologists, pediatricians, pathologists, radiologists, and other allied professionals. Fundamental to pediatric practice is nutrition, growth, and development, which are paramount to pre- and post-transplant management. Some of these long-term issues, and others including quality of life, have been reviewed elsewhere [10].

Conclusion

Although a successful kidney transplant is the pinnacle of end-stage renal disease management, it remains merely a treatment rather than a cure. Graft survival is poorer at the "extremes of childhood" as well as the extremes of life, and the causes are multifactorial. Although the uropathies are represented disproportionally in the etiology of pediatric renal failure, graft outcome overall is as good in this group, although particular attention is required in their pretransplant workup. Attention to detail in the operative procedure is a *sine qua non*. Transition into the adult services can be a trying time for patients and clinicians, and mandates particular vigilance of graft function. The transplanted child, with our current techniques of renal replacement therapy, becomes an adult who will require further renal replacement. Pre-emptive transplantation preserves venous access sites and probably allows for improved graft survival. Living donor kidneys currently have better outcomes than those from deceased donor kidneys. Therefore the "gold" standard for renal replacement in childhood should be a pre-emptive live donor kidney transplant.

References

1 NAPRTCS Annual Report 2006. Available at http://www.naprtcs.org accessed on 23.02.2008.

2 Mahmoud A, Said MH, Dawahra M *et al*. Outcome of preemptive renal transplantation and pretransplantation dialysis in children. *Pediatr Nephrol* 1997;11:537–41.

3 Ishitani M, Isaacs R, Norwood V *et al*. Predictors of graft survival in pediatric living-related kidney transplant recipients. *Transplantation* 2000;70:288–92.

4 Vats AN, Donaldson L, Fine RN, Chavers BM. Pretransplant dialysis status and outcome of renal transplantation in North American children: A NAPRTCS study. *Transplantation* 2000;69:1414–19.

5 Bartosh SM. Donor and recipient characteristics. In *Pediatric Solid Organ Transplantation*. Edited by AH Tejani, WE Harmon, RN Fine. Copenhagen: Munksgaard, 2000: pp. 153–62.

6 Thomas SE, Bunchman TE. Donor and recipient evaluation. In *Pediatric Solid Organ Transplantation*. Edited by AH Tejani, WE Harmon, RN Fine. Copenhagen: Munksgaard, 2000: pp. 163–75.

7 Papalois VE, Najarian JS. Surgical technique and management. In *Pediatric Solid Organ Transplantation*. Edited by AH Tejani, WE Harmon, RN Fine. Copenhagen: Munksgaard, 2000: pp. 176–85.

8 Sheldon CA. Pediatric renal transplantation: Surgical considerations. In *Pediatric Urology*. Edited by JP Gearhart, RC Rink, PDE Mouriquand. Philadelphia: WB Saunders, 2001: pp. 801–27.

9 Dharamsi N, Sheldon C, Goebel J. Renal transplantation. In *Clinical Pediatric Urology*. Edited by SG Docimo, DA Canning, AE Khoury. London: Informa, 2007: pp. 367–86.

10 Alonso MH, Tiao G, Ryckman FC. Renal failure and transplantation. In *Pediatric Surgery and Urology, Long-Term Outcomes*. Edited by MD Stringer, KT Oldham, PDE Mouriquand. Cambridge University Press, Cambridge, 2006: pp. 845–57.

11 UK Transplant. http://www.uktransplant.org.uk accessed on 23.02.2008.

12 McGuire EJ, Woodside JR, Borden TA, Weiss RM. Prognostic value of urodynamic testing in myelodysplastic patients. *J Urol* 1981;126:205–9.

13 Houle AM, Gilmour RF, Churchill BM *et al*. What volume can a child normally store in the bladder at a safe pressure? *J Urol* 1993;149:561–4.

14 Rigamonti W, Capizzi A, Zacchello G *et al*. Kidney transplantation into bladder augmentation or urinary diversion: Long-term results. *Transplantation* 2005;80:1435–40.

15 Mendizabal S, Estornell F, Zamora I *et al*. Renal transplantation in children with severe bladder dysfunction. *J Urol* 2005;173:226–9.

16 Ali-El-Dein B, Abol-Enein H, El-Husseini A *et al*. Renal transplantation in children with abnormal lower urinary tract. *Transplant Proc* 2004;36:2968–73.

17 Adams J, Mehls O, Wiesel M. Pediatric renal transplantation and the dysfunctional bladder. *Transpl Int* 2004;17:596–602.

18 Neild GH, Dakmish A, Wood S *et al*. Renal transplantation in adults with abnormal bladders. *Transplantation* 2004;77:1123–7.

19 Luke PP, Herz DB, Bellinger MF *et al*. Long-term results of pediatric renal transplantation into a dysfunctional lower urinary tract. *Transplantation* 2003;76:1578–82.

20 Crowe A, Cairns HS, Wood S *et al*. Renal transplantation following renal failure due to urological disorders. *Nephrol Dial Transplant* 1998;13:2065–9.

21 Alfrey EJ, Salvatierra O, Tanney DC et al. Bladder augmentation can be problematic with renal failure and transplantation. *Pediatr Nephrol* 1997;11:672–5.

22 John U, Everding AS, Kuwertz-Broking E et al. High prevalence of febrile urinary tract infections after paediatric renal transplantation. *Nephrol Dial Transplant* 2006;21:3269–74.

23 Singh-Grewal D, Macdessi J, Craig J. Circumcision for the prevention of urinary tract infection in boys: A systematic review of randomised trials and observational studies. *Arch Dis Child* 2005;90:853–8.

24 Pape L, Hoppe J, Becker T et al. Superior long-term graft function and better growth of grafts in children receiving kidneys from paediatric compared with adult donors. *Nephrol Dial Transplant* 2006;21:2596–600.

25 Sanni A, Wilson CH, Wyrley-Birch H et al. Donor risk factors for renal graft thrombosis. *Transplant Proc* 2007;39:138–9.

26 De Coppi P, Guiliani S, Fusaro F et al. Cadaver kidney transplantation and vascular anomalies: A pediatric experience. *Transplantation* 2006;82:1042–5.

27 Martinez-Urrutia MJ, Lopez Pereira P, Avila Ramirez L et al. Renal transplant in children with previous inferior vena cava thrombosis. *Pediatr Transplant* 2007;11:419–21.

28 Eneriz-Wiemer M, Sarwal M, Donovan D et al. Successful renal transplantation in high-risk small children with a completely thrombosed inferior vena cava. *Transplantation* 2006;82:1148–52.

29 French CG, Acott PD, Crocker JF et al. Extravesical ureteroneocystostomy with and without internalized ureteric stents in pediatric renal transplantation. *Pediatr Transplant* 2001;5:21–6.

30 Bergmeijer JH, Nijman R, Kalkman E et al. Stenting of the ureterovesical anastomosis in pediatric renal transplantation. *Transpl Int* 1990;3:146–8.

31 Veale JL, Yew J, Gjertson DW et al. Long-term comparative outcomes between 2 common ureteroneocystostomy techniques for renal transplantation. *J Urol* 2007;177:632–6.

32 Surange RS, Johnson RW, Tavakoli A et al. Kidney transplantation into an ileal conduit: A single center experience of 59 cases. *J Urol* 2003;170:1727–30.

33 Nguan CY, Beasley KA, McAlister VC, Luke PP. Treatment of renal transplant complications with a mesh hood fascial closure technique. *Am J Surg* 2007;193:119–21.

34 Sandid MS, Assi MA, Hall S. Intraoperative hypotension and prolonged operative time as risk factors for slow graft function in kidney transplant recipients. *Clin Transplant* 2006;20:762–8.

35 Cecka JM, Gjertson DW, Terasake PI. Pediatric renal transplantation: A review of the UNOS data. *Pediatr Transplant* 1997;1:55–64.

36 Williams AR, Watson AR, Rigg KM. *Paediatric Kidney Transplantation into the Abnormal Urinary Tract: A UK survey on Behalf of the 'Surgical Challenges in Paediatric Transplantation' Forum*. Presented at the 9th Annual Congress of the British Transplantation Society, Edinburgh, 2006.

37 Bartsch L, Sarwal M, Orlandi P et al. Limited surgical interventions in children with posterior urethral valves can lead to better outcomes following renal transplantation. *Pediatr Transplant* 2002;6:400–5.

38 Remorino R, Taylor J. Smoothing things over: The transition from pediatric to adult care for kidney transplant recipients. *Prog Transplant* 2006;16:303–8.

39 Benfield MR, McDonald RA, Bartosh S et al. Changing trends in pediatric transplantation: 2001 annual report of the North American pediatric renal transplant cooperative study. *Pediatr Transplant* 2003;7:321–35.

40 Fuller TF, Deger S, Buchler A et al. Ureteral complications in the renal transplant recipient after laparoscopic living donor nephrectomy. *Eur Urol* 2006;50:535–40.

41 Khauli R. Modified extravesical ureteral reimplantation and routine stenting in kidney transplantation. *Transpl Int* 2002;15:411–14.

42 Lapointe SP, Charbit M, Jan D et al. Urological complications after renal transplantation using ureteroureteral anastomosis in children. *J Urol* 2001;166:1046–8.

43 Smith JM, Stablein D, Singh A et al. Decreased risk of renal allograft thrombosis associated with interleukin-2 receptor antagonists: A report of the NAPRTCS. *Am J Transplant* 2006;6:585–8.

44 Turner-Warwick R, Worth PHC. The Psoas-Hitch procedure for the replacement of the lower third of the ureter. *Br J Urol* 1969;41:701–9.

45 Bromwich E, Coles S, Atchley J et al. A 4-year review of balloon dilation of ureteral strictures in renal allografts. *J Endourol* 2006;20:1060–1.

46 Coulthard MG, Keir MJ. Reflux nephropathy in kidney transplants, demonstrated by dimercaptosuccinic acid scanning. *Transplantation* 2006;82:205–10.

47 Seifert HH, Mazzola B, Zellweger T et al. Ureteral obstruction after dextranomer/hyaluronic acid copolymer injection for treatment of secondary vesicoureteral reflux after renal transplantation. *Urology* 2006;68:203.

VIII Urogenital Tumors

33

Wilms Tumor and Other Renal Tumors

Michael Ritchey and Sarah Conley

Key points

- Preoperative imaging and recognition of vena caval or intracardiac extension of tumor allows for safe surgical planning.

- Large tumors may distort vascular anatomy. Adequate exposure of the renal vessels is crucial to avoid injury to the aorta and its major vessels.

- The most common postoperative complication following surgery for renal tumors is small bowel obstruction.

- Preoperative chemotherapy may decrease the risk of hemorrhage and the incidence of postoperative bowel obstruction due to adhesions.

Introduction

The prognosis of children with renal tumors is now excellent, primarily due to advances in modern chemotherapy. This is most notable for those patients with favorable histology Wilms tumor. Other renal tumors are not as responsive to adjuvant therapies and complete removal of the tumor remains the best chance for success. Even with the remarkable advances in survival from adjuvant therapy, surgery remains an integral part of the multimodality treatment of Wilms tumor. The surgeon has an important role in assessing the extent of the primary tumor, and how the surgery is performed has an impact on the ultimate local tumor stage. This chapter will review the most common complications associated with surgery for renal tumors of childhood and discuss the management of these complications. The majority of literature available regarding complications of renal tumor surgery in children are from patients treated for Wilms tumor; however, the principles discussed below are applicable to other renal tumors.

Pediatric Urology: Surgical Complications and Management. Edited by Duncan T. Wilcox, Prasad P. Godbole and Martin A. Koyle. © 2008 Blackwell Publishing, ISBN: 978-1-4051-6268-5.

Surgical technique: General principles

Primary nephrectomy is the procedure of choice for unilateral tumors. Nephron-sparing surgery has a greater role in the treatment of bilateral Wilms tumor. Partial nephrectomy or tumor enucleation may benefit select cases of unilateral Wilms tumor, although this has been evaluated in a small number of patients [1,2].

All patients should undergo noninvasive imaging prior to surgery with either computed tomography (CT) or magnetic resonance imaging (MRI). These studies provide important information regarding local extent of tumor, such as extension into the inferior vena cava (IVC) and to exclude involvement of the contralateral kidney prior to nephrectomy [3]. Ultrasound is often the first imaging study obtained in a newly diagnosed abdominal mass. It can help differentiate between cystic and solid nature of the tumor, and can also exclude caval thrombus that may be present in 4% of patients [4]. If the IVC cannot be cleared with ultrasound or if there is concern for suprahepatic or intracardiac extension of tumor thrombus echocardiogram, MRI should be performed [5]. Extrinsic compression of the vena cava by the renal mass may simulate intracaval extension [4,6]. CT may be helpful for staging purposes in terms of identifying enlarged lymph nodes, extension of tumor into adjacent organs, or bilateral involvement. However, prospective correlation with imaging and surgical findings has not been reported. Chest CT is recommended to identify pulmonary metastases and can identify some lesions not visible on plain chest radiographs [7].

There are a variety of surgical approaches for performing nephrectomy. Extraperitoneal flank incision should be avoided as it does not allow for proper staging. A transabdominal transperitoneal approach allows for gross inspection and exploration of the abdominal cavity and a generous transverse upper abdominal is most often employed. The type of surgical incision has not been shown to make a difference in terms of operative spillage or incomplete removal of tumor [8]. However, Ritchey *et al.* demonstrated a higher risk for surgical complications with "other incisions" compared to a transverse incision (OR = 5.3, $p = 0.02$) [9]. An increased complication rate has been noted with thoracoabdominal incisions, but this may reflect the selection of this approach for extremely large tumors that may have an inherent increased risk of removal. For patients with intracardiac extension of tumor, a midline abdominal incision with median sternotomy may be the best choice. Cardiopulmonary bypass is often needed in such cases.

Recently, the role of laparoscopic removal of renal tumors in children has been explored. Duarte *et al.* report on eight patients with unilateral nonmetastatic Wilms tumor who had received preoperative chemotherapy prior to laparoscopic nephrectomy [10]. In this small series, there were no conversions to open surgery, no tumor rupture, and no postoperative complications. For the present, it would appear that the role of laparoscopy is for removal of tumors that have been pretreated with chemotherapy. The role of laparoscopic nephrectomy in untreated Wilms tumors will be limited due to the large size of these tumors, risk of tumor spill during removal, and the need for accurate surgical staging that requires removal of the tumor intact. It may find a role in other renal tumors, but differentiation of Wilms tumor from other childhood renal tumors by imaging alone is difficult.

Several aspects of surgical technique should be emphasized. Gentle manipulation of tissue is crucial to avoid tumor rupture with spillage of tumor because of an increased risk of local tumor recurrence when this occurs in children with Wilms tumor [11]. Adequate exposure facilitates staging and allows for inspection of the abdominal contents. Early ligation of the renal vessels before manipulation is recommended and the renal artery should be ligated prior to the renal vein. This will

avoid distension of the vein that can dislodge the ligature. Also, early ligation of the artery may decrease the theoretically increased risk of tumor dissemination. However, in many patients early ligation is not feasible due to the large size of the tumor that obscures the hilar area and the great vessels.

Extension of Wilms tumor into the IVC or right atrium, occurring in 4% and 0.7%, respectively, poses a challenge to the surgeon [4,12]. Obstruction of the hepatic veins may lead to ascites, hepatomegaly, or hepatic dysfunction. Atrial thrombus may present with hypertension or congestive heart failure. Despite adequate preoperative imaging, cases of intracaval or atrial tumor thrombus are still diagnosed intraoperatively. The difficulty of the operation is increased when the diagnosis is missed preoperatively.

In patients with IVC or atrial tumor extension, nephrectomy can be carried out prior to cardiopulmonary bypass and removal of tumor thrombus. Luck *et al.* described their technique of performing median sternotomy and preparation for cardiopulmonary bypass followed by laparotomy and mobilization of the kidney and tumor, leaving the renal vein intact [6]. Atriotomy and removal of all gross tumor through the atriotomy and the renal vein is performed simultaneously. Removal of caval thrombus may be achieved by venacavotomy either with manual extraction or with a Fogarty or Foley balloon catheter. In rare cases of tumor, the thrombus invades the vena cava wall precluding thrombectomy. In this situation, cavectomy is a reasonable surgical alternative [4,13].

For many years, formal exploration of the contralateral kidney was recommended in children with presumed unilateral Wilms tumor [3]. Data from National Wilms Tumor Study (NWTS-4) showed that 7% of contralateral lesions were missed on preoperative imaging [14]. However, extended follow-up of this cohort showed that the overall good outcomes of small contralateral lesions missed on modern day imaging obviates the need for routine contralateral renal exploration [3]. Imaging modalities have continued to improve and even very small lesions should be detected on the preoperative CT or MRI scans.

Complications

In this section we describe the recognition, management, and prevention of intraoperative and postoperative complications of nephrectomy for renal tumors of childhood. Management of complications should be individualized for each child based on the clinical findings.

Table 33.1 Comparison of complication rates from SIOP and NWTSG trials.

	SIOP-93-01	NWTS-5	
Number of patients	360	326	
Complication rate	6.4%	9.8%	($p = 0.12$)
Intraoperative tumor spill	2.2%	15.3%	($p < 0.001$)
Small bowel obstruction	1.1%	4.3%	($p = 0.002$)
Stage III tumors	14.2%	30.4%	($p < 0.001$)
Resection of other organs	6.9%	15.0%	($p < 0.001$)

The overall surgical complication rate of nephrectomy for Wilms tumor appears to have declined over time. In a comparison of the complication rates from NWTS-3 (1979–1987) to NWTS-4 (1986 and 1994), NWTS investigators found the complication rate decreased from 19.8% to 12.7% ($p < 0.001$) [9]. Small bowel obstruction (SBO) and hemorrhage were the most common surgical complications. Factors associated with increased risk of surgical complications included higher local tumor stage, tumor diameter >10 cm, and intravascular extension into the IVC or atrium.

Preoperative chemotherapy may influence surgical complication rates by producing tumor shrinkage. A report from International Society of Pediatric Oncology (SIOP), where nephrectomy was performed after 4 or 8 weeks of chemotherapy, was associated with an overall surgical complication rate of 5% [15]. The most common complication in the SIOP group was SBO. A recent prospective comparison of complications in patients enrolled in the NWTS-5 and the SIOP-93-01 trials demonstrated overall complication rate for the SIOP patients was 6.4% compared to 9.8% in NWST patients ($p = 0.12$) [16] (Table 33.1).There was a decreased incidence of intraoperative tumor spill in the SIOP patients, 2.2%, compared to the NWSTG, 15.3% ($p < 0.001$). There was also a statistically significant decreased incidence of stage III tumors in the SIOP group (14.2%) than in the NWST-5 (30.4%).

Intraoperative complications

Hemorrhage
The incidence of extensive intraoperative hemorrhage has decreased over time from NWTS-3 to NWTS-4

[9]. In NWTS-4 only 1.9% of children had blood loss exceeding 50 ml/kg of body weight compared to 6.0% in NWTS-3 ($p = 0.0003$). Review of the SIOP-9 data showed a 0.33% hemorrhage rate (defined as blood loss over 50 ml/kg) during postchemotherapy nephrectomy [15]. In a prospective analysis comparing complication rates among patients enrolled in SIOP-93 and NWTS-5 trials, there was a significant reduction in rates of intraoperative hemorrhage in the group that received preoperative chemotherapy compared to the group who did not [16]. In addition to a reduction in tumor size following chemotherapy, there is decreased tumor vascularity and thus a decreased risk of intraoperative bleeding.

It is important to recognize that up to 8% of patients with newly diagnosed Wilms tumor may have acquired von Willebrand's disease and preoperative screening is needed [17].

Vascular injury
Iatrogenic injury to the aorta and its major vessels can occur during nephrectomy. Large tumors can distort the anatomy and the great vessels can easily be mistaken for the renal vessels. Vascular injury can be avoided by proper surgical exposure and identification of the aorta, IVC, superior mesenteric artery (SMA), celiac axis, and contralateral renal vessels. Inadvertent ligation of any of these structures could potentially lead to a devastating outcome. Mesenteric vessels may be adherent to the renal hilum. The renal artery should be carefully traced and seen entering the kidney prior to ligation. The surgeon may choose to forgo early ligation of the renal vessels until after mobilization of the tumor if it allows precise identification of the renal vessels.

There are several reports of injury to the SMA, however the actual incidence may be underreported [18]. All patients had left sided tumor where the aorta and its branches lie in close proximity to the tumor, and it occurred in children under 5 years old. In each reported case of iatrogenic SMA ligation, the injury was identified intraoperatively and repaired. None of these children experienced adverse events related to the bowel or vascular anastomosis. The operative management of SMA injury depends on the type of injury. Options for repair include primary end-to-end anastomosis, anastomosis of the cut end of the SMA to the aorta in an end-to-side fashion, or possibly interposition graft if there is inadequate length for direct anastomosis.

Unexplained intraoperative hypotension or cardiac arrest should raise concern for unrecognized vena caval or intracardiac extension of tumor [12]. The tumor thrombus can break off and embolize during the course of nephrectomy. The renal vein and IVC should be palpated prior to manipulation of the tumor to evaluate for the presence of intravascular tumor.

Postoperative complications

Small bowel obstruction

The most common postoperative complication after nephrectomy for Wilms tumor is SBO, occurring in 3–7% of patients [9,15,19]. The majority of cases of SBO occur within the first 100 days after surgery [19]. The most common cause of SBO is bowel adhesions, and less common is intussusception. Factors associated with increased risk of SBO include intravascular tumor extension, resection of other organs, preoperative tumor rupture, residual disease, stage III, and possibly tumor spill. Interestingly, patients who underwent small bowel resection did not have an increased risk of SBO compared to those who underwent resection of other visceral organs. There was no statistically significant difference in the incidence of SBO in patients who received radiation therapy compared to those who did not.

As noted above, the incidence of postoperative SBO is lower when nephrectomy is performed after preoperative chemotherapy. The rate of intestinal intussusceptions was similar between the two groups, but there was a higher rate of obstruction secondary to adhesions in children undergoing primary nephrectomy [16]. One explanation may be that nephrectomy after preoperative chemotherapy requires less extensive dissection.

Surgical techniques thought to reduce the incidence of SBO include gentle handling of the bowel, maintaining a moist serosal surface of the bowel, and avoiding foreign materials on the bowel [19]. Despite adherence to these surgical guidelines, adhesions are thought to form from both an inflammatory and an ischemic process.

Chylous ascites

Disruption or obstruction of lymphatic drainage can lead to chylous ascites. The actual incidence of chylous ascites is unknown [20]. Extended lymph node dissection is not recommended for Wilms tumor, although lymph node sampling is mandatory [11]. Avoiding extended lymphadenectomy may help prevent the formation of chylous ascites. Intraoperatively, care should be taken to ligate any disrupted lymphatics.

Increased abdominal girth and poor feeding should lead to the suspicion of chylous ascites [21]. Diagnosis

is confirmed by evaluation of the white milky fluid obtained during paracentesis or exploratory laparotomy which will reveal a high triglyceride content 2–8 times as great as plasma, specific gravity greater than serum, and protein content >3 gm/dl [22]. Radiographic imaging also plays a role in diagnosis of chylous ascites, however it may be difficult to differentiate chyle from hemorrhage on CT scan [21]. In the supine position, a fluid–fluid level may develop with the nondependent layer consistent with fat density.

Several treatment algorithms for management of postoperative chylous ascites exist in the adult literature, but may not necessarily apply to the pediatric population [22,23]. The initial management of chylous ascites should be conservative, including total parenteral nutrition (TPN) or a medium chain triglyceride (MCT). Small lymphatic leaks usually resolve with conservative management. Occasionally chylous ascites may require surgical intervention, such as direct ligation of leaking lymphatic channels or placement of peritoneovenous shunt. Weiser *et al.* reported on nine children with chylous ascites following surgical treatment for Wilms tumor [20]. Seven patients were treated conservatively and completely resolved in 6–68 days (mean 26). The remaining two patients underwent exploratory laparotomy, one after failed conservative treatment and the other after presenting with increased abdominal girth and signs of an acute abdomen.

Outcomes

Surgeon experience

Surgeon experience may influence complication rates. Results from the NWTS-4 suggested a lower incidence of surgical complications among pediatric surgeons and pediatric urologists than among nonspecialized general surgeons [9]. The prospective study comparing the NWTS and SIOP found a trend toward a lower incidence of complications in more experienced surgeons who had performed >10 nephrectomies for tumor in the previous 2 years.

Bilateral Wilms tumor

Synchronous bilateral Wilms tumor occurs in 4–6% of all patients with Wilms tumor [24]. Surgery for bilateral Wilms tumor has its own unique set of complications. Horwitz *et al.* demonstrated a 15.3% complication rate in their series of 98 children undergoing renal sparing surgery [24]. The most common postoperative complication was SBO in 7 of the 15 patients. The second most common complication was urine leak in four children (4.1%), the result of cutting across the collecting system during partial nephrectomy. Urine leak has been successfully managed with cystoscopic placement of double J stent.

Conclusion

Surgery remains an integral part of the multimodal treatment of Wilms tumor and other non-Wilms tumors of childhood. How the surgery is conducted has a great impact on tumor stage and therefore patient survival. Increased awareness of surgical morbidity has resulted in a decreased overall incidence of complications. Prevention of surgical complications starts with adequate preoperative imaging and sound surgical technique.

References

1 Cozzi DA, Zani A. Nephron-sparing surgery in children with primary renal tumor: Indications and results. *J Urol* 2006;15:3–9.

2 Moorman-Voestermans CGM, Aronson DC, Staalman CR, Delemarre JF, de Kraker J. Is partial nephrectomy appropriate treatment for unilateral Wilms' tumor? *J Pediatr Surg* 1998;33:165–70.

3 Ritchey ML, Shamberger RC, Hamilton T, Haase G, Argani P, Peterson S. Fate of bilateral renal lesions missed on preoperative imaging: A report from the National Wilms Tumor Study Group. *J Urol* 2005;174:1519–21.

4 Ritchey ML, Kelalis PP, Breslow NE, Offord KP, Shochat SJ, D'Angio GJ. Intracaval and atrial involvement with nephroblastoma: Review of National Wilms Tumor Study-3. *J Urol* 1988;140:1113–18.

5 Shamberger RC, Ritchey ML, Haase GM, Bergemann TL, Loechelt-Yoshioka T, Breslow NE *et al.* Intravascular extension of Wilms tumor. *Ann Surg* 2001;234:116–21.

6 Luck SR, DeLeon S, Shkolnik A, Morgan E, Labotka R. Intracardiac Wilms' tumor: Diagnosis and management. *J Pediatr Surg* 1982;17:551–4.

7 Owens CM, Veys PA, Pritchard J, Levitt G *et al.* Role of computed tomography at diagnosis in the management of Wilms' tumour. A study of the United Kingdom Children's Cancer Study Group. *J Clin Oncol* 2002;20:2763–4.

8 Leape LL, Breslow NE, Bishop HC. The surgical treatment of Wilms' tumor: Results of the National Wilms' Tumor Study. *Ann Surg* 1978;187:351–6.

9 Ritchey ML, Shamberger RC, Haase G, Horwitz J, Bergemann T, Breslow NE. Surgical complications after primary nephrectomy for Wilms' tumor: Report from the National Wilms' Tumor Study Group. *J Am Coll Surgeons* 2001;192:63–8.

10 Duarte RJ, Denes FT, Cristofani LM, Vicente OF, Srougi M. Further experience with laparoscopic nephrectomy for Wilms' tumour after chemotherapy. *BJU Intl* 206;98:155–9.

11 Shamberger RC, Guthrie KA, Ritchey ML, Haase GM, Takashima J, Beckwith JB *et al.* Surgery-related factors and local recurrence of Wilms tumor in National Wilms Tumor Study 4. *Ann Surg* 1999;229:292–7.

12 Nakayama DK, Norkool P, deLorimier AA, O'Neill JA, Jr., D'Angio GJ. Intracardiac extension of Wilms' tumor: A report of the National Wilms' Tumor Study. *Ann Surg* 1986;204:693–7.

13 Ribeiro RC, Schettini ST, Abib Sde C, da Fonseca JH, Cypriano M, da Silva NS. Cavectomy for the treatment of Wilms tumor with vascular extension. *J Urol* 2006;176:279–84.

14 Ritchey ML, Green DM, Breslow NB, Moksness J, Norkool P. Accuracy of current imaging modalities in the diagnosis of synchronous bilateral Wilms' tumor: A report from the National Wilms Tumor Study Group. *Cancer* 1995;75:600–4.

15 Godzinski J, Tournade MF, deKraker J, Lemerle J, Voute PA, Weirich A *et al.* Rarity of surgical complications after postchemotherapy nephrectomy for nephroblastoma. Experience of the International Society of Paediatric Oncology-Trial and Study "SIOP-9". *Eur J Pediatr Surg* 1998;8:83–6.

16 Ritchey ML, Godzinski J, Shamberger RC, Haase G, deKraker J, Graf N *et al.* Surgical complications following nephrectomy for Wilms tumor: Prospective study from the National Wilms Tumor Study Group (NWTSG) and the International Society of Pediatric Oncology (SIOP). Unpublished manuscript.

17 Coppes MJ. Serum biological markers and paraneoplastic syndromes in Wilms tumor. *Med Pediatr Oncol* 1993;21:213–21.

18 Ritchey ML, Lally KP, Haase GM, Shochat SJ, Kelalis PP. Superior mesenteric artery injury during nephrectomy for Wilms' tumor. *J Pediatr Surg* 1992;27:612–15.

19 Ritchey ML, Kelalis PP, Etzioni R, Breslow N, Schochat S, Haase GM. Small bowel obstruction after nephrectomy for Wilms' tumor: A report of the National Wilms' Tumor Study-3. *Ann Surg* 1993;218:654–9.

20 Weiser AC, Lindgren BW, Ritchey ML, Franco I. Chylous ascites following surgical treatment for Wilms tumor. *J Urol* 2003;170:1667–9.

21 Aalami OO, Allen DB, Organ CH. Chylous ascites: A collective review. *Surgery* 2000;126:761–78.

22 Leibovitch I, Mor Y, Golomb J, Ramon J. The diagnosis and management of postoperative chylous ascites. *J Urol* 2002;167:449–57.

23 Evans JG, Spiess PE, Kamat AM, Wood CG, Hernandez M, Pettaway CA *et al.* Chylous ascites after post-chemotherapy retroperitoneal lymph node dissection: Review of the M.D. Anderson experience. *J Urol* 2006;176:1463–7.

24 Horwitz JR, Ritchey ML, Moksness J, Breslow NE, Smith GR, Thomas PR *et al.* Renal salvage procedures in patients with synchronous bilateral Wilms' tumors: A report from the National Wilms' Tumor Study Group. *J Pediatr Surg* 1996;31:1020–25.

34

Rhabdomyosarcoma

Barbara Ercole, Michael Isakoff and Fernando A. Ferrer

Key points

- 15–25% of all rhabdomyosarcomas are genitourinary in origin.
- Up to 20% of the time it will be impossible to determine if site is prostate or bladder.
- The treatment paradigm includes primary chemotherapy and radiotherapy after initial biopsy followed by surgery.
- The 6-year overall survival has been reported at 82% for patients with nonmetastatic cancers.
- Treatment complications include inadequate biopsy, postresection positive surgical

margins, rhabdomyoblasts on post-treatment biopsy, hemorrhagic cystitis, bladder dysfunction, general surgical complications, chemotherapy and radiation-related complications, and recurrence.

- Rhabdomyoblasts on post-treatment biopsy do not require exenterative surgery.
- A significant percentage of children may suffer from bladder dysfunction post-treatment.

Introduction

Rhabdomyosarcoma (RMS) is one of the most common soft tissue sarcomas in children and was first described in 1850 by Wiener [1]. In children younger than 15 years, RMS comprises 4–8% of malignant tumors. About 15–25% of all RMSs are genitourinary in origin [2,3]. The category of pelvic RMS describes tumors arising in the bladder, prostate, uterus, and vagina. It does not include the pelvic retroperitoneal space or paratesticular regions. More than 75% of pelvic RMSs involve the bladder/prostate (B/P) [4].

Treatment principles

Initially, management of B/P RMS involved primary resection and/or exenteration combined with

chemotherapy and radiotherapy. Development of multimodal treatments comprising of chemotherapy, radiotherapy, and bladder preservation expanded and progressed with the aid of multicenter trials led by the Intergroup RMS Study. This approach shifted the treatment paradigm to primary chemotherapy and radiotherapy after initial biopsy followed by surgery.

Treatment protocols as delineated by Children's Oncology Group (COG) protocols for RMS are based on risk stratification. Patients are categorized into low risk, intermediate risk, and high risk. Low-risk patients include those with embryonal RMS (including botryoid RMS) occurring at favorable sites (orbit/head/neck, nonparameningeal/GU, nonbladder/prostate, and biliary tract), and embryonal RMS with either completely resected disease or microscopic residual disease at unfavorable sites. Therapy is divided into subsets 1 and 2 based on stage, location, and clinical group. Patients in both subsets receive vincristine, actinomycin D, and cyclophosphamide (VAC) for 4 cycles. Those in subset 1 receive extra 4 cycles of vincristine and actinomycin D, while those in subset 2 continue on 12 weeks of actinomycin D and vincristine.

Pediatric Urology: Surgical Complications and Management. Edited by Duncan T. Wilcox, Prasad P. Godbole and Martin A. Koyle. © 2008 Blackwell Publishing, ISBN: 978-1-4051-6268-5.

Radiation therapy is given at week 13 for those patients who require local control.

Intermediate risk RMS includes most B/P primaries. It is defined as incompletely excised nonmetastatic embryonal, alveolar, or undifferentiated RMS occurring at any unfavorable site, and metastatic embryonal RMS in children <10 years old. In general, complete excision at the initial procedure is impossible. Intermediate risk patients undergo an increased number of second-look operations and exenterative procedures. The COG protocol for intermediate risk patients includes a randomization of standard VAC chemotherapy as used on prior IRS protocols versus VAC alternating with cycles of vincristine/irinotecan, a combination that has been shown to have efficacy in patients with relapsed RMS [5].

High-risk patients have metastatic embryonal tumors at presentation and are older than 10 years. It also includes patients with metastatic alveolar or undifferentiated tumors [6]. Up front complete resection of primary tumor is rarely indicated. Initial biopsy is undertaken to establish diagnosis. Surgical resection is undertaken if metastatic disease is controlled (3–6 months), if biopsy proven residual tumor exists after external beam radiation, or if early local failure occurs after radiation or chemotherapy treatment. Previously unresectable primary tumors may be resected with partial cystectomy after chemotherapy or radiotherapy has caused shrinkage. Consideration for radical exenteration should be given if there is no metastatic disease present after treatment and only local disease remains. Outcome for this group of patients has historically been very poor with <50% of patients surviving 3 years [7]. Therefore, the COG protocol for high-risk patients includes the use of standard VAC in combination with additional multiagent intensive chemotherapy. Alternating dose-intensive compression cycles of vincristine, doxorubicin, cyclophosphamide with ifosfamide, and etoposide are utilized, in addition to an up front window of vincristine and irinotecan. The feasibility and toxicity of the vincristine/irinotecan combination, when given together with radiation therapy, will also be assessed.

Surgical principles

One of the initial goals of early management is preservation of renal function. If the patient presents with obstruction, early decompression is important. Management differs with presentation. If bladder outlet obstruction is present, it is best managed with urethral catheterization. The use of suprapubic drainage has been associated with the potential for tract seeding. Should ureteral obstruction be present, the preferred management is with internal stents. However, in the setting of tumor involvement of the trigone, percutaneous nephrostomy tubes may need to be placed. These may be subsequently internalized.

One of the principal goals of therapy is bladder function preservation. Initial management is with biopsy, delaying definite surgery until after chemotherapy, or after radiation therapy has caused shrinkage of the tumor. However, should complete resection be feasible at time of biopsy with preservation of bladder function, the tumor should be resected in its entirety.

In certain cases initial biopsy is done before establishing a malignant diagnosis. This may result in a situation where gross residual tumor, microscopically positive margins, or margin status is unclear. At this juncture it is recommended that the concept of pretreatment re-excision be applied. In these cases a wide envelope of tissue is removed that includes normal margins. This procedure is done prior to administration of chemotherapy or radiation therapy.

Second look operations are performed to confirm clinical response, evaluate pathological response to therapy, and remove residual tumor in patients who achieve clinical complete or partial response after chemotherapy or radiation therapy. If residual tumor or early failure or progression of disease after therapy is present, anterior exenteration with preservation of the rectum should be considered.

Outcomes

Available literature from IRS I–III states that bladder preservation is possible in approximately 60% of patients [8]. However, it is important to bear in mind that bladder preservation is not synonymous with normal function. Formal urodynamic testing and questionnaires were not performed during this time period [9,10].

The goal of IRS IV (1993–1997) was to improve overall event free survival and bladder preservation rate. Outcomes in patients with B/P RMS were reported by Ardnt et al. in 2004. Records of 88 patients with B/P RMS were reviewed. The majority of these tumors arose from the bladder (70%) and had favorable histology (80%). Seventy-four patients received radiation therapy and all received alkylating-based chemotherapy. The event free survival rate was 77% at a mean of 6.1 years of follow-up. The 6-year overall survival was 82% for patients with nonmetastatic cancers. Of the 55 patients who retained their bladder, 40% had normal function as determined by history [11]. This percentage is lower than that reported in previous IRS studies and suggests underestimation of treatment impact on bladder function [10–12].

Treatment complications/management

Inadequate biopsy

Endoscopic biopsy of the primary lesion is frequently attempted using a pediatric resectoscope or cold-cup biopsy forceps. Because the loop size of the pediatric resectoscope is small, multiple samples may be needed to make an accurate diagnosis. Cautery artifact can mimic spindle cell appearance to the inexperienced examiner or destroy the sample entirely. Low cutting current should therefore be used when taking a loop biopsy. Alternatively, the loop can be used to cut out a wedge of tissue that can subsequently be retrieved [13]. Biopsy should be performed with an experienced onsite pathologist that can evaluate frozen section specimens and guide the surgeon.

If endoscopy reveals no mucosal abnormality, or if endoscopic biopsy is inconclusive, the surgeon should convert to an open biopsy. If laparotomy is performed for biopsy, preliminary evaluation of the pelvic and retroperitoneal nodes at or below the level of the renal arteries should be performed.

Postresection positive surgical margins

Intraoperative frozen section at the time of definitive resection can be difficult to interpret. This becomes a significant issue if up front continent reconstruction is performed at the time of extirpative surgery. Landers *et al.* described the use of Le Bag continent reconstructions in three children one of whom was 26 months. Unfortunately, despite initially negative frozen section analysis, permanent sections revealed residual viable tumor requiring local radiation and chemotherapy [14]. Similarly, Merguerian *et al.* performed reconstruction at the time of cystectomy in their patients, but simultaneously cautioned readers that frozen section is an unreliable predictor of residual disease, several of their patients had residual disease requiring adjuvant therapy or reoperation [15]. In addition, early reconstruction of irradiated tissues may lead to impaired healing and an increase in postoperative complications.

The authors' preference is to delay reconstruction. In cases where positive margins are found on permanent

section consideration must be given to re-excision (when deemed feasible) or local radiotherapy with extended systemic chemotherapy should be given. Estimated volume of residual disease is an important consideration.

Rhabdomyoblasts only on post-treatment biopsy

Maturation of rhabdomyoblasts after chemotherapy has been observed by various investigators, and their clinical significance has been called into question [16]. Atra *et al.* reported a group of patients with residual "rhabdomyoblast" that did not go on to relapse during observation [17]. Subsequently, Heyn reported on 2/14 patients that had maturing cells on post-treatment biopsy that remained in remission [18]. Analysis of postcystectomy specimens has also demonstrated rhabdomyoblasts along with a reduction in cellularity in patients treated with chemotherapy suggesting that this pattern may be indicative of response to therapy. More recently, Chertin and coauthors reported the long-term follow-up of a patient with residual atypical cells after treatment with bladder RMS that has not recurred after 5 years [19].

Ortega *et al.* followed 6 patients with post-treatment biopsy showing mature rhabdomyoblasts [20]. All 6 patients remained free of disease after a follow-up period of 37–237 months. The authors emphasized the importance of correctly identifying mature cells as those with a large smooth solitary nucleus, no significant pleomorphism, no mitotic activity, and the absence of clusters of cells suggestive of growth from a common precursor [20]. Finally, a report by the COG clearly supporting observation for rhabdomyoblasts only has recently been published. Failure after apparent tumor cell maturation on biopsy has been reported; therefore, careful observation of these patients is required [21].

Hemorrhagic cystitis

The risk of hemorrhagic cystitis is related to the use of cyclophosphamide and ifosfamide. These agents are metabolized to form the bladder toxic byproduct acrolein. Fortunately, aggressive hydration and administration of mesna, a compound that binds acrolein, decreases the incidence and severity of this complication [22,23]. Hemorrhagic cystitis can also be due to radiation treatment of the pelvis and may occur years from the time of treatment. Unlike the chemotherapy agents cyclophosphamide and ifosfamide, there are no preventive measures to decrease the incidence of hemorrhagic cystitis from radiation therapy other than modification of the irradiation field and dose.

Hemorrhagic cystitis has been treated successfully utilizing a variety of methods; however, no method has been used consistently or is known to be universally successful. Cases of mild hematuria respond to hydration and diuresis. Should the hematuria be more substantial, the practitioner may have to perform a clot evacuation and initiate continuous bladder irrigation. It is important that the patient be clot free prior to starting continuous bladder irrigation to prevent further clot formation and bladder overdistention. Because of the small urethral diameter in children, clot evacuation may be difficult and alternative approaches utilizing a suprapubic tube or cutaneous vesicostomy have been used in some cases.

Conjugated estrogens, either IV or PO, have been successfully used. Estrogens act by stabilizing the microvasculature [24,25]. Hyperbaric oxygen has also been used in the treatment of radiation-induced hemorrhagic cystitis with a reported response rate range of 78–100% [26,27]. The authors have had success using this modality in several children.

Intravesical installations include aminocaproic acid, alum (aluminum ammonium sulfate or aluminum potassium sulfate), silver nitrate, phenol, and formaldehyde. These are not without side effects. Aminocaproic acid forms hard clots that are not easily flushed and should not exceed 12 g daily due to risk of thromboembolic events [28]. Alum, silver nitrate, phenol, and formaldehyde should be avoided in patients with ureteral reflux due to the possibility of renal failure. Alum acts as an astringent agent [29] and has been associated with systemic toxicity [30]. Some authors have reported limited success with this agent. Silver nitrate causes a chemical coagulation, phenol destroys the urothelium, and while touted as an alternative to formalin its use has been limited [31].

Instillation of formalin at concentrations from 2% to 10% requires general anesthesia but has been reported to be fairly effective. The authors advocate beginning at lower concentrations such as 2–4% [32,33]. Embolization has been successfully used in refractory hemorrhagic cystitis. Side effect of gluteal pain due to occlusion of the superior gluteal artery has diminished with the use of super selective embolization [34–36]. Should all other treatments fail, surgery is reserved as the final option for these patients when hemorrhagic cystitis becomes life threatening. Options include urinary diversion, open packing of the bladder, and cystectomy [37–39]. Urinary diversions may include bilateral percutaneous nephrostomy tubes or ileal loop diversions. The goal of diverting urine from the bleeding mucosa is to decrease the contact time with urokinase to allow hemostasis.

Bladder dysfunction

The true incidence of bladder dysfunction in patients treated for RMS is unknown. It was not until recently that validated questionnaires and urodynamic studies have been used to assess functionality of the bladder. Soler *et al.* reported on 11 patients who were evaluated with urodynamics. Four of the 11 had urodynamic findings of reduced bladder capacity, 2 had over-activity and sensory urgency, 1 patient had sensory urgency, and 1 patient experienced suprapubic pain on filling [10]. Raney *et al.* reported 31% of patients over 6 years had some urinary incontinence as well as 27% of patients undergoing partial cystectomy [40]. Yeung *et al.* reported on a limited number of patients, while not all had urodynamics, it was noted that a significant number of the group studied had bladder dysfunction [12].

These patients are at high risk for bladder dysfunction and thus require close monitoring of both the upper tracts and lower urinary tracts. A sensitive and easy tool to detect bladder dysfunction is the frequency-volume voiding chart. Standardized voiding dysfunction questionnaires can also be helpful. Upper tract US can detect hydronephrosis and postvoid residual evaluation can aid in the assessment of lower tract function. Should any child exhibit an abnormal voiding pattern, they should undergo formal urodynamic testing [12].

Patients demonstrating frequency, urgency may be treated with anticholinergics to relieve symptoms and improve continence, but should have formal lower tract evaluation. For patients with intractable urinary frequency or incontinence bladder augmentation with or without bladder neck reconstruction and catheterizable channel should be considered. In particular, evaluation of the bladder neck competence must be performed as treatment may have affected sphincteric function [41].

Surgical complications in general

Surgery performed for treatment of RMS is associated with early and late effects. Higher complication rates are to be expected in patients with previous radiation and chemotherapy [41]. Urinary diversion carries its own complications namely ureteral obstruction, pouch stones, and cutaneous fistulas. Careful consideration as to which bowel used in a patient with history of pelvic radiation is recommended. In some instances transverse or sigmoid colon may be used for the diversion to avoid irradiated bowl segments. Merguerian *et al.* advocated reconstruction at time of cystectomy, though this carries the possibility of residual disease and subsequently requiring adjuvant therapy or re-operation [15]. Some patients are candidates for definitive continent reconstruction if long-term cure has been achieved, defined as at least 2 years disease-free period, and the patient is motivated and mature enough to perform self-catheterization [42].

Reports by Lerner et al. delineated major early complications of pelvic exenteration to include wound infection (24%), abscess formation (12%), fistula (12%), and malnutrition (12%), whereas late complications include hydronephrosis (35%) and bowel obstruction (24%) [43,44]. Late effects of surgery include loss of sexual function, fertility, and bladder function. There is also the possibility of secondary procedures. The most common secondary procedure is revision of urinary conduit. They also include lysis of adhesions, repair of fistulae, total cystectomy for bleeding or fibrosis, intra-abdominal abscess drainage, colostomy for rectal stricture, augmentation vesicocecoplasty for low-capacity bladder, and lysis of ureteral obstruction [45].

Chemotherapy and radiation-related complications

Multiagent combination chemotherapy continues to be a standard component in the treatment of RMS [6]. However, the utilization of intense chemotherapeutic regimens and radiation therapy carries potential serious acute and long-term toxicities (Tables 34.1 and 34.2).

Table 34.1 Chemotherapy-related complications [6,47–49].

Acute effects	Myelosuppression, bacteremia, renal toxicity, fever, neutropenia, and mucositis
Late effects	Secondary malignancy (i.e. myelodysplasia and leukemia), cardiotoxicity (doxorubicin), and endocrine dysfunction (i.e. gonadal failure, pubertal delay, and GI disorders)

Table 34.2 Radiation-related complications [46–48].

Acute effects	Urinary frequency/urgency, diarrhea, skin irritation, and fatigue
Late effects	Impairment of bone growth, delayed puberty, growth retardation, radiation cystitis, radiation enteritis, fibrosis, incompetent sphincter, rectal stricture, secondary tumors, distal ureteral strictures, and difficult biopsy interpretation

In general, all patients should be screened with periodic physical exams and complete blood counts after completion of therapy. Radiation therapy independently impacts bladder function (low capacity, frequency, urgency) as summarized by Fryer [46] and management would include clean intermittent catheterization or bladder augmentation.

Recurrence

Management of early recurrence includes early local radiation for patients with residual disease and involvement of lymph nodes [50]. Unfortunately, recurrence of RMS after treatment carries with it a poor prognosis. Most relapses occur within 3 years of initial diagnosis. Attempts at prolonging life have included exenteration after chemo/radiation. The estimated 5-year survival rate after relapse is 64% for botryoid embryonal, 26% for other embryonal, and 5% for alveolar or undifferentiated pathology [51].

Conclusion

Despite improved overall survival, children with RMS of the pelvic organs continue to suffer from a wide range of treatment-related side effects and complications. Meticulous follow-up including careful evaluation of bladder function is required to assess the sequela of current therapies.

References

1 Wiener E. Rhabdomyosarcoma. In *Pediatric Surgery*, Edited by JA O'Neil MIRJLG. St. Louis: C.V Mosby, 1998: 431–45.
2 Pappo AS, Shapiro DN, Crist WM, Maurer HM. Biology and therapy of pediatric rhabdomyosarcoma. *J Clin Oncol* 1995;13:2123–39.
3 Shapiro E, Strother D. Pediatric genitourinary rhabdomyosarcoma. *J Urol* 1992;148:1761–8.
4 Hays DM. Bladder/prostate rhabdomyosarcoma: Results of the multi-institutional trials of the Intergroup Rhabdomyosarcoma Study. *Semin Surg Oncol* 1993;9:520–3.
5 Pappo AS, Lyden E, Breitfeld P, Donaldson SS, Wiener E, Parham D *et al.* Two consecutive phase II window trials of irinotecan alone or in combination with vincristine for the treatment of metastatic rhabdomyosarcoma: The children's oncology group. *J Clin Oncol* 2007;25:362–9.
6 Crist WM, Anderson JR, Meza JL, Fryer C, Raney RB, Ruymann FB *et al.* Intergroup rhabdomyosarcoma study-IV: Results for patients with nonmetastatic disease. *J Clin Oncol* 2001;19:3091–102.
7 Breneman JC, Lyden E, Pappo AS, Link MP, Anderson JR, Parham DM *et al.* Prognostic factors and clinical outcomes

in children and adolescents with metastatic rhabdomyo-sarcoma – a report from the Intergroup rhabdomyosarcoma study IV. *J Clin Oncol* 2003;21:78–84.

8 Raney B, Jr., Heyn R, Hays DM, Tefft M, Newton WA, Jr., Wharam M et al. Sequelae of treatment in 109 patients followed for 5 to 15 years after diagnosis of sarcoma of the bladder and prostate. A report from the intergroup rhabdomyosarcoma study committee. *Cancer* 1993;71:2387–94.

9 Ferrer FA. Re: Does bladder preservation (as a surgical principle) lead to retaining bladder function in bladder/prostate rhabdomyosarcoma? Results from Intergroup Rhabdomyosarcoma Study IV. *J Urol* 2004;172:2084.

10 Soler R, Macedo A, Jr., Bruschini H, Puty F, Caran E, Petrilli A et al. Does the less aggressive multimodal approach of treating bladder-prostate rhabdomyosarcoma preserve bladder function? *J Urol* 2005;174:2343–6.

11 Arndt C, Rodeberg D, Breitfeld PP, Raney RB, Ullrich F, Donaldson S. Does bladder preservation (as a surgical principle) lead to retaining bladder function in bladder/prostate rhabdomyosarcoma? Results from intergroup rhabdomyosarcoma study iv. *J Urol* 2004;171:2396–403.

12 Yeung CK, Ward HC, Ransley PG, Duffy PG, Pritchard J. Bladder and kidney function after cure of pelvic rhabdomyosarcoma in childhood. *Br J Cancer* 1994;70:1000–3.

13 Snyder HM, D'Angio GL, Evans AE, Raney RB. Pediatric oncology. In *Campbell's Urology*, Edited by PC Walsh, AB Retik, ED Vaughan Jr. Philadelphia: W.B. Saunders Co., 1998: pp. 2210–56.

14 Lander EB, Shanberg AM, Tansey LA, Sawyer DE, Groncy PK, Finklestein JZ. The use of continent diversion in the management of rhabdomyosarcoma of the prostate in childhood. *J Urol* 1992;147:1602–5.

15 Merguerian PA, Agarwal S, Greenberg M, Bagli DJ, Khoury AE, McLorie GA. Outcome analysis of rhabdomyosarcoma of the lower urinary tract. *J Urol* 1998;160:1191–4.

16 Molenaar WM, Oosterhuis JW, Kamps WA. Cytologic "differentiation" in childhood rhabdomyosarcomas following polychemotherapy. *Hum Pathol* 1984;15:973–9.

17 Atra A, Ward HC, Aitken K, Boyle M, Dicks-Mireaux C, Duffy PG et al. Conservative surgery in multimodal therapy for pelvic rhabdomyosarcoma in children. *Br J Cancer* 1994;70:1004–8.

18 Heyn R, Newton WA, Raney RB, Hamoudi A, Bagwell C, Vietti T et al. Preservation of the bladder in patients with rhabdomyosarcoma. *J Clin Oncol* 1997;15:69–75.

19 Chertin B, Reinus C, Koulikov D, Rosenmann E, Farkas A, Chertin B. Post-chemotherapy microscopic residual prostate rhabdomyosarcoma: Long-term conservative follow-up. *Pediatr Surg Int* 2002;18:68–9.

20 Ortega JA, Rowland J, Monforte H, Malogolowkin M, Triche T. Presence of well-differentiated rhabdomyoblasts at the end of therapy for pelvic rhabdomyosarcoma: Implications for the outcome. *J Pediatr Hematol Oncol* 2000;22:106–11.

21 Arndt CA, Hammond S, Rodeberg D, Qualman S. Significance of persistent mature rhabdomyoblasts in bladder/prostate rhabdomyosarcoma: Results from IRS IV. *J Pediatr Hematol Oncol* 2006;28:563–7.

22 Andriole GL, Sandlund JT, Miser JS, Arasi V, Linehan M, Magrath IT. The efficacy of mesna (2-mercaptoethane sodium sulfonate) as a uroprotectant in patients with hemorrhagic cystitis receiving further oxazaphosphorine chemotherapy. *J Clin Oncol* 1987;5:799–803.

23 Brock N. The development of mesna for the inhibition of urotoxic side effects of cyclophosphamide, ifosfamide, and other oxazaphosphorine cytostatics. *Recent Results Cancer Res* 1980;74:270–8.

24 Heath JA, Mishra S, Mitchell S, Waters KD, Tiedemann K. Estrogen as treatment of hemorrhagic cystitis in children and adolescents undergoing bone marrow transplantation. *Bone Marrow Transplant* 2006;37:523–6.

25 Miller J, Burfield GD, Moretti KL. Oral conjugated estrogen therapy for treatment of hemorrhagic cystitis. *J Urol* 1994;151:1348–50.

26 Chong KT, Hampson NB, Corman JM. Early hyperbaric oxygen therapy improves outcome for radiation-induced hemorrhagic cystitis. *Urology* 2005;65:649–53.

27 Dall'Era MA, Hampson NB, Hsi RA, Madsen B, Corman JM. Hyperbaric oxygen therapy for radiation induced proctopathy in men treated for prostate cancer. *J Urol* 2006;176:87–90.

28 Singh I, Laungani GB. Intravesical epsilon aminocaproic acid in the management of intractable bladder hemorrhage. *Urology* 1992;40:227.

29 Ostroff EB, Chenault OW, Jr. Alum irrigation for the control of massive bladder hemorrhage. *J Urol* 1982;128:929–30.

30 Kanwar VS, Jenkins JJ, III, Mandrell BN, Furman WL. Aluminum toxicity following intravesical alum irrigation for hemorrhagic cystitis. *Med Pediatr Oncol* 1996;27:64–7.

31 Susan LP, Marsh RJ. Phenolization of bladder in treatment of massive intractable hematuria. *Urology* 1975;5:119–21.

32 Efros MD, Ahmed T, Coombe N, Choudhury MS. Urologic complications of high-dose chemotherapy and bone marrow transplantation. *Urology* 1994;43:355–60.

33 Shrom SH, Donaldson MH, Duckett JW, Wein AJ. Formalin treatment for intractable hemorrhagic cystitis: A review of the literature with 16 additional cases. *Cancer* 1976;38:1785–9.

34 Gine E, Rovira M, Real I, Burrel M, Montana J, Carreras E et al. Successful treatment of severe hemorrhagic cystitis after hemopoietic cell transplantation by selective embolization of the vesical arteries. *Bone Marrow Transplant* 2003;31:923–5.

35 McIvor J, Williams G, Southcott RD. Control of severe vesical haemorrhage by therapeutic embolisation. *Clin Radiol* 1982;33:561–7.

36 Palandri F, Bonifazi F, Rossi C, Falcioni S, Arpinati M, Giannini MB et al. Successful treatment of severe hemorrhagic cystitis with selective vesical artery embolization. *Bone Marrow Transplant* 2005;35:529–30.

37 Andriole GL, Yuan JJ, Catalona WJ. Cystotomy, temporary urinary diversion and bladder packing in the management of severe cyclophosphamide-induced hemorrhagic cystitis. *J Urol* 1990;143:1006–7.

38 deVries CR, Freiha FS. Hemorrhagic cystitis: A review. *J Urol* 1990;143:1–9.

39 Garderet L, Bittencourt H, Sebe P, Kaliski A, Claisse JP, Esperou H *et al.* Cystectomy for severe hemorrhagic cystitis in allogeneic stem cell transplant recipients. *Transplantation* 2000;70:1807–11.

40 Raney B, Anderson J, Jenney M, Arndt C, Brecht I, Carli M *et al.* Late effects in 164 patients with rhabdomyosarcoma of the bladder/prostate region: A report from the international workshop. *J Urol* 2006;176:2190–4.

41 Duel BP, Hendren WH, Bauer SB, Mandell J, Colodny A, Peters CA *et al.* Reconstructive options in genitourinary rhabdomyosarcoma. *J Urol* 1996;156:1798–804.

42 Wu HY, Snyder III, HM. Pediatric urologic oncology: Bladder, prostate, testis. *Urol Clin North Am* 2004;31:619–27, xi.

43 Lerner SP, Hayani A, O'Hollaren P, Winkel C, Ohori M, Harberg FJ *et al.* The role of surgery in the management of pediatric pelvic rhabdomyosarcoma. *J Urol* 1995;154:540–5.

44 Michalkiewicz EL, Rao BN, Gross E, Luo X, Bowman LC, Pappo AS *et al.* Complications of pelvic exenteration in children who have genitourinary rhabdomyosarcoma. *J Pediatr Surg* 1997;32:1277–82.

45 Raney B, Jr., Heyn R, Hays DM, Tefft M, Newton WA, Jr., Wharam M *et al.* Sequelae of treatment in 109 patients followed for 5 to 15 years after diagnosis of sarcoma of the bladder and prostate. A report from the Intergroup Rhabdomyosarcoma Study Committee. *Cancer* 1993; 71:2387–94.

46 Fryer CJ. Pelvic rhabdomyosarcoma: Paying the price of bladder preservation. *Lancet* 1995;345:141–2.

47 Navid F, Santana VM, Billups CA, Merchant TE, Furman WL, Spunt SL *et al.* Concomitant administration of vincristine, doxorubicin, cyclophosphamide, ifosfamide, and etoposide for high-risk sarcomas: The St. Jude Children's Research Hospital experience. *Cancer* 2006;106:1846–56.

48 Raney RB, Asmar L, Vassilopoulou-Sellin R, Klein MJ, Donaldson SS, Green J *et al.* Late complications of therapy in 213 children with localized, nonorbital soft-tissue sarcoma of the head and neck: A descriptive report from the Intergroup Rhabdomyosarcoma Studies (IRS)-II and -III. IRS Group of the Children's Cancer Group and the Pediatric Oncology Group. *Med Pediatr Oncol* 1999;33:362–71.

49 Spunt SL, Sweeney TA, Hudson MM, Billups CA, Krasin MJ, Hester AL. Late effects of pelvic rhabdomyosarcoma and its treatment in female survivors. *J Clin Oncol* 2005;23:7143–51.

50 Tefft M, Hays D, Raney RB, Jr., Lawrence W, Soule E, Donaldson MH *et al.* Radiation to regional nodes for rhabdomyosarcoma of the genitourinary tract in children: Is it necessary? A report from the intergroup rhabdomyosarcoma study no. 1 (IRS-1). *Cancer* 1980;45:3065–8.

51 Pappo AS, Anderson JR, Crist WM, Wharam MD, Breitfeld PP, Hawkins D *et al.* Survival after relapse in children and adolescents with rhabdomyosarcoma: A report from the intergroup rhabdomyosarcoma study group. *J Clin Oncol* 1999;17:3487–93.

35

Testicular Tumors

Jonathan H. Ross

Key points

- Inguinal orchiectomy is the standard approach to testicular tumors in adolescents and in children with an elevated AFP level.

- Testis-sparing surgery should be considered in prepubertal patients with a normal AFP level.

- Scrotal violations are probably not critical, but local tumor spillage may require adjuvant treatments.

- The complication of ejaculatory dysfunction following RPLND can be avoided in nearly all patients with a nerve-sparing technique.

- To avoid surgical complications, meticulous technique, protection of retracted viscera, and a working knowledge of vascular surgical techniques are important when undertaking an RPLND.

Introduction

Testis tumors are rare in children and fall into two categories in the pediatric population – prepubertal and postpubertal tumors. Tumors occurring in adolescents are the same as those seen in older adults, with nonseminomatous mixed germ cell tumors (NSMGCT) predominating. Benign tumors are uncommon in this population. The incidence of testis tumors in prepubertal children is 0.5–2.0 per 100,000 children, accounting for only 1–2% of all pediatric tumors [1]. Teratomas are benign in children and nearly all malignant tumors in children are yolk sac tumors. Unlike testicular tumors occurring in adolescents and adults, a large proportion, perhaps even a majority, of prepubertal testis tumors are benign [2,3]. Therefore the management of testis tumors in prepubertal and postpubertal boys differs significantly.

The initial radiographic evaluation of children with a suspected testis tumor is limited. Because many prepubertal testis tumors are benign, a metastatic evaluation is usually deferred until tissue confirmation of the tumor's histology is obtained. However, when a malignancy is suspected (e.g. in children with an elevated alpha-fetoprotein (AFP) level or in adolescents) a computerized tomography (CT) scan of the abdomen may be obtained preoperatively. Imaging of the primary tumor is sometimes helpful. Ultrasonography is most often employed. It is able to distinguish a testicular tumor from a benign extratesticular lesion or from a paratesticular rhabdomyosarcoma. The extent of testicular involvement can also be determined, which is helpful if testis-sparing surgery is being considered. The ultrasonographic appearance of specific testis tumors has been described. Unfortunately, ultrasound findings are too inconsistent to allow a definitive diagnosis.

Tumor markers play an important role in the evaluation and follow-up of childhood testis tumors. AFP is the most important tumor marker in prepubertal patients. AFP levels are elevated in 80–90% of children with a yolk sac tumor, and AFP has a biological half-life of approximately 5 days [4]. It should be kept in mind that AFP levels are normally quite high in infancy. An "elevated" level in a boy less than 1 year of age does not rule out the possibility of a benign tumor, such as teratoma [5]. In addition to AFP, the beta subunit of human chorionic gonadotropin (HCG) is an important marker in adolescent testis tumors, but this is rarely elevated in children

Pediatric Urology: Surgical Complications and Management. Edited by Duncan T. Wilcox, Prasad P. Godbole and Martin A. Koyle. © 2008 Blackwell Publishing, ISBN: 978-1-4051-6268-5.

because the histologic types that lead to elevated human chorionic gonadotropin levels are rarely encountered in prepubertal testis tumors.

Surgical approach

The standard approach to a malignant testis tumor or paratesticular rhabdomyosarcoma is an inguinal orchiectomy. Through an inguinal incision, the spermatic cord is isolated and clamped with a noncrushing clamp. The testis is then delivered into the inguinal incision with the tunica vaginalis intact. Once a testis tumor is confirmed by direct palpation, the cord is ligated and divided at the internal ring.

Increasing consideration has been given to performing testis-sparing surgery for benign testicular tumors [2]. This is particularly attractive in prepubertal patients because more than one-third of tumors are benign in this population. The preoperative evaluation plays a significant role in patient selection for testis-sparing surgery. An elevated AFP level in a child over 1 year of age virtually always reflects the presence of a yolk sac tumor and precludes a testis-sparing approach. However, in infants (who normally have high AFP levels) and older children with a normal AFP, the likelihood of a benign tumor is considerable. This is also true in boys presenting with androgenization. For these patients an inguinal exploration should be considered so that testis-sparing surgery may be performed if a benign histology is confirmed. The initial approach is the same as for an inguinal orchiectomy. Once the testis is delivered into the inguinal incision (the cord having been clamped with a noncrushing clamp), the field is draped off with towels and the tunica vaginalis is opened. The tumor is excised with a margin of normal parenchyma or enucleated and sent for frozen section. If a benign histology is confirmed, then the testicular defect is closed with absorbable suture and the testis is returned to the scrotum. Reports from small series suggest that testis-sparing is safe and effective in preserving testicular tissue with no reports of local recurrence of benign tumors managed in this fashion [6]. If a malignancy is detected, or the frozen section is nondiagnostic, then an orchiectomy is performed.

After orchiectomy, children with malignant testicular tumors or paratesticular rhabdomyosarcoma require additional evaluation and therapy. The type of adjunctive management selected will depend on the histology of the primary tumor and the results of radiographic and biochemical studies. The intensity of follow-up also depends on the malignant potential of the primary

tumor. Prepubertal patients with stage 1 yolk sac tumor whose AFP normalizes postoperatively are managed with observation. Patients with radiographic or biochemical evidence of metastatic disease, and those stage 1 patients who recur on observation, are treated with 3 or 4 cycles of platinum-based multiagent chemotherapy. Retroperitoneal surgery is undertaken only in the rare event of equivocal lymph node involvement on CT scan with normal markers or in the event of a persistent retroperitoneal mass following chemotherapy. Retroperitoneal lymph node dissection (RPLND) is employed more frequently in adolescents with NSMGCT. It may be undertaken in select patients as a staging and therapeutic approach to clinical stage 1 disease or in stage 2 patients with limited retroperitoneal disease. It is also undertaken for patients with a persistent mass following chemotherapy – a more common occurrence in adolescents than in prepubertal patients. RPLND also plays a role in the management of patients with paratesticular rhabdomyosarcoma. It is indicated as a staging procedure in adolescents with clinical stage 1 disease and is also indicated in all patients (prepubertal or postpubertal) with apparent lymphatic involvement on CT scan. From a surgical point of view then, all patients with a testis tumor will undergo an orchiectomy or test-sparing tumor excision and a select group of patients will undergo an RPLND as well.

Orchiectomy: Outcomes and complications

Inguinal orchiectomy provides excellent local control for testicular cancer in prepubertal and postpubertal patients. Local recurrence is extremely rare and occurs almost exclusively in the context of local tumor spillage. Guidelines for the surgical management of testicular cancer have emphasized the importance of avoiding scrotal violation in removing these tumors. Despite this standard, a significant number of patients in single institution reports and in multicenter clinical trials have had scrotal violations occur. Studies in prepubertal and postpubertal patients suggest that these violations do not affect overall survival [7,8]. Scrotal violations occur in three settings. First, someone with a testicular cancer may have had previous unrelated scrotal surgery, such as an orchidopexy for an undescended testicle. These patients may be at risk for inguinal lymphatic spread. While inguinal lymphadenectomy is not recommended, careful observation of the inguinal lymph nodes during evaluation and follow-up is prudent. A second type of scrotal violation involves extracting the tumor intact through a scrotal incision. Finally, patients may have a scrotal violation with potential tumor spillage such as might occur with a transcrotal biopsy or violation of the tumor capsule during a transcrotal excision. Local recurrence in the absence of tumor spillage or violation is exceedingly rare and can occur whether the approach is scrotal or inguinal. An inguinal approach is still recommended as a way to avoid tumor spillage or cutting across tumor that may involve the spermatic cord. However, a scrotal violation in the absence of tumor spillage probably does not require any additional local therapy, though once the error is recognized, a separate inguinal incision should be made to remove that portion of the spermatic cord. If tumor spillage does occur during a scrotal violation, then consideration should be given to hemiscrotectomy or other adjuvant therapy.

Complications following inguinal orchiectomy are rare. Bleeding occasionally occurs and is best prevented by close attention to hemostasis in the soft tissues of the scrotum and appropriate control of the spermatic cord at the internal ring. Bleeding from the spermatic cord can be difficult to control once the cord is divided and retracts into the retroperitoneum. This can be prevented by controlling the cord with a suture ligature and a more proximal free tie. The cord cannot retract from the suture ligature and the more proximal free tie will prevent tracking into the retroperitoneum of any bleeding inadvertently caused by the suture ligature. Following the orchiectomy, the scrotum should be inverted into the inguinal incision for fulguration of any bleeding tissue or vessels. When postoperative bleeding does occur, whether in the scrotum or retroperitoneum, it is best managed conservatively without exploration. In addition to the direct consequences of bleeding, a retroperitoneal hematoma can interfere with the interpretation of staging CT scans since a retroperitoneal hematoma may be confused for adenopathy [9]. When a pelvic mass without higher retroperitoneal involvement is seen on a postorchiectomy CT scan, a retroperitoneal bleed is more likely than metastatic disease. Magnetic resonance imaging can sometimes make the distinction in difficult cases. However, to prevent this confusion it is best to obtain abdominal imaging prior to orchiectomy in cases suspicious for cancer.

RPLND: Outcomes and complications

In 1977, Donahue described the classic suprahilar bilateral retroperitoneal lymph node dissection for testicular cancer [10]. The operation held significant morbidity,

particularly loss of ejaculatory function due to disruption of the lumbar sympathetic chains and hypogastric plexus. However, in the era when chemotherapy and radiation were largely ineffective for metastatic disease, radical surgical clearance was of paramount importance and the associated morbidity was acceptable. Over the years both the effectiveness of chemotherapy and an increased understanding of retroperitoneal neuroanatomy have led to an evolution in the approach to RPLND [11]. Currently, the nerve-sparing technique is employed at most centers for patients with low-stage disease undergoing RPLND – whether unilateral or bilateral (Figure 35.1). Since RPLND is rarely indicated in prepubertal patients, there is no data to support the feasibility of nerve-sparing for this group. For children with paratesticular rhabdomyosarcoma and limited positive retroperitoneal nodes, a modified unilateral template is appropriate. The same is true for children with yolk sac tumor and a persistent mass following chemotherapy. Whether children with more extensive lymphadenopathy should undergo a more extensive bilateral dissection is unclear since there is no data delineating the oncologic benefit in these rare clinical situations. The uncertain oncological benefit must be weighed against the increased morbidity of the more extensive operation. In prepubertal children with yolk sac tumor, normalization of AFP, and an equivocal node(s) on abdominal CT, an excisional node biopsy is adequate for staging purposes. The result of the biopsy will then determine whether adjuvant chemotherapy is indicated. Unless otherwise noted, the discussion below reflects the results for RPLND primarily in adults, which should be similar to those for adolescents with NSMGCT.

The oncological effectiveness of RPLND is reflected in the very low incidence of retroperitoneal recurrence [11–13]. Surgical complication rates of primary RPLND for low-stage disease range from 11% to 32% with lower rates in more recent series [13–15]. In a series of 478 patients treated at Indiana University the most common complication was a superficial wound infection accounting for nearly half of the patients with complications [14]. Most major complications were related to small bowel obstruction (SBO) or atelectasis. Complications were twice as common in patients undergoing a bilateral dissection as those undergoing a unilateral approach. Ejaculation was preserved in 98% of those undergoing a nerve-sparing approach. The more common complications following RPLND in a recent study from Germany are shown in Table 35.1. Other complications occurring in fewer than 1% of patients included late bleeding,

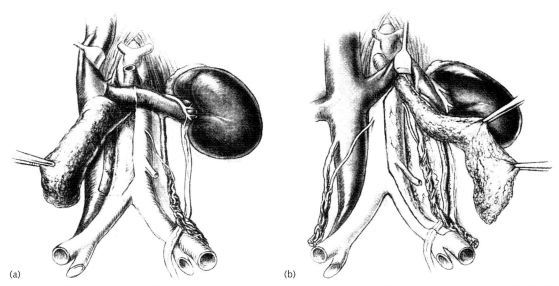

(a)   (b)

Figure 35.1 (a) The right-sided modified unilateral template in which the interaortocaval lymph nodes are included while the left para-aortic lymphatic tissue remains undisturbed. (b) The left-sided modified unilateral template includes the upper interaortocaval group and left para-aortic lymphatic tissues. The lower right para-aortic region remains undisturbed. (Reproduced from Donohue JP and Foster RS, *Urol Clin North Am* 1998;25:461–78, with permission from Elsevier.)

Table 35.1 Complications of RPLND.

Complication	Incidence (%)
Superficial wound infection	5.4
Ileus	2.1
Chylous ascites	2.1
Lymphocele	1.7
Hydronephrosis	1.3

Source: Data from Heidenreich *et al.* [13].

pulmonary embolism, SBO, and deep vein thrombosis (DVT). In this study of nerve-sparing RPLND antegrade ejaculation was preserved in 93%.

Loss of ejaculation/infertility

The key to preserving ejaculation is maintenance of the sympathetic chains which arise behind the vena cava on the right side and dorsolateral to the aorta on the left side (Figures 35.2 and 35.3). The T12–L4 nerve fibers travel anterocaudally to decussate on the anterior surface of the

aorta and form the hypogastric plexus as they course over the aortic bifurcation. The nerve roots should be identified early in the dissection in order to minimize this complication. With nerve-sparing techniques antegrade ejaculation is preserved in nearly all patients (Table 35.2). However, in patients with more advanced disease, this may not be possible. When retrograde ejaculation occurs, it can be treated with a short course of imipramine [16]. Electroejaculation or testis biopsy can also be employed to achieve a pregnancy [17,18].

While nerve-sparing modifications of the RPLND have preserved ejaculation, fertility rates among patients who have undergone an RPLND are affected by other aspects of their treatment and the underlying disease itself. Interestingly, fertility rates are higher among men with stage 1 disease who undergo nerve-sparing RPLND than among those managed on surveillance [19]. This is due to the fact that a higher percentage of men on surveillance ultimately require more intense systemic therapy for recurrence. In men undergoing nerve-sparing RPLND for low-stage disease fertility rates of 75% and 84% have been reported [11,20]. Interpreting fertility results in testis tumor patients following RPLND is difficult since the causes are multifactorial. Following unilateral orchiectomy alone, sperm cell count is highly impaired 1–4 weeks

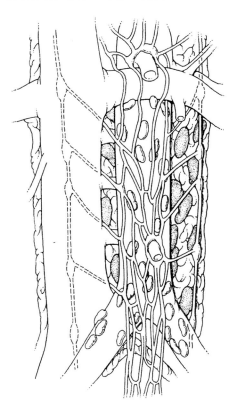

Figure 35.2 A schematic diagram of the lumbar sympathetic nervous system and its relation to the great vessels. Note the sympathetic ganglia L2–L4, the hypogastric plexus and terminal nerve trunks. (Reproduced from Donohue JP and Foster RS, *Urol Clin North Am* 1998;25:461–78, with permission from Elsevier.)

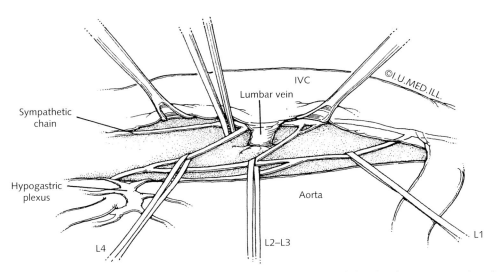

Figure 35.3 The right postganglionic fibers L1–L4 arise from the right sympathetic trunk dorsal to the cava, emerge into the interaortocaval and preaortic area, where they commingle with splanchnic fibers in larger trunks. These are prospectively identified and isolated before lymphadenectomy. (Reproduced from Donohue JP and Foster RS, *Urol Clin North Am* 1998;25:461–78, with permission from Elsevier.)

Table 35.2 Oncologic and ejaculatory results of RPLND.

Study	Type of dissection	Retroperitoneal recurrence (%)	Ejaculation preserved (%)
Weissbach et al. [12]	Bilateral	1.5	34
	Unilateral	2.4	74
Heidenreich et al. [13]	Nerve-sparing (88% unilateral)	1.2	93
Donohue et al. [11]	Unilateral nerve-sparing	0.6	100

after surgery in 60–70% of patients, but improves over 2–3 years. Recovery of spermatogenesis is delayed by a year for those receiving chemotherapy, and high-dose therapy reduces the chances of ultimate recovery [21]. Adults undergoing chemotherapy for testis tumor nearly all become azoospermic, though most recover spermatogenesis within 4 years [22]. Semen cryopreservation should be offered to all postpubertal patients undergoing treatment for testis cancer. Long-term data in children undergoing therapy for testis cancer is sparse. The Intergroup Rhabdomyosarcoma Study Committee reported the long-term health consequences of 86 children treated for paratesticular rhabdomyosarcoma from 1972 to 1984, most of whom had some form of RPLND. Elevated follicle-stimulating hormone or azoospermia occurred in more than half for whom data was available [23].

Bleeding

Major intraoperative bleeding is a rare, but significant problem when it occurs. Surgeons undertaking RPLND must be skilled at basic vascular surgery techniques as a significant percentage of patients will require repair of an intraoperative vascular injury. Repair of inadvertent injuries to the vena cava or aorta can be easily accomplished with fine vascular suture. Inadvertent injuries to the renal arteries can be more problematic occasionally resulting in nephrectomy [24]. Rarely, resection and replacement of portions of the vena cava or aorta may be necessary in patients with advanced disease. Immediate availability of an experienced vascular surgeon is essential when undertaking these more complicated cases.

Ileus/small bowel obstruction

Some degree of ileus is inevitable following a major transperitoneal operation. The risk of prolonged ileus

and SBO may be minimized by limiting manipulation of the bowel. Retractors that lift up and away from the field such as self-retaining Deaver or sweetheart retractors can be helpful. Minimizing the duration of bowel retraction is also important. Self-retaining retractors should be released on a regular basis (e.g. every 45 min) and the bowel examined for impending injury. Once the operation is complete, the bowel should be returned to its normal anatomic position. Some surgeons favor tacking the bowel back in place with absorbable sutures, though the efficacy of this approach is unproven. Prolonged nasogastric (NG) tube drainage has not been shown to be important for preventing prolonged ileus/SBO and the NG tube can be removed on the first postoperative day. Early ambulation may also stimulate bowel activity. SBO may be more common in children. Festen reported a 2.2% incidence of SBO following 1476 abdominal operations in infants and children [25]. Eighty percent of cases occurred within 3 months of surgery and 70% were due to a single adhesive band.

Patients who recover bowel function postoperatively and then re-present weeks or months later with complete bowel obstruction with no flatus or stool should undergo immediate laparotomy. When partial SBO occurs, it can usually be managed conservatively with NG tube suction, intravenous fluids, aggressive monitoring for and correction of electrolyte abnormalities, and serial radiographs [26]. Akgur et al. found that conservative management of SBO in children was successful in 74% of cases. However, these patients were more likely to suffer future recurrent SBO than those managed initially with lysis of adhesions (36% versus 19%) [27]. An elevated white blood cell count with a left shift and persistent localized pain following NG decompression suggest possible compromise of the bowel and early exploration should be considered in those cases.

In addition to SBO, patients presenting with abdominal pain, nausea, and vomiting following RPLND may have pancreatitis. This is presumably secondary to elevation and retraction of the pancreas when obtaining exposure. Serum amylase and lipase should be obtained in patients with persistent symptoms postoperatively.

Deep vein thrombosis

While very rare in children, pulmonary embolism is a potentially fatal complication of RPLND in adults. Most surgeons prefer to avoid the prophylactic use of anticoagulants because of concern for lymphatic leaks and lymphoceles. PAS stockings have been shown to be equally effective for preventing DVTs and should be considered for adolescent patients. For PAS stockings to be effective, it is crucial that the stockings be applied and activated before the induction of anesthesia. They should be maintained postoperatively and early ambulation is encouraged. Frequent physical examination and prompt radiographic evaluation of signs of DVT with early intervention are important for preventing pulmonary embolism.

Chylous ascites

Chylous ascites can be a debilitating complication of RPLND, which usually presents with abdominal distension. The diagnosis can be made by paracentesis. The aspirated fluid will be high in triglyceride, total protein, and cholesterol concentrations and have a cellular differential that is primarily lymphocytes [28]. The complication can be prevented by meticulous attention to hemostasis and control of lymphatic channels. All significant lymphatic vessels should be ligated or clipped. Ligatures should also be applied at the superior and inferior limits of the dissection, particularly where the lymphatic tissue exits the field at the renal hilum. Chylous ascites most commonly occurs in patients with prolonged courses of preoperative chemotherapy and in those with a large intraoperative blood loss – particularly during a postchemotherapy RPLND [29]. Most patients can be managed without surgery. Conservative therapy includes a combination of paracenteses, medium-chain triglycerides, and total parenteral nutrition with a selective use of abdominal drains [29,30]. While occasional patients will respond to observation or dietary changes, most require TPN. With conservative management the ascites will usually resolve within a few months. Use of somatostatins may also be helpful [31]. Those that fail conservative management will require placement of a peritoneovenous shunt. Occasionally early re-exploration and ligation of the offending leak can be

accomplished [32]. Feeding the patient a high-fat diet up to 6h before surgical exploration may facilitate intraoperative identification of the offending leak. There is little information regarding the management of chylous ascites in prepubertal patients, though the same approach used in adults seems reasonable [33].

Surgical approach and morbidity

While an anterior transperitoneal approach is still favored at most institutions, alternative approaches have been employed in an attempt to reduce morbidity. An extraperitoneal approach has been advocated for excision of residual masses following chemotherapy [34]. Reported advantages include the ability to excise coexisting thoracic masses when a thoracoabdominal extraperitoneal approach is used, improved access to nodes above and behind the renal vessels, and a more rapid postoperative recovery. Increasingly popular has been a laparoscopic approach – particularly for primary RPLND in patients with low-stage disease. An initial report of 20 patients in 1994 utilizing a modified unilateral template reported ejaculation in all patients and no retroperitoneal recurrences [35]. However, significant complications, most commonly bleeding, occurred in 30% of patients. In contrast, a 2001 report of 125 patients undergoing laparoscopic RPLND reported only two conversions for bleeding, no major complications, and only 13 minor complications [36]. More recent reports suggest that laparoscopic RPLND utilizing a modified unilateral template and, in some cases, nerve-sparing, can be performed with less morbidity and an improved quality of life compared to open techniques [37,38]. Laparoscopic RPLND has also been performed retroperitoneally [39–41]. Retroperitoneal recurrence is a serious problem and no compromise on the extent of dissection should be accepted to accommodate a laparoscopic approach.

Complications in postchemotherapy RPLND

Not surprisingly, complications are more common in patients undergoing RPLND following chemotherapy for disseminated disease. A report of such patients from Indiana University reported a 30–50% intraoperative complication rate and a 7–14% postoperative complication rate including ascites, wound infection, prolonged ileus, pancreatitis, acute renal failure, and atelectasis

[42]. Patients with higher stage disease had a higher rate of complications and more frequent need for additional intraoperative procedures including nephrectomy, IVC resection, bowel resection, hepatic resection/biopsy, arterial grafting, caval thrombectomy, adrenalectomy, and cholecystecomy. Christmas *et al.* reported on 98 patients undergoing a postchemotherapy RPLND. Some type of vascular procedure was required in nearly all patients including 14 nephrectomies, 35 IMA ligations, 2 aortic grafts, and 2 IVC ligations [43]. Complete macroscopic resection of residual disease was possible in 97% of patients. In another series, 10 of 710 patients undergoing postchemotherapy RPLND required intraoperative or postoperative aortic grafting (for aortic rupture or aortoenteric fistula) [44]. Preemptive intraoperative grafting should be considered when there is extensive subadventitial dissection, a duodenal enterotomy or extensive serosal bowel violation. A 7% rate of caval resection or thrombectomy has been reported in patients undergoing a postchemoterapy RPLND [45]. Not only are complications more common in those undergoing a postchemotherapy RPLND, but also the occurrence of complications in these patients has been shown to adversely affect their disease-free survival [46]. Ejaculatory dysfunction is also more common following postchemotherapy RPLND due to the difficulty in preserving the sympathetic nerves in this group of patients. Among 472 patients undergoing postchemoterapy RPLND, Coogan *et al.* reported that 20% were amenable to a nerve-sparing approach [47]. Seventy-six percent of these patients reported normal ejaculation.

Summary

Orchiectomy and testis-sparing tumor excision are relatively straightforward procedures with low complication rates. However, meticulous hemostasis and adherence to oncological surgical principles are important. RPLND is the operation that carries the greatest risk of complications for patients with testicular cancer. Loss of ejaculation – an expected outcome decades ago – can now be avoided in nearly all patients with low-stage disease. Knowledge and implementation of sound vascular surgical techniques is crucial to anyone undertaking the operation. Chylous ascites, while rare, can be a major complication requiring prolonged management until resolution. Finally, efforts to avoid the complications of any major intraabdominal operation – atelectasis, ileus, SBO, DVT, and PE – should be made.

These efforts include attention to all aspects of preoperative, intraoperative, and postoperative management. Fortunately most patients undergoing operations for testicular tumors are young and otherwise healthy. But complications still occur, particularly in patients undergoing postchemotherapy RPLND.

References

1 Coppes MJ, Rackley R, Kay. Primary testicular and paratesticular tumors of childhood. *Med Pediatr Oncol* 1994;22:329.

2 Ross JH, Rybicki L, Kay R. Clinical behavior and a contemporary management algorithm for prepubertal testis tumors: A summary of the Prepubertal Testis Tumor Registry. *J Urol* 2002;168:1675.

3 Pohl HG, Shukla AR, Metcalf PD *et al.* Prepubertal testis tumors: Actual prevalence rate of histological types. *J Urol* 2004;172:2370.

4 Uehling DT, Phillips E. Residual retroperitoneal mass following chemotherapy for infantile yolk sac tumor. *J Urol* 1994;152:185.

5 Grady R, Ross JH, Kay R. Epidemiologic features of teratomas of the testis in a prepubertal population. *J Urol* 1997;158:1191.

6 Valla S. Testis-sparing surgery for benign testicular tumors in children. *J Urol* 2001;165:2280.

7 Schlatter M, Rescorla F, Giller R *et al.* Excellent outcome in patients with stage I germ cell tumors of the testes: A study of the Children's Cancer Group/Pediatric Oncology Group. *J Pediatr Surg* 2003;38:319.

8 Aki FT, Bilen CY, Tekin MI *et al.* Is scrotal violation per se a risk factor for local relapse and metastases in stage I nonseminomatous testicular cancer? *Urology* 2000;56:459–62.

9 Bochner BH, Lerner SP, Kawachi M *et al.* Postadical orchiectomy hemorrhage: Should an alteration in staging strategy for testicular cancer be considered. *Urology* 1995;46:408–11.

10 Donahue JP. Retroperitoneal lymphadenectomy: the anterior approach including bilateral suprarenal hilar dissection. *Urol Clin North Am* 1977;4:509.

11 Donahue JP, Foster RS. Retroperitoneal lymphadenectomy in staging and treatment – the development of nerve-sparing techniques. *Urol Clin North Am* 1998;25:461–468.

12 Weissbach L, Boedefeld EA, Horstmann-Dubral B. Surgical treatment of stage-I non-seminomatous germ cell testis tumor: Final results of a prospective multicenter trial 1982–1987. *Eur Urol* 1990;17:97–106.

13 Heidenreich A, Albers P, Hartmann M *et al.* Complications of primary nerve sparing retroperitoneal lymph node dissection for clinical stage I nonseminomatous germ cell tumors of the testis: Experience of the German Testicular Cancer Study Group. *J Urol* 2003;169:1710–14.

14 Baniel J, Foster RS, Rowland RG *et al.* Complications of primary tetroperitoneal lymph node dissection. *J Urol* 1994;152:424–7.

15 Moul JW, Robertson JE, George SL *et al.* Complications of therapy for testicular cancer. *J Urol* 1989;142:1491–6.

16 Ochsenkuhn R, Kamischke A, Nieschlag E. Imipramine for successful treatment of retrograde ejaculation caused by retroperitoneal surgery. *Int J Androl* 1999;22:173–7.

17 Chung PH, Palermo G, Schlegel PN *et al.* The use of intra-cytoplasmic sperm injection with electroejaculates from anejaculatory men. *Hum Reprod* 1998;13:1854–8.

18 Ohl DA, Denil J, Bennett CJ *et al.* Electroejaculation following retroperitoneal lymphadenectomy. *J Urol* 1991;145:980–3.

19 Herr HW, Bar-Chama N, O'Sullivan M *et al.* Paternity in men with stage I testis tumors on surveillance. *J Clin Oncol* 1998;16:733–4.

20 Foster RS, McNulty A, Rubin LR *et al.* Fertility considerations in nerve-sparing retroperitoneal lymph-node dissection. *World J Urol* 1994;12:136–8.

21 Fossa SD, Aabyholm T, Vespestad S *et al.* Semen quality after treatment for testicular cancer. *Eur Urol* 1993;23:172–6.

22 Ohl DA, Sonksen J. What are the chances of infertility and should sperm be banked? *Sem Urol Oncol* 1996;14:36–44.

23 Heyn R, Raney RB, Jr., Hays DM *et al.* Late effects of therapy in patients with paratesticular rhabdomyosarcoma. Intergroup Rhabdomyosarcoma Study Committee. *J Clin Oncol* 1992;10:614–23.

24 Morin JF, Provan JL, Jewett MA *et al.* Vascular injury and repair associated with retroperitoneal lymphadenectomy for nonseminomatous germinal cell tumours of the testis. *Can J Surg* 1992;35:253–6.

25 Festen C. Postoperative small bowel obstruction in infants and children. *Ann Surg* 1982;196:580–3.

26 Gingalewski CA. Other causes of intestinal obstruction. In *Pediatric Surgery*, 6th edn. Edited by JL Grosfeld. Philadelphia: Mosby Elsevier, 2006: pp. 1358–68.

27 Akgur FM, Tanyel FC, Buyukpamukcu N *et al.* Adhesive small bowel obstruction in children: The place and predictors of success for conservative treatment. *J Pediatr Surg* 1991;26:37–41.

28 McGahren ED. Ascites. In *Pediatric Surgery*, 6th edn. Edited by JL Grosfeld. Philadelphia: Mosby Elsevier, 2006: pp. 1407–13.

29 Evans JG, Spiess PE, Kamat AM *et al.* Chylous ascites after post-chemotherapy retroperitoneal lymph node dissection: Review of the M. D. Anderson experience. *J Urol* 2006;176:1463–7.

30 Baniel J, Foster RS, Rowland RG *et al.* Management of chylous ascites after retroperitoneal lymph node dissection for testicular cancer. *J Urol* 1993;150:1422–4.

31 Andreou A, Papouli M, Papavasiliou V *et al.* Postoperative chylous ascites in a neonate treated successfully with octreotied: Bile sludge and cholestasis. *Am J Perinatol* 2005;22:401–4.

32 Castillo OA, Litvak JP, Kerkebe M *et al.* Case report: Laparoscopic management of massive chylous ascites after

salvage laparoscopic retroperitoneal lymph-node dissection. *J Endourol* 2006;20:394–6.

33 Allen W, Parrott TS, Saripkin L *et al.* Chylous ascites following retroperitoneal lymphadenectomy for granulosa cell tumor of the testis. *J Urol* 1986;135:797–8.

34 Christmas TJ, Doherty AP, Rustin GJ *et al.* Excision of residual masses of metastatic germ cell tumours after chemotherapy: The role of extraperitoneal surgical approaches. *BJU* 1998;81:301–8.

35 Gerber GS, Bissada NK, Hulbert JC *et al.* Laparoscopic retroperitoneal lymphadenectomy: Multi-institutional analysis. *J Urol* 1994;152:188–91.

36 Janetschek G, Peschel R, Hobisch A *et al.* Laparoscopic retroperitoneal lymph node dissection. *J Endourol* 2001; 15:449–53.

37 Poulaki V, Skriapas K, de Vries R *et al.* Quality of life after laparoscopic and open retroperitoneal lymph node dissection in clinical Stage I nonseminomatous germ cell tumor: A comparison study. *Urology* 2006;68:154–60.

38 Steiner H, Paschel R, Janetschek G *et al.* Long-term results of laparoscopic retroperitoneal lymph node dissection: A single-center 10-year experience. *Urol* 2004;63:550–5.

39 Hsu T, Su L, Ong A. Anterior extraperitoneal approach to laparoscopic retroperitoneal lymph node dissection: A novel technique. *J Urol* 2003;169:258–60.

40 LeBlan E, Caty A, Dargent D *et al.* Extraperitoneal laparoscopic para-aortic lymph node dissection for early stage nonseminomatous germ cell tumors of the testis with introduction of a nerve sparing technique: Description and results. *J Urol* 2001;165:89–92.

41 Rassweiler JJ, Frede T, Lenz E *et al.* Long-term experience with laparoscopic retroperitoneal lymph node dissection in the management of low-stage testis cancer. *Eur Urol* 2000;37:251–60.

42 Mosharafa AA, Foster RS, Koch MO *et al.* Complications of post-chemotherapy retroperitoneal lymph node dissection for testis cancer. *J Urol* 2004;171:1839–41.

43 Christmas TJ, Smith GL, Kooner R. Vascular interventions during post-chemotherapy retroperitoneal lymph-node dissection for metastatic testis cancer. *Eur J Surg Oncol* 1998;24:292–7.

44 Donohue JP, Thornhill JA, Foster RS *et al.* Vascular considerations in postchemotherapy. Retroperitoneal lymph-node dissection: Part II. *World J Urol* 1994;12:187–9.

45 Donohue JP, Thornhill JA, Foster RS *et al.* Vascular considerations in postchemotherapy. Retroperitoneal lymph-node dissection: Part I – Vena cava. *World J Urol* 1994;12:182–6.

46 Spiess PE, Brown GA, Liu P *et al.* Predictors of outcome in patients undergoing postchemotherapy retroperitoneal lymph node dissection for testicular cancer. *Cancer* 2006;107:1483–90.

47 Coogan CL, Hejase MJ, Wahle GR *et al.* Nerve sparing post-chemotherapy retroperitoneal lymph node dissection for advanced testicular cancer. *J Urol* 1996;156:1656–8.

36

Adrenal Tumors

Bruce Broecker and James Elmore

Key points

- Adrenal surgery in children consists of adrenalectomy, performed for removal of an adrenal tumor – benign or malignant.

- The tumors that are encountered in children include adrenal neuroblastoma, pheochromocytoma, and adrenal cortical carcinoma.

- Neuroblastoma is the most common adrenal tumor in children.

- Pheochromocytoma, which may be benign or malignant, and adrenal cortical carcinoma are extremely rare.

- Surgical complications consist of injuries to adjacent organs or structures and the untoward effects of stimulation or removal of a hormonally active gland and/or tumor.

Introduction

Although adrenal tumors in children are rare, several of these tumors are of particular clinical importance. These tumors, which may be benign or malignant, can be hormonally active and infiltrative at times causing dramatic clinical presentations as well as lethal outcomes. As a result, surgery poses a distinct challenge. Removing them without complication requires a firm understanding of adrenal anatomy, with variations, and of adrenal hormonal biochemistry and physiology. Surgical techniques must be particularly meticulous, and recognition of the signs and symptoms of an excess or deficiency of the hormonal products of the adrenal cortex and medulla is essential knowledge. This chapter will summarize some of the important surgical considerations of the most common childhood adrenal tumors.

Adrenal anatomy

The adrenal glands (Figure 36.1) lie within Gerota's fascia and are separated from kidney by a thin layer of

connective tissue. The left adrenal gland is semilunar in shape and lies lateral to the aorta and posterior to the pancreas. The right adrenal gland is pyramidal in shape and lies posterior to the vena cava and superior and medial to the upper pole of the right kidney. Both glands are supplied by paired superior, middle, and inferior adrenal arteries. The superior adrenal artery arises from the inferior phrenic artery, which is a branch of the aorta. The middle adrenal artery arises from the lateral aspect of the aorta near the superior mesenteric artery. The inferior adrenal artery is typically a branch of the main renal artery, though it may also arise from an upper pole renal artery. Venous drainage of each adrenal gland is typically a single vein. The right adrenal vein is short and passes directly into the posterior aspect of the inferior vena cava. Occasionally accessory right adrenal veins are present and join the inferior vena cava superior to the right adrenal vein. The left adrenal vein drains into the superior aspect of the left renal vein.

Adrenal physiology/biochemistry

The adrenal gland consists of a cortex and medulla, which function independently. The cortex makes up approximately 80% of the weight and volume of the adrenal gland and is composed of three distinct zones – an outer zona

Pediatric Urology: Surgical Complications and Management. Edited by Duncan T. Wilcox, Prasad P. Godbole and Martin A. Koyle. © 2008 Blackwell Publishing, ISBN: 978-1-4051-6268-5.

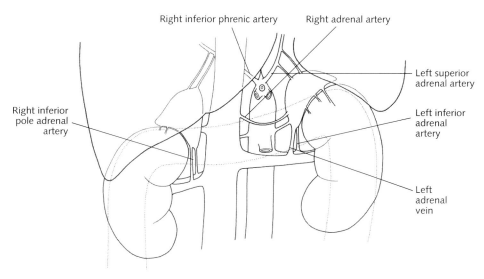

Figure 36.1 Anatomy of the adrenal glands. (Adapted from Hohenfellner R, Fitzpatrick J, and McAninch J (eds), *Advanced Urologic Surgery*, 3rd edn. Oxford: Blackwell Publishing, 2005, with permission from Blackwell Publishing.)

glomerulosa, a middle zona fasciculata, and an inner zona reticularis. These zones are responsible for the production of aldosterone, cortisol, and adrenal androgens, respectively. Adrenal cortisol production is regulated primarily by the pituitary hormone adrenocorticotropic hormone (ACTH). Aldosterone is the major mineralocorticoid produced by the adrenal gland and regulates fluid and electrolyte balance by stimulating sodium retention and potassium and hydrogen ion secretion in the distal convoluted tubule of the kidney. The renin-angiotensin system and plasma potassium concentrations are the principal regulators of aldosterone secretion whereas ACTH and plasma sodium are minor contributors. The major hormones produced by the zona reticularis are dehydroepiandrosterone (DHEA) and androstenedione, both weakly androgenic hormones.

The medulla is composed of specialized neuroendocrine cells, the chromaffin cells, and is richly innervated by preganglionic sympathetic nerves. The adrenal medulla produces the catecholamines epinephrine and norepinephrine from the metabolism of tyrosine. Excitation of the medulla stimulates a discharge of catecholamines from intracellular granules and results in the classically described "fight or flight" response. The physiologic effects of catecholamine release are mediated by alpha- and beta-adrenergic receptors of target organs and tissues and include a rise in blood pressure, tachycardia, sweating, and pupillary dilation.

Adrenal insufficiency: Symptoms

Adrenal insufficiency can occur following bilateral adrenalectomy or unilateral adrenalectomy if the contralateral adrenal gland is absent or nonfunctional. Bilateral adrenalectomy is almost never necessary or performed in children, and adrenal insufficiency is easily avoided by appropriate hormonal replacement. However, unsuspected absence or nonfunction of the contralateral adrenal gland may give rise to acute adrenal insufficiency following unilateral adrenalectomy resulting in "adrenal crisis." The symptoms are well defined and mainly attributable to mineralocorticoid deficiency. Symptoms include hypotension, fever, abdominal pain, nausea, and weakness. Laboratory findings include hyponatremia, hyperkalemia, hypoglycemia, and azotemia. Acute adrenal insufficiency may be difficult to distinguish from septic shock. In Waterhourse–Friderichsen syndrome the two coincide secondary to an overwhelming bacterial infection, classically by *Neisseria meningitidis*, which results in massive bilateral adrenal hemorrhage.

Table 36.1 International Neuroblastoma Staging System (INSS) and Evans' staging system.

Evans' classification	International Neuroblastoma Staging System
Stage I: tumor confined to the organ or structure of origin	Stage 1: localized tumor confined to the area of origin; complete gross excision with or without microscopic residual disease; ipsilateral or contralateral lymph nodes are microscopically negative
Stage II: tumor extending in continuity beyond the organ or structure of origin but not crossing the midline; regional lymph nodes on ipsilateral side may be involved	Stage 2a: unilateral tumor with incomplete gross excision; ipsilateral or contralateral lymph nodes are microscopically negative Stage 2b: unilateral tumor with complete or incomplete gross excision; ipsilateral lymph nodes microscopically positive, contralateral lymph nodes microscopically negative
Stage III: tumor extending in continuity beyond the midline; regional lymph nodes may be involved bilaterally	Stage 3: tumor infiltrating across the midline with or without regional lymph node involvement or unilateral tumor with contralateral lymph node involvement or midline tumor with bilateral lymph nodes involvement
Stage IV: remote disease involving the skeleton, bone marrow, soft tissue, or distant lymph nodes	Stage 4: disseminated tumor to bone, bone marrow, liver, distant lymph nodes, and/or other organs
Stage IVs: Stage I or II except for the presence of remote disease confined to the liver, skin, or bone marrow	Stage 4s: localized primary tumor – stage 1 or 2 – with dissemination limited to liver, skin, or bone marrow

Adrenal hypersecretion: Symptoms

Adrenal hypersecretion as a complication of adrenal surgery can occur during resection of pheochromocytoma and represents an outpouring of catecholamines during surgical manipulation. Symptoms include tachycardia and malignant hypertension.

Proper preoperative preparation of the patient with known pheochromocytoma will substantially reduce the occurrence of these potentially lethal symptoms (see section "Prevention of Complications"). Adrenal hypersecretion also occurs in patients with adrenocortical carcinoma. In children, 95% of these tumors are hormonally active. The most common products are the androgenic hormones leading to virilization. Less commonly they produce glucocorticoids leading to Cushing's syndrome and very rarely aldosterone or estradiol (feminizing) producing tumors have been reported in children.

Specific tumors

Neuroblastoma: Overview

Neuroblastoma is a malignant tumor of neural crest origin and is the most common extracranial solid neoplasm found in children. Most occur between birth and 4 years of age. It accounts for 8–10% of all childhood cancers [1]. The overall incidence of neuroblastoma is approximately 1 case per 10,000 persons, with approximately 525 newly diagnosed cases in the United States each year [2]. Neuroblastoma occurs wherever there are sympathetic ganglia – the neck, thorax, retroperitoneum (abdomen), and pelvis. Approximately 75% of neuroblastomas arise in the retroperitoneum, 50% in the adrenal, and 25% from the paravertebral ganglia [2].

The presenting signs and symptoms are variable and reflect the effect of the tumor, metastatic disease, and/or tumor hormone production. An abdominal mass, malaise, bone pain due to metastasis and anemia reflecting bone marrow involvement are common.

The most common current staging system is the International Neuroblastoma Staging System (INNS), which is based on resectability and has replaced the Evans' system (Table 36.1). One of the significant features in the outcome of patients with neuroblastoma is the fact that the majority present with high-stage disease – 70% have metastatic disease at presentation [2].

Biology of the tumor determines the treatment given with a risk-based approach incorporating the following factors: age, stage, MYC status, histopathology (Shimada classification), and DNA ploidy. Surgery is the foundation of treatment for those with localized disease which, when completely excised, allows an excellent survival [3]. A number of multiagent chemotherapy regimens have been developed to treat high-risk patients. Survival in these patients remains poor, and there is an ongoing search for more effective agents. The role of aggressive surgery in patients with advanced disease is not clear [4].

Neuroblastoma: Surgical complications

There are no studies that systematically and specifically measure the risk of adrenal surgery in children with neuroblastoma. The available literature, however, suggests that a significant degree of morbidity can be expected. Neuroblastoma is an infiltrative tumor arising adjacent to major vascular structures and resection of the tumor inevitably involves significant risk of injury to those structures. Complication rates reported vary widely reflecting not only biologic features such as age, stage, and location of the tumor but also very much the aggressiveness of the surgeon's efforts to achieve a complete resection in advanced tumors and the criteria or definition of a surgical complication. A report by Cantos noted a 67% overall surgical complication rate associated with an intensive treatment protocol for high-risk neuroblastoma but included hypertension, the use of total parenteral nutrition, and the need for pain management consultation among the postoperative complications [5]. The most common complication in this series was hemorrhage requiring transfusion which occurred in 86% patients. Von Schwienitz reported "clinically relevant" surgical complications occurring in 19.2% of 2112 operations for neuroblastoma (all sites), which included hemorrhage (3%), intestinal obstruction (3%), and renal complications (2.3%) [6]. No difference was noted in the incidence of complications when stratified by stage, age, site (abdominal versus thoracic), or initial versus delayed resection. Also of note, 20 surgical complications (1% of all operations) contributed directly to the patient's death. In several smaller series major vascular injury (4%), intestinal infarction, splenic injury (requiring splenectomy), intussusception, and chylous ascites have been reported in the early perioperative period [7].

The kidney appears to be at particular risk in patients with abdominal neuroblastoma, though probably more so with those arising from the sympathetic plexus rather than the adrenal gland itself. Shamberger reported nephrectomy in 52 of 349 (15%) patients who underwent resection of an abdominal neuroblastoma between 1981 and 1991 as part of Pediatric Oncology Group protocols

[8]. In most cases this represented direct involvement of the kidney and/or renal hilum by the tumor but in five cases a preserved kidney was later removed for renal infarction or atrophy. Tanabe *et al.* reported renal impairment in six cases in which an apparently viable kidney remained at the conclusion of surgical removal of an abdominal neuroblastoma [9]. In one of these cases early recognition of impaired blood flow by color Doppler ultrasound was followed by intra-arterial instillation of lipo-prostaglandin E_1 with subsequent preservation of the kidney. In the remaining five recognition was delayed and the kidney atrophied though it was not removed. Ogita also reported a case of renal artery spasm in the solitary remaining kidney following tumor resection, ipsilateral nephrectomy, and para-aortic lymph node dissection (celiac to iliac bifurcation) [10]. This patient developed oliguria and renal failure in the immediate postoperative hours. Angiography at 10 h following surgery revealed complete renal artery obstruction which resolved with intra-arterial administration of lidocaine. Monclair has advocated avoidance of twisting or traction of the renal vessels and prophylactic application of local anesthetic to the renal artery during surgery as well as nephropexy of the fully mobilized kidney as intraoperative methods to minimize risk to the kidney [11].

Long-term complications of both surgical and chemotherapeutic treatments of neuroblastoma may also occur. Koyle *et al.* reported three cases of retroperitoneal fibrosis and four cases of renal cell carcinoma occurring during long-term follow-up of survivors of advanced stage abdominal neuroblastoma [12]. Other reported secondary tumors include pheochromocytoma, leukemia, bone tumors, brain tumors, and thyroid cancer [13–16]. Kiely reported prolonged diarrhea in 30% (23 of 77) patients after excision of advanced abdominal neuroblastoma [17]. The need to do extensive dissection around the celiac and superior mesenteric artery to remove the tumor appeared to increase this risk.

Pheochromocytoma: Overview

Pheochromocytoma is a neuroendocrine tumor that arises from chromaffin cells of the adrenal medulla or other sites where small clusters of chromaffin cells settle embryologically. These extra-adrenal tumors, termed paragangliomas, occur in sympathetic ganglia anywhere between the neck (carotid artery) and pelvis (organ of Zuckerkandl) and even (rarely) in the wall of the urinary bladder and prostate. Only 10% of these tumors occur in childhood but these are characterized by an increased incidence of bilaterality (25–50%), extra-adrenal site

(25–30%), familial pattern (10%), and sustained rather than paroxysmal hypertension (90%). They have a lesser risk of malignancy (3%). Pediatric pheochromocytoma can be found in association with several conditions, including neurofibromatosis, von Hipple–Lindau disease, Sturge–Weber syndrome, and multiple endocrine neoplasia, type 2 (MEN-2).

The clinical symptoms of pheochromocytoma are those due to its elaboration of catecholamines – epinephrine and norepinephrine – which is most commonly sustained and severe hypertension. Treatment of pheochromocytoma is surgical excision of the tumor. This includes the adrenal gland for those arising in this organ.

Pheochromocytoma: Surgical complications

Pheochromocytoma is a rare tumor in children. Consequently there is no large series from which a meaningful estimate of the complications specific to this tumor in childhood can be derived. The adequacy of the preoperative preparation of the patient (see later), the size and vascularity of the tumor as well as the surgical approach will be significant factors in the expected morbidity of the surgical procedure.

Adrenocortical tumors: Overview

Adrenal cortical tumors – adrenal cortical adenoma and adrenal cortical carcinoma – comprise 0.2% of childhood neoplasms and only 6% of tumors arising in the adrenal gland [18]. Most of these tumors are malignant carcinomas but between one-quarter and one-third are adenomas. The mean age of presentation in a review of 209 cases in childhood was 4.63 years [19]. Females predominate by a ratio of between 2:1 and 9:1. In contrast to adult tumors those in children are almost all functional, primarily virilizing. A lesser number have Cushing's syndrome or are mixed. Surprisingly in older studies the diagnosis was frequently delayed and historically the survival has been poor. Hayles *et al.* reported a survival of only 10% among 222 children with tumors of the adrenal cortex [20]. Recent studies have reported survival of approximately 50% [21]. Stage is the most important determining factor in survival. Small (<5 cm, 200 g) have a survival of 90–100% while those with nodal or distant metastasis have <20% survival. Patients <5 years and tumors <9 cm appear to have a better survival than patients who are older or have larger tumors [21]. In the pediatric literature, two series have reported a 30% and 38% tumor response rate to mitotane [22]. Complete surgical removal if possible, however, remains the best hope for cure [21–23].

Adrenocortical carcinoma: Surgical complications

Adrenocortical carcinoma is a very rare tumor in childhood and, as with pheochromocytoma, there is no large series from which to estimate an incidence of complications. Tumor extension into the vena cava occurs in approximately 15% increasing the risk of hemorrhage during surgery. In one series nephrectomy was performed in almost 25% as part of an *en bloc* resection of the tumor [21]. However excision of an adrenocortical tumor does not carry the risk of catecholamine release and severe hypertension which may be seen with pheochromocytoma, reducing those associated risks.

Adrenal surgery: Surgical approach

The surgical approach to the adrenal gland, whether endoscopic or open, should be chosen based on the size of tumor and the degree of local invasion. Several open approaches to resection have been described, each with their own advantages and disadvantages. Classically, a transverse abdominal or chevron incision is used. A longer left adrenal vein which drains into the left renal vein as well as the slightly anterior lie of the left adrenal gland in relation to the kidney makes left adrenalectomy somewhat easier than right adrenalectomy. Regardless of the side, the colon is first mobilized and reflected medially. A right-sided tumor also requires an incision in the posterior peritoneum to reflect the liver cranially. Gerota's fascia is then exposed and the adrenal veins identified. These are doubly ligated and divided. Venous control may be more difficult and hazardous on the right since that adrenal vein is shorter and drains directly into the vena cava. Accessory hepatic veins may also enter the cava in this area. Great care must be taken to prevent avulsion of these vessels and if necessary they may be ligated. Medial and cephalad attachments are then divided to allow greater mobility of the adrenal gland. Lateral attachments are then divided and the gland is dissected from the kidney.

Laparoscopic approaches to the adrenal gland have been utilized for more than a decade in adults and in this population have largely supplanted open surgery. Recent reviews of laparoscopic adrenalectomy performed in adults (various diagnoses) suggests a complication rate of 1–3% for major complications – myocardial events, pneumonia, excess hemorrhage with reoperation – and 15–20% for minor complications [24,25]. Children may be less vulnerable though not immune to the myocardial and cerebral-vascular consequences of severe hypertension which may occur during excision of a pheochromocytoma. However, there are fewer series describing laparoscopic adrenalectomy in children. Most reports are feasibility studies with small numbers with limited follow-up. The largest review of laparoscopic adrenalectomy in children included 20 children who underwent 21 adrenalectomies [26]. Nine of these patients had neuroblastoma and other diagnoses included adrenal hyperplasia, adenomas, and pheochromocytoma. In this series postoperative hospital stay averaged 1.5 days. In addition to a shorter convalescence, laparoscopic approaches are less painful and may allow more rapid delivery of adjuvant chemotherapy [27]. Tumor seeding of trocar sites has been reported and intact removal of the specimen can be done by extending the umbilical trocar site [28]. It should be emphasized that tumor size or the degree of local invasion may prohibit safe laparoscopic excision.

Prevention of complications

Neuroblastoma: Preoperative chemotherapy

Survival in patients with localized neuroblastoma, where complete tumor resection is possible, is good. Unfortunately many patients present with advanced and seemingly unresectable tumors.

Preresection chemotherapy can significantly reduce the size of the tumor and render it resectable. Canete reported shrinkage in 88% of 63 tumors treated with chemotherapy before tumor resection [29]. In another study, gross complete surgical resection was possible in only 24% patients who underwent initial exploration but in 64% patients who underwent delayed exploration [30]. Preresection chemotherapy may also reduce surgical complications. Shamberger reported surgical complications in 8 of 20 patients who underwent initial surgical resection for Evans' stages III and IV neuroblastoma and 0 of 22 in those having delayed resection following multiagent chemotherapy [31]. He also noted that the risk of nephrectomy was significantly higher in those having initial tumor resection (29/116, 25%) compared with those undergoing surgery following induction chemotherapy (23/233, 10%). The larger study by von Schweinitz [6] however demonstrated no difference in the complication rate and Canete [29] found a higher complication rate in those who received preresection chemotherapy versus initial resection. The higher complication rate was attributed to patient/tumor selection – larger and more extensive tumors being those

that were pretreated and subjected to delayed resection. Since none of these studies are randomized the issue is unresolved as is the issue of whether survival is improved by aggressive surgery aimed at complete excision in advanced neuroblastoma.

Based on current available evidence, it seems unwise to sacrifice vital structures at the first exploration, particularly in those with otherwise favorable tumor characteristics. An aggressive effort at complete tumor excision may lead to devascularization and atrophy of the kidney, injury to other organs, and increased blood loss without proven long-term benefit. In these cases an attempt at complete resection can be delayed and addressed at a second or even third exploration with similar survival rates [32–34].

Pheochromocytoma: Preoperative catecholamine blockade

Blockade of the production and effects of catecholamines is an essential step in reducing the metabolic complications of surgery for pheochromocytoma (Table 36.2). As a result of the hemodynamic instability that can be encountered intraoperatively, arterial and central venous lines are crucial for monitoring blood pressure and fluid status. Agents with short half-lives are ideal for correcting acute variations in blood pressure. Sodium nitroprusside is an excellent agent for intraoperative hypertensive episodes given its rapid onset and dissipation.

Preoperatively alpha-adrenergic blockade will lower blood pressure and produce vasodilation allowing plasma volume re-expansion. The long-acting, nonselective alpha-blocker phenoxybenzamine has been the drug of choice [35]. It has significant side effects including somnolence, orthostasis, and stuffy nose. If phenoxybenzamine

Table 36.2 Pharmacologic agents used preoperatively with pheochromocytoma.

Hypertension	Phenoxybenzamine: 10 mg BID up to 40 mg QID (maximum) as needed to normalize BP Metyrosine: 250 mg QID up to 1 g QID (maximum) as needed to normalize BP
Tachycardia	Propranolol (started after alpha-blockade): 10 mg TID up to 80 mg TID (maximum) to control heart rate

is not tolerated, the selective alpha 1 receptor blockers like prazosin, doxazosin, or terazosin can be used [36]. Alpha-blockade not only mutes the intraoperative risk of hypertension but decreases postoperative hypotension which can result from the precipitous removal of alpha-adrenergic stimulation in a severely volume contracted patient. After alpha-blockers are initiated, beta-blockers (propranolol or metoprolol) are added to prevent the reflex tachycardia associated with alpha-receptor blockade. Other authors favor the preoperative use of calcium channel blockers for its myocardial protective effects [37]. The use of alpha-methy-L-tyrosine (metryrosine) which is a competitive inhibitor of tyrosine hydroxylase, the rate limiting enzyme in catecholamine synthesis, has been advocated by others [38,39]. Preoperative use will result in a 50–80% reduction in catecholamine formation.

The preoperative pharmacologic preparation of the patient should be as long as is necessary to achieve a normal blood pressure, pulse, and volume status – generally a minimum of 3–5 days and often 1–2 weeks. Adequate blockade is heralded by the decrease in blood pressure to normal levels and a fall in the hematocrit indicating adequate expansion of blood volume. Because norepinephrine and epinephrine contribute to insulin resistance, patients should be monitored for the development of hypoglycemia in the 48 h after surgery [36].

Conclusion

Given their anatomy and complex physiology, adrenal tumors pose unique surgical challenges. Neuroblastoma, the most common adrenal tumor in children, is typically infiltrative and may involve other major organs and structures. Care must be used in both patient selection and during surgery to prevent injury to these structures and significant blood loss. Pheochromocytomas, with their potential for liberation of excess catecholamines, require unique preoperative and operative considerations. Laparoscopy has replaced open surgery for the management of most adrenal tumors in adults, and in the coming years it can be expected that laparoscopic and robotic techniques will be increasingly applied to childhood adrenal tumors.

References

1 Gurney JG, Ross JA, Wall DA et al. Infant cancer in the US: Histology-specific incidence and trends, 1973 to 1992. *J Pediatr Hematol Oncol* 1996;19:428–32.

2 Alexander F. Neuroblastoma. *Urol Clin North Am* 2000;27:383–92.

3 O'Neill JA, Littman P, Blitzer P et al. The role of surgery in localized neuroblastoma. *J Pediatr Surg* 1985;20:708–12.

4 Kiely E. Radical surgery for abdominal neuroblastoma. *Semin Surg Oncol* 2006;9:489–92.

5 Cantos MF, Gerstle JT, Irwin MS, Pappo A, Farley S, Cheang T et al. Surgical challenges associated with intensive treatment protocols for high risk NBT. *J Pediatr Surg* 2006;41:960–5.

6 von Schweinitz D, Hero B, Berthold F. The impact of radicality on outcome in childhood neuroblastoma. *Eur J Pediatr Surg* 2002;12:402–9.

7 Ikeda H, Suzuki N, Takahashi A, Kuroiwa M, Nagashima K, Tsuchida Y et al. Surgical treatment of neuroblastoma in infants under 12 months of age. *J Pediatr Surg* 1998;33:1246–50.

8 Shamberger RC, Smith EI, Joshi VV, Rao PV, Hayes FA, Bowman LC et al. The risk of nephrectomy during local control in abdominal neuroblastoma. *J Pediatr Surg* 1998;33:161–4.

9 Tanabe M, Ohnuma N, Iwai J, Yoshida H, Takahashi H. Renal impairment after surgical resection of neuroblastoma. *J Pediatr Surg* 1996;31:1252–5.

10 Ogita S, Tokiwa K, Takahashi T. Renal artery spasm: A cause of renal failure following abdominal surgery for neuroblastoma. *J Pediatr Surg* 1989;24:215–17.

11 Monclair T. *Measures to Avoid Kidney Loss during Neuroblastoma Surgery*. Paris: IPSO, 1994 (personal communication).

12 Koyle MA, Hatch DA, Furness PD III, Lovell MA, Odom LF, Kurzrock EA. Long-term urological complications in survivors younger than 15 months of advanced stage abdominal neuroblastoma. *J Urol* 2001;166:1455–8.

13 Fairchild R, Kyner J, Hermreck A et al. Neuroblastoma, pheochromocytoma, and renal cell carcinoma. Occurrence in a single patient. *JAMA* 1979;242:2210–1.

14 Hunger S, Sklar J, Link M. Acute lymphoblastic leukemia occurring as a second malignant neoplasm in childhood: Report of three cases and review of the literature. *J Clin Oncol* 1992;10:156–63.

15 Ben-Arush M, Doron Y, Braun J et al. Brain tumor as a second malignant neoplasm following neuroblastoma stage IV-S. *Med Pediatr Oncol* 1990;18:240–5.

16 Smith M, Xue H, Strong L et al. Forty-year experience with second malignancies after treatment of childhood cancer: Analysis of outcome following the development of the second malignancy. *J Pediatr Surg* 1993;28:1342–8.

17 Rees H, Markley MA, Kiely EM, Pierro A, Pritchard J. Diarrhea after resection of advanced abdominal neuroblastoma: A common problem. *Surgery* 1998;123:568–72.

18 Liou LS, Kay R. Adrenocortical carcinoma in children. *Urol Clin North Am* 2000;27:469–79.

19 Neblett W, Freses-Steed M, Scott H. Experience with adrenocortical neoplasms in childhood. *Am Surg* 1987;53:117–25.

20 Hayles A, Hahn H, Sprague R, Bahn R, Priestly J. Hormone secreting tumors of the adrenal cortex in children. *Pediatrics* 1996;37:19–25.

21 Tucci S, Martins A, Suaid H, Cologna A, Reis R. The impact of tumor stage on prognosis in children with adrenocortical carcinoma. *J Urol* 2005;174:2338–42.

22 Teinturier C, Pauchard MS, Brugieres L *et al.* Clinical and prognostic aspects of adrenocortical neoplasms in childhood. *Med Pediatr Oncol* 1999;32:106–11.

23 Mayer SK, Oligny LL, Deal C *et al.* Childhood adrenocortical tumors: Case series and reevaluation of prognosis – A 24-year experience. *J Pediatr Surg* 1997;32:911–15.

24 Permpongkosol S, Link RE, Su LM, Romero FR, Bagga HS, Pavlovich CP *et al.* Complications of 2775 urologic laparoscopic procedures: 1993 to 2005. *J Urol* 2007;177:580–5.

25 Walz MK, Alesina PF, Wenger FA, Deligiannis A, Szuczik E, Petersenn S *et al.* Posterior retroperitoneoscopic adrenalectomy results of 560 procedure in 520 patients. *Surgery* 2006;140:943–8.

26 Skarsgard ED, Albanese CT. The safety and efficacy of laparoscopic adrenalectomy in children. *Arch Surg* 2005;140:905–8.

27 de Lagausie P, Berrebi D, Michon J, Philippe-Chomette P, El Ghoneimi A, Garel C *et al.* Laparoscopic adrenal surgery for neuroblastoma in children. *J Urol* 2003;170:932–5.

28 Porpiglia F, Fiori C, Tarabuzzi R, Giraudo G, Garrone C, Morino M *et al.* Is laparoscopic adrenalectomy feasible for adrenocortical carcinoma or metastasis? *BJU Int* 2004;94:1026–9.

29 Canete A, Jovani C, Lopez A, Costa E, Segarra V, Fernandez JM *et al.* Surgical treatment for neuroblastoma: Complications during a 15 years' experience. *J Pediatr Surg* 1998;33:1526–30.

30 Matsumura M, Atkinson JB, Hays DM *et al.* An evaluation of the role of surgery in metastatic neuroblastoma. *J Pediatr Surg* 1998;23:448–53.

31 Shamberger RC, Allarde-Segundo A, Kozakewich HP, Grier HE. Surgical management of stage III and IV NBT: Resection before or after chemotherapy. *J Pediatr Surg* 1991;26:1113–7.

32 Haase GM, Wong WY, deLorimier AA, Sather HN, Hammond GD. Improvement in survival after excision of primary tumor in stage III neuroblastoma. *J Pediatr Surg* 1989;24:194–200.

33 Matthay K, Perez C, Seeger RC *et al.* Successful treatment of stage III neuroblastoma based on prospective biologic staging: A children's cancer group study. *J Clin Oncol* 1998;16:1256–64.

34 Rubie H, Michon J, Plantaz D *et al.* Unresectable localized neuroblastoma: Improved survival after primary chemotherapy including carboplatin-etoposide. *Br J Cancer* 1998;77:2310–17.

35 Schiff RL, Welsh GA. Perioperative evaluation and management of the patient with endocrine dysfunction. *Med Clin North Am* 2003;87:393–402.

36 Ross JH. Pheochromocytoma: Special considerations in children. *Urol Clin North Am* 2000;27:393–402.

37 Lebuffe G, Dosseh E, Tek G, Tygat H, Moreno S, Tavernier B *et al.* The effect of calcium channel blockers on outcome following the surgical treatment of phaeochromocytoma and paragangliomas. *Anesthesia* 2005;60:439–44.

38 Perry RR, Keiser HR, Norton JA *et al.* Surgical management of pheochromocytoma with the use of metyrosine. *Ann Surg* 1990;212:621–8.

39 Steinsapir J, Carr AA, Prisant LM *et al.* Metyrosine and pheochromocytoma. *Arch Intern Med* 1997;157:901–6.

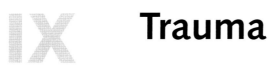

IX Trauma

37

Genital Trauma

Vijaya Vemulakonda and Richard W. Grady

Key points

- Genital trauma is rare in the pediatric population.

- Penile trauma is most commonly iatrogenic.

- Ultrasonography is valuable in the evaluation of scrotal trauma when physical exam is nondiagnostic.

- Examination under anesthesia should be used to fully assess the extent of injury and allow for surgical intervention when necessary.

- Sexual abuse should be considered, especially in cases where the extent of injury is greater than expected from the mechanism of injury.

Introduction

Trauma is the leading cause of death in children. However, genitourinary tract injuries are present in <3% of trauma cases [1]. The majority of these injuries are due to blunt trauma resulting from motor vehicle collisions or sports-related injuries [2]. Iatrogenic injuries are especially prominent in the neonatal period. When evaluating isolated genital trauma, physicians should have a high index of suspicion for sexual abuse. This chapter will review common etiologies for traumatic genital injuries and evaluate current diagnostic and treatment options. We will also discuss potential risk factors and presenting signs of sexual abuse.

Penile injuries

Penile injuries in the neonate are most commonly iatrogenic in nature [2]. Circumcision-related injuries are often due to clamp (e.g. Mogen or Gomco) circumcisions and may range from a mild loss of penile skin (Figure 37.1) to more significant glans, distal urethral, and penile shaft injuries.

Self-inflicted or noniatrogenic pediatric penile injuries are less common. Traumatic injuries include degloving of the penis or penile amputations. Etiologies for injuries include zipper-related injuries, which may result in contusion or pressure necrosis of the prepuce [3]. Tourniquet injuries result from hair wrapping around the penis ("hair tourniquet") [2]. These often lead to preputial edema or inflammation or less commonly causing more significant injury to the corpora or the urethra. In toddlers, falling from toilet seats during toilet training may lead to preputial, glans, or distal shaft contusions or lacerations. These

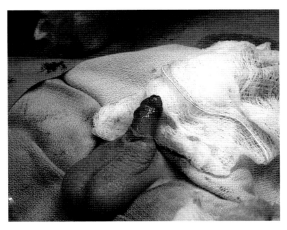

Figure 37.1 Penile degloving injury after Gomco clamp circumcision.

Pediatric Urology: Surgical Complications and Management. Edited by Duncan T. Wilcox, Prasad P. Godbole and Martin A. Koyle. © 2008 Blackwell Publishing, ISBN: 978-1-4051-6268-5.

same injuries may also occur secondary to rubber band powered toys used during bathtub playtime. Rarely, penile amputations may result from dog or other animal bites [4]. Finally, blunt perineal trauma may result in associated high-flow priapism secondary to a traumatic arteriovenous fistula in rare cases [5].

Treatment

Superficial contusions and lacerations are generally managed nonoperatively with topical antibiotic ointments and icepacks where indicated. Empiric antibiotics are commonly used in this situation, including first generations cephalosporins such as cephalexin, to decrease the chance of a secondary cellulitis, although there is little empiric data to support this practice. Where significant penile skin is lost due to neonatal circumcision, full thickness skin grafting of the excised prepuce or shaft skin may be performed in the immediate postinjury period [6]. In cases where the prepuce is not available, healing by secondary intention may result in a satisfactory outcome, although it can involve frequent, often painful, dressing changes [7]. Late complications of these injuries include penile trapping, distal urethral or meatal stenosis, and cosmetic deformities. However, it is remarkable to note how well postcircumcision injuries heal when they occur in the neonatal period and are treated soon after the injuries occur.

Zipper injuries to the uncircumcised penis may be treated with mineral oil to slip the trapped skin from the zipper [3] or by cutting of the median bar of the zipper with bone cutters [8]. These procedures may be performed in the emergency room under local anesthesia, although the use of sedation (typically using an oral benzodiazepine such as midazolam) aids in examination and treatment. Formal conscious sedation is not generally required [2]. In cases of delayed presentation or if less invasive methods are unsuccessful, operative intervention may be required. Devitalized skin should be excised with primary reapproximation of the preputial skin or healing by secondary intention in cases of delayed presentation where contamination is of concern [9].

Although tourniquet injuries are generally superficial, these injuries can extend to the corporal bodies or urethra. Often the initial diagnosis is balanitis or paraphimosis due to associated preputial edema. Examination under anesthesia and removal of the constricting band should be performed immediately upon diagnosis. Localizing the hair can be difficult especially in the case of blond hairs; loupe magnification helps considerably in this situation. Local wound care may be used for isolated skin necrosis.

In more severe cases, early primary repair of corpora cavernosal injuries should be performed to minimize risk of fibrosis and preserve erectile function [2].

Amputation injuries may be managed with reanastomosis up to 8 h after injury [10]. Cook *et al.* have suggested the use of buccal mucosa grafting to reapproximate the coronal sulcus and provide an improved cosmetic result in cases of glans amputation [11]. Partial amputation injuries may be treated nonoperatively with intermittent application of epinephrine-soaked sponges to control hemorrhage in the absence of associated urethral injury. If urethral involvement is present, formal hypospadias repair may be required [6]. As with any amputated body part, the amputated penis should be cooled as quickly as possible (i.e. placing in crushed ice) to reduce ischemic injury.

In cases of genital injury due to dog bite, examination under anesthesia is generally necessary to fully assess the extent of trauma. Broad spectrum antibiotics and tetanus prophylaxis should be administered prior to treatment [4]. Debridement of devitalized tissue and aggressive irrigation of the wound have been shown to reduce the risk of wound infection from 59% to 12% [12]. Split thickness skin grafts should be applied to denuded areas to minimize wound contraction. Investigation for potential abuse or neglect should be initiated in these cases to reduce the risk of future injury [4].

High-flow priapism may be managed nonoperatively, with spontaneous resolution reported within days to weeks after injury [5]. Alternatively, if definitive therapy is desired or conservative measures fail, embolization with autologous clot is the treatment of choice, with preservation of erectile function in 80–100% of patients. However, up to 44% of patients may recur. In cases of recurrence, repeat embolization with nonabsorbable materials may be utilized [13]. Open surgical ligation is a measure of last resort due to the high risk of erectile dysfunction [5].

Scrotal/testicular injuries

Injury of the testis may be associated with straddle injury, including bicycle handlebar injuries, where the testis is forced against the pubic ramus, causing tearing of the tunica albuginea. Injuries may also result from hits or kicks to the scrotum during sporting events or roughhousing. Due to its higher position, the right testis is more prone to injury than the left [14]. Injuries tend to be less common in infants due to the smaller size and increased mobility of the testes during infancy. As a result, significant testicular injury associated with minor trauma in these patients should raise the possibility of intrinsic testicular pathology, including malignancy.

Trauma to the scrotum without underlying testicular injury tends to resolve within a short time. In patients with pain that initially resolves after a short period but recurs after several days, traumatic epididymitis should be considered [15]. However, pain persisting greater than 2 h after trauma is suspicious for more significant testicular injuries, such as testicular torsion or rupture [15,16].

Several case reports have suggested that testicular torsion may be associated with scrotal injury. Cases of delayed testicular torsion following blunt scrotal trauma, sports-related injuries, and bicycle riding have also been reported [17,18]. A history of trauma is the presenting symptom in 4–8% of all cases of testicular torsion [15,19].

Acute scrotal swelling may also be associated with intraperitoneal pathology, such as appendicitis, peritonitis, liver laceration, or splenic rupture [20–22]. Especially in the child with a history of abdominal trauma, scrotal pathology in the absence of scrotal trauma should prompt a more thorough evaluation [22]. In the newborn period, adrenal hemorrhage should also be considered in cases of scrotal swelling and ecchymosis. Retroperitoneal imaging with ultrasonography aids in differentiating this diagnosis from other possible etiologies.

Treatment

If physical examination and/or ultrasound are indeterminate or suggest significant testicular injury, early scrotal exploration is mandatory (Figure 37.2). Early scrotal

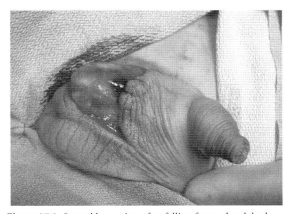

Figure 37.2 Scrotal laceration after falling from a bunk bed without associated testicular injury.

exploration significantly increases the rate of salvage of the injured testis. Rates of salvage in cases of testicular rupture have been reported as high as 90% if performed within 72 h [23]. Early exploration may also lead to decreased convalescent times and reduced risk of infection.

In cases of suspected torsion, early exploration is also recommended. Schuster suggests that testicular salvage rates for torsion increase with earlier exploration, with little benefit seen after 3 days [14]. In contrast, nonoperative management has been associated with an orchiectomy rate of approximately 45% [1]. Animal studies suggest that early application of ice to the scrotum may aid in the preservation of seminiferous tubules in patients with testicular torsion [24].

Cases of isolated hematocele may be followed nonoperatively in the absence of impaired testicular flow. Isolated epididymitis may also be treated with supportive care including scrotal elevation and nonsteroidal medications. In the absence of ischemic changes, testicular fracture without disruption of the tunica albuginea may be observed. If nonoperative management is selected, follow-up with both physical exam and ultrasonography should be used to monitor resolution of the injury.

Vaginal injuries

Vaginal injuries are relatively rare in the pediatric population [25]. The majority of injuries are due to straddle injuries [25]. Straddle injuries may be associated with falls from bicycles, monkey bars, tree limbs, or ladders. Injuries may also be due to foreign body insertion or blunt trauma associated with motor vehicle collision. More rare causes of injury include vaginal hydro-distension during water skiing or jet skiing [26]. Pelvic fractures may result in both penetrating injury due to bone spicules and traction injury due to shear forces [27]. Due to the proximity of the urethra and vagina and the susceptibility of the urethrovaginal septum to injury, traumatic urethral injuries in girls should prompt an evaluation for associated vaginal injuries [28].

Diagnosis

Prompt diagnosis is essential to avoid fistulae, stenosis, or other long-term complications of unrecognized vaginal injuries [29,30]. Physical exam may show evidence of labial bruising, bleeding at the introitus, vulvar edema, or hematuria. Patients associated with pelvic fractures should also be evaluated for urethral injury [25]. Examination in the prone position with the knees to the chest allows for adequate examination of the hymen, vagina, and anus without significant patient discomfort. It may also allow for noninvasive visualization of the cervix [31].

Examination in the emergency room can underestimate the extent of injuries due to several factors. First, lighting is often inadequate. Second, the patient is often unable to relax and fully cooperate with exam. Finally, the discomfort associated with an awake exam may lead to an incomplete evaluation [32]. As a result, although an examination may be attempted with oral or intravenous sedation in the emergency department, an examination under anesthesia is generally necessary to fully evaluate injuries. In their series of 22 patients who had a history of blunt urogenital trauma, Lynch *et al.* found that 76% had significantly greater injuries on EUA than diagnosed in the emergency department. Six patients had associated perianal lacerations, while three had periurethral injuries requiring repair [32]. Based on these findings, exam under anesthesia should be performed when any doubt exists as to the extent of injury.

Treatment

During examination under anesthesia, cystoscopy, vaginoscopy, and rectal exam are performed to fully evaluate associated injuries [1]. Continuous flow of vaginoscopy aids in complete evaluation of the vagina, allows for removal of foreign bodies and for coagulation of isolated mucosal bleeding [33]. Gentle coaptation of the introitus during endoscopic examination with irrigation allows for better distention and visualization of the vaginal vault.

For more extensive vaginal lacerations, primary repair should be performed if possible, as primary repair reduces the rate of vaginal stenosis and urethrovaginal fistulae [28]. Perioperative use of antibiotics may help reduce the risk of secondary infection and wound dehiscence. Vaginal lacerations should be closed in layers with absorbable sutures (Figure 37.3). Postoperative care includes the avoidance of extremely lower extremity abduction, sitz bathing, and the use of topical antibiotic ointments. For injuries that extend into the introitus, the use of permanent monofilament sutures in an interrupted fashion is recommended to reduce the chance of postrepair dehiscence. Long-term follow-up is essential to rule out postpubertal development of vaginal stenosis or hematocolpos, especially in patients with extensive urethrovaginal injuries [34].

Associated rectal injuries

Although rectal injuries are associated with increased morbidity in the adult population, they tend to be rare and less severe in children. In their study of 116 patients ranging from 3 to 13 years old, Onen *et al.* found that prolonged delay in diagnosis and presence of associated anorectal injury significantly increased their postoperative complication rates in patients with traumatic genital injuries. Frequent complications in these patients included wound infection, dehiscence, and fistulae [35]. To minimize these risks, patients with a delayed diagnosis of genital injury with concomitant anorectal injury may require temporary diverting colostomy instead of primary repair of their rectal injury [36].

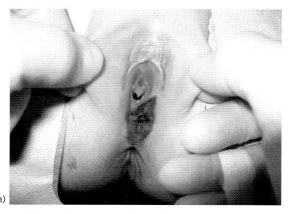
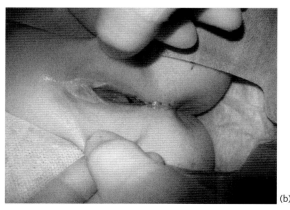

(a) (b)

Figure 37.3 (a) Perineal laceration without associated rectal or hymenal involvement after straddle injury. (b) Postoperative image after multilayered closure with deep vicryl and superficial chromic sutures.

Sexual abuse

Sexual abuse has been defined as "the engaging of a child in sexual activities that the child cannot comprehend, for which the child is developmentally unprepared and cannot give informed consent, and/or that violate the social and legal taboos of society" [37]. It is the most common etiology for genital trauma in the pediatric population [38]. Approximately 10% of all reported child abuse is associated with sexual abuse. It is estimated that 25% of girls and 10% of boys will undergo some form of sexual abuse by the age of 18 years [31]. However, studies suggest that less than 6% of sexual child abuse is reported [39]. Although most victims are female, approximately 15% of reported cases are in boys [1].

Risk factors for abuse include children living without one or both of their natural parents, those living with a stepfather, those with mothers who are disabled or ill, and those whose parents have a significant amount of conflict in their relationship. Paternal violence may also be a risk factor for abuse. However, socioeconomic status, parental education level, and ethnicity are not significant risk factors for abuse [40].

A thorough patient history is essential in evaluating potential abuse. Separate accounts should be obtained from the victim as well as any witnesses and family members present. Children are often reluctant to discuss their experience due to a sense of fear, shame, or guilt [41]. In interviewing the child, a supportive environment should be created, and a thorough history should be obtained using simple, open-ended, nonleading questions. Any spontaneous admission of abuse should be documented using the child's exact words, as these statements may be later accessed in legal proceedings [42]. Once abuse is suspected, child protection services should be contacted to assure protection of the child from potential future abuse. If more intense investigation is required, an individual with experience in this area should be designated to avoid repetitive questioning of the child [31]. Many medical centers have designated health care providers who are part of a child protection program. Their input and expertise can be invaluable in these situations especially in regard to the medicolegal implications in this setting.

Physical exam should include a general physical exam as well as a thorough genital and anal exam. The reliability of the physical exam is dependent on the experience of the physician performing the exam [43]. The exam should include inspection of the thighs, labia, clitoris, urethra, hymen, and posterior fourchette in girls. In boys, the thighs, scrotum, penis, and urethral meatus should be evaluated [31]. Cultures for sexually transmitted diseases should be obtained at time of examination.

All findings should be carefully documented with photographs or drawings if necessary. Thorough documentation is critical and cannot be overemphasized. The use of colposcopy allows for magnification and improved lighting to detect subtle abnormalities [31,44]. It may also allow for simultaneous recording of the examination for documentation purposes. Although most children will tolerate examination in the emergency department, examination under anesthesia should be used if a speculum examination or more invasive evaluation of the urinary tract, vagina, or rectum is required [31,41]. The use of a Wood's lamp to aid in semen detection by UV fluorescence has been described, but is unreliable as a screening tool due to the variability of semen fluorescence with time and the inability to distinguish semen from urine, surgilube, and other commonly used products [45,46].

Findings suspicious for abuse in girls include vaginal discharge and hymenal abnormalities, including attenuation, irregularity, scarring, mounding, or absence [43]. Also suspicious are vulvar and perihymenal erythema, friability or adhesions of the posterior fourchette, and vaginal synechiae. Of note, hymenal bumps, rounding, and notching may be normal variants and are not an indication of abuse in the absence of other findings [44].

In boys, suggestive findings include asymmetric rectal scars or tags, asymmetric rectal folds, venous engorgement, and perineal bruises or abrasions. Isolated rectal injuries, particularly those occurring at the twelve or six o'clock positions, are significantly more common in victims of abuse as compared to those with accidental injuries [38]. However, the majority of children under the age of 10 years who have suffered sexual abuse will have a normal genital examination [44].

Treatment should include management of any physical injuries identified on exam. In addition, social support services and psychiatric treatment should be made available to both the patient and family members.

Conclusion

Because pediatric genital trauma occurs less frequently than adult genital trauma, the involvement of experienced health care providers and subspecialists in the care of these patients is needed to optimize care. The use of adjunct imaging studies such as ultrasonography has greatly improved our ability to accurately diagnose underlying conditions in this group of patients. However, at this time, the standard of care remains examination under anesthesia and surgical exploration when any doubt exists as to the underlying diagnosis, and certainly when surgical intervention will reduce post-trauma morbidity, lead to organ preservation, and reduce long-term complications from these injuries. Although trauma classification systems and algorithms have been developed for urinary tract injuries, few classification systems have been proposed for pediatric genital trauma [35]. Multicenter studies and evaluation of trauma registries are therefore the next logical steps to better elucidate the etiologies and best treatment practices for pediatric genital trauma.

References

1 McAleer IM, Kaplan GW, Scherz HC, Packer MG, Lynch FP. Genitourinary trauma in the pediatric patient. *Urology* 1993;42:563–7.

2 Livne PM, Gonzales ET, Jr. Genitourinary trauma in children. *Urol Clin North Am* 1985;12:53–65.

3 Kanegaye JT, Schonfeld N. Penile zipper entrapment: A simple and less threatening approach using mineral oil. *Pediatr Emerg Care* 1993;9:90–1.

4 Donovan JF, Kaplan WE. The therapy of genital trauma by dog bite. *J Urol* 1989;141:1163–5.

5 Hatzichristou D, Salpiggidis G, Hatzimouratidis K, Apostolidis A, Tzortzis V, Bekos A *et al.* Management strategy for arterial priapism: Therapeutic dilemmas. *J Urol* 2002;168:2074–77.

6 Patel HI, Moriarty KP, Brisson PA, Feins NR. Genitourinary injuries in the newborn. *J Pediatr Surg* 2001;36:235–9.

7 Sotolongo JR, Jr, Hoffman S, Gribetz ME. Penile denudation injuries after circumcision. *J Urol* 1985;133:102–3.

8 Nakagawa T, Toguri AG. Penile zipper injury. *Med Princ Pract* 2006;15:303–4.

9 Mydlo JH. Treatment of a delayed zipper injury. *Urol Int* 2000;64:45–6.

10 Sherman J, Borer JG, Horowitz M, Glassberg KI. Circumcision: Successful glanular reconstruction and survival following traumatic amputation. *J Urol* 1996;156:842–4.

11 Cook A, Khoury AE, Bagli DJ, Farhat WA, Pippi Salle JL. Use of buccal mucosa to simulate the coronal sulcus after traumatic penile amputation. *Urology* 2005;66:1109.

12 Callaham ML. Treatment of common dog bites: Infection risk factors. *JACEP* 1978;7:83–7.

13 Marotte JB, Brooks JD, Sze D, Kennedy, 2nd WA. Juvenile posttraumatic high-flow priapism: Current management dilemmas. *J Pediatr Surg* 2005;40:E25–8.

14 Schuster G. Traumatic rupture of the testicle and a review of the literature. *J Urol* 1982;127:1194–6.

15 Ciftci AO, Senocak ME, Tanyel FC, Buyukpamukcu N. Clinical predictors for differential diagnosis of acute scrotum. *Eur J Pediatr Surg* 2004;14:333–8.

16 Kass EJ, Lundak B. The acute scrotum. *Pediatr Clin North Am* 1997;44:1251–66.

17 King LM, Sekaran SK, Sauer D, Schwentker FN. Untwisting in delayed treatment of torsion of the spermatic cord. *J Urol* 1974;112:217–21.

18 Jackson RH, Craft AW. Bicycle saddles and torsion of the testis. *Lancet* 1978;1:983–4.

19 Seng YJ, Moissinac K. Trauma induced testicular torsion: A reminder for the unwary. *J Accid Emerg Med* 2000;17:381–2.

20 Nagel P. Scrotal swelling as the presenting symptom of acute perforated appendicitis in an infant. *J Pediatr Surg* 1984;19:177–8.

21 Udall DA, Drake DJ, Jr., Rosenberg RS. Acute scrotal swelling: A physical sign of primary peritonitis. *J Urol* 1981;125:750–1.

22 Sujka SK, Jewett TC, Jr., Karp MP. Acute scrotal swelling as the first evidence of intraabdominal trauma in a battered child. *J Pediatr Surg* 1988;23:380.

23 Munden MM, Trautwein LM. Scrotal pathology in pediatrics with sonographic imaging. *Curr Probl Diagn Radiol* 2000;29:185–205.

24 Miller DC, Peron SE, Keck RW, Kropp KA. Effects of hypothermia on testicular ischemia. *J Urol* 1990;143:1046–8.

25 Okur H, Kucikaydin M, Kazez A, Turan C, Bozkurt A. Genitourinary tract injuries in girls. *Br J Urol* 1996;78:446–9.

26 Merritt DF. Vulvar and genital trauma in pediatric and adolescent gynecology. *Curr Opin Obstet Gynecol* 2004;16:371–81.

27 Boos SC, Rosas AJ, Boyle C, McCann J. Anogenital injuries in child pedestrians run over by low-speed motor vehicles: Four cases with findings that mimic child sexual abuse. *Pediatrics* 2003;112:e77–84.

28 Merchant, 3rd, WC, Gibbons MD, Gonzales ET, Jr. Trauma to the bladder neck, trigone and vagina in children. *J Urol* 1984;131:747–50.

29 Pode D, Shapiro A. Traumatic avulsion of the female urethra: Case report. *J Trauma* 1990;30:235–7.

30 Patil U, Nesbitt R, Meyer R. Genitourinary tract injuries due to fracture of the pelvis in females: Sequelae and their management. *Br J Urol* 1982;54:32–8.

31 Hinds A, Baskin LS. Child sexual abuse: What the urologist needs to know. *J Urol* 1999;162:516–23.

32 Lynch JM, Gardner MJ, Albanese CT. Blunt urogenital trauma in prepubescent female patients: More than meets the eye! *Pediatr Emerg Care* 1995;11:372–5.

33 Golan A, Lurie S, Sagiv R, Glezerman M. Continuous-flow vaginoscopy in children and adolescents. *J Am Assoc Gynecol Laparosc* 2000;7:526–8.

34 Thambi Dorai CR, Boucaut HA, Dewan PA. Urethral injuries in girls with pelvic trauma. *Eur Urol* 1993;24:371–4.

35 Onen A, Ozturk H, Yayla M, Basuguy E, Gedik S. Genital trauma in children: Classification and management. *Urology* 2005;65:986–90.

36 Reinberg O, Yazbeck S. Major perineal trauma in children. *J Pediatr Surg* 1989;24:982–4.

37 American Academy of Pediatrics Committee on Child Abuse and Neglect: Guidelines for the evaluation of sexual abuse of children. *Pediatrics* 1991;87:254–60.

38 Kadish HA, Schunk JE, Britton H. Pediatric male rectal and genital trauma: Accidental and nonaccidental injuries. *Pediatr Emerg Care* 1998;14:95–8.

39 Geist RF. Sexually related trauma. *Emerg Med Clin North Am* 1988;6:439–66.

40 Finkelhor D. Epidemiological factors in the clinical identification of child sexual abuse. *Child Abuse Negl* 1993;17:67–70.

41 Giardino AP, Finkel MA. Evaluating child sexual abuse. *Pediatr Ann* 2005;34:382–94.

42 Myers JE. Role of physician in preserving verbal evidence of child abuse. *J Pediatr* 1986;109:409–11.

43 Makoroff KL, Brauley JL, Brandner AM, Myers PA, Shapiro RA. Genital examinations for alleged sexual abuse of pre-pubertal girls: Findings by pediatric emergency medicine physicians compared with child abuse trained physicians. *Child Abuse Negl* 2002;26:1235–42.

44 Emans SJ, Woods ER, Flagg NT, Freeman A. Genital findings in sexually abused, symptomatic and asymptomatic, girls. *Pediatrics* 1987;79:778–85.

45 Santucci KA, Nelson DG, McQuillen KK, Duffy SJ, Linakis JG. Wood's lamp utility in the identification of semen. *Pediatrics* 1999;104:1342–4.

46 Gabby T, Winkleby MA, Boyce WT, Fisher DL, Lancaster A, Sensabaugh GF. Sexual abuse of children. The detection of semen on skin. *Am J Dis Child* 1992;146:700–3.

38

Urinary Tract Trauma

Ashok Rijhwani, W. Robert DeFoor, Jr, and Eugene Minevich

Key points

- The majority of injuries to the kidney are blunt in nature.

- Over the last 20 years, management of most pediatric renal trauma has shifted to a more conservative initial approach.

- Accurate staging is necessary by means of a computed tomography (CT) scan for nonoperative management to be feasible.

- Management goals are to preserve renal tissue and kidney function without significantly increasing morbidity and mortality risks to the child.

- Early complications of renal injury include bleeding, urinoma, infection, devitalized tissue, and renovascular compromise.

- Late complications include hypertension and loss of renal function.

Introduction

Traumatic accidents are responsible for almost half of childhood deaths between the ages of 1 and 14 years. Motor vehicles are most commonly involved, with pedestrian accidents being a leading cause in the 5–9 year age group [1,2]. Injuries to the urinary tract and associated complications remain a source of significant morbidity following trauma in the pediatric age group. The kidney is also the most commonly injured abdominal organ in children.

Renal trauma

The majority (85–97%) of injuries to the kidney are blunt in nature. Penetrating trauma causes 3–15% of renal injury and is responsible for the majority of kidney trauma that requires surgery in children [3]. Some common causes of renal trauma in childhood are presented in Figure 38.1. Organized sports are an uncommon cause of serious renal injury in childhood.

When compared to adults, children are less frequently affected by penetrating injuries. However, the incidence is on the rise, and reviews of firearm injuries in children show a significant rise in deaths due to firearms in recent decades [4]. Gunshot wounds are peculiar because they result in a "blast effect" with widespread damage away from the tract of the projectile. This may result in delayed

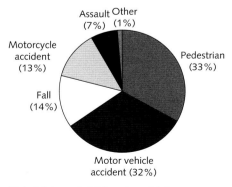

Figure 38.1 Etiology of childhood renal injury.

Pediatric Urology: Surgical Complications and Management. Edited by Duncan T. Wilcox, Prasad P. Godbole and Martin A. Koyle. © 2008 Blackwell Publishing, ISBN: 978-1-4051-6268-5.

tissue necrosis in areas that initially appear viable at the time of surgery. These patients can later present with bleeding, urinary extravasation, and abscess formation.

Imaging and staging

Radiographic imaging must be done efficiently and with accuracy so that important resuscitation measures are not interfered with in any way. Accurate staging is necessary, preferably by means of a spiral computed tomography (CT) scan in major renal injuries for nonoperative management to be feasible. A renal protocol CT scan consisting of noncontrast, contrast, and delayed phases makes it possible to evaluate the renal blood vessels, parenchyma, and the pelvicalyceal system, respectively. Table 38.1 shows the widely accepted grading scale for traumatic renal injuries.

All patients who sustain a penetrating injury to the abdomen, flank, or torso must have further imaging to rule out significant renal injury. Previously, it was recommended that any child with a history of blunt trauma with any amount of hematuria should undergo further imaging. Recently it has been noted that major injuries to the kidney are rare in children following blunt trauma in the absence of multisystem trauma, gross hematuria, or substantial microscopic hematuria (>50 RBC/hpf) at presentation [5,6,7].

Table 38.1 Grading of renal traumatic injuries.

I	Renal contusion or subcapsular hematoma
II	Non-expanding perirenal hematoma, <1 cm parenchymal laceration, no urinary extravasation, all renal fragments viable
III	Non-expanding perirenal hematoma, >1 cm parenchymal laceration, no urinary extravasation, renal fragments may be viable or devitalized
IV	Laceration extending into the collecting system with urinary extravasation, renal fragments may be viable or devitalized or injury to the main renal vasculature with contained hemorrhage
V	Completely shattered kidney, multiple major lacerations of >1 cm associated with multiple devitalized fragments or injury to the main renal vasculature with uncontrolled hemorrhage, renal hilar avulsion

If the CT scan cannot be done because the child needs immediate exploration, then a single-shot intravenous pyelogram (IVP) is recommended. It serves to identify and document a normally functioning contralateral kidney if a situation arises where the involved kidney needs to be removed. A single-shot IVP can also provide important information about the anatomy and function of the involved kidney and limit the amount of exploration necessary. Sonography can also be valuable in the bedside evaluation of the severely injured child.

Initial management and outcomes

Management goals are to preserve renal tissue and kidney function without significantly increasing morbidity and mortality risks to the child. The initial emphasis is on a prompt assessment of the condition concurrent with respiratory and hemodynamic stabilization of the patient.

Blunt injuries are mostly minor in nature and anatomically represented by contusions, minor perirenal fluid collections, and uncomplicated lacerations (grades I–III). They comprise 70–85% of pediatric renal injuries [3]. Management is usually conservative and involves bed rest and observation until gross hematuria clears and limited activity until microhematuria clears. The length of convalescence is from 2 to 6 weeks and is usually free of complications such as loss of renal function, hypertension, or hydronephrosis [8].

The management of major renal injuries (grades IV and V) is controversial and needs to be individualized. Over the last 20 years, management of most pediatric renal trauma has shifted to a more conservative initial approach. Early surgical intervention may lead to increased nephrectomy rates (up to 89%) and subsequent complications [9]. It has been noted that the complication rates are higher for conservative management of parenchymal lacerations of the kidney with significant (>25%) devitalized renal tissue [10,11]. The challenge lies in the early detection and prompt evaluation of the severity of injury. Selective nonoperative management may be appropriate in the hemodynamically stable child, but only after accurate staging of the injury by a CT scan. Most centers have adopted an ICU protocol for children with a severe renal injury undergoing initial conservative management. Bed rest for the first 24–48 h is mandatory as well as continual monitoring of hematocrit, blood pressure, and clinical signs. The risk of bleeding is highest during this time period. Nonoperative management may lead to surgery in up to 50% of patients for complications of trauma such as bleeding, renal infarction, or segmental hydronephrosis [2].

The nephrectomy rate increases if surgery is necessary on other intra-abdominal organs, suggesting that the kidney may be removed as a damage control measure or due to insufficient experience with renal reconstructive techniques. Possibly, under these conditions, potentially salvageable kidneys are sacrificed to control hemorrhage.

Relative indications for exploration are significant urinary extravasation, nonviable renal tissue, arterial injury, and incomplete staging of the injury or significant extrarenal injuries. Partial nephrectomy is the operation of choice in this condition. Surgical management involves the preliminary control of the vessels of the kidney as well as the aorta. This is followed by debridement of devitalized tissue, hemostasis, closure of the collecting system, and repair or coverage of tears in the renal parenchyma. Initial trial of a double-J stent or a nephrostomy tube may be used in children with significant urinary extravasation. Initial conservative management of stable children with grade IV renal injuries has been reported with close CT follow-up to rule out urinoma [3,8].

It is generally accepted that those with major renal injuries such as a vascular pedicle injury or a shattered kidney will require surgery. In most cases these injuries are severe enough to warrant a nephrectomy, particularly considering the high incidence of life-threatening extrarenal injuries that these patients suffer. Results of emergency vascular repair for a pedicle injury or thrombosis in children are usually poor, particularly with the amount of warm ischemia that the kidney undergoes during the resuscitation and evaluation. An attempt at repair is generally limited to extreme situations such as a solitary kidney or bilateral injuries.

The outcome differs between blunt and penetrating injuries. Overall, patients in the penetrating injury group are more severely injured, have a higher 24-h transfusion requirement, and have a higher nephrectomy rate. The rate of surgery is higher in penetrating injury, around 36%, and in contrast to blunt trauma, approximately half of these result in operative repair of the kidney [3,9,12]. Recent large series quote renal salvage rates of more than 98% in pediatric blunt kidney injuries with conservative management and selective surgical exploration when indicated. The expected exploration rate is under 10% [1,3,8]. It is almost universal in grade V injuries and the renal salvage rate in this group of patients is around 30% in the long term [13,14].

Early complications

Bleeding

The risk of bleeding is highest in the first 48 h after the trauma and close observation is necessary during this phase. Strict bed rest and serial hematocrit monitoring is imperative. Observation may be continued if the child is clinically stable and the CT scan shows a stable hematoma (or stable amount of urine extravasation). Bleeding can recur even later and grade IV–V injuries generally need to have a follow-up imaging at around 3–6 months to document complete healing.

If at any time during the course of treatment the child shows signs of hemodynamic instability (hypovolemia with severe hypotension or is unresponsive to packed red cells), then consideration should be given to either surgical exploration or to angiography and embolization. On exploration, expanding pulsatile or uncontained retroperitoneal hemorrhage indicates persistent bleeding. Primary angioembolization has been found to be useful in the treatment of isolated grade IV renal injuries with segmental artery bleeding. It also has a role to play in delayed hemorrhage in grades II–IV renal injuries. It can be done only in a nonrenal failure patient with a definable segmental artery injury.

Urinary extravasation/urinoma

Extravasation of urine is a pointer to major renal injury resulting from a laceration of the renal pelvis, a parenchymal tear extending into the collecting system, a forniceal rupture, or an avulsion of the UPJ. Persistent urine extravasation can lead to urinoma formation, perinephric infection, and renal loss. UPJ disruption is very rare, being associated with forces of rapid deceleration involved in motor vehicle trauma and falls from heights. It is detected when there is major contrast leak in the medial and perirenal areas and the ipsilateral ureter is not visualized. Complete disruption needs immediate operative intervention.

It has been reported that almost 75% of children even with a severe grade IV laceration had spontaneous resolution of the urinoma, therefore a conservative approach has been suggested in these patients [14–16]. Possible long-term complications of a large urinoma include retroperitoneal fibrosis, pelviureteral and infundibular obstruction, infection, and hypertension. Initially children are treated with parenteral antibiotics followed by the appropriate oral antibiotic. Monitoring by CT scan is essential. Symptomatic or worsening urinary extravasation can be managed either by percutaneous drainage of the collecting system or internal (double-J) stenting. It has been recommended that if resolution of extravasation does not occur within 2 weeks of conservative management, then ureteral stenting may be done. These measures have been found to be helpful in this scenario, more than percutaneous drainage of the urinoma itself. Stents may need to be maintained for as long as 10 weeks and bladder drainage for as long as 2–3 weeks. Patients who failed conservative approach with or without endoscopic drainage (less than 10%) require open operative intervention. Half of these operations result in nephrectomy [14,17].

Infection

Perinephric abscess can result from a hematoma, urinoma, or devitalized fragment of kidney. The incidence may be increased by concomitant pancreatic or bowel injuries. It may need intervention either by the percutaneous or open routes to achieve drainage. Sepsis commonly affects those with multiorgan trauma and judicious initial use of antibiotics is advised.

Nonviable tissue

Large devitalized fragments (involvement of 25–50% of affected kidney) are associated with significant complications when managed nonoperatively. Nonviable tissue can result from both blunt and penetrating trauma, and it can lead to short-term complications such as persistent urine leak and abscess (that might require surgical intervention), and in the long term, hypertension [10,11,14,17,18]. Immediate surgery has been shown to reduce the morbidity in these patients. Therefore, it is suggested that renal injuries with large devitalized fragments and associated urine extravasation or a retroperitoneal hematoma to undergo surgical exploration [19]. The surgical procedure of choice is a partial or polar nephrectomy. Delayed necrosis with possible fistula formation is more likely to happen in penetrating trauma especially if it is due to a gunshot. The blast effect may lead to delayed tissue necrosis resulting in bleeding, urine leak, or an abscess in areas which may be viable at time initial presentation.

Renovascular complications

Renal vascular injury has been reported in 9–31% of children with renal trauma, the incidence being nearly twice that seen in adults [20]. Detection of pedicle injuries is generally delayed and repair beyond 14 h reduces the chances of renal salvage. These injuries can involve either main or segmental renal vessels and are classified as avulsions, lacerations, or occlusions (secondary to thrombosis or dissection).

Traumatic occlusion of the main renal artery

Deceleration injuries cause the intima of the main renal artery to rupture, since it is low in elastic fiber content (the muscularis and the adventitia are more flexible). Intimal disruption may create a subintimal false lumen, resulting in decreased renal blood flow, renal ischemia or infarction, hypertension, or arterial occlusion due to a thrombus. This can be diagnosed by prompt CT scan or arteriography. Surgical revascularization may be considered only in hemodynamically stable patients with a warm ischemia time of <5 h [20]. These patients frequently have multiple injuries and the mortality rates are high. Therefore, doing a revascularization procedure is not often practical and a nephrectomy is usually done due to time constraints and to control hemorrhage.

Late complications

Renin-mediated hypertension

Hypertension (early or late) in children with renal injury is rare. It is through activation of the renin angiotensin system from renal ischemia. Overall incidence has been reported 1–2% in large series [20–21, 27–29]. A restrictive fibrous capsule may develop around the injured kidney reducing the renal blood flow by compression of the parenchyma (Page kidney). This is usually due to a prolonged urine leak or an inadequately treated urinoma. Other mechanisms are stenosis or occlusion of the main renal artery or one of its branches or the development of a posttraumatic arteriovenous fistula. Medical management is usually successful but surgery may be necessary. Surgical options include vascular or endovascular reconstructions, capsulotomy, or nephrectomy. Long-term monitoring of blood pressure is recommended.

Loss of renal function

The goal of management of renal injury in children is to preserve functioning renal parenchyma. Renal nuclear scans (DMSA) may be done to document and track recovery. Preservation of renal tissue is less successful in children with renovascular trauma as well as severe concomitant injuries with shock and extensive blood loss. Conservative management of minor renal injuries (grades I–III) usually result in almost complete healing. Grades IV and V show some evidence of volume loss (22% and 50%, respectively) [22,28]. Surgical reconstruction after major blunt or penetrating trauma preserves more than one-third of the kidney in 81% of

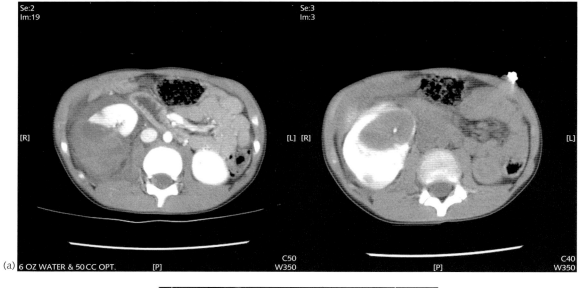

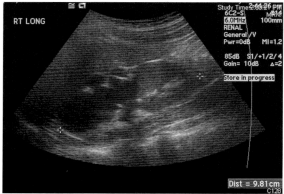

Figure 38.2 (a) Computed tomography scan of right high grade renal laceration with retroperitoneal hematoma in 7 year old boy (left image). Delayed images of same kidney (right image). (b) Ultrasound showing cystic changes in the upper pole of the right kidney 5 years after conservative management of the injury shown above.

cases [21]. The incidence of posttraumatic renal failure is low [28]. It has been reported in 6.4% of patients with renal injury who also have associated renovascular injury [22].

Morphological abnormalities

Conservative management of high-grade renal injuries in children can result in residual morphological changes such as single or multiple scars, cystic lesions with septae or segmental hydronephrosis. Figure 38.2 shows a follow-up ultrasound 5 years after a grade IV renal injury managed

conservatively with urinary diversion by percutaneous nephrostomy.

Ureteral injuries

Ureteral injuries constitute around 3% of genitourinary trauma [22]. Blunt traumatic disruption of the upper ureter and ureteropelvic junction, though very rare, is more common in children than in adults by a ratio of

3:1. They should always be suspected after severe blunt trauma or penetrating injury.

Penetrating injuries are extremely rare in children and are almost always accompanied by injuries to other organs. Gunshot wounds are also rare in children, but the mechanism of injury makes the ureter a target even if it is not in the path of the bullet. Iatrogenic injuries to the ureter have increased since the advent of laparoscopic and ureteroscopic interventions in childhood. They also happen during pelvic surgical procedures. Common injuries are mucosal injury during ureteroscopy with possible ureteral perforation, false passages, complete avulsion, or loss of a ureteral segment.

Diagnosis and management

Initially, these injuries may be unrecognized and a high index of suspicion is required in their evaluation. It is essential to evaluate for ureteral injury in any child with significant blunt abdominal trauma and multiple associated injuries. Though rare in the child, any penetrating injury should be suspected of injuring the ureter as well.

CT scan is the primary method of evaluation in these patients with multiple injuries. Extravasation of contrast may be confined to the medial perirenal space. If a rapid sequence spiral CT is done, then delayed films must be performed. On delayed images there is absence of contrast material in the distal ureter if there is complete ureteral transection. A complete high-dose intravenous urogram can be done in the resuscitation suite. The findings include contrast extravasation, delayed function, or mild ureteral dilation or deviation (Figure 38.3). Retrograde ureterography is probably the most accurate method of assessment of ureteral integrity, but is sometimes not practical in acute trauma. Intraoperative evaluation by inspection of the ureter, with the aid of injection of methylene blue into the collecting system or intravenous indigocarmine can be used.

The timing and type of the intervention depends on proper injury staging, the patient's overall condition, and timing of diagnosis. When recognized early, the ureter should be repaired immediately. Repair should be by means of a tension free, spatulated, anastomosis. If possible, the repair should be wrapped with omentum or retroperitoneal fat. Stent or nephrostomy placement is advised in most cases. Surgical options are direct reanastomosis, ureteral reimplantation (with possible vesico-psoas hitch or Boari flap), transposition of ileum or appendix, transuretero-ureterostomy, and

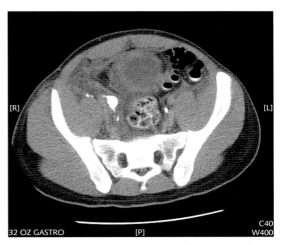

Figure 38.3 Computed tomography scan of right ureteral injury from penetrating trauma in an 11-year-old boy.

autotransplantation of the kidney. Nephrectomy may be done only in a life-threatening situation with a normal contralateral kidney.

If immediate definitive repair is not possible, then one should wait for several months before attempting reconstruction. In case of an unstable patient or if there has been a delay in diagnosis, a temporary diversion may be done. Percutaneous nephrostomy with or without ligation of the ureter or a cutaneous ureterostomy may be done initially for damage control.

Most iatrogenic injuries are diagnosed intraoperatively. Identification of the ureters by passing ureteric catheters prior to a difficult abdominal or pelvic dissection is a valuable aid to prevent these injuries. Passing a safety guidewire prior to ureteroscopy is an essential step, which if omitted, can lead to disaster. Trying to retrieve large fragments of stones without breaking them up can lead to avulsion of the ureter. Most ureteroscopic iatrogenic injuries and their complications can be managed by double-J stenting for a short period of time.

Complications

Urinary extravasation can present as an enlarging flank mass in the absence of signs of bleeding. The initial management of a double-J stent or a percutaneous nephrostomy is appropriate. Urinoma or abscess may be drained percutaneously. Most patients heal without stricturing.

Ureteral injuries especially its delayed diagnosis may be complicated by ureteral strictures. Usually they can be managed by balloon dilatation, internal stenting, or endoureterotomy. Stricture length and duration determine whether conservative management is going to be successful. These methods have a higher failure rate with longer strictures. Previous infection, urine extravasation, and poor blood supply may be factors causing longer strictures. Open or laparoscopic repair if required should be delayed for 1–3 months while infection and inflammation subside.

Hydronephrosis is due to transient obstruction due to contusion or a stricture. Ureteral stenting is usually adequate treatment unless there is a long stricture. Ureterocutaneous and ureterogenital fistulae can occur later in the course of illness and may respond to a period of stenting during which the fistula undergoes spontaneous healing. If stenting with or without proximal diversion is unsuccessful, open repair is needed. Renal failure and anuria may occur in children with bilateral injuries or when a ureter of a solitary kidney is affected. Temporary dialysis with the appropriate drainage procedure may be done.

Bladder injuries

Pediatric bladder injuries are rare and are usually associated with other severe injuries and a high mortality rate. Blunt trauma is the most common cause of bladder injury in children. Inappropriately fastened lap belts increase the risk of this injury. Iatrogenic injury is also known, especially with the increasing use of laparoscopic surgery. Augmented bladders and children with previous pelvic surgery are also at a greater risk. An augmented bladder may perforate spontaneously or with trauma [23].

Bladder rupture may be intraperitoneal or extraperitoneal or a combination of the two. The bladder in a child occupies a more abdominal position when full, in comparison to adults. It is therefore more susceptible to external injury and intraperitoneal rupture accounts for one-third of bladder injuries [24]. Extraperitoneal rupture almost always occurs due to pelvic fracture. It has been reported that bladder injury in children with a pelvic fracture is rare and occurs 1% of the time [25]. This lower incidence in children has been attributed to the elastic nature of a child's pelvis and its attachments.

Diagnosis and management

Diagnosis depends on precise studies including CT scan, cystography, and IVP. The bladder must be adequately filled and oblique as well as post-drainage films should be taken. Currently CT cystography is a very sensitive and specific test. Children with intraperitoneal rupture develop hyponatremia, hypokalemia, elevated serum urea, and creatinine (urea nitrogen rises out of proportion when compared to creatinine), whereas those with extraperitoneal rupture do not do so. Hematuria is a cardinal sign and the patient may be unable to void.

The majority of injuries that present solely with hematuria are bladder contusions and require no specific treatment. Most extraperitoneal injuries may be treated by bladder drainage, either urethral or suprapubic, for 7–10 days. If bladder drainage is not efficient in the first 48 h, then open repair should be done and a suprapubic tube placed. It has been recommended that these tears may be treated by catheter drainage if the urine clears of blood promptly, the catheter drains well, and the bladder neck is not involved in the laceration.

Major extraperitoneal injuries and intraperitoneal injuries are usually treated by primary operative repair. Prophylactic antibiotics need to be started on the day of the injury to prevent infection of the associated pelvic hematoma and continued till 3 days after catheter removal. Major extraperitoneal injuries include open pelvic fracture, rectal perforation (both of which have a high risk of infection when treated conservatively), and bone fragment projecting into the bladder, which is rare. When a laparotomy is done for other associated injuries, it is advised that the bladder be opened and repaired if a bladder injury is suspected. Massive injuries of the bladder and lower ureter are best drained by a temporary diversion. Occasionally nonoperative treatment can be successful in cases of small intraperitoneal bladder tears in children [26]. The treatment consists of bladder drainage, percutaneous intraperitoneal tube drain, and antibiotics in children who present early. Surgery is done in these children if bladder drainage is inadequate, there is prolonged drainage from the peritoneal drain, or if the clinical situation deteriorates. A follow-up cystogram must be obtained 10–14 days after the injury in case of conservative management or 7–10 days after bladder repair. Only then the bladder catheter is removed.

If there is involvement of the bladder neck, trigone, prostate, or vagina in the injury, immediate formal repair of all these structures is necessary. This type of injury is more common in children and early repair prevents complications. A small vaginal injury may be left open. A large laceration may need repair through the opening in the bladder. The bladder is then drained by both urethral and suprapubic tubes. Placing omentum between the bladder and vaginal repairs may reduce the risk of fistula formation.

Complications

Complications of bladder perforations include clot retention, ileus, pelvic abscess, and urinary fistula. Other complications are urge incontinence and areflexic bladder that might require intermittent catheterization. Bladder stones may occur from retained sutures. Pseudodiverticulum can occur due to a bony spike. Acute complication of intraperitoneal rupture is peritonitis, which can be fatal. Late complications of bladder repair are rare. Acute, self-limiting urinary frequency is common. Bladder neck injuries can result in bladder neck stricture and urinary incontinence. In females they can also result in stress incontinence, sexual dysfunction, and vesicovaginal fistula. Impotence in males is related to wide separation of the pubic bones.

References

1 Buckley JC, McAninch JW. The diagnosis, management, and outcomes of pediatric renal injuries. *Urol Clin North Am* 2006;33:33–40, vi.

2 Schafermeyer R. Pediatric trauma. *Emerg Med Clin North Am* 1993;11:187–205.

3 Buckley JC, McAninch JW. Pediatric renal injuries: Management guidelines from a 25-year experience. *J Urol* 2004;172:687–90,discussion 690.

4 Deaths resulting from firearm- and motor-vehicle-related injuries – United States, 1968–1991. *Morb Mortal Wkly Rep* 1994;43:37–42.

5 Cass AS. Blunt renal trauma in children. *J Trauma* 1983;23:123–7.

6 Carpio F, Morey AF. Radiographic staging of renal injuries. *World J Urol* 1999;17:66–70.

7 Morey AF, Bruce JE, McAninch JW. Efficacy of radiographic imaging in pediatric blunt renal trauma. *J Urol* 1996;156:2014–18.

8 Broghammer JA, Langenburg SE. *et al.* Pediatric blunt renal trauma: Its conservative management and patterns of associated injuries. *Urology* 2006;67:823–7.

9 Wright JL, Nathens AB. *et al.* Renal and extrarenal predictors of nephrectomy from the national trauma data bank. *J Urol* 2006;175:970–5,discussion 975.

10 Husmann DA, Gilling PJ. *et al.* Major renal lacerations with a devitalized fragment following blunt abdominal trauma: A comparison between nonoperative (expectant) versus surgical management. *J Urol* 1993;150:1774–7.

11 Moudouni SM, Patard JJ. *et al.* A conservative approach to major blunt renal lacerations with urinary extravasation and devitalized renal segments. *BJU Int* 2001;87:290–4.

12 Kuan JK, Wright JL. *et al.* American Association for the Surgery of Trauma Organ Injury Scale for kidney injuries predicts nephrectomy, dialysis, and death in patients with blunt injury and nephrectomy for penetrating injuries. *J Trauma* 2006;60:351–6.

13 Margenthaler JA, Weber TR, Keller MS. Blunt renal trauma in children: Experience with conservative management at a pediatric trauma center. *J Trauma* 2002;52:928–32.

14 Rogers CG, Knight V. *et al.* High-grade renal injuries in children: is conservative management possible? *Urology* 2004;64:574–9.

15 Alsikafi NF, McAninch JW. *et al.* Nonoperative management outcomes of isolated urinary extravasation following renal lacerations due to external trauma. *J Urol* 2006;176:2494–7.

16 Matthews LA, Smith EM, Spirnak JP. Nonoperative treatment of major blunt renal lacerations with urinary extravasation. *J Urol* 1997;157:2056–8.

17 Meng MV, Brandes SB, McAninch JW. Renal trauma: Indications and techniques for surgical exploration. *World J Urol* 1999;17:71–7.

18 Husmann DA, Morris JS. Attempted nonoperative management of blunt renal lacerations extending through the corticomedullary junction: The short-term and long-term sequelae. *J Urol* 1990;143:682–4.

19 Falcone RA, Jr., Luchette FA. *et al.* Zone I retroperitoneal hematoma identified by computed tomography scan as an indicator of significant abdominal injury. *Surgery* 1999;126:608–14,discussion 614–15.

20 Haas CA, Dinchman KH. *et al.* Traumatic renal artery occlusion: A 15-year review. *J Trauma* 1998;45:557–61.

21 Wessells H, Deirmenjian J, McAninch JW. Preservation of renal function after reconstruction for trauma: Quantitative assessment with radionuclide scintigraphy. *J Urol* 1997;157:1583–6.

22 Armenakas NA, Current methods of diagnosis and management of ureteral injuries. *World J Urol* 1999;17:78–83.

23 DeFoor W, Tackett L. *et al.* Risk factors for spontaneous bladder perforation after augmentation cystoplasty. *Urology* 2003;62:737–41.

24 Corriere JN, Jr., Sandler CM. Bladder rupture from external trauma: Diagnosis and management. *World J Urol* 1999;17:84–9.

25 Tarman GJ, Kaplan GW. *et al.* Lower genitourinary injury and pelvic fractures in pediatric patients. *Urology* 2002;59:123–6,discussion 126.

26 Osman Y, EI-Tabey N. *et al.* Nonoperative treatment of isolated posttraumatic intraperitoneal bladder rupture in children: is it justified? *J Urol* 2005;173:955–7.

27 Montgomery RC, Richardson JD, Harty JI. Posttraumatic renovascular hypertension after occult renal injury. *J Trauma* 1998;45(1):106–10.

28 Keller MS. *et al.* Functional outcome of nonoperatively managed renal injuries in children. *J Trauma* 2004;57(1):108–10; discussion 110.

29 El-Sherbiny MT. *et al.* Late renal functional and morphological evaluation after non-operative treatment of high-grade renal injuries in children. *BJU Int* 2004;93(7):1053–6.

Surgery for Urinary and Fecal Incontinence

39

Augmentation Cystoplasty

Prasad P. Godbole

Key points

- Preoperative workup and a multidisciplinary approach is key to the success of an augmentation cystoplasty.
- The timing of surgery should be dictated by the compliance and understanding of the child and carers.
- In case of deteriorating upper tracts and unfavorable child and social situation, alternative urinary diversion procedures may be considered.

- Bowel preparation is not always necessary.
- The main complications are related to the reservoir; namely, mucus and stone formation, urinary tract infections, rupture, metabolic, and development of malignancy.
- Lifelong surveillance and support of children with an augmentation cystoplasty is essential.

Introduction

Augmentation cystoplasty is aimed at achieving a low-pressure reservoir of adequate capacity primarily to protect the upper tracts and secondarily to achieve continence [1]. This technique finds use predominantly in children with a neurogenic bladder due to spinal dysraphism, anorectal malformation, tumors, or spinal cord injury as well as in children with nonneurogenic bladder dysfunction (Hinman bladder). Emptying of the reservoir is by clean intermittent catheterization urethrally or via a continent catheterizable conduit. This chapter deals with the preoperative workup, surgical techniques, complications, and management of augmentation cystoplasty.

Surgical techniques

Various segments of the gastrointestinal tract have been used to augment the bladder from stomach, ileum, colon,

and composite grafts [2]. The principal drawback of this is the close contact of urothelium and urine to gastrointestinal mucosa and its consequences [3]. A dilated ureter may be used in the form of a ureterocystoplasty in selected cases [4]. Autoaugmentation or detrusor myotomy alone has also been described [5]. The various techniques and their outcomes are discussed below.

Outcomes

The main aim of an augmentation cystoplasty is to provide a capacious reservoir that can store urine at low pressures (compliant), thereby preventing deterioration of the upper tracts. The other aim is to achieve continence. Hence, the outcome measures by which the various techniques can be compared are directly related to the above. Further outcome measures include long-term effects of augmentation cystoplasty including mucus formation, urinary tract sepsis, stone formation, and development of malignancy. Although bladder neck surgery is closely related to augmentation cystoplasty and the continence mechanism, this is described in subsequent chapters and is excluded from this discussion. The outcomes are tabulated in Table 39.1.

Pediatric Urology: Surgical Complications and Management. Edited by Duncan T. Wilcox, Prasad P. Godbole and Martin A. Koyle. © 2008 Blackwell Publishing, ISBN: 978-1-4051-6268-5.

Table 39.1 Outcomes of augmentation cystoplasty.

Technique	Ileo/colocystoplasty	Gastrocystoplasty	Ureterocystoplasty	Autoaugmentation
Outcome				
Mucus [6]	Common problem	Decreased mucus production	No	No
Stone [7]	Up to 20%	Lower incidence		
UTI [8]	Up to 20%	Up to 20%		
Metabolic [9]	Hyperchloremic metabolic acidosis. Not significant if normal kidneys at outset.	Decreased chloride absorption	No	No
Malignancy [10]	Currently rare. Histological changes at anastomotic line noted in experimental studies.	Not documented although DNA-ploidy abnormalities noted along anastomotic line on flow cytometry.	No	No
Rupture [11]	10% in one series	Can occur	Can occur	Can occur
Capacity of reservoir [8]	Significant increase	Significant increase	Improvement in carefully selected cases	Up to 93% no improvement in urodynamic parameters
Compliance [8]	Significant improvement	Significant improvement	Improvement in carefully selected cases	Poor on long-term follow-up
Continence [8]	Up to 96% improvement/ resolution in one series	Up to 89% continence	Good medium-term results in up to 90%	Poor in long term
Upper tracts [8]	As above	Stable in up to 91%	Stable	Deterioration in over 50%
Other		Patch contraction, ureteral obstruction. Hematuria dysuria syndrome in up to 25%. Long-term complications greater than enterocystoplasty in one series.	High reaugmentation rate of 82–91% where case selection is inappropriate, ureteral necrosis.	Not shown to be useful with respect to continence and urodynamic parameters.

Complications

Complications may occur at any stage following an augmentation cystoplasty and are discussed below.

Intestinal obstruction

This may occur in up to 10% of children following an augmentation cystoplasty [12]. Several series have demonstrated an incidence of approximately 3% of mechanical bowel obstruction following augmentation cystoplasty with a higher incidence of up to 10% after gastrocystoplasty [13–16]. It may occur early or late. The author has noted that in some children an ileus may develop approximately 4–5 days after surgery after a period of relatively normal enteral intake (unpublished observations). The cause of this phenomenon is not known. Comparing the incidence of intestinal complications after augmentation cystoplasty with an ileal conduit, it is apparent that the comparative incidence is significantly lower in the former (10% versus up to 70%) [17]. There are dangers during relaparotomy as failure to identify the vascular pedicle may result in its inadverdent division.

Mucus production

Mucus production can be problematic for years after an augmentation cystoplasty. Experimental studies suggest maximal mucus production with a colocystoplasty and to a lesser degree by the ileum and minimal mucus production by the stomach [18,19]. Mucus production may prevent adequate drainage of the neobladder via the catheter thereby predisposing to infections and stone formation.

Urinary tract infection

This occurs in approximately 20% of children with an augmentation cystoplasty [8,20]. Rink and colleagues report an incidence of symptomatic lower urinary tract infections in 22.7% of ileocystoplasties, 17.3% of sigmoid cystoplasties, and 8% of gastrocystoplasties [8]. The incidence of febrile UTIs has been reported in upto 10–15% of children [8]. Urinary stasis secondary to inadequate drainage, mucus production, and intermittent catheterization predispose to Urinary tract infections (UTIs) [21]. True UTIs needing treatment need to be differentiated from bacteruria without symptoms which is almost inevitable following an augmentation cystoplasty in patients performing intermittent catheterization.

Stone formation

Urinary stasis, mucus production, UTIs, foreign bodies such as a suture or staple may predispose to stone formation. This may occur in 18–50% patients in several large series [7,22–25]. The incidence of stone formation is much less with gastrocystoplasty presumably due to the acid millieu compared to ileocystoplasty [26]. The risk may be increased by the addition of a bladder neck procedure or a catheterizing abdominal wall conduit [24].

Metabolic

The metabolic consequences of an augmentation cystoplasty depend on the segment of bowel used and the duration of contact between urine and the bowel mucosa. This occurs as a result of the bowel segment maintaining its physiological absorptive and secretory properties. With an ileocystoplasty or colocystoplasty,

chloride ions from the urine are absorbed in exchange for bicarbonate ions from the bowel lumen. Other ions such as ammonium, hydrogen, and organic acids are also readily absorbed by the bowel mucosa. This results in a hyperchloremic metabolic acidosis [27] which is compensated by hyperventilation. Where the renal function is normal at the outset, patients do not generally have a problem with these metabolic changes. In cases of an acute acid load, hydrogen ions are secreted in the distal tubule. Normally, chronic acid loads are dealt with by secretion of large amounts of ammonium in the distal tubule. However in cases of an augmentation cystoplasty, the ammonium is reabsorbed thereby negating this effect. Inorganic salts or bony buffers may therefore be released to handle this chronic acid load. Hence, bone demineralization and impaired linear growth could occur and has been demonstrated in experimental studies [28,29]. While there are several series that support this concept [30,31], other authors have not shown any difference in linear growth with or without an augmentation cystoplasty [32].

Other substances may also be reabsorbed across the intestinal mucosa. Phenytoin absorption may need an alteration in dosage schedule [33]. Glucose absorption across the mucosa may give misleading results on a urine glucose analysis [34]. False positive pregnancy tests have also been reported [35].

With a gastrocystoplasty, the gastric mucosa secretes chloride and hydrogen ions thereby potentially leading to a hypochloremic metabolic alkalosis [36]. The gastric segment has therefore been recommended in children with renal impairment [37,38]. Discontinuation of alkalinization therapy following a gastrocystoplasty has been reported [16] although recent studies have demonstrated no beneficial effect of a gastrocystoplasty in the face of an acute acid load [39].

The aciduria and hematuria dysuria syndrome can affect up to 25% of patients with a range of 9–70% in various series [16,40,41]. The incidence is higher in children with a sensate urethra as opposed to insensate urethra [41]. The symptoms are as a result of the irritation of the native urothelium by acidic urine.

Malignancy

Much of the work regarding malignancy developing at the suture line has been done in ureterosigmoidostomies with a mean latency period of over 20 years from surgery to development of malignancy. As follow-up after augmentation cystoplasty is comparatively short, it is difficult to predict the potential for development of malignancy in this group. There have been numerous reports of malignancy developing along the suture line following cystoplasty [42–45], the earliest being at 4 years following surgery [43]. Dysplasia and metaplasia along the suture line has also been noted in experimental studies [46].

Rupture

Perforation of an augmented bladder is a well recognized complication [11,20,47,48]. In our institute, we have seen this mainly in the adolescent age group who have not catheterized for a significant period of time and then have sustained relatively innocuous trauma. Other postulated contributing mechanisms include ischemia, overdistention, poorly compliant hyperreflexic bladder, and sepsis [49,50]. A leak may occur early following an enterocystoplasty and may be due to a technical error or delayed healing. The reported incidence of rupture is up to 10% [11]. In one series, it has been shown that sigmoid cystoplasties had a higher incidence of rupture compared to gastrocystoplasty or ileocystoplasty [51]. However, this has not been seen in other series where ileocystoplasties had a higher incidence of perforation [52].

Redo augmentation

The aims of an augmentation cystoplasty are to achieve a low pressure compliant capacious reservoir with limited contractility. Detubularization of the bowel segment to be used has been standard practice. Several studies have demonstrated that ileum is the most compliant segment of bowel [53–55]. Despite detubularization, persistent contractions generating high pressures may occur. In our experience, this has been more in the sigmoid cystoplasties compared to ileocystoplasties. Other series have shown less contractility with ileum as compared to sigmoid or cecum [56,57]. Gastric patch also demonstrates similar contractility [58,59]. Secondary augmentations as a result of this persistent contractility have been done in order of decreasing frequency in colocystoplasties, gastrocystoplasties with ileocystoplasty requiring the least in the way of redo augmentation [60].

Ventriculoperitoneal shunt complications

An augmentation cystoplasty is commonly performed in the myelodyplasia population who have a functioning ventriculoperitoneal shunt *in situ*. Recent series have shown a shunt infection rate varying between 0% and 20% following augmentation cystoplasty [61,62]. Revision shunt surgery for distal end blockage has been recorded, but the incidence of this is not higher in those children who have not had an augmentation cystoplasty [61]. The Indiana experience [61] suggests that the rate of shunt infection is low (2% in this series) provided meticulous attention is paid to the intraoperative and perioperative details.

Prevention of complications

An augmentation cystoplasty is a major reconstructive procedure that should only be performed if and when the patient (where applicable) and carers are fully conversant and compliant with the postoperative and long-term management. Preventing complications of this procedure starts well before contemplating surgery.

Preoperative evaluation

Thorough evaluation by a specialist nurse who is part of a multidisciplinary team is essential. This evaluation consists of assessing current management of the bladder (CIC or diapers/pads), possibility of performing clean intermittent catheterization (CIC) by the patient/carers, dexterity of the patient, body habitus of the patient etc. The assessment should also include a subjective impression of the compliance and understanding of the patient/carers toward this procedure. In our institute, the specialist nursing team would carry out this assessment and also use audiovisual aids to help in understanding of the patient/carers. The families are then invited to a meeting with the surgeon and the rest of the multidisciplinary team to discuss the technicalities of the surgery, the risks and complications, and reinforce the postoperative management. An augmentation is performed only when the multidisciplinary team feel that the patient/carers will be able to follow the postoperative regime. Other urinary diversions as alternatives to an augmentation are also discussed so that a fully informed decision can be made.

Imaging techniques

Full formal urodynamic assessment including appearances of the bladder neck, leak point pressures , maximum cystometric capacity, detrusor activity, and maximum pressure is essential to determine the optimum procedure to be performed. At this time, presence or absence of vesicoureteric reflux can also be documented as well as its grade. We perform the videourodynamics off anticholinergics such as oxybutinin/tolterodine to give an accurate picture of the bladder dynamics. A baseline urinary tract ultrasound is also necessary as is functional imaging Dimercaptosuccinic acid (DMSA)/ Mercapto acetyl triglycine 3 (MAG 3) for baseline function.

Other investigations

Where renal function is compromised, a recent glomerular filtration rate (GFR) is essential. Renal biochemistry and hematology is checked preoperatively and blood is made available for the day of surgery. A preoperative urine is checked for culture/sensitivity and any active infection treated appropriately.

Marking the site

Where a concomitant catheterizable conduit (Mitrofanoff/Monti) or an Antegrade continental enemat (ACE) conduit is to be created, the site for either/both these stomas should be marked to ensure that they are appropriately placed and easily accessible. This is more so for patients who are in wheelchairs or those whose body habitus precludes them from having the stomas sited in the usual position.

Preoperative preparation

There is no standardized preoperative preparation for an augmentation cystoplasty. All patients are starved appropriately. In our institute, we advise a low residue diet 48 h prior to surgery and clear fluids the day before surgery. Where ileum (the author's preference) is to be used, no specific bowel preparation is used. In a recent study of the role of bowel preparation prior to augmentation cystoplasty, it was demonstrated that there was no significant difference in outcome measures such as time to full feeds, incidence of sepsis, and UTI with or without bowel preparation [63]. If colon/ileocecum is to be used, bowel preparation with Golitely/Kleen Prep or Oral Picolax may be used. Oral antibacterials commencing 24 h prior to surgery are used in some centers. We use a combination of Cefuroxime and Metronidazole at induction of anesthesia. If there is an active UTI, it is aggressively treated and surgery delayed until it is controlled.

Intraoperative management

The principles underlying a successful augmentation are good exposure, careful and delicate handling of tissues, a secure anastomosis (both bowel and the enterocystoplasty), choice of appropriate segment of bowel, prevention of potential internal herniae, and good postoperative drainage. The first step is the extraperitoneal mobilization of the bladder down to the level of the ureteric orifices. The bladder may be opened in the coronal or sagittal plane from one ureteric orifice to the other. Failure to do so may result in an hourglass constriction of the neobladder. The patch or reconfigured segment is sutured on with absorbable sutures. The peritoneal opening is closed to extraperitonealize the neobladder, the theoretical advantage being that of a leak being isolated to the extraperitoneal space if it should occur. This is not mandatory. The ureters are not routinely stented in our institute unless they have been reimplanted. Good drainage is obtained by one or two large bore catheters (the author uses a 16F Foley catheter along with a second 14F catheter via the Mitrofanoff conduit if present). Some surgeons use perivesical drain/s.

Postoperative management
Early postoperative management

Intravenous antibiotics are continued for 48 h or longer if enteral intake has not resumed. With an ileocystoplasty, in the author's experience, normal enteral intake is resumed in 48 h. To prevent blockage of catheters with blood or mucus, some authors advocate a continuous bladder irrigation for 24–48 h. In our institute, we maintain adequate hydration or even overhydration to maintain the urine output at 2 ml/kg/h for at least 48 h. In cases of children with compromised renal function, close attention to fluid balance and input from a pediatric nephrologist is essential. Both Foley catheters are periodically flushed to ensure patency. If a catheter is not draining, the smaller bore catheter is flushed (usually the Mitrofanoff) allowing the effluent to drain out along the gradient through the larger bore catheter. Patients are usually discharged by the end of a week with all catheters on free drainage. Prior to discharge, carers are taught the technique of flushing of catheters and have open access to the wards/specialist nurses in case of problems.

Further postoperative management

Bladder washouts are continued at a variable frequency depending on the amount of troublesome mucus. The author continues oral chemoprophylaxis till the first office visit at 3 months with an ultrasound scan. Further management depends on routine evaluation of the upper tracts, close liasion between the families and the multidisciplinary team via the specialist nurses with appropriate and proactive intervention if complications arise.

Management of complications

Intestinal obstruction

There should be a low threshold for surgical intervention after a period of conservative management with nil per orally (NPO), intravenous fluids, nasogastric decompression, and intravenous antibiotics. The appropriate surgical procedure may be carried out depending on the findings at laparotomy.

Mucus/UTI/stones

Bacteruria itself does not require treatment as this is inevitable. A pure growth of an organism in an unwell child should prompt aggressive treatment with intravenous antibiotics. Bladder drainage should be by an indwelling catheter with frequent washouts/irrigation if necessary. Hyaluronic acid has been used with some success in children with recurrent UTIs following augmentation cystoplasty (author, unpublished observations). Stones in the augmented bladder may be tackled by several techniques including open surgery or minimally invasive techniques [64,65]. Complete stone clearance is the aim whichever technique is chosen.

Metabolic

Acidosis may be managed by oral bicarbonate supplements. Regular monitoring of growth parameters and cooperation with a pediatric nephrologist is helpful in managing the metabolic sequelae of augmentation cystoplasty.

Rupture

This is usually a dramatic occurrence. Initial management should include full resuscitation and stabilization of the child prior to transfer to a tertiary unit. Imaging techniques in the form of an ultrasound and CT with contrast will confirm the diagnosis. Alternatively, an ultrasound scan finding of free fluid in the abdomen and pelvis combined with the history and clinical findings may be sufficient to make a presumptive diagnosis. A small amount of free fluid in the pelvis in an otherwise stable patient without features of peritonism may allow for conservative management with an indwelling catheter and intravenous antibiotics. A cystogram may be considered for confirmation of the diagnosis although the author has not always found this helpful. In peritonitic patients, a laparotomy is required with closure of the perforation.

Ventriculoperitoneal shunt sepsis

This may be manifest by neurological signs only or associated with or without a pyrexia or pyrexia alone. Confirmation is by culture of the cerebrospinal fluid (CSF) from a shunt tap. If shunt sepsis is confirmed, exteriorization of the shunt is necessary and treatment with culture sensitive antibiotics. In our institute, the shunt is reinteriorized after three successive negative CSF cultures. In cases of shunt malfunction secondary to a CSF collection in the abdomen, relocation of the shunt is required.

Conclusion

An augmentation cystoplasty is a major undertaking with potential risks and complications. All families and carers should be made aware of these before proceeding to surgery. Surgery should be performed after adequate preoperative preparation and with attention to detail. A multidisciplinary approach is essential throughout the child's journey.

References

1 Rink RC, Yerkes EB, Adams MC. Augmentation cystoplasty. In *Pediatric Urology*, Edited by Gearhart J, Mouriquand P, Rink R. Philadelphia: WB Suanders, 2001: pp. 961–79.

2 Shokeir AA, Shamaa M, el-Mekresh MM, el-Baz M, Ghoneim MA. Late malignancy in bowel segments exposed to urine without fecal stream. *Urology* 1995;46:657–61.

3 Ferris DO, Odel HM. Electrolyte pattern of blood after bilateral ureterosigmoidostomy. *JAMA* 1949;142:634.

4 Husmann DA, Snodgrass WT, Koyle MA, Furness PD, 3rd, Kropp BP, Cheng EY *et al.* Ureterocystoplasty: Indications for a successful augmentation. *J Urol* 2004;171:376–80.

5 Gurocak S, De Gier RP, Feitz W. Blader augmentation without integration of intact bowel segments: Critical review and future perspectives. *J Urol* 2007;177:839–44.

6 Gough DCS, Guys JM. Enterocystoplasty. In *Pediatric Neurogenic Bladder Dysfunction*, Edited by Esposito C, Guys JM, Gough DCS, Savanelli A. Heidelberg: Springer-Verlag, 2006: pp. 235–40.

7 Hendren WH, Hendren RB. Bladder augmentation: Experience with 129 cases in children and young adults. *J Urol* 1999;144:445–53.

8 Rink RC, Hollensbe D, Adams MC. Complications of augmentation in children and comparison of gastrointestinal segments. *AUA update series* 1995;14:122–28.

9 Nurse DE, Mundy AR. Metabolic complications after cystoplasty. *Br J Urol* 1985;63:165–70.

10 Smith P, Hardy GJ. Carcinoma occurring as a late complication of ileocystoplasty. *Br J Urol* 1971;43:576–9.

11 Krishna A, Gough DCS, Fishwick J, Bruce J. Ileocystoplasty in children. Assessing safety and success. *Eur Urol* 1995;31:62–7.

12 McDougal WS. Use of intestinal segments and urinary diversion. In *Campbells Urology*, 7th edn. Edited by Walsh PC, Retik AB, Vaughn ED, Jr., Wein AJ. Philadelphia: WB Saunders, 1998: pp. 3121–61.

13 Mitchell ME, Piser JA. Intestinocystoplasty and total bladder replacement in children and young adults: Follow up in 129 cases. *J Urol* 1987;138:579–84.

14 Gearhart JP, Albertsen PC, Marshall FF *et al.* Pediatric applications of augmentation cystoplasty: The Johns Hopkins experience. *J Urol* 1986;136:430.

15 Hollensbe DW, Adams MC, Rink RC *et al.* Comparison of different gastrointestinal segments for bladder augmentation. *Proceedings of the Annual Meeting of the American Urological Association, Washington DC,* 1992.

16 Leonard MP, Dharamsi N, Williot PE. Outcome of gastrocystoplasty in tertiary pediatric urology practice. *J Urol* 2000;164:947.

17 Shapiro SR, Lebovitz R, Colodny AH. The fate of 90 children with an ileal conduit urinary diversion 10 years later. *J Urol* 1975;114:289–93.

18 Kulb TB, Rink RC, Mitchell ME. Gastrocystoplasty in azotemic canines. *Proceedings of the Annual Meeting of the American Urological Association, North Central section, Ranchos Las Palmos, CA,* 1986.

19 Murray K, Nurse D, Mundy AR. Secreto-motor function of intestinal segments used in lower urinary tract reconstruction. *Br J Urol* 1987;60:532.

20 Krishna A, Gough DC. Evaluation of augmentation cystoplasty in childhood with reference to vesicoureteric reflux and urinary tract infection. *Br J Urol* 1994;74(4):465–8.

21 Woodhouse CRJ. The infective, metabolic and histological consequences of enterocystoplasty. *Eur Urol Update* 1994;3:10–15.

22 Blyth B, Ewalt DH, Duckett JW, Snyder HM, III. Lithogenic properties of enterocystoplasty. *J Urol* 1992;148:575.

23 Palmer LS, Franco I, Kogan SJ *et al.* Urolithiasis in children following augmentation cystoplasty. *J Urol* 1993;150:726.

24 Kronner KM, Casale AJ, Cain MP *et al.* Bladder calculi in the pediatric augmented bladder. *J Urol* 1998;160:1096.

25 Mathoera RB, Kok DJ, Mijman RJ. Bladder calculi in augmentation cystoplasty in children. *Urology* 2000; 56:482–7.

26 Kaefer M, Hendren WH, Bauer SB *et al.* Reservoir calculi: A comparison between reservoirs constructed from stomach and other enteric segments. *J Urol* 1998;160:2187.

27 Koch MO, McDougal WS. The pathophysiology of hyperchloremic metabolic acidosis after urinary diversion through intestinal segments. *Surgery* 1985;98:561.

28 Koch MO, McDougal WS. Bony demineralization following ureterosigmoid anastomosis. An experimental study in rats. *J Urol* 1988;140:856.

29 Bushinsky DA. Net calcium efflux from live bone during chronic metabolic but not respiratory acidosis. *Am J Physiol* 1989;256:F836.

30 Hafez AT, McLorie G, Gilday D *et al.* Long term evaluation of metabolic profile and bone mineral density after ileocystoplasty in children. *J Urol* 2003;170:1639–41.

31 Vajda P, Pinter AB, Harangi F, Farkas A, Vastyan A, Oberritter Z. Metabolic findings after colocystoplasty in children. *Urology* 2003;62:542–6.

32 Gerharz EW, Preece M, Duffy PG, Ransley PG, Leaver R, Woodhouse CR. Enterocystoplasty in childhood: A second look at the effect on growth. *BJU Int* 2003;91:79–83.

33 Savarirayan F, Dixey GM. Syncope following ureterosigmoidostomy. *J Urol* 1969;101:844.

34 Sridhar KN, Samuell CT, Woodhouse CR. Absorption of glucose from urinary conduits in diabetics and non diabetics. *BMJ* 1983;287:1327.

35 Nethercliffe J, Trewick A, Samuell C, Leaver R, Woodhouse CR. False positive pregnancy tests in patients with enterocystoplasties. *BJU Int* 2001;87:780–2.

36 Piser JA, Mitchell ME, Kulb TB *et al.* Gastrocystoplasty and colocystoplasty in canines: The metabolic consequences of acute saline and acid loading. *J Urol* 1987;138:1009.

37 Adams MC, Mitchell ME, Rink RC. Gastrocystoplasty: An alternative solution to the problem of urological reconstruction in the severely compromised patient. *J Urol* 1988;140:1152–6.

38 Ganesan GS, Mitchell ME, Adams MC *et al.* Use of the stomach for the reconstruction of the lower urinary tract in patients with compromised renal function. *Proceedings of the Annual Meeting of the American Academy of Pediatrics, Section on Urology, New Orleans,* October 1991.

39 De Freitas, Filho LG, Carnevale J, Leao JQ, Schor N, Ortiz V. Gastrocystoplasty and chronic renal failure: An acid base metabolism study. *J Urol* 2001;166:251–4.

40 Mingin GC, Stock JA, Hanna MK. Gastrocystoplasty: Longer term complications in 22 patients. *J Urol* 1999;162:1122–5.

41 Plaire JC, Snodgrass WT, Grady RW, Mitchell ME. Long term follow up of hematuria-dysuria syndrome. *J Urol* 2000;164:921.

42 Lane T, Shah J. Carcinoma following augmentation ileocystoplasty. *Urol INt* 2000;64(1):31–2.

43 Carr LK, Herschorn E. Early development of adenocarcinoma in a young woman following augmentation cystoplasty for undiversion. *J Urol* 1997;157:2255.

44 Gregoire M, Kantoff P, DeWolf WC. Synchronous adenocarcinoma and transitional cell carcinoma of the bladder associated with augmentation: Case report and review of the literature. *J Urol* 1993;149:115.

45 Barrington JW, Fulford S, Griffiths D, Stephenson TP. Tumors in bladder remnant after augmentation enterocystoplasty. *J Urol* 1997;157:482.

46 Little JS, Jr., Klee LW, Hoover DM, Rink RC. Long term histopathological changes in rats subjected to augmentation cystoplasty. *J Urol* 1994;152:720–4.

47 Elder JS, Snyder HM, Hulbert WC, Duckett JW. Perforation of the augmented bladder in patients undergoing clean intermittent catheterization. *J Urol* 1988;140:1159.

48 Rushton HG, Woodard JR, Parrott TS *et al.* Delayed bladder rupture after augmentation enterocystoplasty. *J Urol* 1988;140:344.

49 Crane JM, Scherz HS, Billman GF, Kaplan GW. Ischemic necrosis: A hypothesis to explain the pathogenesis of spontaneously ruptured enterocystoplasty. *J Urol* 1991;146:141.

50 Anderson PAM, Rickwood AMK. Detrusor hyperreflexia as a factor in spontaneous perforation of augmentation cystoplasty for neuropathic bladder. *Br J Urol* 1991;67:210.

51 Pope JC, Albers P, Rink RC *et al.* Spontaneous rupture of the augmented bladder: From silence to chaos. *Proceedings*

of the Annual Meeting of the European Society for Pediatric Urology, Istanbul, Turkey, April 1999.

52 Bauer SB, Hendren WH, Kozakewich H *et al.* Perforation of the augmented bladder. *J Urol* 1992;148:699.

53 Goldwasser B, Webster GD. Augmentation and substitution enterocystoplasty. *J Urol* 1986;135:215.

54 Rink RC, McLaughlin KP. Indications for enterocystoplasty and choice of bowel segment. *Probl Urol* 1994;89:389–403.

55 Studer UE, Zingg EJ. Ileal orthotopic bladder substitutes. What we have learned from 12 years experience with 200 patients. *Urol Clin North Am* 1997;24:781–93.

56 Sidi AA, Reinberg Y, Gonzalez R. Influence of intestinal segment and configuration on the outcome of augmentation enterocystoplasty. *J Urol* 1986;136:1201.

57 Goldwasser B, Barrett DM, Webster GD *et al.* Cystometric properties of ileum and right colon after bladder augmentation, substitution or replacement. *J Urol* 1987;138:1007.

58 Atala A, Bauer SB, Hendren WH *et al.* The effect of gastric augmentation on bladder function. *J Urol* 1993;149:1099.

59 Ngan JHK, Lau JLT, Lim STK *et al.* Long term results of antral gastrocystoplasty. *J Urol* 1993;149:731–4.

60 Pope JC IV, Keating MA, Casale AJ, Rink RC. Augmenting the augmented bladder: Treatment of the contractile bowel segment. *J Urol* 1998;160:854–7.

61 Yerkes EB, Rink RC, Cain MP, Luerssen TG, Casale AJ. Shunt infection and malfunction after augmentation cystoplasty. *J Urol* 2001;165:2262–4.

62 Pinto K, Jerkins GR, Noe HN. Ventriculoperitoneal shunt infection after bladder augmentation. *Urology* 1999;54:356–8.

63 Gundeti MS, Godbole PP, Wilcox DT. Is bowel preparation required before cystoplasty in children? *J Urol* 2006;176:1574–6.

64 Lopez PJ, Kellett MJ, Duffy PG. Percutaneous nephrolithotomy and laparoscopic management of urinary tract calculi. In *Pediatric Endourology Techniques*, Edited by Godbole P. London, UK: Springer-Verlag, 2007: pp. 101–6.

65 Mills JN, Barqawi AB, Chacko J, Koyle MA. Minimally invasive management of calculi in augmented/neuropathic bladders. In *Pediatric Endourology Techniques*, Edited by Godbole P. London, UK: Springer-Verlag, 2007: pp. 110–15.

40

Appendicovesicostomy and Ileovesicostomy

Martin Kaefer

> **Key points**
>
> - The success of a continent catheterizable channel depends on a flap-valve mechanism, a low-pressure storage of urine in the reservoir, adequate backing to the channel, and an intravesical length to tube diameter of 4:1 to 5:1.
> - The appendix is the most commonly used channel followed by the transverse
>
> tubularized ileal segment with similar continence outcomes.
> - Difficulties in catheterizing the conduit due to kinking or stomal stenosis, stomal incontinence, and stones are the commonest complications needing surgical intervention.

Introduction

The initial concept of a continent catheterizable channel and the subsequent utilization of this technique has dramatically improved the quality of life of many children with bladder dysfunction [1]. Following Mitrofanoff's initial experience, in which the appendix was implanted to create a flap-valve mechanism in the bladder, many other structures have been utilized as the efferent channel [2]. Advances in our knowledge of bladder function and structural characteristics of the channel have led to a better understanding of the complications that can result from this technique. Success of the procedure appears to be largely independent of underlying urologic disease, age of the patient, and specific configuration of the urinary storage reservoir.

Ideally, all patients should be able to achieve social continence using modern methods of continent urinary reconstruction. However, not all patients have the physical or cognitive ability to perform clean intermittent catheterization (CIC). Additionally, patients who have undergone reconstruction may fail to demonstrate the adequate compliance with CIC required to maintain

healthy intravesical pressures. In these patients the incontinent ileovesicostomy (i.e. ileal chimney) can prove invaluable.

This chapter will focus on the most common problems that arise following creation of both continent catheterizable and incontinent channels and provide an approach to the management of these complications.

Surgical techniques

General

There are several factors that appear to be critical to the success of the continent catheterizable channel. From a mechanical standpoint, continence depends on a flap-valve mechanism in which there is maintenance of a positive pressure gradient between the lumen of the efferent limb and the reservoir [3]. To achieve this, the channel should consist of a supple tube which is tunnelled submucosally and achieves an intravesical length to tube diameter of between 4:1 and 5:1 [4]. A urodynamic assessment of the efferent limb in 21 patients revealed that continence was generally achieved if the functional profile length (i.e. distance over which conduit pressure exceeds reservoir pressure) was greater than 2.0 cm [5]. The wall of the reservoir should be of adequate thickness to provide

Pediatric Urology: Surgical Complications and Management. Edited by Duncan T. Wilcox, Prasad P. Godbole and Martin A. Koyle. © 2008 Blackwell Publishing, ISBN: 978-1-4051-6268-5.

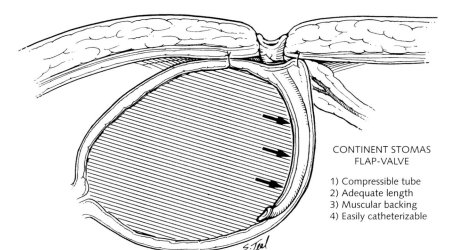

CONTINENT STOMAS
FLAP-VALVE

1) Compressible tube
2) Adequate length
3) Muscular backing
4) Easily catheterizable

Figure 40.1 The flap-valve mechanism.

adequate support of the tube as it is compressed by intravesical forces (Figure 40.1). The ability to store an adequate volume of urine at low intravesical pressure is a necessity due to the fact that excessively high intravesical pressures can cause a technically adequate channel to leak (just as high intravesical pressures can cause an otherwise adequate ureterovesical junction to reflux) [6].

Anatomic characteristics of the tube are predictive of whether the channel will function adequately. The conduit should have a constant diameter throughout its length (at least 10 French) and have a predictable, healthy blood supply. It must be of sufficient size to achieve adequate tunnel length and traverse the abdominal wall. The appendix and transversely tubularized bowel segments (TTBS, otherwise known as Yang–Monti channels) appear to be the best substrates due to the fact that they meet these criteria [2,7,8]. Other conduits including ureter, vas deferens, Meckel's diverticulum, Fallopian tube, tubularized stomach, and foreskin are either frequently unavailable (in the case of ureter) or have proven far less reliable for various reasons and therefore will not be discussed further in the context of this chapter [9–13]. The geometric relationships that exist between the conduit, reservoir, fascia, and skin also play an important roles in determining the success of the channel and will be discussed further in the appropriate sections of the text.

Continent channels

The conduit

When a healthy appendix exists, care must be taken to preserve its mesenteric blood supply. If the appendix is

not deemed of adequate length, methods for cecal extension/tubularization can be utilized [14,15]. If a suitable appendix is not available or a decision has been made to use it for a concomitant MACE procedure then the TTBS technique can provide a uniformly suitable conduit for the efferent limb mechanism. For this procedure a 2.5 cm segment of ileum (or colon) is subtracted from the fecal stream [7]. The bowel segment is then opened along the antimesenteric boarder and subsequently tubularized in a transverse fashion over a catheter. This technique provides a tube with a centralized mesentery (Figure 40.2a). Anatomic considerations may dictate the need for a conduit with an offset mesentery. In these cases the bowel segment is opened closer to one side of the mesentery than the other (Figure 40.2b). Two techniques have been described to create a longer channel for individuals with a thick abdominal wall. Monti described the use of a tandem tube in which two conduits were anastomosed to each other with interrupted absorbable sutures [7] (Figure 40.2c). Irregularities at the anastomotic site may result in difficulties with catheterization. The alternative technique of the Spiral Monti as described by Casale allows for the construction of a long tube with a more uniform, smooth lumen [16] (Figure 40.3).

Implantation

As previously noted, a firm reservoir wall is needed to provide adequate support of the channel so that intravesical pressure can compress the conduit [3]. The preferred site for implantation is therefore the native bladder wall. If native bladder wall is not available then tunnelling into a tenia of the colon or the wall of a gastric augmentation is

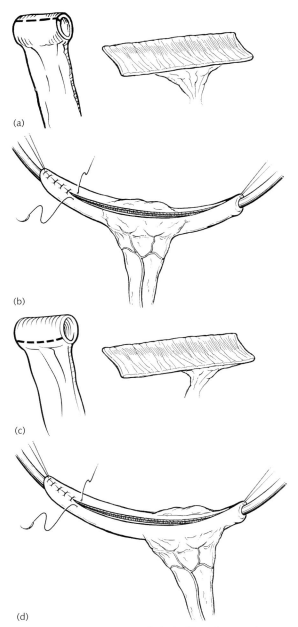

(d)

Figure 40.2 (a) Transverse tubularized bowel segment, incision; (b) transverse tubularized bowel segment, central mesentery; (c) transverse tubularized bowel segment, incision for off center mesentery; and (d) transverse tubularized bowel segment, off center mesentery. (© IUSM Visual Media.)

the next best option. Although an antireflux technique can be created between the conduit and the ileum, the thinness of the ileal muscle wall may result in suboptimal transmission of intravesical pressure to the tube. The conduit

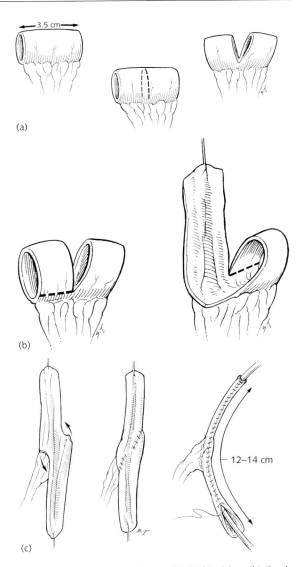

Figure 40.3 (a) Casale Spiral Monti, initial incision; (b) Casale Spiral Monti, subsequent incisions; and (c) Casale Spiral Monti, completed. (© IUSM Visual Media.)

can be implanted into the reservoir using either an intravesical or extravesical technique as long as the submucosal tunnel is of adequate length.

Once the conduit is implanted into the reservoir an appropriate location for its exit from the abdomen is determined. Many factors help determine the optimal location for stoma creation in a given individual. First, a location must be chosen that will allow for a straight trajectory through the abdominal wall. Second, the reservoir

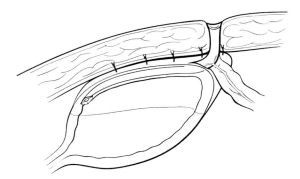

Figure 40.4 Proper anatomic relationships of conduit to bladder and abdominal wall. (© IUSM Visual Media.)

must be fixed with permanent sutures at the point of exit of the conduit from the reservoir to the anterior abdominal wall (Figure 40.4). Failure to achieve these two goals will result in kinking of the tube at various degrees of bladder filling. Thickness of the abdominal wall relative to the length of the conduit may also play a role in deciding the stoma site. The umbilicus, because it is the shortest course between the abdominal skin and peritoneum, is a unique location for catheterizable stoma placement. A stoma placed in this site is appealing, as it allows the cosmetic (and possibly image) advantage of hiding the stoma more readily than in other abdominal locations. Finally, manual dexterity, patient preference, and gender must be considered when choosing the stoma location. Mitrofanoff himself raised a concern regarding the stretching/kinking of an umbilical-based conduit during pregnancy [17]. Anchoring of the appendix at the umbilicus also has the potential to tether the bladder making it more difficult to safely retract away from the uterus during a C-section delivery.

Stoma

The stoma itself can be created using a number of techniques. The anastomosis at the skin level should be performed in the absence of tension so as to avoid any compromise to the conduit's blood supply. Early descriptions of the technique proposed excising a circular skin segment, slightly wider than the conduit itself, and anastamosing it flush to the skin [1,2]. Various techniques have subsequently been championed which are believed to decrease subsequent stomal stenosis rates. Each method consists of developing a skin flap that maximizes the diameter of the junction between the skin and conduit. Included among these are the V- or U-shaped flap advancement into a spatulated conduit, VQZ-plasty and

VQ-plasty [17–22]. Another potentially useful method for minimizing stomal stenosis with appendicovesicostomies is to harvest the appendix with a small cecal cuff [23].

Incontinent ileovesicostomy: The ileal chimney

The incontinent ileovesicostomy is an excellent surgical option that provides safe evacuation of urine from the bladder in patients who are not suitable candidates for continent urinary reconstruction [24,25]. This operation can dramatically simplify the care of patients with poor dexterity, impaired cognitive function and individuals who prove to be poorly compliant with catheterization schemes required to maintain low intravesical pressures. In contrast to ileal loop diversion, this technique does not require construction of uretero-ileal anastomoses and preserves the antirefluxing mechanism by leaving the ureters within the bladder. For this procedure a segment of ileum with adequate mobility to reach the bladder and the abdominal wall is subtracted from the fecal stream. The proximal end is anastomosed widely to the dome of the bladder and the distal end brought out as a budded stoma [26].

Outcomes

Continent catheterizable channels

Continence achieved with a Mitrofanoff tube is greater than 90% in most published series. Continence results appear to be independent of whether appendix or a segment of transverse tubularized bowel is utilized for the conduit. In Mitrofanoff's original series of patients treated between 1976 and 1984, 23 patients underwent creation of a continent catheterizable conduit (20 constructed from appendix). Mean patient age at surgery was 8 years and 4 months (range 3–16) and mean follow-up was 20 years (range 15–23). Bilateral upper tract deterioration was found in 10 cases secondary to elevated intravesical pressures. Bladder stones were found in 5 patients while complications directly related to the conduit included stomal stenosis or persistent leakage in 11 cases [17].

In Monti's series of 55 conduits (7 tandem channels: 48 single Yang–Monti channels) created using the TTBS technique, 91% continence was reported. After an average follow-up of <7 months, only one patient required a revision for stomal stenosis. Five patients experienced incontinence. One patient was rendered dry by adjustment of the catheterization routine, while the four others required two open revisions and two endoscopic procedures [4].

Castellan *et al.* reported three experiences with 45 Monti urinary channels (4 tandem, 41 single), with mean follow-up of 38 months. Overall, stoma-related problems were noted in approximately 20% of patients. Three patients developed complete fibrosis of the channel while another three experienced stomal incontinence. Difficulties with catheterization were noted in four patients with one undergoing stomal revision [27].

Narayanaswamy *et al.* reported their results with 94 continent catheterizable conduits, of which 25 were Monti channels (tandem/single 17:8). Mean follow-up was 2.1 years. Fifteen (60%) patients had problems with catheterization, with stenosis of the conduit, diverticular pouch formation, or both occurring in 13 of these patients. Out of six to seven patients with pouch formation had a double Monti. The authors reported no difference in stomal stenosis rates between appendiceal channels and Monti channels [19].

Finally, a recent study from Indiana University comparing the Monti Procedure to the Spiral Monti Procedure revealed a 98% continence rate. Surgical revision of the conduit was required in 19% of patients (9% stomal revisions, 10% subfascial revisions). The only significant difference noted between the two procedures was a higher incidence of subfascial revisions for umbilical stomas in both groups. The need for subfascial revision was highest in the spiral Monti channels placed in the umbilicus.

Incontinent ileovesicostomy

Leng *et al.* reviewed their experience in 25 men and 13 women with a mean age of 44.9 years who underwent incontinent ileovesicostomy. Mean follow-up was 52 months. Before ileovesicostomy the incidence of serious complications associated with an indwelling catheter was significant, including poor bladder compliance in 50% of cases, urosepsis in 45%, hydronephrosis in 21%, renal struvite calculi in 18%, urethrocutaneous fistula in 18%, autonomic dysreflexia in 13%, and bladder calculi in 2%. After conversion >80% of this high-risk population maintained a normal upper urinary tract and normal bladder storage compliance. Other complications including stomal stenosis, loop stricture, and bladder calculi were noted in up to 5% of patients [25].

Recently, this technique has been described in a cohort of 17 children [26]. Average age at time of operation was 14.1 years. Average follow-up was >2 years, seven children underwent the procedure due to a primary inability to perform CIC while 10 required the procedure secondary to poor compliance with CIC following continent urinary reconstruction. Renal function stabilized in all patients. No patient had developed intravesical calculi. Despite its apparent high success rate, others have reported that subsequent excessive weight gain can result in angulation of the channel resulting in reduced efficiency of drainage.

Complications

General

Complications can generally be minimized if proper catheterization techniques are utilized. Although the mucosa of the bowel makes lubrication theoretically unnecessary, generous utilization of lubricant is recommended. The author will have his patients fill a 5 ml syringe with lubricant and gently instill this directly into the stoma prior to catheterization to maximally lubricate the channel.

When difficulty with catheterization is encountered families are told to contact their physician immediately so that a catheter can be placed across the channel. Failure to place a catheter across the site may allow the traumatized site to fibrose. The surgeon should have a low threshold for utilizing flexible endoscopy to evaluate the channel in these cases. Multiple unsuccessful attempts to place a catheter may simply extend the area of trauma. Our recommendation is to then leave the catheter secured in place for 1 week. This will allow most false passages or edema to resolve before catheterization resumes and hence minimizes the chance of exacerbating the injury.

Stomal stenosis

Stomal stenosis is the most common complication of the Mitrofanoff procedure with reported rates ranging between 8% and 40% [9,23,27–31]. Stenosis generally appears to occur within the first 2 years following the initial surgery [23,28,32]. However, one report has demonstrated that this complication can occur as late as 15 years following the procedure emphasizing the continued need for close follow-up of this patient population [17]. Initially it was felt that the well-constructed TTBS may have a theoretical advantage over the appendix in that the luminal diameter could be determined by the surgeon. This is in contrast to the appendix in which the luminal diameter is fixed and generally between 10 and 12 Fr. However, most studies have shown that the incidence of stomal stenosis does not differ significantly between TTBS and appendiceal conduits.

The use of a hydrophilic catheter can allow for continued use of the stoma that has experienced a degree of

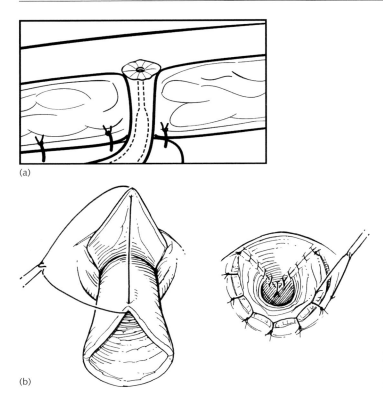

(a)

(b)

Figure 40.5 (a) Stomal stenosis and
(b) technique of repair of stomal stenosis.
(© IUSM Visual Media.)

stenosis. Simple dilation can be enough but often recurrence will require surgical revision. Injections of triamcinolone around the stoma or topical steroid application have been used in an attempt to limit the local inflammatory response that likely plays a role in stenosis [33]. Definitive treatment of stomal stenosis involves the creation of a new laterally based V- or U-shaped flap, division of the stomal cicatrix along its most lateral edge, and creation of a widely spatulated anastomosis (Figure 40.5). A catheter is generally left in place for 3 weeks before catheterization is restarted.

Subfascial conduit complications

If one is able to pass a catheter at the level of the stoma yet unable to advance the catheter into the reservoir, one of several conduit-based complications may exist either individually or in combination.

Kinking of the channel is one of the more common subfascial problems. This most commonly occurs when there has been poor fixation of the reservoir to the posterior rectus sheath. As a result the bladder moves during filling, altering the angle at which the channel enters into the conduit (Figure 40.6). This problem can initially be overcome if one can decompress the bladder by placing

a urethral catheter. In patients with an altered or obliterated bladder neck who experience acute urinary retention secondary to difficulty catheterizing the channel, an 18 ga needle can be placed suprapubically to decompress the reservoir. After the bladder has been decompressed the angulation of the channel relative to the reservoir is often reduced and a catheter can be placed easily across the conduit. The long-term solution to the problem of conduit kinking may be to catheterize more often and not allow the reservoir to overfill. Persistence of the problem may require reoperation to more securely anchor the bladder to the fascia.

Conduit redundancy is another common etiology for catheterization difficulties. This generally occurs when the surgeon has left a portion of the catheterizable channel unsupported during the original procedure (Figure 40.7a). As a result of cumulative minor difficulties with catheterization, the channel becomes stretched and tortuous making future catheterizations progressively more challenging. For this reason we have generally advocated bringing the conduit to a right lower quadrant location unless the reservoir is of sufficient size to extend up to the umbilicus. Conduit redundancy can often be resolved by freeing-up the channel and putting it on

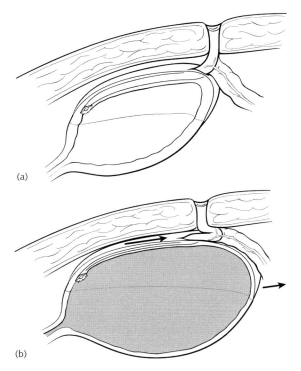

Figure 40.6 (a) Channel course in unanchored bladder and (b) channel angulation with bladder filling as a result. (© IUSM Visual Media.)

additional stretch to straighten its course (Figure 40.7b). However, the continued presence of an unsupported free intraperitoneal segment of the conduit leaves the patient vulnerable to recurrence of difficulties with conduit redundancy.

False passages can occur in combination with kinking and/or conduit redundancy or in a well-supported conduit. In either case the management is to place a catheter across the site and allow the tube ample time to heal before future attempts at catheterization are attempted. Even full thickness perforations can be successfully managed conservatively if no gross periconduit contamination has occurred.

Stomal incontinence

Incontinence through the efferent conduit may be the result of an inadequate flap-valve mechanism, high intravesical pressures or a combination of these two factors. Proper determination of cause is essential in determining the appropriate surgical treatment. Urodynamic evaluation with the catheter preferentially placed through the native bladder neck will establish bladder compliance

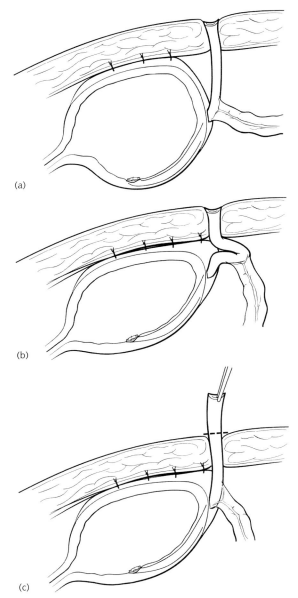

Figure 40.7 (a) Channel redundancy – long extravesical course of channel to the abdominal wall; (b) kinking of the redundant channel; and (c) technique for repair of channel redundancy. (© IUSM Visual Media.)

and determine the conduit leak point pressure. A poorly compliant reservoir should be properly addressed with anticholinergic medication and/or bladder augmentation. An inadequate tunnel can be corrected by submucosal injection of biomaterial [34]. The biomaterial can be injected transvesically in the same fashion as the

STING procedure is carried out. If the urethra has been surgically modified, the material can be injected via the conduit with the bulking agent delivered submucosally at the 6 o'clock position. When this minimally invasive technique is utilized, the bladder should be drained by a route other than the channel so as to avoid the catheter molding the polymer. If the bulking agent is unsuccessful in resolving the incontinence then an open surgical procedure to re-establish a proper valve mechanism is indicated.

Stones

Urinary stasis is a well-known etiologic factor for stone formation throughout the urinary tract. Most patients with neuropathic bladder dysfunction and many patients with anatomic abnormalities of the bladder or bladder outlet (i.e. bladder exstrophy and posterior urethral valves, respectively) do not have the ability to spontaneously empty their bladder to completion. These patients are hence more prone to urinary stasis with subsequent precipitation of urinary solutes and creation of an environment amenable to bacterial overgrowth. Bladder stones have been reported with increased frequency in augments with coexistent bladder outlet resistant procedures and/or catheterizable abdominal wall stomas [35–37]. In one series patients with an abdominal stoma had a >4-fold higher risk of developing reservoir calculi if the patient emptied via and abdominal wall stoma versus the native urethra (66% versus 15%). The incorporation of a gastric segment when an abdominal stoma is created may decrease the risk of calculus formation [35]. Leng et al. reported the development of stones in approximately 5% of patients following creation of an ileal chimney. In contrast, Kaefer et al. found no cases of stone formation in patients who irrigated their conduit daily using a catheter placed via the ileal segment into the bladder [26].

Methods for bladder stone removal include open cystolithotomy, percutaneous cystolithotomy and endoscopic cystolithotomy via the efferent conduit. Evacuation of stones from the bladder that is drained by the ileal chimney is straightforward. The large diameter of the conduit allows for easy passage of endoscopic equipment into the bladder and removal of stones intact from the bladder. In contrast, although it may be tempting to attempt stone removal via a continent efferent conduit, any manipulation of the conduit does carry with it the potential for injury and other options should be strongly considered, if there is any difficulty passing endoscopic equipment or the stone is of significant size.

Perhaps the most important aspect of managing bladder calculi in patients following genitourinary reconstruction is the prevention of further stones. The patient and parents must clearly understand that there is a high probability of stone recurrence if measures are not taken to reduce risk factors. A number of series have demonstrated a clear reduction in bladder calculi when a postaugmentation bladder irrigation protocol is instituted following bladder augmentation or creation of an ileal chimney [35,37,38]. Hensle et al. compared the incidence of stone formation in two distinct patient groups following bladder augmentation. Of 91 patients who did not perform postaugmentation irrigation, 39 (41%) developed bladder calculi with a mean time to presentation of 30 months. In contrast, only 3 of 42 (7%) patients who did perform postaugmentation irrigation developed reservoir calculi with a mean time to presentation of 26 months.

Therefore, lifelong daily bladder irrigation of the bladder is imperative to evacuate all mucous. Mitrofanoff emphasized the importance of creating a continent catheterizable channel of large caliber so as to allow more rapid drainage and minimize the chances of leaving residual urine within the bladder. In patients with continent catheterizable stomas mucous may build up in the most dependent portion of the bladder. If the bladder neck is still accessible, it may be of benefit to periodically irrigate via the more gravity-dependent bladder neck to minimize buildup of mucous.

References

1 Kaefer M, Retik AB. The mitrofanoff principle in continent urinary reconstruction. *Urol Clin North Am* 1997;24:795–811.
2 Mitrofanoff P. Trans-appendicular continent cystostomy in the management of the neurogenic bladder [French]. *Chirurgie Pediatrique* 1980;21:297–305.
3 Hinman F, Jr. Functional classification of conduits for continent diversion. *J Urol* 1990;144:27–30.
4 Monti PR, de Carvalho JR, Arap S. The monti procedure: Applications and complications. *Urology* 2000;55:616–21.
5 Watson HS, Bauer SB, Peters CA et al. Comparative urodynamics of appendiceal and ureteral Mitrofanoff conduits in children. *J Urol* 1995;154:878–82.
6 Duckett JW, Snyder 3rd, HM. Use of the Mitrofanoff principle in urinary reconstruction. *Urol Clin North Am* 1986;13:271–4.
7 Monti PR, Lara RC, Dutra MA et al. New techniques for construction of efferent conduits based on the Mitrofanoff principle. *Urology* 1997;49:112–5.

8 Yang W. Yang needle tunneling technique in creating antire-fluxing and continent mechanisms. *J Urol* 150:830–4.

9 Duckett JW, Lotfi AH. Appendicovesicostomy (and variations) in bladder reconstruction. *J Urol* 1993;149:567–9.

10 Mor Y, Kajbafzadeh AM, German K *et al*. The role of ureter in the creation of Mitrofanoff channels in children. *J Urol* 1997;157:635–7.

11 Perovic S. Continent urinary diversion using preputial penile or clitoral skin flap. *J Urol* 1996;155:1402–6.

12 Gotsadze D, Pirtskhalaishvili G. Meckel's diverticulum as a continence mechanism. *J Urol* 1998;160:831–2.

13 Bihrle R, Klee LW, Adams MC *et al*. Early clinical experience with the transverse colon-gastric tube continent urinary reservoir. *J Urol* 1991;146:751–3.

14 Bruce RG, McRoberts JW. Cecoappendicovesicostomy: Conduit-lengthening technique for use in continent urinary reconstruction. *Urology* 1998;52:702–4.

15 Cromie WJ, Barada JH, Weingarten JL. Cecal tubularization: Lengthening technique for creation of catheterizable conduit. *Urology* 1991;37:41–2.

16 Casale AJ. A long continent ileovesicostomy using a single piece of bowel. *J Urol* 1999;162:1743–5.

17 Liard A, Seguier-Lipszyc E, Mathiot A *et al*. The Mitrofanoff procedure: 20 years later. *J Urol* 2001;165:2394–8.

18 Keating MA, Rink RC, Adams MC. Appendicovesicostomy: A useful adjunct to continent reconstruction of the bladder. *J Urol* 1993;149:1091–4.

19 Narayanaswamy B, Wilcox D, Cuckow P *et al*. The yang-monti ileovesicostomy a problematic channel? *BJU Int* 2001;87:861.

20 Kajbafzadeh A, Chubak N. Simultaneous malone antegrade continence enema and mitrofanoff principle using the divided appendix report of a new technique for prevention of stoma complications. *J Urol* 2001;165:2404.

21 Khoury AE, Van Savage JG, McLorie GA *et al*. Minimizing stomal stenosis in appendicovesicostomy using the modified umbilical stoma. *J Urol* 1996;155:2050–1.

22 Glassman D, Docimo S. Concealed umbilical stoma long-term evaluation of stomal stenosis. *J Urol* 2001;166:1028.

23 Harris CF, Cooper CS, Hutcheson JC *et al*. Appendicovesicostomy: The mitrofanoff procedure – A 15-year perspective. *J Urol* 2000;163:1922–6.

24 Schwartz SL, Kennelly MJ, McGuire EJ *et al*. Incontinent ileovesicostomy urinary diversion in the treatment of lower urinary tract dysfunction. *J Urol* 1994;152:99–102.

25 Leng WW, Faerber G, Del Terzo M *et al*. Long-term outcome of incontinent ileovesicostomy management of severe lower urinary tract dysfunction. *J Urol* 1999;161:1803–6.

26 Kaefer M, Molitierno J, Misseri R *et al*. *The Ileal Chimney: A Versatile Alternative to Continent Urinary Reconstruction in Children*. Presented at the 2007 meeting of the American Academy of Pediatrics, San Fransisco, California.

27 Castellan MA, Gosalbez R, Labbie A *et al*. Outcomes of continent catheterizable stomas for urinary and fecal incontinence: Comparison among different tissue options. *BJU Int* 2005;95:1053–7.

28 Woodhouse CR, MacNeily AE. The mitrofanoff principle: Expanding upon a versatile technique. *Br J Urol* 1994;74:447–53.

29 Sumfest JM, Burns MW, Mitchell ME. The mitrofanoff principle in urinary reconstruction. *J Urol* 1993;150:1875–7, discussion 1877–8.

30 Van Savage JG, Khoury AE, McLorie GA *et al*. Outcome analysis of mitrofanoff principle applications using appendix and ureter to umbilical and lower quadrant stomal sites. *J Urol* 1996;156:1794–7.

31 Cain MP, Casale AJ, King SJ *et al*. Appendicovesicostomy and newer alternatives for the Mitrofanoff procedure: results in the last 100 patients at riley children's hospital. *J Urol* 1999;162:1749–52.

32 Thomas JC, Dietrich MS, Trusler L *et al*. Continent catheterizable channels and the timing of their complications. *J Urol* 2006;176:1816–20, discussion 1820.

33 Snodgrass W. Triamcinolone to prevent stenosis in mitrofanoff stomas. *J Urol* 1999;161:928.

34 Gosalbez R, Jr., Wei D, Gouse A. Refashioned short bowel segments for the construction of catheterizable channels (the Monti procedure): Early clinical experience. *J Urol* 1998;160:1099–1102.

35 Kaefer M, Hendren WH, Bauer SB *et al*. Reservoir calculi: A comparison of reservoirs constructed from stomach and other enteric segments. *J Urol* 1998;160:2187–90.

36 Kronner KM, Casale AJ, Cain MP *et al*. Bladder calculi in the pediatric augmented bladder. *J Urol* 1998;160:1096–8, discussion 1103.

37 Hensle TW, Bingham J, Lam J *et al*. Preventing reservoir calculi after augmentation cystoplasty and continent urinary diversion: the influence of an irrigation protocol. *BJU Int* 2004;93:585–7.

38 Brough RJ, O'Flynn KJ, Fishwick J *et al*. Bladder washout and stone formation in paediatric enterocystoplasty. *Eur Urol* 1998;33:500–2.

41

Surgical Management of the Sphincter Mechanism

Juan C. Prieto and Linda A. Baker

Key points

- Outcome analyses are confounded by the lack of randomized, controlled trials, limited preoperative/postoperative assessment of bladder physiology, and poor standardization of outcomes measures, given the multifactorial nature of the problem.

- The highest urinary continence rate (85–96%) is achieved with the artificial urinary sphincter (AUS) in long-term studies. However, significant rates of AUS removal, AUS revision, and bladder deterioration dampens enthusiasm.

- Minimally invasive outpatient bulking agent injection achieves dryness or improvement in 40–50% at >1.5-year follow-up with very few complications.

- In long-term follow-up, bladder neck sling procedures have 70–80% success rates in neurogenics.

- In long-term follow-up, Young–Dees–Leadbetter (YDL) bladder neck reconstructions have 70–80% success rates in exstrophy–epispadias patients.

- Continence can be achieved surgically; however, it may be at the expense of augmentation cystoplasty and multiple procedures.

- Proper preoperative patient selection and meticulous surgical technique can decrease complications and improve outcomes.

- Close urodynamic follow-up is required in all patients to monitor for detrusor and upper tract deterioration. This deterioration may not be associated with incontinence.

Introduction

Urinary incontinence in children is common, affecting approximately 20% of 4–6 year old children [1]. Several factors participate in the dynamic process of urinary continence, including urine volume, bladder physiology (capacity, compliance, stability, and evacuation), and bladder outlet physiology (pelvic floor support and a coordinated sphincter mechanism). Sphincter resistance should be higher than intravesical pressure to achieve continence, thus management of the sphincter mechanism is only one component of the equation. Pediatric urologists often treat challenging congenital defects with

sphincter incompetence, such as neurogenic bladder, cloacal exstrophy, classic bladder exstrophy (BE), epispadias, cecoureterocele, urethral duplication, ectopic ureters, or common cloaca. Multiple medical and surgical treatment options exist to cure outlet incompetence, indicating that one simple solution does not cure all. The timing, indications, approach and management of these interventions are controversial. This chapter will focus upon the outcomes and complications of surgical techniques to increase bladder outlet resistance.

Surgical techniques

Four surgical strategies that enhance sphincter mechanism resistance without complete obstruction include bladder neck bulking agents, bladder neck sling, artificial urinary sphincter (AUS), and bladder neck reconstruction

Pediatric Urology: Surgical Complications and Management. Edited by Duncan T. Wilcox, Prasad P. Godbole and Martin A. Koyle.
© 2008 Blackwell Publishing, ISBN: 978-1-4051-6268-5.

(BNR). Criteria for surgical enhancement of bladder outlet resistance are controversial but some include low detrusor leak point pressures ($\leqslant$25–45 cm H_2O), an open bladder neck during filling at low detrusor pressures, striated sphincter denervation, and clinical evidence of stress urinary incontinence. In general, when the patient has diminished bladder capacity (<50–60% of expected bladder capacity), impaired compliance, or severe detrusor instability, concomitant augmentation cystoplasty should be considered (as discussed in Chapter 39). In contrast, bladder neck closure may be performed when there is no hope for the bladder neck and urethra as a controllable conduit for urine egress.

In all series, the primary outcome is urinary continence. However, the evaluation of surgical outcomes of therapy for sphincter mechanism incompetence is confounded by the lack of randomized, controlled trials, limited preoperative/postoperative assessment of bladder physiology, and poor standardization of outcomes measures. Published series have varied reporting, including outcomes as dry/improved/wet, minutes of dryness, stress incontinence, or nocturnal wetness. Thus, the definition of success must be critically assessed in each series. Meta-analyses from published series are even impossible since individual patient details, such as pathology, adjunctive medical, or surgical therapy, are not traceable in most published series. In essence, we are limited to assessing outcomes from the largest patient series with multiple etiologies for their urinary incontinence.

Bladder neck bulking agents

Berg and Politano first reported periurethral injections of polytetrafluoroethylene (PTFE) (Teflon®) for the treatment of pediatric urinary incontinence in 1973 [2,3]. Since then, other bulking agents, including glutaraldehyde cross-linked bovine collagen (Contigen®, Zyplast®) [4], polydimethylsiloxane (PDMS, Macroplastique®) [5], and dextranomer/hyaluronic acid copolymer (Dx/HA,

Deflux®) [6] have been used transurethrally. The ideal bulking agent is nonmigratory, nonallergenic, nonmutagenic, nonimmunogenic, and easily injected. Due to safety concerns (Table 41.1) and decreased long-term success rates, most of the first bulking agents used are currently obsolete. Presently, the most frequent agents used in urinary incontinence in children are PDMS and Dx/HA.

Bulking agents could be considered as initial therapy for sphincter incompetence since they are less invasive, carry lower morbidity, generate lower costs, and can be performed as an ambulatory procedure. For transurethral leak, the cystoscope can be inserted retrograde transurethrally or antegrade via continent catheterizable channel or suprapubic access, permitting multiple injections until bladder neck/urethral coaptation is achieved [13].

Outcomes

Outcomes by duration of follow-up

Long-term follow-up of 49 patients who received PDMS injections demonstrated that the initial 68% success rate at 6 months deteriorated to 47% (33% complete continence rate and 14% significant improvement rate) at a mean follow-up of 6 years [14]. Similarly, long-term follow-up of Dx/HA bladder neck injection in 61 children by Lottmann et al. demonstrated a decrease in the continence rate (dryness or significant improvement) from 70% at 6 months to 50% during the first 18 months. The success rate stabilizes approximately 40% at up to 7 years of follow-up [12]. In summary, most studies show that as the duration of follow-up lengthens after injection therapy, early good continence rates exhibit a slow continuous loss down to ~40% at approximately 18 months follow-up.

Outcomes by sex

At 1 month follow-up of 61 patients with mixed pathologies, Lottmann et al. observed 54% of males and 60% of females treated with Dx/HA were dry or improved. Two

Table 41.1 Complications specific to bulking agent used.

Agent	Complication	Current status	Reference
PTFE	Particle migration (lung, brain)	Abandoned	[7,8]
PDMS (silicone)	Teratogenicity; particle migration; nonbiodegradable	Limited use	[9,10]
Collagen	Volume loss; allergenic; not latex-free	Abandoned; requires preoperative hypersensitivity testing	[11]
Dextranomer/HA	None currently reported	Used	[12]

males with improved continence became dry at puberty [12]. Similarly, even at 6 years mean follow-up, Guys *et al.* found gender to have no influence on continence in 49 children treated with PDMS [14]. Thus, gender has no significant effect on short- or long-term outcome [15].

Outcomes by pathology (neurogenic versus nonneurogenic/structural)

Outcomes by pathology are somewhat difficult to assess, given published series are not well controlled for bladder functional parameters. Early short-term series with small patient numbers suggested a poorer outcome in neurogenic patients. In one of the largest series to date with mean follow-up of 28 months, Lottmann *et al.* reported 48% and 53% dryness or improvement rates in neurogenic and BE patients, respectively [12]. Burki *et al.* reviewed 52 patients with exstrophy–epispadias at mean follow-up of 4.6 years, finding epispadic patients were more likely to benefit from PDMS injection than exstrophy patients. However, Dyer found 100% failure rate in BE patients treated with Teflon or Dx/HA [16]. At 3 years mean follow-up on 19 neurogenic children who received collagen injection, no patients were dry and only 37% remained improved [11]. In 2006, Guys *et al.* reported on 41 neurogenics treated with PDMS, finding that bladder hyperactivity has no influence on long-term results if medically controlled. Thus patient selection will impact outcomes analyses, as patients with uncontrolled detrusor overactivity and poor bladder compliance would be poor candidates for bulking agents.

Outcomes by bulking agent employed

As seen in Table 41.2, long-term success rates with PDMS and Dx/HA, the two most commonly employed bulking agents, are comparable at 40–50%.

Outcomes of repeat bulking agent injections

Multiple injections of bulking agents have yielded dryness or improvement in 37% at best [12,18] with three injections predicting outcome [15]. Theoretical concerns with the formation of bladder neck scar tissue complicating future BNRs has not been substantiated [16].

Outcomes by timing of open bladder neck reconstructive surgery:

By pooling data from six published series with various pathologies and bulking agents, Nelson and Park observed no difference in dryness or improvement whether injection therapy was administered before or after open bladder neck surgery [19].

A secondary outcome measure of bulking agent injection therapy has been increase in bladder capacity in small bladders. Some have reported it ineffective in 5 neurogenics [20] and in 13 BE [16]. However, a mean capacity increase of ~50% at >2 years follow-up was observed in 5 of 6 exstrophy–epispadias patients after collagen injection [21] and in 12 of 18 patients after Dx/HA injection [12].

In conclusion, long-term studies of patients without uncontrolled detrusor overactivity and poor bladder compliance show 40–50% dryness or improvement [12,14,15]. While dry is infrequently achieved, bulking agent injection may provide a better dry interval. Hopefully as experience grows, future studies will identify patient subgroups most likely to benefit from bulking agent treatment. Preoperative counseling should include realistic expectations.

Complications

As previously mentioned, some reported complications are specific to the bulking agent used (Table 41.1). Complications reported from bulking agent general use of bulking agent are unusual but can include temporary dysuria, cystitis, pyelonephritis, and epididymo-orchitis

Table 41.2 Long-term outcomes of the use of bulking injectable materials for urinary incontinence in children.

Author	Material used	Number of patients	Complete continence rate (%)	Improved continence rate (%)	Overall continence rate (%)	Mean follow-up duration (years)
Burki *et al.* (2006) [17]	PDMS	52	17	33	50	4.6
Guys *et al.* (2006) [14]	PDMS	49	33	14	47	6
Lottmann *et al.* (2006) [12]	Dx/HA	61	Not described	Not described	40	7

[12]. Collagen injection calcification has been noted in 13% at 8.8 years postinjection [22]. More serious complications include single reports of bladder perforation, bladder stone, perineal abscess (Figure 41.1), and gluteal hematoma, urinary retention [12,23], and detrusor deterioration (decreased capacity and compliance) with or without vesicoureteral reflux (VUR) hydroureteronephrosis in 10–27% [12,20,24]. Lottmann observed this despite all patients being on clean interhittent catherization (CIC) and anticholinergics. Thus, long-term close urodynamic follow-up is mandated.

As most of these complications are rare, no studies exist which compare surgical methods to minimize complications. However, various authors have made recommendations. In order to prevent infections, prophylactic antibiotics should be used and sterile urine cultures should be documented prior to any procedure. Formal antibiotic treatment is advisable up to 5–7 days postinjection. To avoid catheterization at the implant site and to prevent urinary retention, some place a suprapubic catheter for at least 5 days postoperatively [12,14].

Bladder neck sling

In 1982, Woodside and Borden initially reported the bladder neck sling for the treatment of urinary incontinence in children [25]. Since then, various types of tissue or material have been used to create bladder neck wraps or slings, including autologous materials (gracilis muscle, tensor fascia lata, rectus fascia, detrusor muscle, etc.), synthetic products (PTFE membrane (Gore-tex), vicryl mesh, silicon elastomers, porcine-derived small intestinal submucosa (SIS)), and cadaveric fascias. Via retropubic, posterior or transvaginal approaches, slings, and wraps

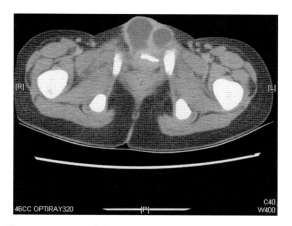

Figure 41.1 Perineal abscess formation after bladder neck Deflux injection. (Photograph courtesy of Dr. Rafael Gosalbez.)

are surgically placed around the urethra at the bladder neck with suspension to the ventral abdominal wall.

Outcomes
Outcomes by duration of follow-up
The continence rates of sling procedures do not seem to demonstrate a severe duration of follow-up effect. Castellan and Gosalbez have reported on their cohort of neurogenics with augmentation cystoplasty, reporting 93% continence at 3 years and 88% continence at 4.6 years mean follow-up [26,27].

Outcomes by sex
Early reports had noted poor sling success in males; however, a meta-analysis and a recent report note an 78–87% continence rate in a mixed population of males studied [26,28]. In a limited study, ambulatory neuropathics males may have less success than nonambulatory males or females irrespective of ambulatory status [29].

Outcomes by pathology (neurogenic versus nonneurogenic/structural)
Fascial sling procedure is more commonly performed over AUS on patients with low outlet resistance and neurogenic bladder, who will undergo bladder augmentation and in whom volitional voiding is not expected. In this context, most pediatric urologists agree that the goal of the bladder neck sling is to achieve bladder neck suspension along with obstructive coaptation. Thus, the patient empties his bladder only by CIC either per urethra or through a continent stoma. No studies have reported continence outcomes in other patient subgroup populations than neurogenics.

Outcomes by sling/wrap material employed
At 5 years follow-up, 13 of 14 patients were dry after bladder wall wraparound sling with augmentation [30]. SIS has demonstrated success rates equivalent to autologous fascia in short-term follow-up [29,31]. PTFE sling in 19 patients had good early success but erosion necessitated sling removal in 14 [32].

Outcomes by sling/wrap technique performed
Some series suggest that circumferential wrap with suspension improves outcomes [33]; however series are small. Currently no head-to-head comparisons exist of the various methods.

Outcomes with or without simultaneous bladder augmentation
Meta-analysis of multiple series shows that simultaneous bladder augmentation has been reported in 55–100%

of patients who achieve urinary continence after sling procedure [34]. The most extensive follow-up series of bladder neck sling with bladder augmentation was presented by Castellan *et al.* in 2005 [26]. They followed 58 patients for mean 4 years with neurogenic bladder who all underwent bladder augmentation over a period of 4 years (mean = 4.16 years). They achieved good operative results (complete passive continence for periods of 4–6 h during the day and 6–8 h at night) in 51 (88%)

patients. Since bladder neck slings only increase bladder outlet resistance up to 20 cm H_2O, it is possible that the concomitant bladder augmentation may count for a considerable part on this high continence rate.

A recent report by Snodgrass addresses this by performing sling and appendicovesicostomy without augmentation in 30 neurogenic patients. Eighty-three percent achieved satisfactory continence (<2 damp pads/day) at mean 22 months follow-up. Twenty-seven

Table 41.3 Reported complications from bladder neck sling/wrap procedures.

Complication	Most susceptible	Treatment	Prevention	Reference
Wound dehiscence/infection	Obese	Antibiotics, wound care	Antibiotics, nutritional support	[34]
Sling slippage	Females	Reoperation	Suture fixation	[26,34]
Sling erosion	Males and females	If synthetic, sling removal	Meticulous surgical dissection and correct sling tension; antibiotics; minimal catheter trauma	[32]
Retracted urethral meatus complicating self-urethral catheterization	Females	Create continent catheterizable channel at surgery	Close attention to severity of suspension	[27]
Bladder neck occlusion	Males and females	Continent catheterizable channel	Minimize bladder neck dissection at sling placement	[26]
Organ perforation (ureter, vagina, rectum)	Males and females; prior surgical patients	Repair and diversion if needed	Meticulous surgical technique	[34]
Pelvic abscess		Postoperative antibiotics; drainage	Preoperative antibiotics	[34]
Difficulty with endoscopic manipulations	Females	Endoscopic manipulation via percutaneous bladder access	Close attention to severity of suspension	[34]
Intraoperative bleeding from the venous plexus of Santorini	Males and females	Surgical hemostasis	Properly place incisions in the endopelvic fascia. Do not place them too close to the bladder neck or too distal on the urethra/prostate	[27]
Erectile dysfunction secondary to periprostatic nerve injury	Males	Erectile dysfunction treatment alternatives	Preserve Denonvillier's fascia; pass sling lateral	[28,39]
Bladder and/or upper tract deterioration	Males and females	CIC + anticholinergics versus bladder augmentation	Proper preoperative patient selection and management; close monitoring	[34,35]

percent developed worsening bladder urodynamics which was successfully medically treated in seven and required augmentation in one [35].

Sling/wrap conclusion
In conclusion, large series of bladder neck slings are sparse. Unfortunately, most lack long-term follow-up, which is crucial to assess morbidity such as bladder and upper tract deterioration. Overall, urinary continence rates oscillate from 40% to 100% [29,33,34,36–39].

Complications
Overall, sling/wrap complications occur at a relatively low rate but some are associated with significant morbidity (Table 41.3). The revision rate of sling procedures is 15–73%, depending on the material used [32,34].

Artificial urinary sphincter
AUS was first successfully used in correcting neurogenic urinary incontinence in 1973 by Scott *et al.* [40]. Technical improvements have been made and the currently used AMS 800 model (American Medical Systems, Minnetonka, MN) was introduced in 1983. A limited number of centers have experience with the surgical placement of the AUS in pediatric patients, who advise implanting the cuff at the bladder neck since the prepubertal male corpus spongiosum is thin. Implantation requires meticulous adherence to surgical protocol. To minimize intraoperative blood loss, Gonzalez *et al.* encourages male AUS placement at prepuberal age since Santorini's plexus is not very prominent [41]. Some groups [27,42] prefer the posterior approach to the bladder neck area, as described by Lottmann *et al.* [43], while others prefer the anterior approach [44].

All surgeons agree that proper patient selection is crucial to achieve success with the AUS without danger. The ideal AUS patient has neurogenic sphincteric incompetence with preserved normal bladder capacity and compliance. Compared to the other surgical options for sphincteric incompetence, AUS offers the major advantage of potentially preserving volitional voiding, noted in 25–68% of implanted patients [45–47].

Outcomes
When reporting urinary continence rates, authors will report overall continence and continence in patients with an intact AUS. This refers to the fact that 9–23% of patients implanted will need to have the AUS removed (Table 41.4). Thus, this outcome is best reported in both ways so there is no over inflation of the perceived benefit.

Outcomes by duration of follow-up
Intact AUS continence rates seem basically stable over time despite improvements in the AUS device implanted. Continence rates in series with shorter follow-up are 85–97% in children with intact AUS, while series with ≥5 years of follow-up report continence rates of 84–100% in the same category of patients and overall continence rate of 80–90% [34,41,45–49]. However, overall continence rates do decrease with duration of follow-up primarily due to the fact that most AUS removals occur in the first 3 years after implantation.

Outcomes by sex or age at implantation
Some have found superior outcomes in males when compared to females. However, at 7.6 years mean follow-up, Castera and Podesta found 83% of 23 females had a functioning original device and were dry (>4 h) [50]. Similarly, the Indiana group found the AUS to be equally versatile in 93 males and 41 females [51]. Concerning age at implantation, Kryger *et al.* found no difference in the number of AUS removals, continence, revision rate, augmentations, complications, or upper tract changes when 21 prepubertal versus 11 postpubertal patients were compared at 15.4 years mean follow-up [52].

Outcomes by pathology (neurogenic versus nonneurogenic/structural)
As seen in Table 41.4, overall continence and continence with an intact AUS was 75% and 96%, respectively in series consisting primarily of neuropathics ($n = 383$). Comparing this to the only series of 23 pure nonneuropathics [47], rates appeared lower in this group (70% and 80%, respectively).

In all five patients with traumatic posterior urethral disruption causing sphincteric incompetence, the AUS eroded into the bladder neck and/or rectum at mean of 3 years [53]. Four of five BE patients implanted developed cuff erosion [49]. In contrast, erosion occurred in only 3 of 23 (13%) nonneurogenic patients with prior bladder neck surgery in Ruiz's series [47]. Thus, further evidence is needed to assess whether prior bladder neck surgery is associated with poor AUS outcomes.

Outcomes with or without simultaneous bladder augmentation
Published series have not separately reported urinary continence rates with or without bladder augmentation. This is likely due to the high continence rates with intact AUS. However, the fact that ~25% of unaugmented patients require post-AUS augmentation

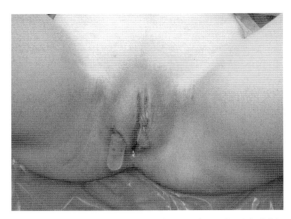

Figure 41.2 Erosion of AUS control pump from the right labia. (Photograph courtesy of Dr. Rafael Gosalbez.)

(Table 41.4)highlights the contribution of bladder instability to incontinence.

Complications
Intraoperative complications
Bladder or vaginal perforations can be primarily closed but urethral perforations can lead to early cuff erosion and incontinence. AUS implantation must be abandoned if bowel injury occurs. All particulate matter should be flushed from the connecting tubing to minimize the chance of AUS malfunction.

Postoperative complications
Mechanical and nonmechanical complications equally contribute to the need for surgical revision.

Mechanical complications
AUS component malfunctions (defective or ruptured pump, pressure-balloon reservoir rupture, cuff leak) and surgical problems (pump migration, cuff migration, improper cuff size) require reoperation to revise the AUS (Figure 41.2). Fluid leakage, abdominal or perineal trauma, or deteriorated areas of the silicone walls may cause AUS malfunctioning [47]. Activation/deactivation system problems are less frequent and could also lead to AUS replacement. Patient growth may require AUS resizing, requiring surgical revision, but this has not been uniformly noted [34,45]. Overall mechanical malfunctions necessitate revision in 20–30% of implanted patients [42,47].

Nonmechanical complications
AUS infection can present early or late and necessitates AUS removal. Early infections of Staphylococcus are primarily caused by intraoperative infection. Thus, to help achieve sterile urine, skin and sphincter placement,

prophylactic antibiotics, mechanical bowel preparation, and postoperative 24 h intravenous antibiotics have been recommended in order to diminish the risk of infection. Late infections are from uropathogens. Fortunately infection rates are <5% in pediatric series [34] and do not seem to be increased by CIC. When AUS and augmentation cystoplasty are done simultaneously, some but not all groups have seen increased frequency of urinary tract infections (UTIs) from 20% to 50% [55–57]. However, there are other groups that find it safe [34,42,58]. The former groups advocate for the use of strict selection criteria to minimize the use of concomitant bladder augmentation with AUS placement, reducing morbidity and infection rates.

Cuff erosion occurs in 5–25% of all implants [47] and may be increased in patients who have had prior bladder neck surgery. However, this is not a strict contraindication to AUS implantation. CIC is not a risk factor for erosion.

Difficult CIC via urethra may necessitate surgical creation of a Mitrofanoff channel.

Bladder calculi can form whether AUS placement is associated or not with bladder augmentation and require surgical or endoscopic removal [41].

Loss of bladder compliance and/or increased bladder instability has been found in 20% of AUS patients in long-term follow-up [49,51]. Possible theories to explain this phenomenon are: dynamic natural history of the meningomyelocele (MMC), spinal cord tethering, non adherence to CIC, recurrent UTI, patient selection bias (failure to exclude severe detrusor hyperreflexia or low bladder compliance), and no systematic urodynamic evaluation pre and postoperatively [34,42,59]. Despite a detailed analysis, Lopez Pereira and colleagues were unable to preoperatively identify urodynamic criteria that predicted bladder function behavior after AUS placement [42].

Upper tract deterioration After AUS implantation, hydronephrosis (10–20% [41,49]), pyelonephritis, and renal failure (0–11% [45]) have been observed. Upper urinary tract deterioration may be part of the natural history of MMC; however, AUS may impose a significant fixed low outlet resistance that can predispose the upper urinary tract to deterioration if bladder compliance worsens, or if the patient fails to adhere to CIC. Furthermore, Credé maneuver to void may generate a tremendous high intravesical pressure that could potentially be transmitted to the upper urinary tract as well. Therefore, life-long evaluation every 6–12 months with renal and bladder ultrasound, urodynamics, and renal function tests should be performed in

Table 41.4 Meta-analysis of pediatric AUS series.

Series	Number of patients in follow-up (M:F)	Mean age (year)	Indications for surgery	Number of removed AUS	Continent (% all implanted:% with intact AUS)	CIC with AUS (%)	Follow-up (year)	Number of patients with pre-AUS or simultaneous bladder augmentation	Number of patients requiring post-AUS bladder augmentation
Primarily Neuropathic									
Levesque et al. (1996)* [45]	54 (34:20)	~11	Neuropathic (49), exstrophy–epispadias (4), other (1)	13	32 (59%:78%)	NA	13.7	8	15
Kryger et al. (1999)* [41]	32 (25:7)	9.9	Neuropathic (28), other (4)	13	18 (56%:95%)	12 (63%)	15.4	2	7
Castera et al. (2001) [54]	49 (39:10)	14	Neuropathic (38), exstrophy (7), trauma (4)	10	33 (67%:85%)	26 (53%)	7.5	11	2
Hafez et al. (2002)* [49]	79 (63:16)	11.7	Neuropathic (74), exstrophy (5)	16	57 (72%:90%)	36 (57%)	12.5	4	2
Herndon et al. (2003)* [51]	134 (93:41)	10	Neuropathic (107), exstrophy (21), other (6)	30	115 (86%:92%)	64 (57%)	7.0	57	40
Lopez Pereira et al. (2006) [42]	35 (22:13)	14.4	Neuropathic (35)	3	32 (91%:100%)	29 (91%)	5.5	13	7
Total	383 (276:107)		Neuropathic (331), exstrophy–epispadias (37), other (15)	85 (22%)	287 (75%:96%)	167/257 (65%)		95 (25%)	73 (25% of unaugmented patients required post-AUS augment)
Nonneuropathics									
Ruiz et al. (2006)* [47]	23 (19:4)	8.1	Bladder exstrophy (12), rectourethral/vesical fistula (7), epispadias (4)	3 (erosion) (13%)	16 (70%:80%)	6 (31%)	6.6	6 (26%)	1 (4%)

*Several models of AUS were implanted in this series.

order to identify bladder dynamic changes and/or deterioration of the upper urinary tract [42]. Management of bladder compliance deterioration and/or instability includes: anticholinergics, spinal cord de-tethering, or augmentation cystoplasty as needed [49]. Overall augmentation rate in patients receiving AUS is 44%, of which 43% are performed after the AUS (Table 41.4). Unfortunately, Herndon noted 12 bladder perforations in 10 augmented patients after AUS implantation [51] thus augmentation is not a cure-all.

AUS revision or removal
Mechanical and nonmechanical complications lead to the need for AUS surgical revision or AUS removal, the greatest downside to the AUS. Several factors have been associated with a high AUS removal/revision rate, including prior AUS erosion, previous bladder neck surgery, positive urine culture within 24 h of the AUS placement, intraoperative bladder or urethral injury, difficult catheterization, previous radiation therapy, placement of the sphincter around the bulbous urethra, and balloon pressure of >70 cm H_2O [34,41,45,60,61]. Surgical revision rates have decreased, when older models are compared with the AS 800, decreasing from 20–30% to 16–23% of patients [34,51]. With the AS 800, revision was performed every 44.3 patient-years [52]. By our meta-analysis, 22% of AUS devices require removal (Table 41.4). Overall 10-year survival of the AUS was 70–80% [45,49].

In summary, advancements in the design of AUS, better patient selection criteria, and meticulous aseptic surgical technique have lowered the AUS revision/removal rate [51]. Despite reoperation rates at 17–35% and removal rates at 9–23%, the continence rate (85–95%) for AUS operations is high and patient satisfaction excellent. While the opportunity for volitional voiding is a major advantage, bladder deterioration with upper tract sequelae is a significant threat (20–30%) which requires close life-long monitoring.

Bladder neck reconstruction

Surgeries for BNR either (1) increase the length and reduce the caliber of the urethra (Young–Dees–Leadbetter (YDL) procedure) or (2) create a flap valve mechanism (e.g. Kropp procedure, Pippi Salle procedure). Theoretically, the first surgical principle preserves the ability to void spontaneously while the second one does not.

YDL BNR

In 1919, Young described a surgical technique in which posterior bladder neck tissue was dissected, and its caliber

reduced to the size of the silver probe to enhance low urinary outlet resistance. Later, Dees (1949) [62] and Leadbetter (1964) [63] revised this technique by excising more tissue up to the level of the trigone and performing higher ureteral reimplantations, tubularization of the trigone, and BNR suspension. Several authors have added modifications to the original technique, including Tanagho (1969) [64], Mollard *et al.* (1980) [65], Koff (1990) [66], Jones *et al.* (1993) [67], Surer *et al.* (2001) [68], and Gosalbez *et al.* (2001). Use of a silicone sheath about the bladder neck has been abandoned due to high erosion rates [34]. The YDL technique was initially conceived with the idea of reconstructing the bladder neck in bladder exstrophy–epispadias patients who theoretically have normal innervated bladders and potential for voiding. However, the YDL BNR requires sufficient bladder capacity and compliance, as some capacity will be lost with the BNR.

Kropp and Pippi Salle BNR

The two most common flap valve operations that require CIC for bladder emptying are the Kropp procedure (1986) [69] and the Pippi Salle procedure (1994) [70]. In flap valve operations, a rectangular anterior bladder wall flap is based on the bladder neck. The Kropp tubularizes it and tunnels it submucosally on the trigone. In order to avoid difficult catheterizations encountered with the Kropp tube, Belman and Kaplan (1989) [71], Snodgrass (1997) 72, and Koyle (1998) have proposed important modifications to the original technique. The Pippi Salle requires cephalad bilateral ureteral reimplantation. Then, the untubularized anterior bladder wall flap is sewn to a rectangular trigonal strip, creating the bladder tube. Since a considerable amount of the anterior bladder wall is used for urethral lengthening, it is generally necessary to perform concomitant augmentation cystoplasty.

Outcomes
Outcomes by BNR type and by pathology (exstrophy–epispadias complex (EEC) versus neurogenic)
YDL BNR + EEC
YDL has achieved success rates of 30–80% in BE patients. Some authors state that approximately 40–79% of patients will undergo an additional procedure to achieve satisfactory dryness in a long-term follow-up [15]. It is important to emphasize that early successful initial bladder closure of BE reduces the chances of bladder augmentation in the future and favors the possibility of volitional voiding. Jeffs' staged reconstruction of BE patients (bladder closure – first 48 h of life, epispadias repair – 9–18 months old, and BNR at 3–4 years old) has achieved

continence rates of 36–90% [15]. Surer *et al.* reported 83% continence rate in 68 classic BE patients who underwent YDL. All of them were voiding per urethra without the need for bladder augmentation or CIC [68]. On the other hand, Mouriquand *et al.* reported lower continence rates (dryness >3 h) in 105 BE (45%) and epispadias (52%) patients who underwent YDL modified by Mollard (mean follow-up of 11 years) [73]. Baka-Jabubiak *et al.* analyzed 73 boys with bladder exstrophy/epispadias complex who underwent simultaneous bladder neck and epispadias repair, resulting in better continence rates (classic exstrophy, 75%; epispadias, 89%) [74].

YDL BNR + neurogenics
In comparison, Leadbetter and Tanagho and Donnahoo *et al.* found lower success (68%) when YDL procedure is performed in neurogenic bladder patients [34,75].

Kropp BNR + neurogenics
Regarding the Kropp procedure, several authors have published consistent continence rates between 77% and 81% in up to 5 years of follow-up [34]. Snodgrass found 91% continence rate (dryness for at least 3 h) in 23 patients who underwent the simplified Kropp procedure described by Belman and Kaplan (mean follow-up 23 months) [72].

Pippi Salle BNR + neurogenics
Several series using the Pippi Salle procedure (Rink *et al.*, [76] Mouriquand *et al.*, [73] Koyle *et al.*, Hayes *et al.*, [77] Pippi Salle *et al.*, [78]) have shown 77% overall continence rate defined as dryness >4 h. However, high proportion of patients in these series underwent concomitant augmentation cystoplasty which in fact contribute to a higher successful continence rate.

Complications
Loss of bladder capacity and compliance
For all BNR, one of the greatest concerns is the reduction of bladder capacity secondary to the use of bladder tissue to build flaps or tubes and reduction of bladder compliance if the bladder outlet is sufficient. A minimum of 20 ml of bladder capacity is used to perform BNR. Only about a quarter of patients with BE may maintain normal detrusor function after BNR [79]. Some techniques have been developed as modifications of the original YDL to preserve bladder capacity by using less bladder wall.

YDL
The most common complication after YDL is elevated post void residuals +/− urinary retention. Surgical

BNR may result in scar tissue formation and/or trigonal innervation damage, resulting in voiding difficulties. This can cause overflow incontinence, especially if the bladder capacity/compliance is reduced for age. Thus, some patients will need to perform CIC via the YDL BNR, which can be difficult due to tortuosity or stricturing. Other reported complications include recurrent UTIs, epididymo-orchitis, referred pain to the glans penis, and complete bladder outlet obstruction.

Kropp
Complications described after Kropp procedure are: difficult catheterization (28–45%), new onset vesicoureteral reflux (22–42%), peritonitis secondary to bladder rupture (38%), febrile UTI (38%), and struvite calculi (33%). In Snodgrass series, postoperative VUR was quite high (50%), so he recommended to leave the posterior bladder wall open and flat when receiving the bowel segment in order to prevent lateral retraction of the ureters from closure of the bladder edges over the detrusor muscle [72]. A rare complication is necrosis of the Kropp tube, presumably secondary to ischemia [34].

Pippi Salle
Complications with the Pippi Salle procedure are urethrovesical fistula (12–17%), new onset VUR (12–17%), bladder calculi (12%), and difficult catheterization (15%) [34].

Conclusions

Currently, there is no "ideal" surgical technique for sphincteric incompetence in children, given their life-long needs. Management of the sphincteric mechanism will remain a surgical challenge as long as complication rates, reoperation rates, and bladder augmentation rates remain high.

References

1 Sureshkumar P, Craig JC, Roy LP, Knight JF. Daytime urinary incontinence in primary school children: A population-based survey. *J Pediatr* 2000;137:814–18.
2 Berg S. Polytef augmentation urethroplasty. Correction of surgically incurable urinary incontinence by injection technique. *Arch Surg* 1973;107:379–81.
3 Politano VA, Small MP, Harper JM, Lynne CM. Periurethral teflon injection for urinary incontinence. *J Urol* 1974;111:180–3.
4 Wan J, McGuire EJ, Bloom DA, Ritchey ML. The treatment of urinary incontinence in children using glutaraldehyde cross-linked collagen. *J Urol* 1992;148:127–30.

5 Duffy PG, Ransley PG. Endoscopic treatment of urinary incontinence in children with primary epispadias. *Br J Urol* 1998;81:309–11.

6 Lottmann HB, Margaryan M, Bernuy M, Rouffet MJ, Bau MO, El-Ghoneimi A, Aigrain Y, Stenberg A, Lackgren G. The effect of endoscopic injections of dextranomer based implants on continence and bladder capacity: A prospective study of 31 patients. *J Urol* 2002;168:1863–7,discussion 1867.

7 Malizia AA, Reiman HM, Myers RP, Sande JR, Barham SS, Benson RC, Jr. Dewanjee MK, Utz WJ. Migration and granulomatous reaction after periurethral injection of polytef (Teflon). *JAMA* 1984;251:3277–81.

8 Claes H, Stroobants D, Van Meerbeek J, Verbeken E, Knockaert D, Baert L. Pulmonary migration following periurethral polytetrafluoroethylene injection for urinary incontinence. *J Urol* 1989;142:821–2.

9 Henly DR, Barrett DM, Weiland TL, O'Connor MK, Malizia AA, Wein AJ. Particulate silicone for use in periurethral injections: Local tissue effects and search for migration. *J Urol* 1995;153:2039–43.

10 Tamanini JT, D'Ancona CA, Netto NR. Macroplastique implantation system for female stress urinary incontinence: Long-term follow-up. *J Endourol* 2006;20:1082–6.

11 Block CA, Cooper CS, Hawtrey CE. Long-term efficacy of periurethral collagen injection for the treatment of urinary incontinence secondary to myelomeningocele. *J Urol* 2003;169:327–9.

12 Lottmann HB, Margaryan M, Lortat-Jacob S, Bernuy M, Lackgren G. Long-term effects of dextranomer endoscopic injections for the treatment of urinary incontinence: An update of a prospective study of 61 patients. *J Urol* 2006;176:1762–6.

13 Yucel S, Baker LA. Bladder outlet injection for urinary incontinence. In *Pediatric Endourology Techniques*, Edited by PP Godbole. London: Springer-Verlag, 2007: pp. 85–91.

14 Guys JM, Breaud J, Hery G, Camerlo A, Le Hors H, De Lagausie P. Endoscopic injection with polydimethylsiloxane for the treatment of pediatric urinary incontinence in the neurogenic bladder: Long-term results. *J Urol* 2006;175:1106–10.

15 Burki T, Hamid R, Duffy P, Ransley P, Wilcox D, Mushtaq I. Long-term followup of patients after redo bladder neck reconstruction for bladder exstrophy complex. *J Urol* 2006;176:1138–41,discussion 1141–2.

16 Dyer L, Franco I, Firlit CF, Reda EF, Levitt SB, Palmer LS. Endoscopic injection of bulking agents in children with incontinence: Dextranomer/hyaluronic acid copolymer versus polytetrafluoroethylene. *J Urol* 2007;178:1628–31.

17 Burki T, Hamid R, Ransley PG, Mushtaq I, Duffy PG. Injectable polydimethylsiloxane for treating incontinence in children with the exstrophy-epispadias complex: long-term results. *BJU Int* 2006;98:849–853.

18 Guys JM, Fakhro A, Louis-Borrione C, Prost J, Hautier A. Endoscopic treatment of urinary incontinence: Long-term evaluation of the results. *J Urol* 2001;165:2389–91.

19 Nelson CP, Park JM. Endoscopic treatment of incontinence in pediatric patients. In smith's Text book of Endourology, 2nd ed. Edited by A.D. Smith Hamilton, Ontario: BC Decker Inc, 2006, pp 787–793.

20 Chernoff A, Horowitz M, Combs A, Libretti D, Nitti V, Glassberg KI. Periurethral collagen injection for the treatment of urinary incontinence in children. *J Urol* 1997;157:2303–5.

21 Caione P, Lais A, de Gennaro M, Capozza N. Glutaraldehyde cross-linked bovine collagen in exstrophy/epispadias complex. *J Urol* 1993;150:631–3.

22 Knudson MJ, Cooper CS, Block CA, Hawtrey CE, Austin JC. Calcification of glutaraldehyde cross-linked collagen in bladder neck injections in children with incontinence: A long-term complication. *J Urol* 2006;176:1143–6,discussion 1146.

23 Cole EE, Adams MC, Brock JW. Outcome of continence procedures in the pediatric patient: A single institutional experience. *J Urol* 2003;170:560–3,discussion 563.

24 Halachmi S, Farhat W, Metcalfe P, Bagli DJ, McLorie GA, Khoury AE. Efficacy of polydimethylsiloxane injection to the bladder neck and leaking diverting stoma for urinary continence. *J Urol* 2004;171:1287–90.

25 Woodside JR, Borden TA. Pubovaginal sling procedure for the management of urinary incontinence in a myelodysplastic girl. *J Urol* 1982;127:744–6.

26 Castellan M, Gosalbez R, Labbie A, Ibrahim E, Disandro M. Bladder neck sling for treatment of neurogenic incontinence in children with augmentation cystoplasty: Long-term followup. *J Urol* 2005;173:2128–31, discussion 2131.

27 Gosalbez R, Castellan M. Defining the role of the bladder-neck sling in the surgical treatment of urinary incontinence in children with neurogenic incontinence. *World J Urol* 1998;16:285–91.

28 Nguyen HT, Bauer SB, Diamond DA, Retik AB. Rectus fascial sling for the treatment of neurogenic sphincteric incontinence in boys: Is it safe and effective? *J Urol* 2001;166:658–61.

29 Misseri R, Cain MP, Casale AJ, Kaefer M, Meldrum KK, Rink RC. Small intestinal submucosa bladder neck slings for incontinence associated with neuropathic bladder. *J Urol* 2005;174:1680–2,discussion 1682.

30 Albouy B, Grise P, Sambuis C, Pfister C, Mitrofanoff P, Liard A. Pediatric urinary incontinence: Evaluation of bladder wall wraparound sling procedure. *J Urol* 2007;177:716–19.

31 Colvert JR, 3rd, Kropp BP, Cheng EY, Pope JCt, Brock JW, 3rd, Adams MC, Austin P, Furness PD, 3rd Koyle MA. The use of small intestinal submucosa as an off-the-shelf urethral sling material for pediatric urinary incontinence. *J Urol* 2002;168:1872–5,discussion 1875–6.

32 Godbole P, Mackinnon AE. Expanded PTFE bladder neck slings for incontinence in children: The long-term outcome. *BJU Int* 2004;93:139–41.

33 Bugg CE, Jr, Joseph DB. Bladder neck cinch for pediatric neurogenic outlet deficiency. *J Urol* 2003;170:1501–3,discussion 1503–4.

34 Kryger JV, Gonzalez R, Barthold JS. Surgical management of urinary incontinence in children with neurogenic sphincteric incompetence. *J Urol* 2000;163:256–63.

35 Snodgrass WT, Elmore J, Adams R. Bladder neck sling and appendicovesicostomy without augmentation for neurogenic

incontinence in children. *J Urol* 2007;177:1510–14, discussion 1515.

36 Elder JS. Periurethral and puboprostatic sling repair for incontinence in patients with myelodysplasia. *J Urol* 1990;144:434–7,discussion 443–4.

37 Austin PF *et al.* Advantages of rectus fascial slings for urinary incontinence in children with neuropathic bladders. *J Urol* 2001;165:2369–71,discussion 2371–2.

38 Decter RM. Use of the fascial sling for neurogenic incontinence: Lessons learned. *J Urol* 1993;150:683–6.

39 Dik P, Van Gool JD, De Jong TP. Urinary continence and erectile function after bladder neck sling suspension in male patients with spinal dysraphism. *BJU Int* 1999;83:971–5.

40 Scott FB, Bradley WE, Timm GW. Treatment of urinary incontinence by implantable prosthetic sphincter. *Urology* 1973;1:252–9.

41 Kryger JV, Spencer Barthold J, Fleming P, Gonzalez R. The outcome of artificial urinary sphincter placement after a mean 15-year follow-up in a paediatric population. *BJU Int* 1999;83:1026–31.

42 Lopez Pereira P, Somoza Ariba I, Martinez Urrutia MJ, Lobato Romero R, Jaureguizar Monroe E. Artificial urinary sphincter: 11-year experience in adolescents with congenital neuropathic bladder. *Eur Urol* 2006;50:1096–101,discussion 1101.

43 Lottmann H, Traxer O, Aigrain Y, Melin Y. Posterior approach to the bladder for implantation of the 800 AMS artificial sphincter in children and adolescents: Techniques and results in eight patients. *Ann Urol (Paris)* 1999;33:357–63.

44 Gonzalez R. Current status of AUS placement in pediatric patients. In *Dialogues in Pediatric Urology*, 2007: p. 2.

45 Levesque PE, Bauer SB, Atala A, Zurakowski D, Colodny A, Peters C, Retik AB. Ten-year experience with the artificial urinary sphincter in children. *J Urol* 1996;156:625–8.

46 Gonzalez R, Merino FG, Vaughn M. Long-term results of the artificial urinary sphincter in male patients with neurogenic bladder. *J Urol* 1995;154:769–70.

47 Ruiz E, Puigdevall J, Moldes J, Lobos P, Boer M, Ithurralde J, Escalante J, de Badiola F. 14 Years of experience with the artificial urinary sphincter in children and adolescents without spina bifida. *J Urol* 2006;176:1821–5.

48 Venn SN, Greenwell TJ, Mundy AR. The long-term outcome of artificial urinary sphincters. *J Urol* 2000;164:702–6, discussion 706–7.

49 Hafez AT, McLorie G, Bagli D, Khoury A. A single-centre long-term outcome analysis of artificial urinary sphincter placement in children. *BJU Int* 2002;89:82–5.

50 Castera R, Podesta M. The artificial urinary sphincter in female pediatric patients. In *Dialogues in Pediatric Urology*. 2007: pp. 3–4.

51 Herndon CD, Rink RC, Shaw MB, Simmons GR, Cain MP, Kaefer M, Casale AJ. The Indiana experience with artificial urinary sphincters in children and young adults. *J Urol* 2003;169:650–4,discussion 654.

52 Kryger JV, Leverson G, Gonzalez R. Long-term results of artificial urinary sphincters in children are independent of age at implantation. *J Urol* 2001;165:2377–9.

53 Ashley RA, Husmann DA. Artificial urinary sphincters placed after posterior urethral distraction injuries in children are at risk for erosion. *J Urol* 2007;178:1813–15.

54 Castera R, Podesta ML, Ruarte A, Herrera M, Medel R. 10-Year experience with artificial urinary sphincter in children and adolescents. *J Urol* 2001;165:2373–2376.

55 Strawbridge LR, Kramer SA, Castillo OA, Barrett DM. Augmentation cystoplasty and the artificial genitourinary sphincter. *J Urol* 1989;142:297–301.

56 Light JK, Lapin S, Vohra S. Combined use of bowel and the artificial urinary sphincter in reconstruction of the lower urinary tract: Infectious complications. *J Urol* 1995;153:331–3.

57 Theodorou C, Plastiras D, Moutzouris G, Floratos D, Mertziotis N, Miliaras S. Combined reconstructive and prosthetic surgery in complicated lower urinary tract dysfunction. *J Urol* 1997;157:472–4.

58 Gonzalez R, Nguyen DH, Koleilat N, Sidi AA. Compatibility of enterocystoplasty and the artificial urinary sphincter. *J Urol* 1989;142:502–4,discussion 520–1.

59 Light JK, Pietro T. Alteration in detrusor behavior and the effect on renal function following insertion of the artificial urinary sphincter. *J Urol* 1986;136:632–5.

60 Simeoni J, Guys JM, Mollard P, Buzelin JM, Moscovici J, Bondonny JM, Melin Y, Lortat-Jacob S, Aubert D, Costa F, Galifer B, Debeugny P. Artificial urinary sphincter implantation for neurogenic bladder: A multi-institutional study in 107 children. *Br J Urol* 1996;78:287–93.

61 Aliabadi H, Gonzalez R. Success of the artificial urinary sphincter after failed surgery for incontinence. *J Urol* 1990;143:987–90.

62 Dees JE. Congenital epispadias with incontinence. *J Urol* 1949;62:513–522.

63 Leadbetter GW, Jr. Surgical Correction of Total Urinary Incontinence. *J Urol* 1964;91:261–266.

64 Tanagho EA, Smith DR, Meyers FH, Fisher R. Mechanism of urinary continence. II. Technique for surgical correction of incontinence. *J Urol* 1969;101:305–313.

65 Mollard P. Bladder reconstruction in exstrophy. *J Urol* 1980;124:525–529.

66 Koff SA. A technique for bladder neck reconstruction in exstrophy: the cinch. *J Urol* 144:546–549; discussion 562–543, 1990.

67 Jones JA, Mitchell ME, Rink RC. Improved results using a modification of the Young-Dees-Leadbetter bladder neck repair. *Br J Urol* 1993;71:555–561.

68 Surer I, Baker LA, Jeffs RD, Gearhart JP. Modified Young–Dees–Leadbetter bladder neck reconstruction in patients with successful primary bladder closure elsewhere: A single institution experience. *J Urol* 2001;165:2438–40.

69 Kroop KA, Angwafo FF. Urethral lengthening and reimplantation for neurogenic incontinence in children. *J Urol* 1986;135:533–536.

70 Salle JL, de Fraga JC, Amarante A, Silveira ML, Lambertz M, Schmidt M, Rosito NC. Urethral lengthening with anterior bladder wall flap for urinary incontinence: a new approach. *J Urol* 1994;152:803–806.

71 Belman AB, Kaplan GW. Experience with the Kropp anti-incontinence procedure. *J Urol* 1989;141:1160–1162.

72 Snodgrass W. A simplified Kropp procedure for incontinence. *J Urol* 1997;158:1049–52.

73 Mouriquand PD, Bubanj T, Feyaerts A, Jandric M, Timsit M, Mollard P, Mure PY, Basset T. Long-term results of bladder neck reconstruction for incontinence in children with classical bladder exstrophy or incontinent epispadias. *BJU Int* 2003;92:997–1001,discussion 1002.

74 Baka-Jakubiak M. Combined bladder neck, urethral and penile reconstruction in boys with the exstrophy–epispadias complex. *BJU Int* 2000;86:513–18.

75 Donnahoo KK, Rink RC, Cain MP, Casale AJ. The Young–Dees–Leadbetter bladder neck repair for neurogenic incontinence. *J Urol* 1999;161:1946–9.

76 Rink RC, Adams MC, Keating MA. The flip-flap technique to lengthen the urethra (Salle procedure) for treatment of neurogenic urinary incontinence. *J Urol* 1994;152:799–802.

77 Hayes MC, Bulusu A, Terry T, Mouriquand PD, Malone PS. The Pippi Salle urethral lengthening procedure; experience and outcome from three United Kingdom centres. *BJU Int* 1999;84:701–705.

78 Salle JL, McLorie GA, Bagli DJ, Khoury AE. Urethral lengthening with anterior bladder wall flap (Pippi Salle procedure): modifications and extended indications of the technique. *J Urol* 1997;158:585–590.

79 Diamond DA, Bauer SB, Dinlenc C, Hendren WH, Peters CA, Atala A, Kelly M, Retik AB. Normal urodynamics in patients with bladder exstrophy: Are they achievable? *J Urol* 1999;162:841–4,discussion 844–5.

42

Surgery for Fecal Incontinence

W. Robert DeFoor, Jr, Eugene Minevich,
Curtis A. Sheldon and Martin A. Koyle

Key points

- Fecal incontinence and constipation must be addressed concurrently with management of the neuropathic bladder.

- All medical options including combinations of laxatives and high retrograde enemas must be exhausted before offering the MACE procedure.

- In general, the MACE procedure is performed concurrently with urinary tract reconstruction,

  but may be considered as an isolated procedure if urinary continence and the upper urinary tracts are stable on medical therapy.

- Stomal-related complications are the most common postoperative problems.

- Serious complications are rare but when present can lead to life-threatening clinical situations.

Introduction

Management of the neuropathic bladder in children with complex urologic abnormalities such as myelomeningocele involves addressing coexistent bowel dysfunction. Thus, fecal incontinence in this population is often left to the pediatric urologist to manage. Therefore it is incumbent for reconstructive surgeons to understand and be aware of the medical as well as surgical management options and their complications.

The Malone antegrade continence enema (MACE) is a surgical procedure that has been widely utilized since its first description in 1990 [1]. Its simplicity is based on three well-established surgical principles as summarized by Malone and Koyle [2]:

1 The Mitrofanoff principle to afford a continent catheterizable conduit.

2 Complete colonic emptying can produce fecal continence.

3 Complete colonic emptying can be achieved by antegrade colonic irrigation.

After an MACE is created, patients perform intermittent catheterization through a continent catheterizable channel to administer antegrade enemas to facilitate colonic washout and improve or achieve fecal continence. The simplicity of the procedure and its high success rates have led to high patient satisfaction and improved quality of life. However, as with any reconstructive procedure, patient selection is important and awareness of potential complications and their management is paramount.

Surgical indications and patient selection

Patients may be offered the MACE procedure after all conservative measures at fecal continence have been initiated and found unsuccessful. In patients with retentive pathology from a neuropathic etiology, this may include a combination of oral laxatives as well as a high retrograde enema program. In general, the procedure is performed in conjunction with reconstruction of the urinary tract but it may also be performed as an isolated surgical procedure if the patient is stable from a urinary

Pediatric Urology: Surgical Complications and Management. Edited by Duncan T. Wilcox, Prasad P. Godbole and Martin A. Koyle. © 2008 Blackwell Publishing, ISBN: 978-1-4051-6268-5.

continence and upper urinary tract standpoint. Patient selection is important as it has been shown previously that patients with chronic idiopathic constipation have worse outcomes with the MACE procedure [3]. In general, patients with neuropathic bowel or anorectal malformations are those most likely to have a successful outcome following the procedure, although recent series have reported improved outcomes in functional slow-transit constipation [4]. Another important consideration is the age of the patient. It has been recommended that only patients over 5 years old be considered candidates for the procedure due to the difficulty in having younger children sit on the toilet for up to 1 h before complete emptying has occurred [5].

Operative technique

Once the decision has been made to proceed with the MACE procedure, a careful discussion of the procedure, site of the stoma, and recovery is necessary. A review of the complications as well as the expectations regarding the success rates of the procedure is also imperative. An aggressive bowel preparation including polyethylene glycol and retrograde enemas is performed generally as an inpatient on the day prior to the procedure. Often patients with severe retentive pathology from myelomeningocele will benefit from starting clear liquids and high-dose laxatives and enemas in the 2 days prior to coming to the hospital. Broad spectrum antibiotics to cover bowel flora are administered on call to the operating room.

The initial operative technique included a dismemberment of the appendix from the cecum and reversing it prior to implantation into the submucosa of the cecum to create a flap valve [1]. Current techniques leave the appendix *in situ* and construct the continence mechanism by applying a cecal wrap or by laying the appendix in a submucosal tunnel along one of the tenia [6]. The free end of the appendix is then brought to the abdominal wall either in the right lower quadrant or to the umbilicus. If the appendix is sufficiently long, it can be split to perform a Mitrofanoff neourethra for concomitant urinary tract reconstruction. If the majority of appendiceal length is necessary for the neourethra, then it may be lengthened using a stapling device (Figure 42.1) [7]. If the appendix is not available, a Monti technique may be necessary to create a conduit from either small or large bowel [8]. Our preference is to create the channel using an antireflux procedure but the literature is not conclusive that this is necessary.

Postoperatively, a catheter is maintained within the conduit for 4 weeks if the native appendix was used and 6 weeks if a Monti conduit was required. Irrigations with mineral oil and saline are begun in the hospital once the patient's bowel function returns. Our preference is to perform an exam under anesthesia with endoscopy of the channel prior to removal of the indwelling tube to ensure adequate healing. This also helps assess the proper size and type of catheter needed for intermittent cannulation. The patients then generally stay in the hospital for a period of observation for catheterization teaching and monitoring.

Newer techniques have been described using a purely laparoscopic approach when concomitant urinary

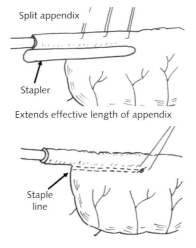
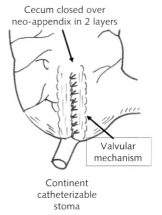

Figure 42.1 Split appendix technique for concomitant MACE and Mitrofanoff neourethra.

Split appendix

Stapler

Extends effective length of appendix

Staple line

Cecum closed over neo-appendix in 2 layers

Valvular mechanism

Continent catheterizable stoma

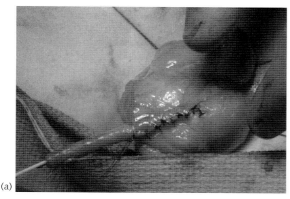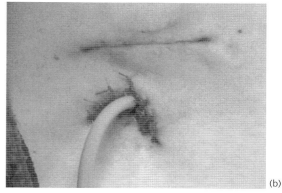

(a)   (b)

Figure 42.2 (a) Extracorporeal construction of a continence mechanism for an isolated MACE procedure. (b) Completed right lower quadrant MACE stoma through small Gibson incision.

reconstruction is not indicated [9]. This can be performed with or without a continence mechanism, although the long-term durability of using the native appendico-cecal valve for continence is unknown. Laparoscopic mobilization of the cecum, appendix, and ascending colon are performed and the spatulated free end of the appendix is brought to a rounded or V-shaped skin flap. The proximal appendix can be imbricated for a conti-nence mechanism either extra- or intracorporeal, but may be technically easier and faster extracorporeally by bringing the cecum up through the fascial incision below the skin flap [10]. A modified laparoscopic approach can also be employed using a small Gibson incision in the right lower quadrant after laparoscopic localization and mobilization (Figure 42.2a and 42.2b).

An additional option is a percutaneous cecostomy with exchange to a cecostomy button once the tract has matured [11]. This can be performed in interventional radiol-ogy under fluoroscopic or computed tomography guid-ance or during colonoscopy similar to the technique for inserting a percutaneous endoscopic gastrostomy (PEG). If the procedure is successful in achieving fecal conti-nence and the patient desires a more definitive option, then the patient can be converted to a formal catheteri-zable conduit.

Outcomes

Since the first description of the procedure in 1990 by Malone and colleagues, outcomes from more than a dozen pediatric series have been published in the literature. Most investigators report a highly successful procedure that

Table 42.1 Classification of results of the MACE procedure.

Full success	Totally clean or minor rectal leakage on the night of the washout
Partial success	Clean but significant rectal leakage, occasional major leak, still wearing protection, but perceived by the parent or child to be improved
Failure	Regular soiling or constipation persisted, no perceived improvement, procedure abandoned, usually to a colostomy

Source: Adapted from Curry *et al.* [5].

improves fecal continence and enhances the quality of life in most patients [12]. A classification system for assess-ing surgical outcomes has been proposed (Table 42.1) [5]. The overall success rate for achieving fecal continence in neuropathic bowel and anorectal malformations is almost 80% (Table 42.2) [6]. Partial success will occasionally be seen with complete daytime continence but mild leakage overnight. There may be some rectal leakage a few hours after irrigation but this is rarely a major problem. It is quite rare to have no improvement after an MACE proce-dure, but a salvage diverting colostomy in these cases has occasionally been necessary [13].

It is important, however, to discuss with the patient and family preoperatively that the irrigation regimen and composition may require some fine-tuning post-operatively to obtain the optimum results and often this involves a period of several months. This discussion early in the counseling process helps to manage expectations

Table 42.2 Surgical outcomes based on primary diagnosis.

Diagnosis	Full success	Partial response	Failure
Myelomeningocele	63	21	16
Anorectal malformation	72	17	11
Hirschsprung's Disease	82	9	9
Constipation	52	10	38
Miscellaneous	44	25	31

Source: Adapted from Curry *et al.* (1999).

Table 42.3 ACE stomal stenosis rates.

Series	Year	Patients (N)	Follow-up (years)	Stomal stenosis N (%)
Barqawi	2004	53	4.0	14 (26)
Cascio	2004	37	NR	4 (11)
Herndon	2004	168	2.3	10 (6)
Tackett	2002	45	2.2	10 (22)
Marshall	2001	32	1.5	16 (50)
Curry	1999	273	2.4	82 (30)
Driver	1998	29	2.3	11 (38)
Hensle	1998	27	NR	5 (19)
Wilcox	1998	36	3.3	8 (22)
Levitt	1997	20	NR	2 (10)
Ellsworth	1996	18	0.5	2 (11)
Griffiths	1995	21	NR	5 (24)
Koyle	1995	22	NR	3 (14)
Squire	1993	25	1.1	5 (20)
Total		806		177 (22)

Source: Adapted from DeFoor [24].

to avoid early disappointment and resultant noncompliance. The dwell time between beginning the irrigation and colonic emptying initially may be as long as an hour but as the bowel dilatation improves with better management, this time may decrease slowly over time. In some cases it may be possible to ultimately decrease the frequency of irrigations to every other day with maintenance of continence.

Various irrigation regimens have been described using saline as well as tap water with equally good results [14]. Our initial routine is 1.5 teaspoons of table salt in 1 l of tap water with an initial volume of 30 ml/kg up to a maximum of 1 l. Sometimes patients will need an additional component to their regimen including stool softeners and cathartics. The diet may also need to be addressed by increasing bulking agents and fiber to optimize the success rate.

Complications

Reports of surgical complications have been low. These include short-term postoperative complications inherent in all abdominal surgery such as wound infections and adhesive small bowel obstruction. Long-term, chronic problems mainly involve stomal and catheterization difficulties. Isolated case reports of major morbidity and mortality secondary to metabolic abnormalities have been published but are considered quite rare.

Stomal complications

A commonly reported long-term complication in published series has been stenosis of the conduit at the level of the skin [15–23]. A review of the experience of 12 institutions as well as the results of a United Kingdom questionnaire (Table 42. 3) revealed a range 6–50%

(mean 22%) [24]. The etiology of stomal stenosis is most likely multifactorial. Factors such as obesity and vascular compromise have been suggested. The rate is higher than for similarly constructed Mitrofanoff neourethral conduits perhaps due to the fact that it is cannulated much less often. Older patients with presumably less parental supervision were felt to be at a higher risk in a review from Barqawi *et al.* [25]. A significant difference in stenosis rates by type of channel (appendiceal versus re-configured ileum) has not been shown [13].

Initial treatment options for patients having difficulty with catheterization include dilatation either in the office with sequential soft catheters or in the operating room with rigid sounds or a balloon. An indwelling catheter is then maintained for a short period before allowing the re-institution of catheterization. Patients will occasionally report some mild crusting around the stoma site that appears to narrow the opening and make catheterization difficult or painful. We instruct the parents to moisten the stoma with a warm washcloth for a few moments prior to catheterization to facilitate initial entry of a well-lubricated catheter.

On occasion, it may be necessary to change the catheter to an olive tip or coudée catheter to help in initial navigation of the stoma. Hydrophilic catheters

(Lo-Fric®, Astra-Tech) can be helpful in patients with recurrent problems cannulating the stoma. These catheters are expensive, however, and letters of medical necessity are often required for third-party payors. One caution that has been raised with hydrophilic catheters is that they tend to dry after being left inside a conduit for an extended period and may be somewhat difficult to remove. In general, parents are instructed to remove the catheter after instillation (usually <10–15 min) so this has not been a major concern.

If dilatation either in the office or under anesthesia is unsuccessful in managing stenosis then formal operative revision can be performed as an outpatient procedure. The technique we employ most commonly has been to create a rounded skin flap adjacent to the stoma and incise the stoma down to healthier-appearing tissue. The skin flap is then anastomosed to the conduit with interrupted absorbable 4-0 polyglactic acid suture. An indwelling catheter is maintained for approximately 4 weeks and removed in the office. Patients with recurrent stenosis are asked to calibrate the stoma more frequently. This often can be coordinated with their clean intermittent catheterization schedule. We have found triamcinolone cream (0.1%) applied to the stoma can be helpful in mild stenosis and for preventing recurrence after dilatation.

For intractable stomal stenosis that recurs despite the above measures, an indwelling gastrostomy button held in place with a Foley type balloon is an alternative to further surgery and allows the continuation of the enema regimen. Discomfort from the appliance can be problematic if it is in the path of the waistband. The buildup of granulation tissue as well as local skin irritation and infection may need to be occasionally addressed. In older children with myelomeningocele and obesity, the button may need to be specially ordered to a specific size and also up-sized when significant weight changes occur to avoid skin breakdown.

Metabolic abnormalities

Iatrogenic metabolic complications of enema administration in children have been well described. Most are associated with hypertonic phosphate enemas [26]. The majority seems to be recognized and treated without subsequent major morbidity. Risk factors include children on long-term therapy due to atonic or neurogenic colonic abnormalities, as well as those with chronic renal insufficiency, although complications have been seen in otherwise normal children. Water toxicity from high colonic tap water enemas has been reported, although a large series from Indiana has been published regarding the

safety of tap water for ACE irrigations [14]. The authors warned that periodic electrolyte evaluation is warranted and that patients using a home water softening system should be alerted to only utilize untreated water. A case of fatal hypernatremia was reported in a 4-year-old boy with VATER syndrome by Schreiber and Stone that was felt to be due to variations in the amount of table salt used for the enema solution combined with recurrent anal stenosis [27].

As mentioned above, our practice has been to use isotonic saline (approximately 1.5 teaspoons table salt in 1 l of tap water) for irrigations with an initial volume of 30 ml/kg up to a maximum of 1 l. The regimen is then adjusted individually based on clinical response. Patients with anorectal malformations should be monitored closely for anal stenosis. Acute viral illnesses such as gastroenteritis with dehydration should prompt clinical and electrolyte evaluation in patients using an MACE with deferment of the irrigations while ill. Patients experiencing abdominal cramping with irrigation should be first evaluated for impaction but the composition of the irrigant should be re-evaluated, particularly if additional ingredients such as phosphate have been added to the regimen.

Rare complications

Isolated reports in the literature have presented patients with rare but devastating complications. Tackett *et al.* described a patient with anal stenosis who developed peritonitis and lower extremity vascular compromise from severe constipation and required emergency total colectomy due to colonic vascular congestion [13]. A cecal volvulus in one patient requiring a hemi-colectomy was reported by Herndon *et al.* [28]. Other investigators have reported cecal-flap necrosis and gangrenous channels [29]. Perforation of the channel with intra-abdominal instillation of irrigant has been reported as a rare complication with potentially morbid sequelae [30]. Seven cases were identified out of 187 consecutive MACE procedures. Figure 42.3a shows free air after a traumatic perforation of the channel and Figure 42.3b shows a contrast study of the MACE documenting no extravasation from the colon. Most were seen within the first few months after the procedure, and endoscopic management with placement of a catheter over a guidewire was a successful treatment if recognized early. Once endoscopic access is obtained, a contrast study is helpful to evaluate for bowel perforation. Wide spectrum antibiotics and inpatient observation with bowel rest is recommended until the patient is clinically

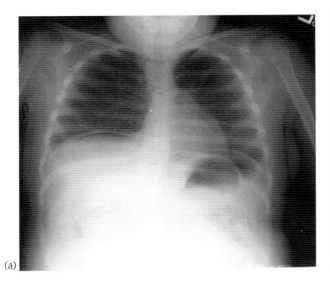

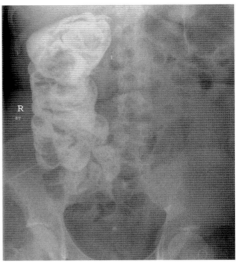

(a)   (b)

Figure 42.3 (a) Free sub-diaphragmatic peritoneal air visible after traumatic catheterization of MACE stoma resulting in channel perforation. (b) Negative contrast study of colon after endoscopic access obtained to rule out bowel perforation.

asymptomatic but immediate exploration may be warranted if peritoneal signs are present.

Conclusion

MACE procedures are successful procedures for improving or resolving intractable fecal incontinence in complex pediatric urologic patients. The procedure can be performed in conjunction with urinary tract reconstruction or as an isolated procedure with low morbidity. The main complications are stomal-related problems and difficulty with catheterization. However, major life-threatening issues can arise and must be recognized and promptly treated.

An organized infrastructure employing experienced nurse practitioners is vital to maintain close contact with these patients while providing families with ready access for questions and problems. At each clinic visit, reinforcement of proper technique and documentation of the irrigation solution and catheterization schedule should be performed. It should not need to be stressed that these patients require lifelong meticulous follow-up with continuous re-evaluation of the home routine and the clinical results.

References

1 Malone PS, Ransley PG, Kiely EM. Preliminary report: The antegrade continence enema. *Lancet* 1990;336:1217–18.

2 Koyle M. Malone PS. The Malone antegrade continence enema (MACE). In *Clinical Pediatric Urology*. Edited by AB Belman, LR King, SA Kramer. London: Martin Dunitz Ltd, 2002: pp. 529–36.

3 Marshall J, Hutson JM. *et al.* Antegrade continence enemas in the treatment of slow-transit constipation. *J Pediatr Surg* 2001;36:1227–30.

4 King SK, Sutcliffe JR. *et al.* The antegrade continence enema successfully treats idiopathic slow-transit constipation. *J Pediatr Surg* 2005;40:1935–40.

5 Curry JI, Osborne A, Malone PS. How to achieve a successful Malone antegrade continence enema. *J Pediatr Surg* 1998;33:138–41.

6 Koyle M, Malone PS. The Malone antegrade continence enema (MACE). In *Clinical Pediatric Urology*. Edited by SG Docimo, DA Canning, AE Khoury. London: Informa Healthcare, 2007: pp. 947–56.

7 Sheldon CA, Minevich E, Wacksman J. Modified technique of antegrade continence enema using a stapling device. *J Urol* 2000;163:589–91.

8 Yerkes EB, Rink RC. *et al.* Use of a Monti channel for administration of antegrade continence enemas. *J Urol* 2002;168:1883–5, discussion 1885.

9 Casale P, Grady RW. *et al.* A novel approach to the laparoscopic antegrade continence enema procedure: Intracorporeal and extracorporeal techniques. *J Urol* 2004;171:817–19.

10 Frimberger D, Kropp BP. Laparoscopic and minimally invasive approaches to the MACE procedure. In *Dialogues in Pediatric Urology: The Malone Antegrade Continence Enema Revisited*. Edited by M Koyle, PS Malone. Beverly, MA: Society for Pediatric Urology, 2006: pp. 1–11.

11 Duel BP, Gonzalez R. The button cecostomy for management of fecal incontinence. *Pediatr Surg Int* 1999;15:559–61.

12 Yerkes EB, Cain MP. *et al.* The Malone antegrade continence enema procedure: Quality of life and family perspective. *J Urol* 2003;169:320–3.

13 Tackett LD, Minevich E. *et al.* Appendiceal versus ileal segment for antegrade continence enema. *J Urol* 2002;167:683–6.

14 Yerkes EB, Rink RL. *et al.* Tap water and the Malone antegrade continence enema: A safe combination? *J Urol* 2001;166:1476–8.

15 Curry JI, Osborne A, Malone PS. The MACE procedure: Experience in the United Kingdom. *J Pediatr Surg* 1999; 34:338–40.

16 Driver CP, Barraw C. *et al.* The Malone antegrade colonic enema procedure: Outcome and lessons of 6 years' experience. *Pediatr Surg Int* 1998;13:370–2.

17 Cascio S, Flett ME. *et al.* MACE or caecostomy button for idiopathic constipation in children: A comparison of complications and outcomes. *Pediatr Surg Int* 2004; 20:484–7.

18 Ellsworth PI, Webb HW. *et al.* The Malone antegrade colonic enema enhances the quality of life in children undergoing urological incontinence procedures. *J Urol* 1996; 155:1416–18.

19 Griffiths DM, Malone PS. The Malone antegrade continence enema. *J Pediatr Surg* 1995;30:68–71.

20 Koyle MA, Kaji DM. *et al.* The Malone antegrade continence enema for neurogenic and structural fecal incontinence and constipation. *J Urol* 1995;154:759–61.

21 Levitt MA, Soffer SZ, Pena A. Continent appendicostomy in the bowel management of fecally incontinent children. *J Pediatr Surg* 1997;32:1630–3.

22 Squire R, Kiely EM. *et al.* The clinical application of the Malone antegrade colonic enema. *J Pediatr Surg* 1993;28:1012–15.

23 Wilcox DT, Kiely EM. The Malone (antegrade colonic enema) procedure: Early experience. *J Pediatr Surg* 1998;33: 204–6.

24 Defoor W. ACE Complications. In *Dialogues in Pediatric Urology: The Malone Antegrade Continence Enema Revisited.* Beverly, MA: Society for Pediatric Urology, 2006: pp. 10–11.

25 Barqawi A, de Valdenebro M. *et al.* Lessons learned from stomal complications in children with cutaneous catheterizable continent stomas. *BJU Int* 2004;94:1344–7.

26 Harrington L, Schuh S. Complications of Fleet enema administration and suggested guidelines for use in the pediatric emergency department. *Pediatr Emerg Care* 1997;13:225–6.

27 Schreiber CK, Stone AR. Fatal hypernatremia associated with the antegrade continence enema procedure. *J Urol* 1999;162:1433,discussion 1433–4.

28 Herndon CD, Rink RC. *et al.* In situ Malone antegrade continence enema in 127 patients: A 6-year experience. *J Urol* 2004;172:1689–91.

29 Hensle TW, Reiley EA, Chang DT. The Malone antegrade continence enema procedure in the management of patients with spina bifida. *J Am Coll Surg* 1998;186:669–74.

30 Defoor W, Minevich E. *et al.* Perforation of Malone antegrade continence enema: Diagnosis and management. *J Urol* 2005;174:1644–6.

Index

A

abdominal wall, 187–188
  thickness, 316, 317, 318
abdominoscrotal hydroceles, 164
ACE, *see* angiotensin converting enzyme (ACE)
acetaminophen, 30
aciduria dysuria syndrome, 309
ACTH, *see* adrenocorticotropic hormone (ACTH)
ADH, *see* antidiuretic hormone (ADH)
adolescents
  idiopathic strictures in, 106
  inguinal hernia operation in, 165
  RAP technique for, 147
  testicular torsion in, 178
  testis size in, 194
  testis tumors, 269
adrenalectomy, 279
  laparoscopic, 282–283
adrenal glands
  anatomy of, 278, 279
  hypersecretion, 280
  insufficiency, 279
  laparoscopic approaches, 282
  physiology/biochemistry of, 278–279
  surgery, complications of, 279–280
  surgical approach to, 282–283
adrenal tumors
  adrenocortical, 282
  neuroblastoma, 280–281
  pheochromocytoma, 281–282
adrenocortical carcinoma, 282
adrenocorticotropic hormone (ACTH), 279
adults
  airway complications during anesthesia in, 37
  botulinum-A toxin benefits in detrusor hyperactivity in, 109
  ESWL in, 125
  euvolemic hyponatremia in, 31
  incidence of conscious awareness in, 38
  incidence of malignant hyperthermia (MH) in, 38
  intraoperative bleeding in, 55
  laparoscopy of, 27
  orchidopexy results, 172
  PCNL complications in, 128
  peripheral nerve injury during anesthesia in, 38
  protein metabolism after trauma in, 26
  testis size in, 194
  thermoregulation in, 26
AFP, *see* alphafetoprotein (AFP)
AIS, *see* androgen insensitivity syndrome (AIS)
aldosterone, 24–25, 279
allantois, 93
alpha-adrenergic blockade, 283–284
alphafetoprotein (AFP) levels, 269
alpha-methy-L-tyrosine (metryrosine), 284

ambiguous genitalia, 218
  genital surgery for, 221–222
aminocaproic acid, 265
Amplatz wire, 121
amputation, *see* traumatic amputation
analgesia, 39–40, 126
anastomosis, 69, 311
  arterial, 249
  donor-recipient, 248
  endoscopic stapled, 135
  extravesical, 250
  nephrostogram for, 78
  in RAP, 146, 149
  recipient ureter distal in patient, 75
  series of ureteroureteric, 251
  in TUU, 73–74, 77
  urethral and venous, 214
  urethroplasty, 103, 106
  in U-U, 73, 77
  vascular, 249, 252
Anderson–Hynes dismembered pyeloplasty, 58, 61
  modern presentations and outcomes of, 60
androgen insensitivity syndrome (AIS), 218, 219
anejaculation, 215
anesthesia
  caudal, 164
  complications, 37–38
  general, 117, 125, 132
  local, 39–40, 118
angiotensin converting enzyme (ACE), 24
  conduit, 311
  stomal stenosis rates, 339
ANP, *see* atrial natriuretic peptide (ANP)
anterior urethral valves (AUV), 105–106
  see also urethral valves
antibiotics
  perioperative use of, 292
  prophylactic, 327, 330
antibody induction agents, 249
anticholinergics, 109, 113, 157, 327
  for hematuria and bladder spasms, 70
antidiuretic hormone (ADH), 41
  and water balance, 25, 29–30
antireflux technique, 317
anuria, 69, 70
  obstructive, 103, 104
appendicectomy, laparoscopic, 132, 135
appendicovesicostomy, 146, 158
appendix
  dismemberment of, 337
  implantation, 315
appendix technique, split, 337
arteriovenous fistula (AVF), 241
  establishment of, 242
artificial urinary sphincter (AUS)
  component malfunctions, 330

  implantation, 329, 330
  intraoperative complications of, 330
  postoperative complications of, 330, 332
  revision or removal, 332
  in treatment of neurogenic urinary incontinence, 329
atelectasis, 50
atrial natriuretic peptide (ANP), 25
AUS, *see* artificial urinary sphincter (AUS)
Automated Endoscopic System for Optimal Positioning (AESOP), 145
autonomic nervous system (ANS), 23
AUV, *see* anterior urethral valves (AUV)
AVF, *see* arteriovenous fistula (AVF)
azoospermia, 172

B

Bailez technique, 184
Balanitis xerotica obliterans (BXO), 202, 207
biopsy
  in B/P RMS, 262, 263
  cold-cup forceps of, 264
  endoscopic, 264
  inadequate, 264
  intraoperative, 207
  from kidney pre-implantation, 249
  laparotomy for, 264
  open, 264
  rhabdomyoblasts only on post-treatment, 264
  transcrotal, 271
bladder
  see also bladder neck bulking agents; bladder neck slings
  augmentation, 84, 85, 86, 87, 327, 328, 329–330
  calculi, 129, 330
  capacity and compliance in BNR, loss of, 333
  characteristics, 248
  compliance, loss of, 330
  compliance deterioration, management of, 332
  decompression procedures, 113
  dehiscence, 85
  drainage, 56
  dysfunctions, 104, 105, 109, 153, 154, 234, 265
  enlargement surgery, 109
  flap-valve mechanism in, *see* flap-valve mechanism in bladder
  injuries, 157, 190, 302, 303
  leaks, 153, 154, 155, 157
  malignancy, 87
  neck surgery, 102, 104, 108
  neoplasia, 83
  neurogenic, 68, 75, 76
  pathology, 74, 75
  perforation of, 310
  preservation, 262, 263
  prolapse, 94

spasms, 69, 108
stomal narrowing in, 159
stones, 303
bladder exstrophy
    see also epispadias-exstrophy complex
        (EEC)
    classic, 324
    repairing of, 83–84
    untreated, 84
bladder-level surgery, 52–53
bladder neck (BN), 53, 86
    endoscopic injection of, 86
bladder neck bulking agents, 325–327
bladder neck reconstruction (BNR), 86, 332–333
bladder neck slings, 327–329
bladder neck surgery, 307
bladder outlet obstruction (BOO), 94
blind balloon insufflation, 133
blind-ending testicular vessels, 183, 184
blood
    screening tests, 42
    transfusion complications of, 41–42
    vessels perforation, 134
blunt renal injuries, 297
    outcomes of, 298
BMA, *see* British Medical Association (BMA)
BNR, *see* bladder neck reconstruction (BNR)
bowel
    injuries, 49–50, 188
    ischemia, 167
    perforation, 134, 142
    segments, 33–34, 310
brachial plexus, 38
British Medical Association (BMA), 13
buccal grafting, 208–209
buccal mucosa, in phalloplasty, 215
bugbee electrodes, 101, 102, 103
bulking agents, 112, 113, 114, 325, 326
bupivacaine, 118
BXO, *see* Balanitis xerotica obliterans (BXO)
Byar's flaps, 205

C

CAH, *see* congenital adrenal hyperplasia (CAH)
calcium, 33, 34
    hydroxyapatite, 111, 112
calcium oxalate monohydrate, 126
canalicular testes, 173, 184
    see also testes
Cantwell-Ransley repairing technique, 84, 88
carbon dioxide (CO_2)
    insufflation pressure, 140
    pneumoperitoneum, 133–134
cardiac surgery, 8–10
cardiopulmonary bypass, 258
carrell patch, *see* common vessel patch
Carter–Thompson fascial closure device, 189
Casale spiral Monti, 316, 317, 319
catecholamines, 22–23, 279, 280, 283–284
catheterizable channel, continent, *see* continent
        catheterizable channel
catheterization, 113, 251, 263, 307, 309, 336, 339
catheters, 302, 309, 337
    see also transurethral catheter
    blockage of, 311
    central venous, 133, 241
    complications of central venous, 242
    drainage, 122, 123
    drainage of bladder, 155, 159
    dual lumen hemodialysis, 242
    Foley, 124, 152–153, 157, 185, 311

holders, adhesive, 118
    hydrophilic, 319, 339–340
    indwelling, 319, 339, 340
    for intermittent cannulation, 337
    Navarre, 118–119
    nephrostomy, 128, 129
    for PD, 243
    PD, problems with, 244, 245
    percutaneous nephrostomy, 119, 123
    snare, 121, 122, 123
    soft, 339
    torque on, 242
    ureteral, 153, 154, 155, 159
    ureteric, 301
    urethral, 154, 155, 157
    urinary, 190, 249
    used in diagnostic imaging, 206
    used in intraoperative evaluation, 206
    watertight closure for removal of, 157
    well-lubricated, 339
    whistle tip ureteric, 141
caudal analgesia, 40
caudal anesthesia, 164
caudal migration of the implant, 114
caudal regression syndrome, 109
cefuroxime, 311
central pontine myelinolysis (CPM), 30
central venous catheter, 133, 241
    complications of, 242
cephalexin, 290
Chagas disease, 41
chemotherapy, 262
    complication rates in patients with, 265
    complications in post, RPLND, 275–276
    effectiveness of, 271
    maturation of rhabdomyoblasts, 264
    modern in Wilms tumor, 257
    modern preoperative, 258, 259
    modern preoperative, incidence of SBO after,
        260
    multiagent, 281
    platinum-based multiagent, 270
    preoperative, 283
    preoperative and chylous ascites, 275
    and radiation-related complications, 266
    randomization of standard VAC, 263
    recovery of spermatogenesis, 274
    systemic, 264
chevron incision, 282
Chiba needles, 118, 122, 124
chloride ions, 309
cholinesterase, 38–39
CHPE, *see* Council for Healthcare Regulatory
        Excellence (CHPE)
chronic allograft nephropathy (CAN), 250, 251
chylous ascites, 260, 275
CIC, *see* clean intermittent catheterization (CIC)
circumcision-related injuries, 289
    treatment of, 290
CJD, *see* Creutzfeldt-Jakob disease (CJD)
clean intermittent catheterization (CIC), 84, 315,
        327, 330, 332, 333
    management of, 310
    urinary continence by, 233, 234
clinical audit
    data used for, 4–5
    good practices in, 6
    reasons for, 3–4
    and research, 3
clitoral surgery, 222
clitoroplasty, 224, 225, 227

cloaca, 93
    see also persistent cloaca
cloacal exstrophy, 120, 213
CMO, *see* Chief Medical Officer (CMO)
coagulating diathermy current, 102, 104
Cohen cross-trigonal technique, 67, 68, 114
cold-cup forceps of biopsy, 264
cold knife resection, 102, 103, 104
Colling's Knife, 103, 104
colocystoplasty, metabolic consequence of, 309
color Doppler ultrasonography (CDU), 193–194
compartment syndrome, 89
complete primary repair of bladder exstrophy
        (CPRE), 84, 86, 87
compressive perirenal hematomas, 141
computed tomography (CT), 122, 269
    cystography, 302
    for fluid collection diagnosis, 122
    follow-up, 298
    reconstructed, 249
    for staging purposes, 257–258
    in testicular tumors, 270, 271
    for urachal anomaly, 93
    in ureteral injuries diagnosis, 301
Congenital adrenal hyperplasia (CAH)
    clitoral surgery for, 226
    vaginoplasty for, 226, 227
continent catheterizable channel, 315–316, 318,
        336
    complications of, 319–322
continent urinary diversions, 84
contralateral reflux, 53
    postoperative, 70–71
contrast materials, 118, 121
controlateral de novo reflex, 115
cord lipomas, 166
corneal abrasion, 38
corpus spongiosum, 105
corticotrophin-releasing factor (CRF), 22
costospinal angle, 140
Council for Healthcare Regulatory Excellence
        (CHPE), 15–16
Cowper's glands, 105
CPM, *see* central pontine myelinolysis (CPM)
CPRE, *see* complete primary repair of bladder
        exstrophy (CPRE)
Creutzfeldt-Jakob disease (CJD), 41, 42
CRF, *see* corticotrophin-releasing factor (CRF)
Crushing's syndrome, 282
cryptorchidism, 170, 171, 177, 183
    see also testes
cutanous ureterostomy, 69
cyclophosphamide, 264
cystectomy, time of, 264
cystic dilatation, 105
cystine, 126
cystogram, 128
    posoperative, 71
cystoplasty
    aim of, 307, 310
    complications of, 308–310
    management of complications of, 311–312
    metabolic consequences of, 309
    in myelodyplasia population, 310
    outcome measures of, 307–308
    prevention of complications of, 310–311
    surgical techniques of, 307
cystoscopy, 73, 77, 94
cystourethrogram, voiding, 112, 115, 155
cystourethroscope, 102
cysts, renal, 54–55

D

Dartos flaps, 202
da Vinci surgical system, 145, 146, 147, 148
Davis ureterotomy, 58, 59
Davydov procedure, *see* laparoscopic procedures
dehiscence, glans, 202, 205, 207
dehydroepiandrosterone (DHEA), 279
delayed graft function (DGF), 249
  risk factors for, 250
demyelination, 30
detrusorrhaphy, 153
detrusors
  botulinum-A toxin benefits for, 109
  defect closure, 155
  fibrosis, 113
  overactivity, 109
  sphincter dysynergia, 109
  tunnel formation, 153
devascularization, of distal ureter, 69, 70
dextranomer, subureteral injection of, 71
dextranomer/hyaluronic acid copolymer (Dx/
    HA), 325
  long-term follow-up of, 325
dextranomer/hyaluronic acid injections, 111,
    114, 153
  see also subureteric injections
  complications with, 115
diathermy
  hook electrode, 102
  in inguinal herniotomy, 165
  injury during laparoscopy, 134
diathermy valve ablation, 102
  urethral strictures from, 103, 104
dicalcium phosphate dihydrate, 126
  dilators, 220
  see also vaginal dilation
dissection during laparoscopy, 139, 140
  operative incidents related to, 142
distal hydroceles, 289
diuresis, postobstructive, 33, 104
diverticulectomy, 105
diverticulum, 202, 205, 207
DMSA nuclear renograms, 55
donor kidneys, 248
donor-recipient anastomosis, 248
Doppler ultrasound, 242, 249, 281
dormia basket, 149
double-J stent, 298, 299, 301
  see also stents
  placement, 120, 121, 122
  placement during PCNL, 129
  removal, 123
drainage catheters, 122, 123
  see also catheters
dumbbell hernias, 164, 165
duplex kidneys, 52, 53, 54–55
dupytren, 164
DVT, preventing, 275
Dx/HA, *see* dextranomer/hyaluronic acid
    copolymer (Dx/HA)
dysplasia, renal, 53, 103

E

edema, 164
  mild dilation due to transient, 72
  preputial, 289
  prevention from, 69
EEC, *see* epispadias-exstrophy complex (EEC)
ejaculation, 88
ejaculation/infertility, loss of

key to preserving, 272
and nerve-sparing technique, 272
and RPLND, 271
elective conversion to open surgery, 136–137
electrodes
  bugbee, 101, 102, 103
  diathermy hook, 102
  insulated wire, 102
  loop, 101
electrohydraulic lithotripters, 127
electrolyte therapy, 29
electrosurgery risks during laparoscopy, 134
embolization, 265
  percutaneous, 195
emergency conversion to open surgery, 136–137
emphysema, subcutaneous, 134
endoscopes
  8F, 102
  McCarthy panendoscope, 101, 102
  staples, 135
  suturing, 135, 136
endoscopic ablation, *see* endoscopy
endoscopic therapy, 112, 113
  failures of, 114
  outcomes for persisting reflux after ureteral
      reimplantation, 114
  reflux resolution rate after, 115
endoscopy
  ablation of posterior urethral valves, 101–105
  management of ureterocele, 107–108
  puncture, 107
  ureterocele incision, 107
end-stage renal disease (ESRD), 103
enemas, 225
  hypertonic phosphate, 340
  iatrogenic metabolic complications of, 340
  retrograde, 336, 337
energy sources during laparoscopy, risks from,
    134
enteric wall hematomas, 126
enterocystoplasty, 158, 310
enterotomy sites closure, 135
epididymitis, traumatic, 291
epidural analgesia
  complications incidence in UK, 39–40
epigastric arteries, 165, 166
epispadias, repairing of, 84
epispadias-exstrophy complex (EEC)
  anatomical reconstruction of, 83–84
  complications, 84–89
epithelium, 93, 94
erectile implants, 216
erectile tissue, of corpora, 229
ergonomics alignment in laparoscopy,
    132–133
erythema, 93, 96
Esposito, C., 187, 197
ESRD, *see* end-stage renal disease (ESRD)
estrogens, conjugated, 265
ESWL, *see* extracorporeal shockwave lithotripsy
    (ESWL)
EuroSCORE, 5, 8–9
euvolemic hyponatremia, 31
extirpative surgery, time of, 264
extracorporeal shockwave lithotripsy (ESWL),
    125–126
extraperitoneal flank incision, 258
extrarenal fluid collection, 128
extratesticular lesion, 269
extrusion of cuff, 245
exufflation, laparoscopic, 141

F

fascia, 93
fascial abnormalities, 88–89
fecal continence, 233
  conservative measures at, 336
  MACE for management of, *see* malone
      antegrade continence enema (MACE)
  overall success rate for achieving, 338
fecundity, in female patients, 88
feeding tubes, 154
femoral hernia, 164–165
  see also hernia
8F endoscope, 102
  see also endoscopes
Fenger technique, 58
fertility outcomes
  after orchidopexy, 171–172, 175, 177
  varicoceles, 193, 194
fibrin glue, 135, 177, 244
fibrosis, 128
  of urachus during embryonic development, 93
firearm injuries, 296
fistulas
  cause and origin of, 202
  diagnosis of, 205
  reoperation of, 206
  ureterovesical, 70
fistulogram, 95
fixed neck positions, 136
flank incisions, 60, 61
flap valve mechanism, 315, 316
  inadequate, 321
fluid balance, 24–25
fluid collections
  complication of PCNL, 128
  requiring percutaneous drainage, 122–123
fluoroscopy, 73, 242
  C-arm fluoroscopy, 124
  for fluid collection diagnosis, 122
  for precutaneous nephrostomy, 118
Fogarty balloon catheter ablation technique, 102
Foley catheter, 124, 152–153, 185, 311
  see also catheters
  drainage, 70, 157
  transurethral, 53
Foley Y-plasty, 58
formalin installations, 265
Fowler–Stephens orchidopexy, 170, 172, 173–174,
    177, 184, 185, 190
  see also orchidopexy
  success rates for, 186, 187
frusemide, 249
fungal infections of urinary tract, 108
  see also urinary tract infections
funnel plots, 9

G

gadolinium (Gd)-enhanced MRI, 176
gait abnormalities, 89
gas embolism, 133
gastric inhibitory peptide (GIP), 24
gastrocystoplasty, 33, 308, 309, 310
gastrointestinal complications, 37–38
general anesthesia, 117, 125, 132
  see also anesthesia
General Medical Council (GMC), 15
  guidance for doctors, 13
genital complications, 87–88
genital injuries
  degloving of penis, 289

due to dog bite, treatment of, 290
penile amputations, 289
penile amputations, treatment of, 289
sexual abuse as etiology for, 293
genital skin, 202
genital surgery, reconstructive, 218
see also vaginoplasty
genitography, 225
genitoplasty, 88
genitourinary RMS, 262
genitourinary tract injuries, 289
germ cells maturation, 171, 172
Gerota's fascia, 147, 148, 278, 282
GFR, *see* glomerular filtration rate (GFR)
GH, *see* growth hormone (GH)
GHRH, *see* growth hormone releasing hormone
(GHRH)
GHRIP, *see* growth hormone releasing inhibitory
peptide (GHRIP)
GIP, *see* gastric inhibitory peptide (GIP)
glansplasty, 205, 206–207
Glans wings, 205
see also glansplasty
Glenn-Anderson technique, 67, 114, 154
glomerular filtration rate (GFR), 29, 33
glomerulosa, outer zona, 278–279
glucagon, 23
gluconeogenesis, 23, 26
glutaraldehyde cross-linked bovine collagen, 325
GMC, *see* General Medical Council (GMC)
GnRH tests, 194
gonadal vessels
injuries, 189–190
transaction, 173–174
graft function, deterioration in, 252
graft perfusion, assessment of, 251
graft survival in kidney transplant, 250–251
graphical techniques for audit data analysis, 9
groin incision, 178
growth hormone (GH), 24
growth hormone releasing hormone (GHRH), 24
growth hormone releasing inhibitory peptide
(GHRIP), 24
gubernaculum, 184, 189
guide wires placement, 127

H
Harmonic Scalpel, 55, 141
Hasson's technique, 147
health care regulators, 4
Health Service Commissioner, 14
Heineke–Mikulicz technique, 58
hematocele, cases of isolated, 291
hematomas, 122, 126, 298, 299
compressive perirenal, 141
in inguinal herniotomy, 165
scrotal, 172, 173, 178
hematuria, 109, 126, 127, 135, 185, 297, 302
cases of mild, 265
in ureteral reimplantation, 69
hematuria dysuria syndrome, 309
heminephrectomy
see also nephrectomy
basic surgical principles of, 55
in duplicated collecting system, 54
ischemic changes during, 56
laparoscopic, 54, 55
retroperitoneoscopic, 54
upper pole, 52–53
retroperitoneoscopic, 146
heminephroureterectomy, 146, 155

hemodialysis, 241–243
hemolysis, 32
hemolytic incompatibility, 42
hemolytic reactions, severe acute, 42
hemoptysis, 126
hemorrhage, 141, 259, 281
abdominal wall, 188
during nephrectomy, 49
during partial nephrectomy, 55
hemorrhagic cystitis, 264–265
hemostasis, 134, 250
during laparoscopy, 140–141, 142
hernia
dumbbell, 164, 165
femoral, 164–165
incarcerated, 163, 164, 166
incisional, 51, 159
inguinal, 88
inguinal, after laparoscopic orchidopexy, 191
inguinal, repair of, *see* inguinal hernia repair
missed, 165, 166
sliding, 164
herniotomy
inguinal, *see* inguinal hernia repair
laparoscopic, 163, 164, 165, 167
hindgut, 93
hinman bladder, *see* nonneurogenic bladder
homemade dilating balloon catheters, 147
hormone manipulation, 170
human chorionic gonadotropin (HCG), 269
hyaluronic acid, 312
subureteral injection of, 71
hyaluronic acid injections, 153
hydroceles
abdominoscrotal, 164
formation in varicocele repair surgery,
196–198
during inguinal herniotomy, 164, 166
residual, 166–167
hydrodistension implantation technique,
111–112, 114
see also subureteric injections
hydrogen ions, 309
hydronephrosis, 119, 126, 139, 142, 149, 265, 302
moderate, 71
patients improvement in, 61
progressive, 68
severe, 71
stents fo worse, 61
hydrophilic catheters, 319, 339–340
hydrophilic guidewire, 242
hydrothorax, 129
hydroureteral nephrosis, 70
hydroureteronephrosis, 68
hyperbaric oxygen, 265
hyperchloremic metabolic acidosis, 309
hyperkalemia, 32–33
hypernatremia, 31
hypertension, 299
hypertonic phosphate enemas, 340
hypervolemic hyponatremia, 31
hypogastric artery, 93
hypokalemia, 32
hyponatremia, 30, 40–41
hypospadias repair, 106
see also urethroplasty
hypotension, 250
intraoperative, 259
hypothalamus
and ADH, 25
and GHRH, 22

impulses, 22
release of CRF from, 22
hypothermia, 133–134
hypotonic fluid, 29
for hyponatremia, 30
hypotrophy, testicular, 194, 197
hypovolemia, 250

I
iatrogenic injuries, 259, 289, 301, 302
iatrogenic trauma, 308
idiopathic strictures, 106
ifosamide, 264
ileal chimney, *see* incontinent ileovesicostomy
ileal cystoplasty, 158
ileocystoplasty, 309, 310
ileus, 159
after laparoscopic orchidopexy, 191
after nephrectomy, 50
ilioinguinal blocks, 55
ilioinguinal nerve, 174, 176
in inguinal herniotomy, 166
immune response, postsurgery, 26
immunosuppression, 248, 251
immunosuppressive steroids, 249
impalpable testes, 170, 176
see also testes
outcomes for, 173–174
incarcerated hernia, 163, 164, 166
incisional hernia, 51
incomplete valve ablation, 103
incontinence, 86–87, 102
urinary, 103–104, 107
incontinent ileovesicostomy
mean follow-up in, 319
outcomes of, 319
surgical techniques for, 318
incontinent urinary diversions, 84
Indiana pouch, 84
indigo carmine, 93
inferior mesenteric artery, 74, 78
inferior vena cava (IVC), 257, 258, 259
informed consent in laparoscopy, 138
infundibulum, 128
inguinal hernia, 88
after laparoscopic orchidopexy, 191
inguinal hernia repair, 163–167
inguinal herniotomy, *see* inguinal hernia repair
inguinal orchidopexy, 172, 173
see also orchidopexy
inlay grafting, 208
inrad needles, 118
insufflation complication in laparoscopy,
133–134, 140
insulated wires
ablation, complications in, 103
electrode, 102
insulin-like growth factor-1 (IGF-1), 24
intergroup RMS Study, trials by, 262
interleukin-2 antagonists, 252
intermittent catheterization, 251
International Neuroblastoma Staging System
(INSS), 280
International Normalized Ratio, 117
International Society of Pediatric Oncology
(SIOP), 259
interventional radiology, 117–124
intestinal obstruction, 308–309
management of, 311–312
Intestinal vaginoplasty, 220
see also vaginoplasty

intra-abdominal testes, 170, 171, 173
  see also testes
    surgical techniques for orchidopexy of, 177
    vanished, 176
intraoperative complications in nephrectomy for
      Wilms tumor, 259–260
intraureteral injections, with hydrodistension,
      112, 115
intravenous fluids, 40–41
intravenous pyelogram (IVP), 77, 297
intravesical installations, 265
intravesical ureteroceles, 107
introitus, coaptation of, 292
inversion, testicular, 174
ipsilateral incisions, 184, 185
ipsilateral testes, 193
ipsilateral ureteral system, 155
ipsilateral ureteroureterostomy (U-U), 73, 74–78
IRS, I-III states, literature from, 263
IRS, IV goal of, 263
IRS, protocols *versus* VAC, 263
ischemia, 167
    male genital, 87
    ureteral trunk, 75
ischemic complications, vaginal, 235–236
ischemic necrosis, 75
ISNA (Intersex Society of North America), 224,
      228
isosulfan blue, 196
Ivanissevich, 196
IVC, *see* inferior vena cava (IVC)
IVP, *see* intravenous pyelogram (IVP)

J
Jackson-Pratt drains, 74
JJ-catheter complications, 149
JJ stenting for primary obstructive megaureters,
      108
Jones incisions, 183
jugular vein, circulation in right internal, 242
jugular vein stenosis, 243

K
kayexalate, *see* sodium polystyrene sulfonate
Keith needles, 189
keloids, 165
ketamine, 135
kidney infections, 86
kidneys, 247–250
    multicystic dysplastic, 139, 191
    percutaneous access of, 145
    transplant, *see* kidney transplant
kidney transplant
    complications of, 251–253
    curved iliac fossa incision in, 249
    graft survival in, 250–251
    medical and surgical workup, 247
    outcome of, 250–251
    pre-emptive, 247
    pretransplant surgery in, 248
    techniques of, 248–250
    transperitoneal approach, 249
    urological workup of, 247–248
kidney trauma, *see* renal trauma
kinking ureters, 150
Kropp procedure for BNR, 332, 333
KTP laser ablation, 102
kyphosis, 159

L
labia minora, 228
labioplasty, 228

lacerations, vaginal, 292
LAP, *see* laparoscopic pyeloplasty (LAP)
laparoscopically retrieved kidneys, 248
laparoscopic herniotomy, 163, 164, 165
    see also inguinal hernia repair
    complications of, 167
laparoscopic/laparoscopic assisted techniques,
      243–244
    advantages of, 245
laparoscopic orchidopexy
    see also orchidopexy
    complications in, 187–189
    diagnostic, 183–184, 191
    pelvic visualization during, 189
    success rates for, 186–187
    surgical techniques for, 184–185
    timing of, 186
laparoscopic percutaneous extraperitoneal
      closure (LPEC), 167
laparoscopic pyeloplasty (LAP), 146–147
laparoscopic surgery
    vs. open surgery, 27
laparoscopy, 138–142
    appendicectomy, 132, 135
    conversion to open nephrectomy, 48
    herniotomy, *see* laparoscopic herniotomy
    history of, 132
    inadvertent injuries during, 134–135
    injury and trauma to surgeon, 135–136
    insufflation during, 133–134
    for lower urinary tract, 152–159
    in lower urinary tract, *see* laparoscopy in lower
          urinary tract
    optimizing performance, 136–137
    orchidopexy, *see* laparoscopic orchidopexy
    port site herniation during, 133
    procedures, 132–133
    pyeloplasty, 135
    retroperitoneal complications in, 135, 136
    rules for safe, 137
    testicular autotransplantation, 174, 175
    testicular mobility, 177
    tissue approximation during, 135
    for urachal remnant, 94
    varicocele ligation, 197, 198
    vascular clamp, 140
laparotomy, 133, 134, 183, 188
    for biopsy, 264
laryngospasm, 37
laser ablation, 102
laser fiber lithotripters, 127, 128
latency period, 309
latex allergy, 89
laxatives, 336, 337
leak point pressure, 248
le bag continent reconstructions, 264
Leydig cell function, 172, 194, 196
Lichen sclerosis, 106
Lich Gregoir laparoscopy, 153
Lich-Gregoir technique, 68
Lich-Gregoir UNC, modified, 251, 252
lidocaine, 118
lipoma of cord, 166
lithotomy, dorsal, 73
lithotripsy, 127
    transurethral, 129
lithotripters, 125, 127, 128
litigation
    for poor surgical outcomes, 14–15
local anesthesia, 39–40, 118
loin incisions, 48, 51
loop electrodes, 101
Lords method, 164

lumbar veins, 49
lumbodorsal fascia, 147
lumbotomy, dorsal, 48, 61
Lyme disease, 41
lymphatic sparing approach, 196, 197, 198
lymphoceles, 122, 251, 252
    drainage, 123

M
MACE, *see* malone antegrade continence enema
      (MACE) procedure
magnetic resonance imaging (MRI), 176, 257
maladaptive behavior, 38
malaria, 41
malfunctions of AUS components, 330
malignancy, 309–310
malignant hyperthermia (MH), 38
Malone antegrade continence enema (MACE)
      procedure, 316, 336–339
management golas, in renal injury, 297–298
mannitol, 249
master–slave telerobotic systems, 145
Mathieu flip-flap, 207
McCarthy panendoscopes, 101, 102
McEvedy technique, 165
McIndoe-Reed procedure, 220–221
McVey repair, 167
meatal stenosis, 202, 205, 206–207
Meckel's diverticulectomy, 135
medial instrument ports, 147
median umbilical ligament, 93
media response, in surgical outcomes, 16
medium chain triglyceride (MCT), 260
medulla, 278–279
megaureters, 68–69
    primary obstructive, 108, 154
menarche, 235
mesenteric artery, inferior, 74, 78
metabolic response to surgery, 22–24
metabolism, of protein, 26
metastasis, 135
methylene blue, 93, 141
metronidazole, 311
metryrosine, *see* alpha-methy-L-tyrosine
      (metryrosine)
micromosquito forceps, 178
micropuncture techniques, 118, 119
microscopic hematuria, 126
microsurgical subinguinal ligation for
      varicoceles, 196
microsurgical vasovasostomy, 178
microvascular orchidopexy, 172, 174, 175, 177
    see also orchidopexy
voiding cystourethrogram (VCUG),
      102
    syringocele diagnosis by, 105
micturation
    due to hypospadias surgery, 209
midline incisions
    in patients with narrow subcostal angle, 48
Mitchell BNR, 86
Mitrofanoff, P., 315, 318
Mitrofanoff channel, 86, 87, 235, 319, 339
modern staged repair of bladder exstrophy
      (MSRE), 86
modified venous valvulotome, 102
monofilament absorbable sutures, 165
monopolar cautery, 149
monorchia, 175
Monti conduits, 318, 337
Monti sigmoid vesicostomy, 158
Monti technique for MACE, 337

Monti urinary channels, 318–319
morphological abnormalities in renal trauma, 300
MRI, *see* magnetic resonance imaging (MRI)
MSRE, *see* modern staged repair of bladder exstrophy (MSRE)
mucus production after cystoplasty, augmentation, 309
management of, 312
multicystic dysplastic kidneys, 139, 191
multidisciplinary team, for clinical audit, 6
myelomeningocele, 68

N
naloxone, 39
NAPRTCS review, 250
narcotic infusions following laparoscopy, 135
National Health Service (NHS), 13, 14, 16
of UK, 5, 6
national Wilms tumor study (NWTS), 258–259
Navarre catheters, 118–119
Nd-YAG laser ablation, 102
necrosis
ischemic, 75
testicular, 196, 198
needled conduits in small children, 241
Neisseria meningitidis, 279
neobladders, 120
neoinguinal hiatus, 185, 189
neomeatus, *see* meatal stenosis
neonatal period, iatrogenic injuries in, 289
treatment of, 290
neophallus, 214
neoplasia, bladder, 83
neourethral stricture, 86
neovagina, creation of, 219–220
nephrectomy
complications, in open, 49–51
conversion from laparoscopic approach to, 48
drainage, percutaneous, 142
partial, 138, 139, 141
primary, 257–259
rates in renal trauma, 297, 298
surgical approaches to kidney, 47–49
total, 138, 139, 140–141
in ureteral injuries, 301
for ureteral stumps, 155
nephrolithotomy, 123–124
catheters, 128, 129
percutaneous (PCNL), 127, 128–129
nephron-sparing surgery
treatment of bilateral Wilms tumor, 257
nephroscopes, flexible, 128
nephrosis, hydroureteral, 70
nephrostogram, antegrade
for patency of anastomosis., 78
nephrostomy
percutaneous, 117–120
tube placement, 118, 119, 121
nephrostomy tubes, 62, 69, 70
use in Anderson–Hynes technique, 60
nephroureterectomy, 139, 155
partial, 53
see also partial nephrectomy
nephroureterostomy tubes, 124
Nerve damage, iatrogenic, 236
nerve-sparing surgery, *see* testis-sparing surgery
neural tube defects, 109
neuroblastoma, 280–283
neurogenic bladder, 68, 75, 76, 109, 307
neurological complications, 38
neurovascular bundle, 225, 229
neurovesical dysfunction, in cloaca, 233

Nissen's fundoplication, 27
nonabsorbable sutures, 165, 167
noninvasive imaging in renal tumors, 257
nonionic contrast materials, 118
nonmechanical complications of AUS, 330, 332
nonneurogenic bladder, 307
nonpalpable testes, 175–176
see also testes
laparoscopic orchidopexy for, 183–184
nonseminomatous mixed germ cell tumors (NSMGCT), 269
retroperitoneal lymph node dissection (RPLND), 270
nonsteroidal anti-inflammatory drugs (NSAID), 39
NPSA, *see* National Patient Safety Authority (NPSA)
NWTSG trials, comparison of complication rates from SIOP and, 259

O
obstetric complications
in females with EEC, 88
obstructive anuria, 103
prevention of, 104
oliguria, 69, 70
obstructive, 103, 104
omental herniation, 189
omental ischemia, 167
omentectomy, 243, 245
omentum, 133
omnitract, 249
omphalomesenteric duct, 94
onlay prepucial flap, 203
open surgery, 129, 134, 151, 153, 154
conversion to, 127, 128
elective *versus* emergency conversions to, 136–137
excision of urachal remnants, 156
irrigation in, 159
versus laparoscopic surgery, 27
therapy, 111
open ureteroneocystostomy, 114
opioids, 30, 39
optical urethrostomy, 207
optic trocars, 132
orchidectomy, 170, 177, 178
orchidopexy, 170
complications of, 174–178
Fowler-Stephens, 170, 172, 173–174, 177, 184, 185, 186, 187, 190
inguinal, 172, 173
laparoscopic, *see* laparoscopic orchidopexy
microvascular, 172, 174, 175, 177
outcomes for, 170–172
preperitoneal, 173
redo, 178, 179
scrotal, 170, 172, 173
staged, 170, 172, 173, 174, 184, 187
success rates for different types of, 172
surgical techniques for, 176–177
for undescended testicle, 270
orchiectomy, inguinal, 270–271
organic acids, 309

P
pain management, complications of, 39–40
Palomo procedure, 196, 197, 198
palpable testes, 170
see also testes
orchidopexy for, 172
palpable varicoceles, 193
pampiniform plexus, 193, 196

pancreatic fistula, 50
papaverine, 141
paracetamol, 39
paragangliomas, 281
paratesticular rhabdomyosarcoma, 269
orchiectomy, inguinal in, 270–271
role of RPLND in management of patients with, 270
RPLND for, 271
parenchyma
localized ischemia in, 56
renal, 55
transected, 54, 55, 56
upper moiety function to, 53
upper pole, 77
partial nephrectomy, 52–55, 257
partial nephroureterectomy, 53
Passerini-Glazel genitoplasty, 227, 228
PAS stockings, 275
patch graft, 106
patency of the central veins, 242
patent processus vaginalis (PPV), 163, 164, 172, 176
patent urachus, 92, 93, 94, 95, 156
patient–controlled analgesia, 39
patient preparation before surgery, 117
patients in RMS, 262–263
PCNL, *see* percutaneous nephrolithotomy (PCNL)
PD, *see* peritoneal dialysis (PD)
Pediatric Perioperative Cardiac Arrest Registry (POCA), 37
PEEP, *see* positive end expiratory pressure (PEEP)
peeping testes, 184
pelvic diaphragm, 93
pelvic osteotomy, 89
pelvis drainage in RAP, 149
penile degloving, 88
Penile ejaculation complications, 215
Penile inadequacy, 213
penile injuries, 289–290
penile nerves, dorsal, 214
penile prosthesis, 214
penile reattachment, 213
see also Phalloplasty
penile shaft, 213
penile skin, loss of, 289
penile stiffener, for sexual penetration, 214
penile stump, tailoring of, 213
penrose drain, 59, 62, 73, 74, 75
percutaneoulsy placed lines in hemodialysis, 241–242
percutaneous embolization/sclerotherapy, 195
percutaneous fluid collection drainage, 122–123
percutaneous nephrolithotomy (PCNL), 127, 128–129
percutaneous nephrostomy, 117–120, 123
Perez-Castro irrigation pump, 127, 128
perineal urethrostomy, 102
perinephric abscess, 299
perinephric tissue, 248
perirenal retroperitoneal fluid collections, 128
perirenal (subcapsular) hematoma, 126
peritoneal dialysis (PD), 243–245, 249
peritoneal incisions, 189–190
peritoneal perforation, 140, 142
peritoneum, 93
periurethral injections of polytetrafluoroethylene (PTFE), 325
Persistent cloaca
anatomy of cloaca channel, 232
fecal continence in, 233

Persistent cloaca (*Contd.*)
  gynecological problems in, 234
  ischemic complications in, 235–236
  MRI scan of, 235
  nerve damage due to, 234–235
  neurovesical dysfunction in, 233
  renal abnormalities in, 233
  stenosis in, 235
  urinary continence in, 233–234
Phallic reconstruction, *see* phalloplasty
Phalloplasty
  benefits of, 216
  complication rate of, 215
  cosmetic and functional requirements for, 213
  fistulas due to, 215
  sexual functions due to, 214–215
  stenosis due to, 215
  use of buccal mucosa in, 214
  use of penile stiffener in, 214
  use of radial forearm flap in, 213, 214
  use of skin grafts in, 214
  use of transurethral catheter in, 214
Phallus, *see* neophallus
pheochromocytoma, 280, 281–284
pigtail stents, 155
Pippi Salle procedure for BNR, 332–333
pneumoperitoneum, 132, 140, 159, 184
  insufflation complication in laparoscopy,
    133–134
pneumothorax, 134, 140, 242
  during nephrectomy, 50
pneumovesical ureter reimplantation, 146
pneumovesicum, 154
POCA, *see* Pediatric Perioperative Cardiac Arrest
  Registry (POCA)
Politano-Leadbetter ureteroneocystostomy, 67,
  68
polydimethylsiloxane, 111, 115, 325
  long-term follow-up of, 325
polytetrafluoroethylene, 111
  complications with, 115
  subureteric injections of, 112, 113
polyuria, 104
port site herniation, 133, 142
positioning-related injuries, 187
posterior urethral valves (PUV), 101–105, 251
  see also urethral valves
postobstructive diuresis, 33, 104
postoperative complications in nephrectomy for
  Wilms tumor, 259–260
postoperative management, 311
postpubertal testis tumors
  human chorionic gonadotropin (HCG) as
    markers in, 269
  management of, 269
  role of inguinal orchiectomy, 270
  studies in patients of, 270
postresection positive surgical margins, 264
potassium balance, disorders, 31–32
potassium ions (K$^+$), 25
pre-ESWL inserted J-stents, 126
Prentiss maneuver in orchidopexy, 177, 178
  see also orchidopexy
preoperative evaluation, 310–311
preoperative preparation for augmentation
  cystoplasty, 311
preperitoneal approach to hernia repair, 163, 164
preperitoneal insufflation, 187
prepubertal testis tumors, 269–270
preputial edema, *see* edema, preputial
pressure, intravesical, 315, 316, 321

pressure, leak point, 248
pressure injuries, 147, 148
pressure sores, 89
priapism, high-flow, 290
primary nephrectomy, *see* nephrectomy, primary
primary obstructive megaureters, 108, 154
primary resection, 262
Prince–Scardino vertical flaps, 58, 59
prophylactic ureteral stenting, 125, 126
  see also stenting
prophylaxis, 88
prostate biopsies, 145
protein metabolism, 26
prune belly syndrome, 93, 96, 174
PSARVUP, *see* posterior sagittal anorecto
  vaginourethroplasty (PSARVUP)
pseudodiverticulum, 303
psoas muscles, 149
psychosocial problems
  in children with exstrophy, 89
PTFE, *see* periurethral injections of
  polytetrafluoroethylene (PTFE)
Pudendal nerve, 225
PUJ, *see* pyeloureteric junction (PUJ)
PUJ obstruction, 135
PUM procedure, *see* urogenital mobilization
purse-string sutures, 164, 167
PUV, *see* posterior urethral valves (PUV)
pyelonephritis, 126, 127, 152
  xanthogranulomatosis, 139
pyeloplasty, 120, 139
  see also robotic assisted pyeloplasty (RAP)
  dismembered, 141
  laparoscopic, 135
  procedure-related complications, 148–149
  redopyeloplasty, 150
  for ureteropelvic junction obstruction, 58–65
pyeloureteric junction (PUJ), 52

R
Radial forearm flap, for phalloplasty, 213, 214
radially dilating ports, 133
radially dilating trocar systems, 184, 185
radial nerve injury, 135–136
radiation therapy, 262, 263, 264
  and chemotherapy complications, 266
  complication rates in patients with, 265
radionuclide scan, 59
radiopaque ruler, 121
radio therapy, *see* radiation therapy
RAP, *see* robotic assisted pyeloplasty (RAP)
RBUS, *see* renal/bladder ultrasound (RBUS)
reconstructive bladder surgery, laparoscopic, 139,
    141, 157–159
  complications, 159
  surgical outcomes, 158
rectal injuries, 292
  in adults and morbidity, 292
  intraoperative, 228
rectum, 93
recurrence in RMS, management of, 266
redo lines in hemodialysis, 242
redo orchidopexy, 178, 179
  see also orchidopexy
redopyeloplasty, 150
"refluo" technique, 174
reimplantations
  open techniques of, 113
  ureteral, 114
"relaxing" incisions, 189

renal abnormalities in cloaca patients, 233
renal artery, traumatic occlusion of, 299
renal biochemistry, checking, 311
renal/bladder ultrasound (RBUS), 77
renal colic, 54–55
renal cysts, 54–55
renal damage, 86
renal dilation, 124
renal dysplasia, 103
renal failure, 103
  after nephrectomy, 50
  incidence, 105
  prevention of, 104
renal function, 55
  developmental changes in, 29
  effect of ESWL on, 126
  loss of, 299–300
  postoperative improvement in, 59
  stabilization of, 59
renal hilum, 248
renal moiety, 53, 55
renal nuclear scans (DMSA), 299
renal pelvis, 118, 119, 128
renal reconstructive techniques, 298
renal replacement therapy, *see* kidney transplant
renal sparing surgery, complication rate in, 260
renal transplantation, 103
renal trauma, 296
  causes of, 296
  early complications of, 298–299
  etiology of childhood, 296
  grading of scales of, 297
  hypertension, 299
  ICU protocol for management of, 297
  imaging and staging in, 296
  late complications of, 299–300
  major, 298
  management goals of, 297–298
  morphological abnormalities in, 300
  nephrectomy rates, 297, 298
  outcomes of, 297–298
  penetrating trauma, 296
  renal function in, loss of, 299–300
  renal vascular injury in, 299
  surgical complication rates, 297
renal tumors
  cystic and solid nature of, 257
  inferior vena cava (IVC), 257
  laparoscopic removal of, 258
  outcomes of, 260–261
  prognosis of children with, 257
  responsive to adjuvant therapies, 257
  role of imaging study in, 257–258
  role of noninvasive imaging, 257
  role of surgeon in, 257
  surgical techniques for removal of, 257–258
  surgical techniques for removal of,
    complications associated with, 258–261
renal vein
  lumbar veins drain into, 49
  retraction during nephrectomy, 48
renal vein misidentification, 141
renin–angiotensin system, 24, 279
renovascular complications, 299
resection, primary, 262
resectoscope, 264
  loops, 103, 104
reticularis, inner zona, 279
retractile testes, 175
retrocatheters, ureteral, 153
retrograde stents, 120, 121

see also stents
retroperitoneal approach
  to nephrectomy, 47–48
  to RAP, 147, 148, 149, 150
retroperitoneal hematoma, 271
retroperitoneal inflammation, 139
retroperitoneal laparoscopic access, 132, 133
retroperitoneal ligation, 196–197, 198
retroperitoneal lymph node dissection (RPLND)
  in adolescents with NSGCT, 270
  bilateral, 271, 272
  and bleeding, 274
  chylous ascites following, 275
  complications in postchemotherapy, 275–276
  complications of, 271–272
  fertility rates in patients undergoing, 272
  and loss of ejaculatory function, 271
  oncological effectiveness of, 271
  oncologic and ejaculatory results of, 274
  outcomes of, 271–272
  pulmonary embolism in adults undergoing, 275
  role in management of patients with paratesticular rhabdomyosarcoma, 270
  small bowel obstruction (SBO) in, 271
  unilateral, 271, 272
retroperitoneoscopy, 139
  complications after, 135, 136, 142
  conversion in, 48
  heminephrectomy, 146
  redo, 141–142
Retzius space, 93, 94
rhabdomyoblasts, 264
rhabdomyosarcoma (RMS)
  biopsy in, 262, 263
  B/P, *see* bladder/prostate(B/P) RMS
  category of pelvic, 262
  chemotherapy and radiation-related complications in, 266
  embryonal, 262–263
  and genitourinary, 262
  goals of management of, 263
  and malignant tumors, 262
  management of recurrence in, 266
  outcomes of, 263–264
  paratesticular, *see* paratesticular rhabdomyosarcoma
  patients with relapsed, 263
  principal goals of therapy in, 263
  surgical complications in, 265–266
  surgical principles, 263
  treatment complications, 264–266
  treatment complications, management of, 264–266
  treatment principles of, 262–263
  treatment protocols from children's oncology group (COG), 262–263
risk-adjustment algorithm, 8
risk averse behavior, 9
risk differentiation in patients, 9
RMS, *see* rhabdomyosarcoma (RMS)
robotic arms movements, 147, 148
robotic-assisted laparoscopy
  see also robotic surgery
  extravesical ureteral reimplantation, 152–154
robotic assisted pyeloplasty (RAP), 146–147
  see also robotic surgery; pyeloplasty
  complications, 148–149, 150
  surgical outcomes, 149–150
robotic surgery
  see also robotic assisted pyeloplasty (RAP)

history of, 145
less-reported applications of, 146
master–slave telerobotic systems, 145
procedure-related complications, 148–149
robotic-assisted laparoscopy, 152–154
robot-related complications, 147–148
robot-related complications, 147–148
Rokitansky syndrome, 218, 219
rotator cuff injury, 136
routine fluid, 29
routine stenting in ureteroscopy, 128
RPLND, *see* retroperitoneal lymph node dissection (RPLND)
rupture, incidence of, 310
  management of, 312

S
sacrocolpopexy
  for uterine prolapse, 88
sclerotherapy for varicoceles
  see also varicoceles
  antegrade scrotal, 195–196, 198
  percutaneous, 195
scrotal "Bianchi" approach, 163, 164
scrotal/testicular injuries, 290
  causes of, 290
  rate of salvage of, 291
  and testicular torsion, 291
  treatment of, 291
scrotal violations in removing testis tumors, 270–271
scrotum
  exploration, initial, 175
  hematomas, 172, 173, 178
  nubbins, 175
  orchidopexy, 170, 172, 173
    see also orchidopexy
  orthotopic position, 184
  puncture, 197
  sclerotherapy for varicoceles, antegrade, 195–196, 198
  testicle delivery into, 185, 190, 191
  trauma to, 291
scrotum-first approach, 175, 178
secondary vaginoplasty, for stenosis, 226–227
  see also vaginoplasty
seldinger technique, 241–242
sepsis, 94, 127
  intraperitoneal, 142
serosal tears, 188, 198
Sertoli cell function, 172
  impairment, 194
serum sodium, 30, 31
sevoflurane, 38
sexual abuse, 293
sexual dysfunction, 88
Sexual function, 209
sheath reimplant, 74
shock wave energy, 125, 126
shock wave lithotripsy (SWL), 124
shoulder strain injury, 136
shunt infection rates, 310
sigmoid cystoplasties, incidence of rapture, 310
silk sutures, 165
sinus, urogenital, 93
skin flaps, 207, 208, 229, 236
skin grafts, 214
  for neovaginal creation, 220
sliding hernia, 164
small bowel obstruction (SBO), 259, 260, 261, 271, 274–275

snake wrist technology, 148
snare catheters, 121, 122, 123
  see also catheters
sodium, regulation of, 24–25
sodium and water balance, disorders, 29–30
sodium concentration in urine, 30
sodium deficit, 30
sodium polystyrene sulfonate, 32–33
spermatic pedicle injuries, 190
spermatogenesis, recovery of, 274
sphincteric incontinence, 104
sphincter mechanism incompetence
  artificial urinary sphincter (AUS) to enhance resistance of, 324, 329–332
  bladder neck bulking agents to enhance resistance of, 324, 325–327
  bladder neck sling to enhance resistance of, 324, 327–329
  BNR to enhance resistance of, 324, 332–333
  bulking agents as initial therapy for, 325
spontaneous vaginal deliveries, 88
staged orchidopexy, 170, 172, 173, 174, 184, 187
  see also orchidopexy
staghorn stone cases, 125, 126, 128
staging in renal trauma, 297
staphylococcus, infections of, 330
staphylococcus aureus, 95
stay sutures, 150
steinstrasse, 126
stenosis
  see also vaginal stenosis
  of conduit, 339–340
  juglar vein, 243
  renal artery, 251
  renal artery, effect on deterioration in graft function, 252
  secondary vaginoplasty for, 226–227
  stomal, 69
  ureteric, 251
  ureteric, management of, 252
stenotic area coverage, 121
stents, 121
  double-J, 298, 299, 301
  migration during ureteroscopy, 127
  pigtail, 155
  placement during RAP, 149
  retrieval of, 121–122, 123
  ureteric, placement of, 120–121
  urethral, 202
stereoscopic video imagery, 148
steroids, 225
STING procedure, 321
stoma, 318
  in MACE procedure, site of, 337
stomal complications, 339–340
stomal incontinence, 321–322
stomal narrowing in bladder, 159
stomal stenosis, 69, 319–320
stoma-related problems, 318–319
stone disease
  see also stones
  bladder stones, 129
  in developing countries, 129
  ESWL for, 125–126, 129
  open surgery for, 129
  PCNL for, 127, 128–129
  ureteroscopy for, 126–128
stone formation, 309
  management of, 312

stone-free rates
see also stone disease; stones
after ESWL, 125, 126, 129
after PCNL, 126
after ureteroscopy, 126
stones, 322
see also stone disease
bladder, 129
burden, 128
composition, 126, 129
location, 126
migration, 126, 127
size, 125
stone-street, 126
straddle injuries, 291
strangulation for inguinal hernia repair, 164
stranguria, 205, 206
stricture, neourethral, 86
stricturotomy, 106
subcutaneous cuff, 244
subcutaneous emphysema, 134
subdartos pouch, 176, 177, 178, 185
subfascial conduit complications, 320–321
subinguinal microsurgical ligation for
varicoceles, 196
submucosal tunnel, 67, 68.69
subureteric injections, 111, 253
comparison with hydrodistension technique,
112
complications in, 114–115
in duplicated ureteral systems, outcomes
after, 113
initial treatment failure, outcomes after, 114
in neuropathic bladders, outcomes after,
113–114
for patients with VUR, 76, 78, 94
in single ureteral systems, outcomes after,
112–113
for VUR, 78
superior mesenteric artery (SMA), 259
suprainguinal ligation for varicoceles, 196–197
surgeon, target organ, and monitor alignment,
132–133
surgeon-controlled systems, automated, 145
surgeons
experience, 260
litigation against, 14–15
perspective of poor surgical outcomes, 15–16
surgical exploration in PD, 244
surgical indications and patient selection in
MACE procedure, 336–337
surgical ligation, 195
surgical outcomes
disclosure of, 12–14
hospital's perspective, 16
information to patients for clinical audit, 3
patient's perspective, 14–15
surgeon's perspective, 15–16
surgical team training, laparoscopy, 138–139
surgical techniques, 67–68
for orchidopexy, 176–177
outcomes of, 68
suture fixation at orchidopexy, 177
sutures
absorbable, 155, 165, 167
endoscopic, 135, 136
fixation at orchidopexy, 177
interrupted vicryl, 166
laparoscopic, 140, 141
mattress, 177
nonabsorbable, 165, 167
purse-string, 164, 167

in RAP, 146, 150
transfixion, 164
suxamethonium, 38–39
syringocele, 105
system troubleshooting in robotic
surgery, 148

T
tandem tube, 316
teflon, subureteric injections of, 112, 113, 114
telepresence surgery, 145
telerobotic systems, master-slave, 145
teratoma tumors in children, 269
testes
ascending, 176
atretic, 184
atrophy, see testicular atrophy
atrophy in, 193, 194
blind-ending vessels, 183, 184
canalicular, 173, 184
cryptorchid, 171, 177
ectopic, 191
growth arrest in, 194
hypotrophy in, 194, 197
impalpable, 170, 173–174, 176
injuries, 194
intra-abdominal, 170, 171, 173, 176, 177
ipsilateral, 193
necrosis, 196, 198
nonpalpable, 175–176
nonpalpable, laparoscopic orchidopexy for,
183–184
palpable, 170, 172
peeping, 184
position, role in orchidopexy, 171
prosthesis, 178
retractile, 175
size, 194
torsion, 178
torsion during laparoscopic orchidopexy, 191
testicle delivery into scrotum, 185, 190, 191
testicular atrophy
in inguinal herniotomy, 167
in laparoscopic orchidopexy, 186, 187, 189
in scrotal orchidopexy, 173, 179
varicoceles related, 193, 194
testis-sparing surgery, 269
for benign testis tumors, 270
fertility rates in, 272
and loss of ejaculation, 272
role of preoperative evaluation in, 270
testis tumors, 269–271
testosterone stimulation, preoperative, 206
tetrafluoroethylene paste, 111
thermoregulation, 26–27
thoracoabdominal approach, 48
thoracoabdominal incisions, complications rate
in, 258
thrombosis, 55, 248
deep vein, 275
graft, 252
risk factors for, 250
vascular, 251
thrombus, removal of, 258
TIP, see tubularized incised plate (TIP)
tissue engineering, 213
tissue retrieval bags, 135
TNF, see tumor necrosis factor (TNF)
Toilet training, 205
torque, 242
total body water (TBW), 30
total nephroureterectomy, 139

total parenteral nutrition (TPN), 260
total urogenital sinus mobilization (TUM), 233,
234
tourniquet injuries, 289
treatment of, 290
transabdominal approaches to nephrectomy, 48
transabdominal transperitoneal approach, 258
transient hydroureteronephrosis (HUN), 86
transperitoneal approach, 249
to RAP, 147, 148, 149
transperitoneal laparoscopy, 139, 140, 153
transperitoneal ring closure, 163, 164
transplantation, renal, 103
transureteroureterostomy, 71, 73–74
outcomes for, 74–76
transurethral catheter, 214
transurethral cystoscopy, 68
transurethral incision, 105
transurethral lithotripsy, 129
transurethral prostatic resection, 145
transurethral subureteric injection, 111
transversalis fascia, 93
transversely tubularized bowel segments (TTBS)
technique, 316, 317
traumatic amputation, 213
traumatic genital injuries, *see* genital injuries,
traumatic
Trendelenburg position, 184, 191
triamcinolone, injections of, 319, 320
trigone, 107, 109
trocars, 132, 140, 147
obturators, 185
placement in abdomen, 188
radially dilating, 184, 185
tubed drainage, complications in, 62–63
tubularized incised plate (TIP), 202–203
reoperation, modification for, 207
tubularized prepucial flap, 203–205
TUM, *see* total urogenital sinus mobilization
(TUM)
tumor enucleation, *see* partial nephrectomy
tunica albuginea calcification, 177
Tunica vaginalis, 206, 207, 209
TUU, *see* transureteroureterostomy

U
UK Transplant Registry 2005, 103
ultrasonic scalpel, 141
renal/pelvic, 225
for urachal anomaly, 93
ultrasound, Doppler, 242, 249
ultrasound guidance
for fluid collection diagnosis, 122
for percutaneous nephrostomy, 118
for Whitaker test, 124
ultrasound localization of veins, 242
umbilical arteries, 93
umbilical cord, 94
patent opening inferior to, 945
umbilical erythema, 96
umbilical fluids, analysis of, 93–94
umbilical ports, 133
umbilicovesical fascia, 93
unilateral adrenalectomy, 279
UPJ, *see* ureteropelvic junction (UPJ)
UPJ, avulsion of, 298
UPJ obstruction, *see* ureteropelvic junction
(UPJ) obstruction
upper respiratory tract infection (URI), 37
urachal abscess, 95
urachal anomalies
clinical, 93

complications of, 94
diagnosis of, 93–94
historical incidence of, 92
management of, 94–96
outcomes of, 94
prevalence of, 92–93
urachal cyst, 92, 156
CT scan evaluation of, 96
diagnosis of, 93, 94–95
treatment of, 95
ultrasound image of, 96
urachal remnant
asymptomatic, 94
excision, 156
laparoscopic management of, 156–157
urachal sinus, 92, 93, 95–96
urachus, 93, 156
ureteral avulsion, 127
ureteral catheters, 153, 154, 155, 159
ureteral duplication, 113
ureteral excision, 154
ureteral injuries, 301–302
ureteral leaks, 155
ureteral obstruction, 70, 129, 175
due to subureteric injections, 115
ureteral perforation, 127
ureteral peristalsis, 114
ureteral reflux, patients with, 265
ureteral reimplantation
early postoperative complications, 69–70
failed, 75
laparoscopic, 152–155
late postoperative complications, 70
outcomes of endoscopic treatment for
persisting reflux after, 114
in patients with, 74
persistence of VUR after, 68
postoperative reflux, 70–71
postreimplantation follow-up, 71
surgical intervention in, 67
techniques for, 67–68
ureteral retrocatheters, 153
ureteral stenosis, 115
ureteral stents, 68, 69
ureteral strictures, 155
ureteral stumps, 53–54
endoscopic management of, 155–156
ureteral success after subureteric injections, 114
ureteral trauma, 127, 128, 129
ureterectomy, 155
ureteric catheters, 301
ureteric complications, 251
management of, 252
ureteric leak, management of, 252
ureteric stent placement, 120–121
see also stents
uretero-hydronephrosis, 55
ureteroneocystostomy (UNC), 249
external, 250
level of, 251
methods to perform, 250
modified Lich-Gregoir, 251, 252
open, 114
ureteroneocystotomy, 71
ureteropelvic junction (UPJ)
obstruction, 58, 64, 65, 118, 119, 146
reconstruction of traumatic disruption in, 146
ureteroplasty, balloon, 121, 122
uretero-pyeloneostomy, 58
ureteroscopy, 124, 126–128
ureterosigmoidostomies, 309
ureterosigmoidostomy (USO), 84

ureterostomy, cutaneous, 69
ureteroureteric anastomoses, 251
uretero–vesical junction obstruction, 103
JJ stenting for, 108
ureter reimplantation, 120, 121, 123
urethra, 53, 213
catheter, 105
dilatation, 106
fistula, 105
stenting, 108
strictures, see urethral strictures
valves, see urethral valves
urethral catheterization, 263
urethral catheters, 154, 155, 157
urethral dilation, 207
urethralgia posterior, 106
urethral strictures
as complication in PUV ablation, 102, 103, 104
etiology of, 106
surgical techniques and outcomes, 106
urethral valves, 105–106
advancements in treatment, 101
urethrocutaneous fistula, formation, 85–86
urethroplasty, 105, 106
anastomotic, 106
causes and origins of complications in,
201–202
diagnosis of complications in, 205–206
outcome of surgery due to, 209
reoperation, principles and techniques of,
206–209
surgical complications of, 202–205
urethroscopic interventions, 126
urethrotomy, 106
perineal, 102
visual internal, 103, 106
urethrovaginal fistula, 229, 235
urethrovaginal septum, loss of, 88
URI, see upper respiratory tract infection (URI)
urinalysis, 70, 71
urinary tract infections
as complication of ESWL, 126
as complication of ureteroscopy, 127
urinary bladder, 93
urinary catheter, 190, 249
urinary complications, during repairing of EEC,
85–87
urinary diversion, 84, 117, 119
urinary extravasation, 105
in renal trauma, 298–299
urinary incontinence, 107
see also incontinence
AUS in treating neurogenic, 329
bladder neck sling for treatment of, 327
bulking agents in treatment of, 325
due to urethral valve ablation, 103–104
Dx/HA for treatment of, 325
factors responsible for, 324
long-term outcomes of the use of bulking
injectable materials for, 326
PTFE for treatment of, 325
urinary leakage
from anastomosis, 74
during partial nephrectomy, 54
prevention of, 55–56
prolonged, 129
at U-U site, 78
urinary obstruction, 86, 153
urinary retention, 109
urinary sodium concentration, 30
urinary stasis, 322
urinary tract

effects of an abnormal lower, 247, 248–251
upper deterioration, 330, 332
urinary tract infections, 85, 86, 103, 309
due to subureteral injections, 115
frequency of, 330
fungal, 108
management of, 312
prevention of, 104
recurrent, 251
risk factor for, 248
ureteral stumps management in, 155
with VUR, 152
urinary tract outflow obstruction, lower, 101
urine bladder, 221–222
urine leak, 142, 299
urine sterilization, preoperative, 126
urinomas, 54, 105, 119, 142
drainage of, 122–123
due to ischemic necrosis, 75
formation of, 77
postoperative, 122
prevention of, 55
transient postoperative, 74
urodynamics, 234
evaluation, 87
urodynamic studies, 248
uroflowometry, 205–206
urogenital mobilization, 228–229
urogenital sinus (UGS)
anomalies of, 224
length of, 225
separation of vagina from, 229
urologist, 123, 124
communication between radiologist and, 121
uropathies, 247, 250
bladder characteristics in children, 248
uterine prolapse, 88
Uterus, obstructed, 234, 235
UTI, see urinary tract infections
U-U, see ipsilateral ureteroureterostomy (U-U)

V
vaginal agenesis, congenital
diagnostic complications of, 219
vaginal dilation for, 219–220
vaginal dilation, nonsurgical, 219–220
vaginal injuries, 291–292
vaginal stenosis
complications due to genital surgery, 222
due to McIndoe-Reed procedure, 221
vaginoplasty
see also neovagina
for ambiguous genitalia, 221–222
assessment of, 219
complications of, 219
cosmetic appearance after, 221
intestinal, 220
pregnancy and delivery after, 235
preventing complications of, 229
psychological outcomes of, 222
psychosocial aspects of, 227, 228
sexual function due to, 222
surgical outcomes and complications due to,
226–228
urinary complications due to, 221–222
vaginoscopy, continuous flow of, 292
valsalva maneuver, 193, 194
valves, urethral, see urethral valves
valvotomes, 102
vanishing testis syndrome, 175, 176
variable life-adjusted display plots, 9
varicocelectomy, 193, 196

varicoceles, 193
    classification of, 193
    classification of intervention methods, 195
    comparison of intervention methods, 199
    complications in repair, 197–198
    diagnosis of, 193–194
    indications for repair of, 194
    prevalence with age, 193
    recurrent, 198, 199
    surgical techniques for, 164, 195–197
    testicular hypotrophy incidences in, 194, 197
    testicular injuries in, 194
vasal injury, 167
vasal mobilization, 174
vascular anastomosis, 249
vascular anatomy, 48, 247
vascular control in laparoscopy, 140–141
vascular injuries during laparoscopic
        orchidopexy, 188
vascular injury, 259–260
vas deferens injuries, 190
vasospasm, 141
vasovasostomy, microsurgical, 178
VATER syndrome, 340
V-18 control wires, 121, 123
VCUG, see voiding cystourethrogram (VCUG)
Vecchietti procedure, see laparoscopic
        procedures
vena cava, 48, 49a
venous bleeding in intraoperative hemorrhage, 49
venous catheter, central, 241
venous drainage, 248
venous hemorrhage, 49
ventriculoperitoneal shunt, 158, 159
ventriculoperitoneal shunt complications, 310
    confirmation of, 312
    management of, 312
Veress needles, 132, 133, 140, 184, 187
verumontanum, 102
vesicostomy, 101, 102, 235
    for bladder drainage, 68

Monti sigmoid, 158
vesicourachal diverticulum, 92, 94, 96
vesicoureteric reflux (VUR), 52, 67, 73, 77,
        112–114, 128, 152, 248
    after surgery, 76, 78
    as complication in AUV, 105
    as complication in endoscopic ureteroceles
        management, 107
    management of, 155, 252
Vibratory sensation, complications in, 226
video-urodynamics, see radiographic screening
vincristine, actinomycin d, and
        cyclophosphamide (VAC)
    chemotherapy, 263
    cycles of, 262–263
VCUG, see Voiding cystourethrogram (VCUG)
voiding cystourethrogram, 112, 115, 155
voiding cystourethrogram (VCUG), 77
    for urachal anomaly, 93
voiding dysfunction, 68
    transient, 70
voiding dysfunctions, 107
    in laparoscopic ureteral reimplantation, 153,
        154
vomiting
    during anesthesia, 37–38
    opioids for, 39
VQZ-plasty, 318
VUR, see vesicoureteral reflux (VUR);
        vesicoureteric reflux (VUR)

W
water balance and sodium, disorders, 29–30
waterhourse-friderichsen syndrome, 279
whistle tip ureteric catheter, 140–141
Whitaker test, 124
Wilms tumor
    bilateral, complication rate in surgery of,
        260–261
    extended lymph node dissection for, 260
    extension into IVC, 258

laparoscopic removal of unilateral
        nonmetastatic, 258
modern chemotherapy in, 257
nephrectomy for, 258
nephrectomy surgical complication rates,
        259–261
nephron-sparing surgery in treatment of
        bilateral, 257
role of partial nephrectomy in unilateral, 257
wound, after nephrectomy
    bulge, 51
    infection and dehiscence, 50
wound cellulitis, 172, 173
wounds in inguinal herniotomy
    cosmesis, 164
    infections, 165, 166

X
xanthogranulomatosis pyelonephritis, 139
XGP nephrectomy, 49
    see also nephrectomy

Y
Yang-Monti channels, see transversely
        tubularized bowel segments (TTBS)
yolk sac tumors, 269, 270
    AFP levels in, 269
    RPLND for, 271
Young-Dees-Leadbetter, procedure for BNR,
        86, 332
    outcomes by exstrophy-episadias complex
        (EEC) and, 332–333
    outcomes by neurogenica and, 333

Z
zero-point movement system, 148
ZEUS telemanipulators, 145
zipper-related injuries, 289
    treatment of, 290